HEALTH PSYCHOLOGY

HEALTH PSYCHOLOGY

JANE OGDEN

SEVENTH EDITION

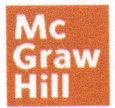

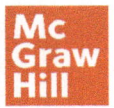

Open University Press
McGraw Hill
Unit 4,
Foundation Park
Roxborough Way
Maidenhead
SL6 3UD

email: emea_uk_ireland@mheducation.com
world wide web: www.openup.co.uk

First edition published 1996
Second edition published 2000
Third edition published 2003
Fourth edition published 2007
Fifth edition published 2012
Sixth edition published 2019
First published in this seventh edition 2023

Executive Editor: Beth Summers
Editorial Assistant: Hannah Jones
Production Coordinator: Hannah Cartwright
Marketing Manager: Ros Letellier
Text Design by Kamae Design
Cover Design by Adam Renvoize

A catalogue record of this book is available from the British Library

ISBN-13: 9780335251865
ISBN-10: 0335251862
eISBN: 9780335251872

Library of Congress Cataloging-in-Publication Data
CIP data applied for

Typeset by Straive

G11248   ACL   2025

Brief table of contents

Detailed table of contents

List of figures and tables

FIGURES

TABLES

List of abbreviations

ADL	activity of daily living
AIDS	acquired immune deficiency syndrome
APT	adaptive pacing therapy; adjuvant psychological therapy
AVE	abstinence violation effect
BDI	Beck depression inventory
BMI	body mass index
BSE	breast self-examination
CAD	coronary artery disease
CBSM	cognitive behavioural stress management
CBT	cognitive behavioural therapy
CHD	coronary heart disease
CIN	cervical intraepithelial neoplasia
CMV	cytomegalovirus
COPD	chronic obstructive pulmonary disease
CR	conditioned response
CS	conditioned stimulus
D&C	dilatation and curettage
DAFNE	dose adjustment for normal eating
DEBQ	Dutch Eating Behaviour Questionnaire
ERPC	evacuation of the retained products of conception
FAP	familial adenomatous polyposis
FH	familial hypercholesterolaemia
GAS	general adaptation syndrome
GCT	gate control theory
GHQ	General Health Questionnaire
GSR	galvanic skin response
HAART	highly active anti-retroviral therapy
HADS	hospital anxiety and depression scale
HAPA	health action process approach
HBM	health belief model
HPA	hypothalamic-pituitary-adrenocorticol
HRT	hormone replacement therapy
IPA	interpretative phenomenological analysis
IPQ	illness perception questionnaire
IPQR	revised version of illness perception questionnaire
LISRES	life stressors and social resources inventory
MAT	medication adherence training
MHLC	multidimensional health locus of control
MI	motivational interviewing, myocardial infarction

MPQ	McGill Pain Questionnaire
MACS	Multi Centre AIDS Cohort Study
NHP	Nottingham Health Profile
NHS	National Health Service
NKCC	natural killer cell cytotoxicity
OCD	obsessive compulsive disorder
PDA	personal digital assistant
PROMS	patient reported outcome measures
PFSQ	parental feeding style questionnaire
PMT	protection motivation theory
PNI	psychoneuroimmunology
PSE	present state examination
PSS	perceived stress scale
PTSD	post-traumatic stress disorder
SEIQoL	schedule for the individual quality of life
SES	socioeconomic status
SEU	subjective expected utility
SIP	Sickness Impact Profile
SLQ	Silver Lining Questionnaire
SOS	Swedish Obese Subjects study
SRE	Schedule of Recent Experiences
SRRS	social readjustment rating scale
STD	sexually transmitted disease
TOP	termination of pregnancy
TPB	theory of planned behaviour
TRA	theory of reasoned action
UR	unconditioned response
US	unconditional stimulus
WHO	World Health Organization
WRAP	Women, Risk and AIDS Project

WHY I FIRST WROTE THIS BOOK

I first wrote this book in 1995 after several years of teaching my own course in health psychology. The texts I recommended to my students were by US authors and this was reflected in their focus on US research and US health care provision. In addition, they tended to be driven by examples rather than by theories or models, which made them difficult to turn into lectures (from my perspective) or to use for essays or revision (from my students' perspective). I decided to write my own book to solve some of these problems. I wanted to supplement US work with that from my colleagues in the UK, the rest of Europe, New Zealand and Australia. I also wanted to emphasize theory and to write the book in a way that would be useful. I hope that the first six editions have succeeded.

AIMS OF THIS NEW SEVENTH EDITION

Over the years this book has grown as I have added in new theories and research and responded to reviewers' feedback. While my aim was always to write a straight forward and user-friendly book, overtime I felt it became unwieldy and too complicated so the sixth edition was a complete rewrite to make the book more focused with a better structure and clearer emphasis on theory and evidence throughout. I also wanted to encourage critical thinking with a separate section on critical thinking for each chapter. But time moves on and, as I write this, the world is becoming a different place with different levels of awareness and different concerns. I am a white heterosexual female Professor from the UK and while I always thought I was very aware of the privileges that came with my position, the past few years have made me realize how naïve I was being! I have learned about the difference between being 'not racist' and 'anti-racist'; I have reflected upon my own 'white privilege'; I have increasingly recognized how 'colonized' our curriculum is; I have maintained my position as a feminist while watching my son (now 22) exist in the complex world of men and seen how difficult it can be to navigate masculinity; I have supported students as they have negotiated their own gender identity; and I have listened to my students, my children, my children's friends and my friends' children as both gender and sexuality have become increasingly fluid. In this seventh edition I have done my best to reflect some of these changes. I hope that this doesn't seem like tokenism but I am sure that this will improve and evolve in future editions. The seventh edition therefore includes the following changes:

Case studies: There is a case study at the start of each chapter to illustrate how the key theories and ideas are relevant to everyday life. These could be used for discussion by lecturers and should help students relate to the material being presented. I hope that these now reflect greater diversity.

Through the eyes of health psychology: Each case study is accompanied by a section to show how a health psychologist could analyse the case study using health psychology ideas.

Critical approaches to health psychology: Together with the 'Thinking critically about . . . .' section in chapter 1 and the separate critical sections at the end of each chapter, I have now added a new section in each chapter called 'Critical approaches to Health Psychology'. This addresses the biases within our discipline in terms of fundamental assumptions reflected in our use of WEIRD populations for our studies and the implications of this for issues such as ethnicity, gender, sexuality, power and culture and the ways in which this underpins the research we do and the theories we develop and test. This new section also explores other key assumptions of our discipline such as the relationship between the individual, the social and the political and between the mind and the body.

Behaviour change: The biggest development in health psychology since this book was first published is the shift in emphasis from predicting behaviour to changing behaviour. Chapter 7 covers the theories and evidence relevant to behaviour change and includes an expanded section on integrated approaches and the drive to develop a new science of behaviour change.

More (and less) common chronic illnesses: There are many chronic illnesses and health psychology is relevant to them all. In this edition I have still focused in Chapters 12 and 13 on HIV/AIDS, cancer, coronary heart disease and obesity but have attempted to highlight how all our research is relevant to a multitude of other chronic conditions such as diabetes, chronic fatigue syndrome and asthma together and have added new focused sections on four less common chronic conditions: Ménière's disease, spinal cord injury, Mild Traumatic Brain Injury and fibromyalgia.

Gender and health: This chapter provides a broader perspective on gender and health and now covers men, women and LGBTQ+ health related issues.

Sexual behaviour: This chapter has also been updated to include a greater emphasis on LGBTQ+ issues in the context of sexual health.

COVID: Since the last edition, the COVID pandemic has happened. I have reflected this where relevant throughout the book but have a separate section on health inequalities and COVID in Chapter 14.

Hybrid/online learning: As a result of COVID, teaching has changed and many of us are involved in hybrid and/or online learning. Hopefully this book will aid this new approach to learning but I have included a new separate section to address this in Chapter 1.

The use of figures and images: I have used far more figures and images throughout to try to make the book more visual. Hopefully this will bring health psychology to life and emphasize how psychological factors are relevant to our daily existence whether we are healthy or not.

Updated throughout: As with the other editions this seventh edition has been updated throughout to reflect recent theories and evidence.

This edition still contains a number of familiar features:

Learning objectives: Each chapter has seven clear learning objectives which are set out at the start of the chapter and then reflected in seven different sections.

Further reading: to recommend to students

Essay questions: for essays, discussion or to structure thinking

For discussion questions: to generate debate in class

An Online Learning Centre website accompanies this edition with useful materials for students of health psychology and their lecturers, including PowerPoint presentations, artwork and more.

Being critical of . . . As with the previous edition this seventh edition encourages critical thinking throughout in terms of design, measures, sample, theory and the notion of truth.

THE STRUCTURE OF THE SEVENTH EDITION

Health psychology focuses on health and illness as a continuum which is reflected in the four parts of this book.

PART 1: THE CONTEXT OF HEALTH PSYCHOLOGY

Chapter 1 explores the main perspectives of health psychology and outlines the aims and structure of this book. In particular, it describes how health psychology differs from clinical psychology and draws upon four frameworks: the biopsychosocial model of health; health as a continuum; the direct and indirect pathways between psychology and health; and a focus on variability. It then highlights the key theories in health psychology. This first chapter next describes how to think critically about the discipline with a focus on theory, methods, design and measurement. It then concludes with a look at how people work within the discipline.

PART 2: HEALTH BELIEFS, BEHAVIOUR AND BEHAVIOUR CHANGE

Central to understanding health and illness is the role of beliefs and behaviour. Chapter 2 describes a number of theories of health beliefs with a focus on individual beliefs, stage models, social cognition models and integrated models. Chapters 3–6 then focus on individual behaviours and describe theories and research which have explored why people do or do not behave in healthy ways. The key behaviours addressed are smoking, drinking and other addictions (Chapter 3), eating behaviour (Chapter 4), exercise (Chapter 5) and sex (Chapter 6). The last chapter in Part 2 then addresses health promotion and theories of behaviour change and explores the ways in which interventions have been developed to encourage people to become more healthy. This is a vast literature and Chapter 7 highlights behaviour change strategies derived from theories such as learning and cognitive theory, affect and integrated models.

PART 3: BECOMING ILL

The next stage along the continuum from health to illness addresses the early factors involved when becoming ill. Chapter 8 describes illness cognitions and ways in which people perceive symptoms and develop representations of their illness. It then addresses theories of coping with illness and the role of both illness cognitions and coping in predicting patient health outcomes. Chapter 9 explores the ways in which individuals come into contact with the health care system. First it examines the mechanisms involved in help-seeking, such as symptom perception and the costs and benefits of visiting a doctor. Next it describes the research on screening, whereby people are drawn into health care even in the absence of any symptoms. Theories and research related to communication in the consultation, with an emphasis on decision-making and how health professionals develop a diagnosis are then discussed. Finally, the chapter explores the issues relating to adherence and how psychological factors such as illness and health beliefs predict whether or not a patient behaves in the way recommended by the health care team. Chapter 10 then describes theories of stress, the ways in which stress can cause illness and how this link can be influenced by psychological and physiological variables.

PART 4: BEING ILL

Following along the continuum is the next stage: being ill. Chapter 11 describes theories of pain and approaches to pain management. It also highlights the important role of the placebo effect and the possible mechanisms behind this process. Chapters 12 and 13 then focus on specific chronic illnesses and assess how the many psychological constructs and theories addressed in the book so far relate to the onset, progression and outcomes of HIV, cancer (Chapter 12), obesity and coronary heart disease (Chapter 13). These chapters also discuss how the key psychological factors such as health beliefs and behaviours, illness cognitions, adherence, coping and social support also relate to all other chronic conditions such as asthma, diabetes and arthritis and include focused sections on four less common conditions: fibromyalgia, Ménière's disease, spinal cord injury and Mild Traumatic Brain Injury. Part 4 then explores the role of health status and quality of life in patient outcomes (Chapter 14) and concludes with a focus on gender and health (Chapter 15) which highlights the role of gender in symptoms, illness and life expectancy with a focus on gender-specific conditions and issues specific to men, women and the LGBTQ+ community.

Guided Tour

CHAPTER OVERVIEW

This chapter offers a broad introduction to
a brief background to health psychology an
and a more traditional biomedical model. It
terms of a biopsychosocial model, health an
indirect pathways between psychological fa
variability. Next the chapter explores key t
frame research and develop and test interve
critically about health psychology with a fo
The chapter also describes the ways in whi

CASE STUDY

Sanjay is 75 years old and has lung cancer.
used to smoke over at the park with the ciga
He worked for many years as a hospital por
outside with his mates. It gave them a break f
ful. He married Saara when he was 25. Saara
smoking but when he became moody and irr
in the house. Sanjay always had a cough, wh

Figures and Tables

Clear and well-represented tables and figures
throughout the book provide up-to-date information and data in a clear and easy-to-read
format.

SOME CRITICAL QUESTIONS

When reading or thinking about the theories
following questions:

• How important are our beliefs compared t
• Can we really measure what someone beli
• To what extent are our beliefs captured b

Title Page

Each chapter is structured around 7 learning
objectives which are listed on the title page
for each chapter for quick and easy reference
to specific topics. The Chapter Overview
section then describes the chapter in more
detail. The title page also has a topic specific
Case Study describing a person with a health
issue relevant to that chapter. It also has a
section entitled 'Through the Eyes of Health
Psychology' which illustrates how health psychology would make sense of the case study
drawing upon key constructs and theories.

Learning Objectives

To understand:

1. The Background to
   Health Psychology
2. What Is Health
   Psychology?
3. The Focus of Health
   Psychology
4. Key Theories

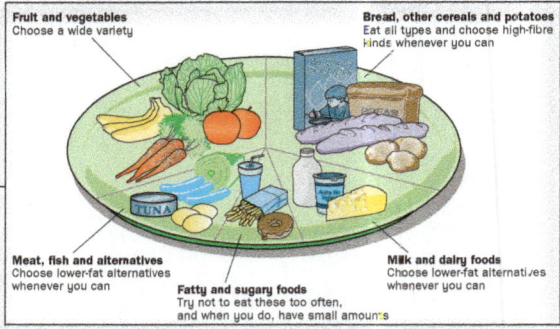

Thinking Critically About. . .

Each chapter ends with a feature called 'Thinking
Critically about. . .' which starts with 'Some
Critical Questions' to encourage you to pause
for thought and reflect on health psychology
research. It then has a detailed section called
'Some Problems with. . .', which outlines key problems with the theories, constructs and methods
covered in the chapter. Finally, it has a section
called 'Critical Health Psychology' which explores
some of the assumptions of the discipline relating
to issues such as the populations we study and
the questions we ask and how this is often underpinned by WEIRD research with a colonial focus.

To Conclude

A wrap-up of the main themes to emerge from the chapter and a useful revision tool to recap the material in a topic area.

TO CONCLUDE

Health psychology explores how a nu
illness and emphasizes four framework
being on a continuum, the direct and in
problem of variability. This book covers
basis for a complete course for students
those both within psychology and in oth
and dieticians.

QUESTIONS

1 To what extent does health psychology c
   health and illness?
2 Why do health psychologists consider he
3 Is the biopsychosocial model a useful per
4 What problems are there with dividing up
   indirect and direct pathways?
5 What factors could explain variability be

Questions

Short questions to test your understanding and encourage you to consider some of the issues raised in the chapter. A useful means of assessing your comprehension and progress.

For Discussion

A discussion point for a seminar or group work, or to form the basis of an essay.

FOR DISCUSSION

Consider the last time you were ill (e.g. fl
factors other than biological ones may have

FURTHER READING

Kaptein, A and Weinman, J. (eds) (2010)
This edited collection provides further deta
tral to health psychology.

Michie, S. & Abraham, C. (eds) (2004) *He*
This edited collection provides a detailed a
chartered health psychologist in the UK. Ho
to anyone interested in pursuing a career in

Further Reading

A list of useful essays, articles, books and research which can take your study further. A good starting point for your research for essays or assignments.

Glossary

At the end of the text there is a brief glossary of the commonly used terms in health psychology methodology.

Methodology glossary

B

Between-subjects design: this involves making comparisons between different groups of subjects; for example, males versus females, those who have been offered a health-related intervention versus those who have not.

C

Case-control design: this involves taking a group of subjects who show a particular characteristic

Longitudinal de
ables at a basel
at a later point
or cohort desig

P

Prospective des
jects over a pe
tudinal or coho

Technology to Enhance Learning and Teaching

Visit www.mcgraw-hill.co.uk/textbooks/ogden today

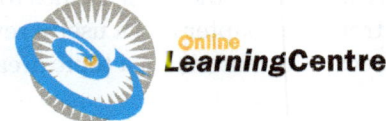

Online Learning Centre (OLC)

After completing each chapter, log on to the supporting Online Learning Centre website. Take advantage of the study tools offered to reinforce the material you have read in the text, and to develop your knowledge in a fun and effective way.

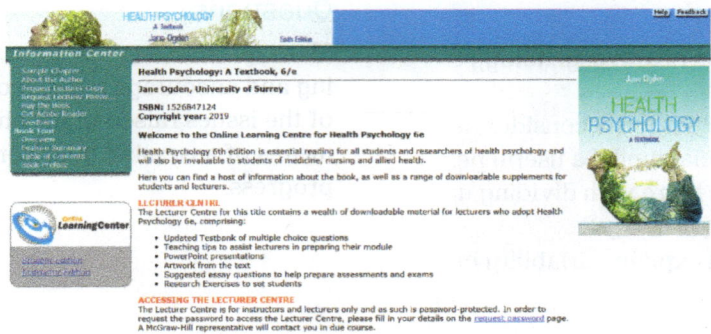

Resources for students include:

- Useful weblinks to extra health psychology resources online
- Searchable online glossary
- Chapter overviews

Also available for lecturers:

- New Test Bank of multiple choice questions
- Teaching tips to assist lecturers in preparing their module
- PowerPoint presentations for use in class or as handouts
- Artwork from the text
- Suggested essay questions to help prepare assessments and exams

Visit www.mheducation.co.uk/textbooks/ogden7 today

Create & Custom Publishing

It's easy to create your perfect
customised reader

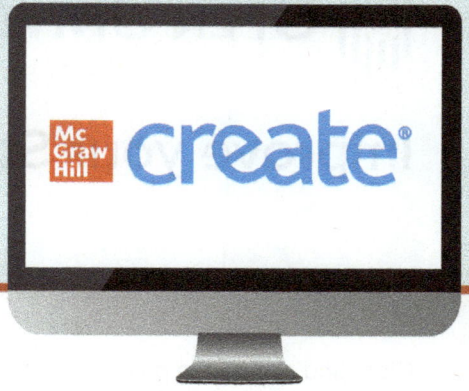

At McGraw-Hill it's easy to create a bespoke reading
resource for our students right from the comfort of your desk.

Using our tool Create you can browse and select material from our extensive library of texts and collections
and if desired, you can even include your own materials, which can be organised in the order in which you'd
like your students to work from them.

Available in both print and eBook format, you can offer your students a learning solution that
works best for them, in addition you can add digital materials to go alongside your reader too.

What are the benefits of having a custom reader?

- You have one **tailor-made** learning resource
- **McGraw-Hill are here to support you** throughout your custom journey
- Students get **value for money**; they only need to purchase & read the required course material
- **Convenient** and students can easily find resources **all in one place**
- Students are **more prepared** for class

How do I Get Started?

1 **Find** and **Select** your content in **Create**

2 **Arrange** and **Integrate** your own content

3 **Personalise** your design and **Choose** the format

Learn more
https://www.mheducation.co.uk/higher-education/services/creating-custom-publishing

Contact the Team
marketing.emea@mheducation.com

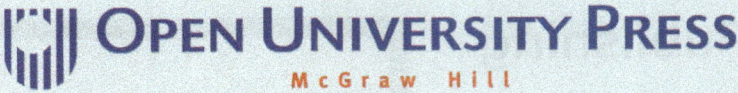

OPEN UNIVERSITY PRESS
McGraw Hill

Improve your Study, Research & Writing Skills

Clear and accessible guides on improving your reading, writing and researching skills. From undergraduate level to career researcher, we have a book to help you with your study and academic progression.

Our Study Skills books are packed with practical advice and tips that are easy to put into practice and will really improve the way you study.

- Develop your study skills
- Learn how to undertake a research project
- Enhance your academic writing and avoid plagiarism
- Learn effective ways to prep for exams
- Improve time management
- Increase your grades
- Get the job you want!

Discount Code: OPENUP20

Special Offer!

As a valued customer, buy online and receive **20% off** any of our Study Skills books by entering the above promo code.

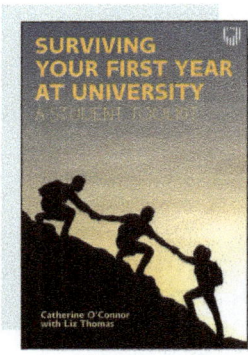 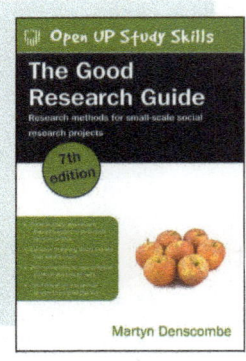 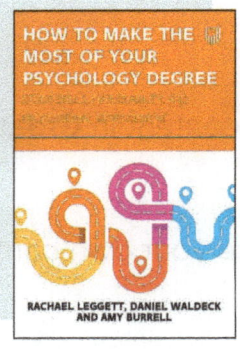 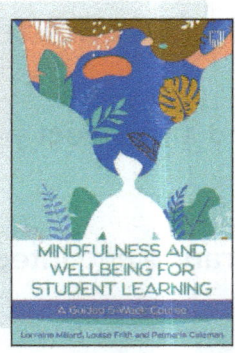

Acknowledgements

My thanks again go to my students and colleagues over the years for their comments, feedback and research input. For this edition I am particularly grateful to Sophia Quirke-McFarlane for helping me with the updating process. And, as ever, I am eternally grateful to Harry and Ellie for giving me that work–life balance and for being a wonderful source of meaning and fun. In the past I have written this book in the evenings when they have gone to bed and have been grateful for stricter bedtimes. Now that they are grown up and independent, and I am in my new phase of life, I have written this in and around the edges of enjoying everything that life in your fifties seems to bring! Which, by the way, for those of you not there yet, is great!

The publishers would also like to thank the reviewers who commented on the previous edition and gave their time and expertise to provide helpful and constructive feedback. Their advice and suggestions were extremely helpful in shaping the seventh edition. The reviewers were:

Elaine Walklet, University of Worcester

Francis Quinn, The Robert Gordon University

Jacqueline Davies, University of London City

Jennie Todd, University of Essex

Katrina Forbes-Mckay, Robert Gordon University

Katy Tapper, University of London City

Liz Whelen, University of Chester

Mioara Cristea, Heriot Watt University

Michael Smith, Northumbria University

Rebecca Jayne Stack, Nottingham Trent University

Stephan Dombrowski, University of Stirling

Susan Faulkner, University of South Wales

Steve Hosier, Bangor University

Floor Kroese, Utrecht University

Mark Tarrant, University of Exeter Medical School

Richard Cooker, Aston University

David Hevey, Trinity College Dublin

Sally Adams, University of Bath

Lynn Myers, Brunel University

Krishna Bhatti, Coventry University

Liz Whelen, University of Chester

Eimear Lee, Anglia Ruskin University

Molly Byrne, National University of Ireland Galway

Shaun Speed, University of Manchester

James Byron-Daniel, University of the West of the England

Paul Kocken, Erasmus University Rotterdam

Gulcan Garip, University of Derby

Wendy Maltinsky, University of Stirling

Finally, every effort has been made to contact copyright holders to secure permission to republish material in this textbook, and to include correct acknowledgements where required. The publishers would be happy to hear from any copyright holders whom it has not been possible for us to contact.

All photographs are © Jane Ogden unless otherwise stated.

PART ONE

The Context of Health Psychology

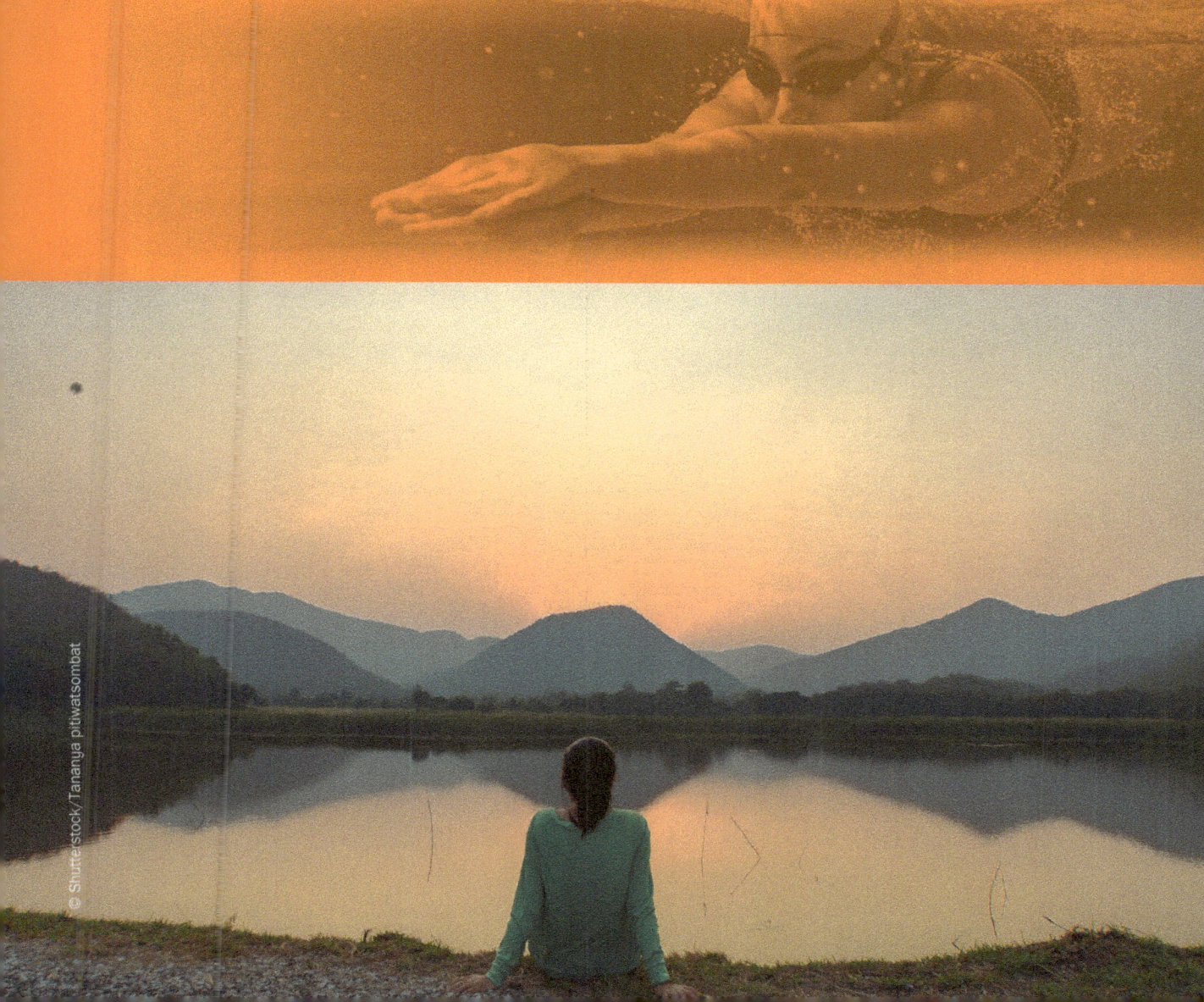

1

Introduction to Health Psychology: Theories and Methods

Learning Objectives

To understand:

1. The Background to Health Psychology
2. What Is Health Psychology?
3. The Focus of Health Psychology
4. Key Theories
5. Thinking Critically About Health Psychology
6. Working in Health Psychology
7. The Aims of this Book

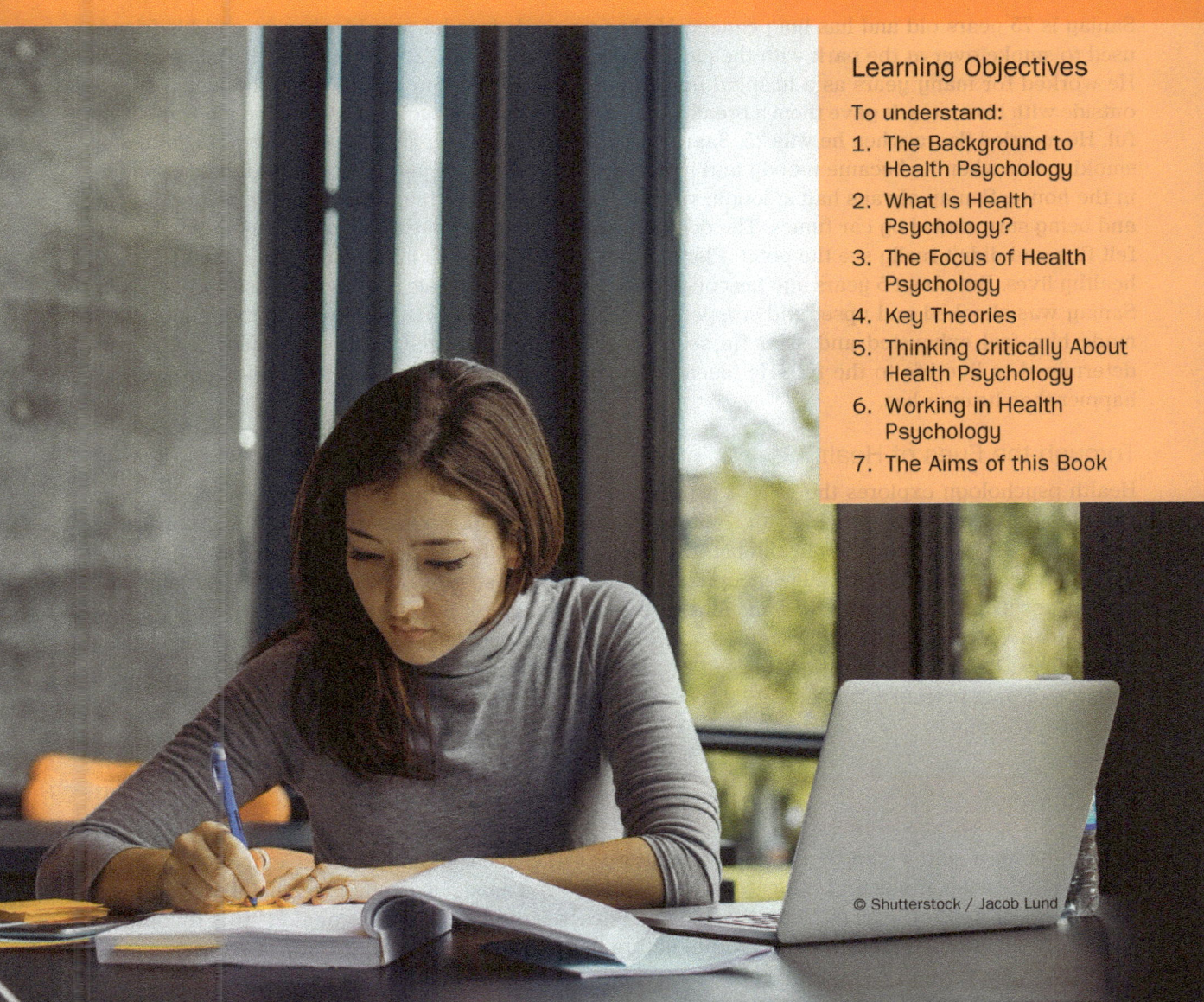

© Shutterstock / Jacob Lund

CHAPTER OVERVIEW

This chapter offers a broad introduction to the discipline of health psychology. First, it provides a brief background to health psychology and highlights differences between health psychology and a more traditional biomedical model. It then describes the focus of health psychology in terms of a biopsychosocial model, health and illness as being on a continuum, the direct and indirect pathways between psychological factors and health and the emphasis on explaining variability. Next the chapter explores key theories used in health psychology as a means to frame research and develop and test interventions. The chapter then describes how to think critically about health psychology with a focus on methods, measures, data analysis and theory. The chapter also describes the ways in which people work in health psychology: either in research, teaching, consultancy or as a practitioner. Finally, this chapter outlines the aims of this textbook and describes how the book is structured.

CASE STUDY

Sanjay is 75 years old and has lung cancer. He has smoked since he was 14 when he and his friends used to smoke over at the park with the cigarettes he 'found' in his father's pockets. It was great fun. He worked for many years as a hospital porter and was allowed 'fag breaks' when he would smoke outside with his mates. It gave them a break from work and time to laugh even when the job was stressful. He married Saara when he was 25. Saara was a nurse at the hospital. She encouraged him to stop smoking but when he became moody and irritable she gave up and just insisted that he didn't smoke in the house. Sanjay always had a cough, which he put down to asthma caused by growing up a city and being surrounded by car fumes. The doctor suggested that he give up smoking but Sanjay always felt fine and didn't really see the point. Plenty of people had smoked in his family and lived long and healthy lives. But about 5 years ago his cough got worse and after tests he was diagnosed with cancer. Sanjay was shocked and upset and stopped smoking immediately. He has had chemotherapy which made him feel exhausted and sick. He seems to be responding well to the treatment and is now determined to live life to the full. He has started cycling and walking more often and says he feels happier than he ever has.

Through the Eyes of Health Psychology. . .

Health psychology explores the role of psychological factors in physical health across the life span and along the continuum from health to illness. Sanjay's story illustrates the multitude of constructs covered in this book, including health beliefs (smoking is fun), health behaviours (fag breaks), behaviour change (started cycling), illness cognitions (it's asthma), stress (at work), coping (smoking with mates), social support (Saara), chronic illness (cancer), quality of life (feeling sick) and gender issues (being with mates at work). It illustrates some of the reasons people behave as they do and the ways in which illness can impact upon their lives. It also highlights the impact of others in what we do and think in terms of peer pressure, role models and social support. These factors make up the essence of what health psychology is.

1 THE BACKGROUND TO HEALTH PSYCHOLOGY

During the nineteenth century, modern medicine was established. 'Man' (the nineteenth-century term) was studied using dissection, physical investigations and medical examinations. Darwin's thesis, *The Origin of Species,* was published in 1856 and described the theory of evolution. This revolutionary theory identified a place for man within nature and suggested that we are part of nature, that we developed from nature and that we are biological beings. This was in accord with the biomedical model of medicine, which studied man in the same way that other members of the natural world had been studied in earlier years. This model described human beings as having a biological identity in common with all other biological beings.

THE TWENTIETH CENTURY

Throughout the twentieth century there were challenges to some of the underlying assumptions of biomedicine which emphasized an increasing role for psychology in health and a changing model of the relationship between the mind and body.

Psychosomatic Medicine

The earliest challenge to the biomedical model was psychosomatic medicine. Towards the end of the nineteenth century, Freud described a condition called 'hysterical paralysis', whereby patients presented with paralysed limbs with no obvious physical cause and in a pattern that did not reflect the organization of nerves. Freud argued that this condition was an indication of the individual's state of mind and that repressed experiences and feelings were expressed in terms of a physical problem. This explanation indicated an interaction between mind and body and suggested that psychological factors may not only be consequences of illness but may contribute to its cause. This led to the development of psychosomatic medicine at the beginning of the twentieth century in response to Freud's analysis of the relationship between the mind and physical illness.

Behavioural Medicine

A further discipline that challenged the biomedical model of health was behavioural medicine, which has been described by Schwartz and Weiss (1977) as being an amalgam of elements from the behavioural science disciplines (psychology, sociology, health education) and which focuses on health care, treatment and illness prevention. Behavioural medicine was also described by Pomerleau and Brady (1979) as consisting of methods derived from the experimental analysis of behaviour, such as behaviour therapy and behaviour modification, and involved in the evaluation, treatment and prevention of physical disease or physiological dysfunction (e.g. essential hypertension, addictive behaviours and obesity). It has also been emphasized that psychological problems such as neurosis and psychosis are not studied within behavioural medicine unless they contribute to the development of illness. Behavioural medicine therefore included psychology in the study of health and departed from traditional biomedical views of health by not only focusing on treatment, but also focusing on prevention and intervention. In addition, behavioural medicine challenged the traditional separation of the mind and the body.

WHAT IS THE BIOMEDICAL MODEL?

The biomedical model of medicine can be understood in terms of its answers to the following questions:

- *What causes illness?* According to the biomedical model of medicine, diseases either come from outside the body, invade the body and cause physical changes within the body, or originate as internal involuntary physical changes. Such diseases may be caused by several factors such as chemical imbalances, bacteria, viruses and genetic predisposition.
- *Who is responsible for illness?* Because illness is seen as arising from biological changes beyond their control, individuals are not seen as responsible for their illness. They are regarded as victims of some external force causing internal changes.
- *How should illness be treated?* The biomedical model regards treatment in terms of vaccination, surgery, chemotherapy and radiotherapy, all of which aim to change the physical state of the body.
- *Who is responsible for treatment?* The responsibility for treatment rests with the medical profession.

- *What is the relationship between health and illness?* Within the biomedical model, health and illness are seen as qualitatively different – you are either healthy or ill, there is no continuum between the two.

- *What is the relationship between the mind and the body?* According to the biomedical model of medicine, the mind and body function independently of each other. This is comparable to a traditional dualistic model of the mind–body split. From this perspective, the mind is incapable of influencing physical matter and the mind and body are defined as separate entities. The mind is seen as abstract and relating to feelings and thoughts, and the body is seen in terms of physical matter such as skin, muscles, bones, brain and organs. Changes in the physical matter are regarded as independent of changes in state of mind.

- *What is the role of psychology in health and illness?* Within traditional biomedicine, illness may have psychological consequences, but not psychological causes. For example, cancer may cause unhappiness but mood is not seen as related to either the onset or progression of the cancer.

2 WHAT IS HEALTH PSYCHOLOGY?

Health psychology is probably the most recent development in this process of including psychology in an understanding of health. It was described by Matarazzo (1980: 815) as 'the aggregate of the specific educational, scientific and professional contribution of the discipline of psychology to the promotion and maintenance of health, the promotion and treatment of illness and related dysfunction'. Health psychology again challenges the mind–body split by suggesting a role for the mind in both the cause and treatment of illness, but differs from psychosomatic medicine and behavioural medicine in that research within health psychology is more specific to the discipline of psychology.

Health psychology can be understood in terms of the same questions that were asked of the biomedical model:

- *What causes illness?* Health psychology suggests that human beings should be seen as complex systems and that illness is caused by a multitude of factors and not by a single causal factor. Health psychology therefore attempts to move away from a simple linear model of health and claims that illness can be caused by a combination of biological (e.g. a virus), psychological (e.g. behaviours, beliefs) and social (e.g. employment) factors.

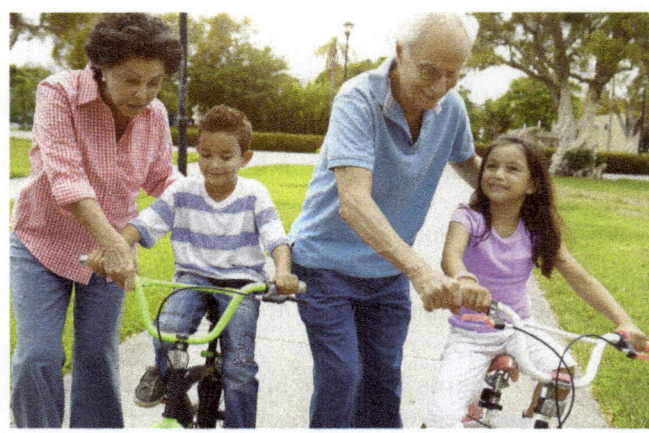

Health behaviour can be encouraged by family

SOURCE: © Shutterstock / Monkey Business Images

- *Who is responsible for illness?* Because illness is regarded as a result of a combination of factors, the individual is no longer simply seen as a passive victim. For example, the recognition of a role for behaviour in the cause of illness means that the individual may be held responsible for their health and illness.

- *How should illness be treated?* According to health psychology, the whole person should be treated, not just the physical changes that have taken place. This can take the form of behaviour change, encouraging changes in beliefs and coping strategies, and compliance with medical recommendations.

- *Who is responsible for treatment?* Because the whole person is treated, not just their physical illness, the patient is therefore in part responsible for their treatment. This may take the form of responsibility to take medication and/or responsibility to change their beliefs and behaviour. They are not seen as a victim.

- *What is the relationship between health and illness?* From this perspective, health and illness are not qualitatively different, but exist on a continuum. Rather than being either healthy or ill, individuals progress along this continuum from health to illness and back again.

- *What is the relationship between the mind and the body?* The twentieth century saw a challenge to the traditional separation of mind and body suggested by a dualistic model of health and illness, with an increasing focus on an interaction between the mind and the body. This shift in perspective is reflected in the development of a holistic or a whole-person approach to health. Health psychology therefore maintains that the mind and body interact.

- *What is the role of psychology in health and illness?* Health psychology regards psychological factors not only as possible consequences of illness but as contributing to it at all stages along the continuum from healthy through to being ill.

WHAT ARE THE AIMS OF HEALTH PSYCHOLOGY?

Health psychology emphasizes the role of psychological factors in the cause, progression and consequences of health and illness. The aims of health psychology can be divided into (1) understanding, explaining, developing and testing theory, and (2) putting this theory into practice.

1 *Health psychology aims to understand, explain, develop and test theory by:*

  A Evaluating the role of behaviour in the aetiology of illness. For example:
- Coronary heart disease is related to behaviours such as smoking, food intake and lack of exercise.
- Many cancers are related to behaviours such as diet, smoking, alcohol and failure to attend for screening or health check-ups.
- A stroke is related to smoking, cholesterol and high blood pressure.
- An often overlooked cause of death is accidents. These may be related to alcohol consumption, drugs and careless driving.

  B Predicting unhealthy behaviours. For example:
- Smoking, alcohol consumption and high fat diets are related to beliefs.
- Beliefs about health and illness can be used to predict behaviour.

  C Evaluating the interaction between psychology and physiology. For example:
- The experience of stress relates to appraisal, coping and social support.
- Stress leads to physiological changes which can trigger or exacerbate illness.
- Pain perception can be exacerbated by anxiety and reduced by distraction.

  D Understanding the role of psychology in the experience of illness. For example:
- Understanding the psychological consequences of illness could help to alleviate symptoms such as pain, nausea and vomiting.
- Understanding the psychological consequences of illness could help alleviate psychological symptoms such as anxiety and depression.

  E Evaluating the role of psychology in the treatment of illness. For example:
- If psychological factors are important in the cause of illness, they may also have a role in its treatment.

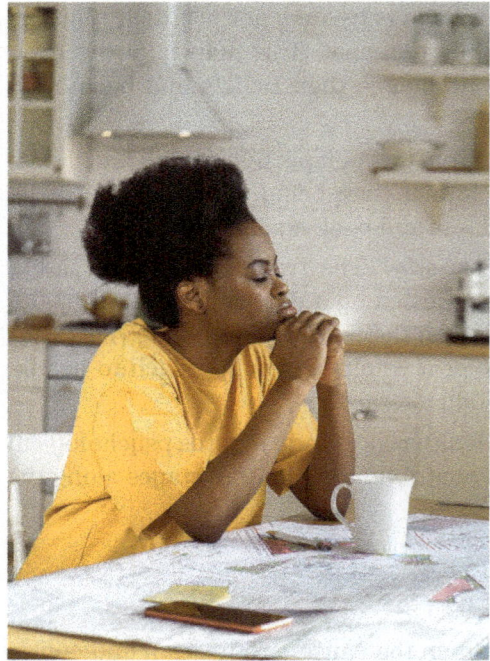

Illness can be prevented by reducing stress

SOURCE: © Shutterstock/DimaBerlin

- Changing behaviour and reducing stress could reduce the chances of a further heart attack.
- Treatment of the psychological consequences of illness may have an impact on longevity.

2 *Health psychology also aims to put theory into practice. This can be implemented by:*

A Promoting healthy behaviour. For example:

- Understanding the role of behaviour in illness can allow unhealthy behaviours to be targeted.
- Understanding the beliefs that predict behaviours can allow these beliefs to be targeted.
- Understanding beliefs can help these beliefs to be changed.

B Preventing illness. For example:

- Changing beliefs and behaviour could prevent onset of illness.
- Modifying stress could reduce the risk of a heart attack.
- Behavioural interventions during illness (e.g. stopping smoking after a heart attack) may prevent further illness.
- Training health professionals to improve their communication skills and to carry out interventions may help to prevent illness.

CLINICAL PSYCHOLOGY VERSUS HEALTH PSYCHOLOGY

Both clinical psychology and health psychology are concerned with the role of psychological factors in the development and experience of health. The focus of clinical psychology, however, tends to be mental health with an emphasis on mental health conditions such as anxiety, depression, psychosis, eating disorders, self-harm and obsessive compulsive disorder (OCD). In contrast, health psychology addresses physical health problems such as obesity, diabetes, cancer, heart disease, asthma and HIV/AIDS. Further, while clinical psychology uses approaches such as cognitive behaviour therapy (CBT), family therapy and psychotherapy to help treat patients, health psychology draws upon constructs such as sense making, illness cognitions, appraisal, social support, beliefs and behaviour change to understand illness onset and progression and to develop interventions to improve patient health outcomes. There are clearly, however, strong crossovers between clinical and health psychology and the distinction between the two can seem somewhat artificial, particularly given the increasing focus on a holistic approach and the interaction between mind and body. For example, those with a physical health problem such as cancer or HIV may well also have associated mental health issues such as anxiety. Likewise, those with a mental health issue such as psychosis or anxiety may well also have physical health problems such as obesity or diabetes or report unhealthy behaviours such as smoking or having a poor diet. To reflect this crossover, therefore, many clinical psychologists are also trained in health psychology and may use their clinical training within a health psychology domain. Further, the research literature often now focuses on the notion of complex conditions, co-morbidities or multi-morbidities to reflect the coexistence of physical and mental health problems. For simplicity, however, it is best to consider clinical psychology as concerned with the mental health components and health psychology as concerned with the psychology aspects of physical health components but to acknowledge that in reality these two components of health are not as discrete as often presented. The differences between clinical and health psychology are shown in Figure 1.1.

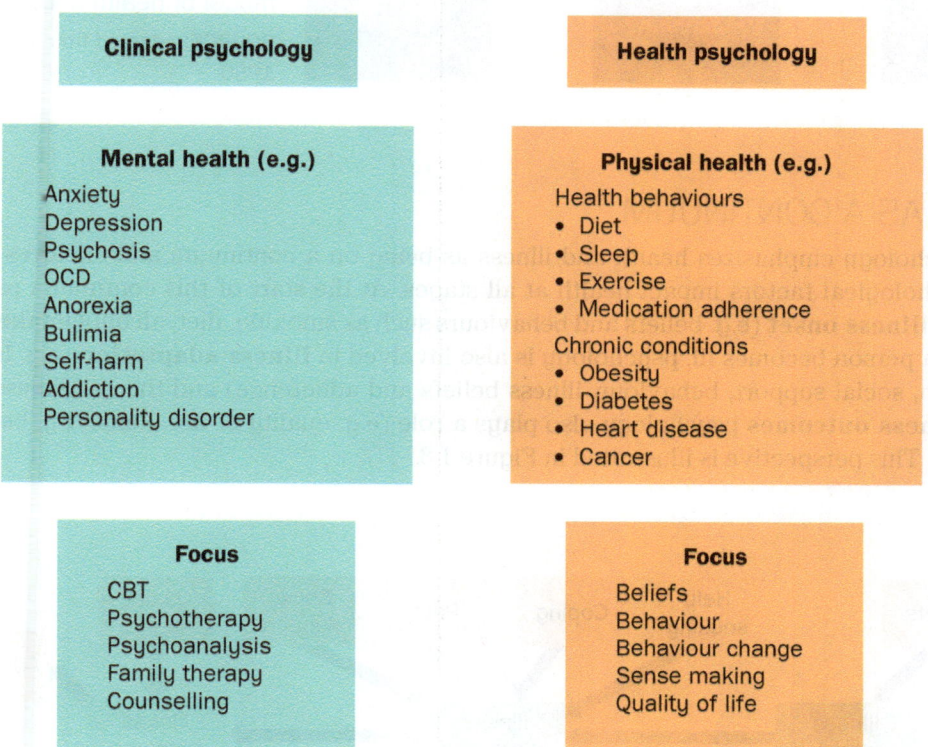

Figure 1.1 Clinical psychology versus health psychology

3   THE FOCUS OF HEALTH PSYCHOLOGY

Health psychology draws upon four key frameworks in its analysis of health and illness. These are the biopsychosocial model of health, health as a continuum, the direct and indirect pathways between psychology and health, and a focus on variability. These will now be described.

THE BIOPSYCHOSOCIAL MODEL

The biopsychosocial model was developed by Engel (1977; see Figure 1.2) and represented an attempt to integrate the psychological (the 'psycho') and the environmental (the 'social') into the traditional biomedical (the 'bio') model of health as follows: (1) the *bio* contributing factors included genetics, viruses, bacteria and structural defects; (2) the *psycho* aspects of health and illness were described in terms of cognitions (e.g. expectations of health), emotions (e.g. fear of treatment) and behaviours (e.g. smoking, diet, exercise or alcohol consumption); (3) the *social* aspects of health were described in terms of social norms of behaviour (e.g. the social norm of smoking or not smoking), pressures to change behaviour (e.g. peer group expectations, parental pressure), social values on health (e.g. whether health was regarded as a good or a bad thing), social class and ethnicity.

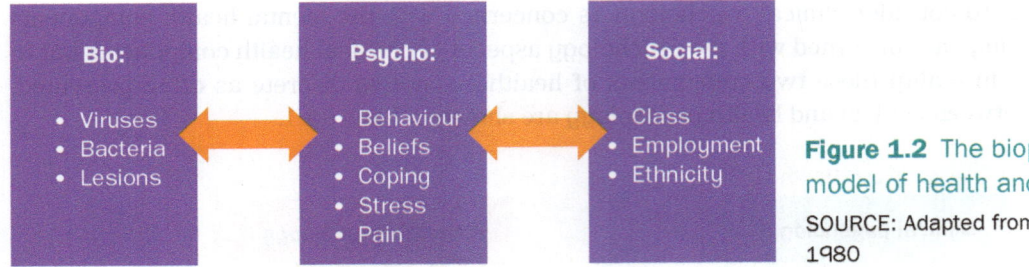

Figure 1.2 The biopsychosocial model of health and illness

SOURCE: Adapted from Engel, 1977, 1980

HEALTH AS A CONTINUUM

Health psychology emphasizes health and illness as being on a continuum and explores the ways in which psychological factors impact health at all stages. At the start of this continuum psychology is involved in **illness onset** (e.g. beliefs and behaviours such as smoking, diet, alcohol intake and stress). Then once a person becomes ill, psychology is also involved in **illness adaptation** (e.g. help seeking, coping, pain, social support, behaviour, illness beliefs and adherence) and then as illness progresses towards **illness outcomes** psychology also plays a role (e.g. quality of life, longevity, behaviour and adherence). This perspective is illustrated in Figure 1.3.

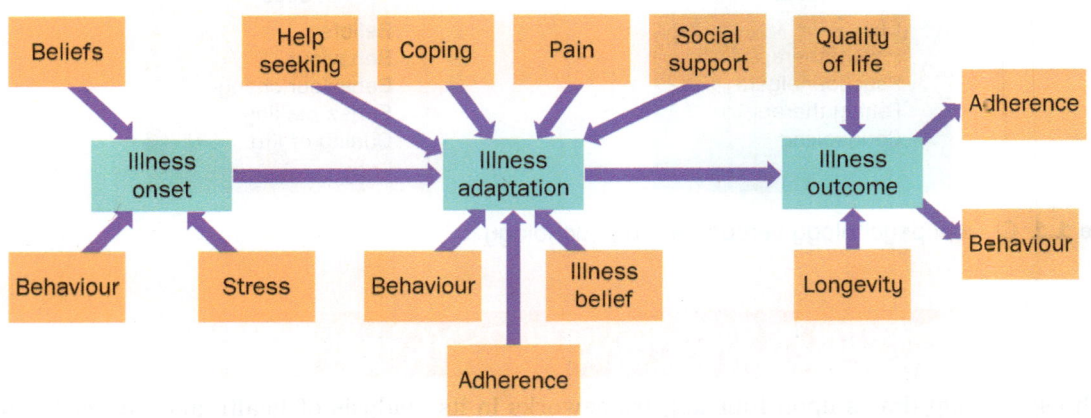

Figure 1.3 Health as a continuum and psychology throughout the course of illness

THE RELATIONSHIP BETWEEN PSYCHOLOGY AND HEALTH

Health psychologists consider both a direct and indirect pathway between psychology and health. The direct pathway is reflected in the physiological literature and is illustrated by research exploring the impact of stress on illnesses such as coronary heart disease and cancer. From this perspective, the way a person experiences their life ('I am feeling stressed') has a direct impact upon their body which can change their health status. The indirect pathway is reflected more in the behavioural literature and is illustrated by research exploring smoking, diet, exercise and sexual behaviour. From this perspective, the way a person thinks ('I am feeling stressed') influences their behaviour ('I will have a cigarette') which in turn can impact upon their health. The direct and indirect pathways are illustrated in Figure 1.4.

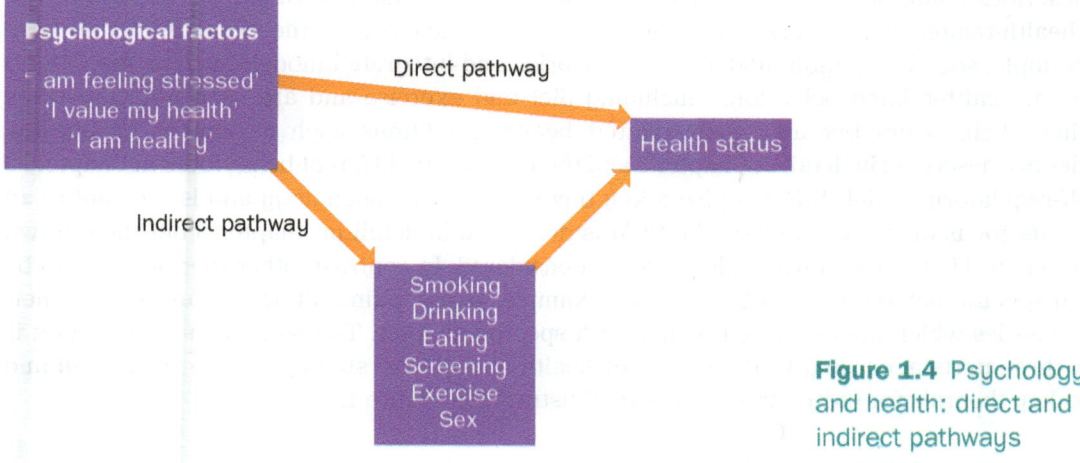

Figure 1.4 Psychology and health: direct and indirect pathways

A FOCUS ON VARIABILITY

Health and illness vary along a number of domains including geographical location, time, social class and gender. Health psychology explores this variability with a focus on the role of behaviour. However, there is also variability between *people* and this is also the focus of health psychology. For example, two people might both know that smoking is bad for them but only one stops smoking. Similarly, two people might find a lump in their breast but only one goes to the doctor. Further, two people might both have a heart attack but while one has another attack in six months' time, the other is perfectly healthy and back to work within a month. This variability indicates that health and illness cannot only be explained by illness severity (i.e. type of cancer, severity of heart attack) or knowledge (i.e. smoking is harmful), but that other factors must have a key role to play. For a health psychologist, these factors are central to the discipline and include a wide range of psychological variables such as cognitions, emotions, expectations, learning, peer pressure, social norms, coping and social support. These constructs are the nuts and bolts of psychology and are covered in the chapters in this book. The notion of variability is shown in Figure 1.5.

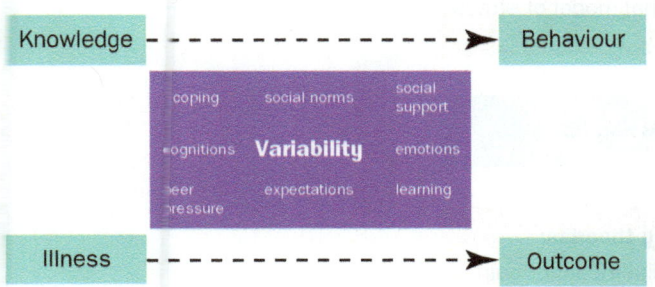

Figure 1.5 A focus on variability: It takes more than knowledge and illness type to explain the variability in behaviour and illness

4 KEY THEORIES

Theories are used to underpin research and frame and test interventions. Health psychology is a magpie discipline and 'steals' its theories from other psychological perspectives. For example, it uses learning theory with its emphasis on associations and modelling; social cognition theories with their emphasis on beliefs and attitudes; stage theories with their focus on change and progression; decision-making theory highlighting a cost–benefit analysis and the role of hypothesis testing; and physiological theories with their interest in biological processes and their links with health. Further, it utilizes many key psychological concepts such as stereotyping, self-identity, risk perception, self-efficacy and addiction.

This book describes many of these theories and explores how they have been used to explain health status and health-related behaviours. Some theories are relevant across the breadth of the discipline. For example, social cognition models, stage theories and integrated models such as the COM-B model focus on health-related behaviours including diet and exercise and are used not only when exploring these behaviours but also their related health conditions such as cancer or obesity. These theories are described in detail in Chapter 2 and then applied to different behaviours in Chapters 3 to 7. The self-regulatory model (SRM) is also a key theory in health psychology and is relevant to all illnesses with its focus on sense making. The SRM is described in detail in Chapter 8 but then drawn upon in Chapters 9, 11, 12 and 13 when illnesses are considered. In contrast, other theories tend to be used to study specific behaviours or illnesses. For example, stress, pain and health status have their own unique theories which are described within each specific chapter. The remainder of this book is divided into three parts according to the stages of health and illness: staying well, becoming ill and being ill. The key theories for these three stages are illustrated in Figure 1.6.

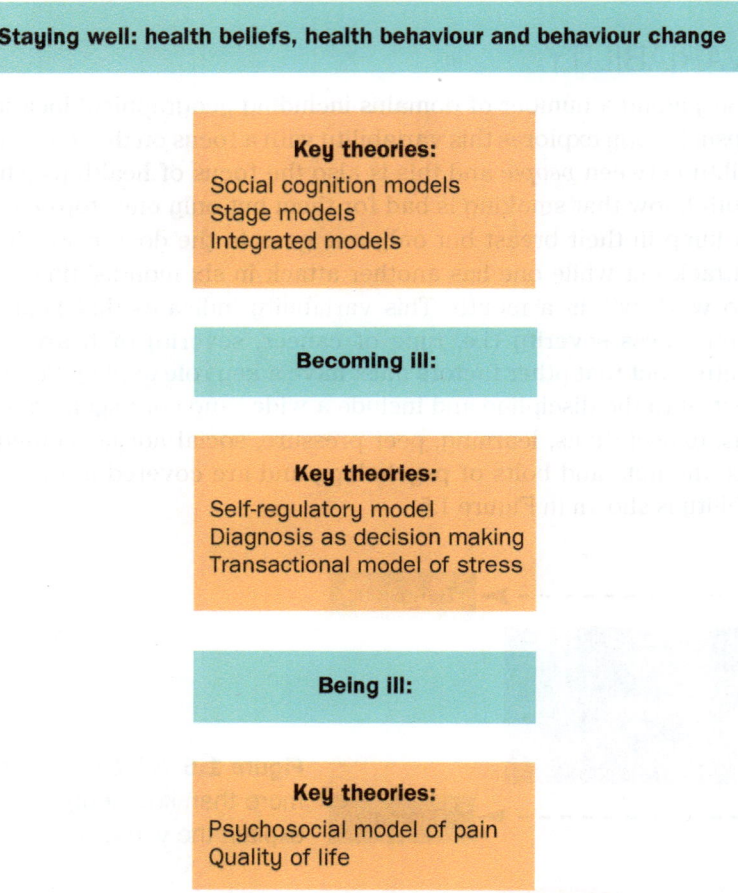

Staying well: health beliefs, health behaviour and behaviour change

Key theories:
Social cognition models
Stage models
Integrated models

Becoming ill:

Key theories:
Self-regulatory model
Diagnosis as decision making
Transactional model of stress

Being ill:

Key theories:
Psychosocial model of pain
Quality of life

Figure 1.6 Key theories in health psychology

If you want a short cut to understanding health psychology I would recommend that you learn one theory relevant to health behaviours (e.g. the health belief model, the theory of planned behaviour or the COM-B) and one theory relevant to sense making and chronic illness (e.g. the self-regulatory model). But if you want to become a skilled and broad-based health psychologist, and as cross-fertilization is often the making of good research and practice, I would recommend becoming familiar with the wealth of theories we use, thinking critically about these theories and drawing upon whichever approach makes the most sense to whatever question you are trying to answer.

5   THINKING CRITICALLY ABOUT HEALTH PSYCHOLOGY

BEING CRITICAL

For years I have told my students to think more critically. But for years I didn't really explain what this meant or what to do. So what does 'being critical' mean? When an article is published and presented in columns, with an 'academic'-looking font, complex tables and figures, a long list of references and a number of senior-sounding authors, it is easy to accept it as 'true'. Becoming critical is about developing the confidence to question a paper to see whether it really makes sense and whether the conclusions are justified. At one level, being critical may be quite simple in terms of exploring issues such as sample size (is it representative?), the measures used (are they valid?), the statistical tests employed (are they the right ones?) or the chosen research design (can they make causal conclusions from a qualitative study?). But at a more sophisticated level, being critical also means thinking about the theories being tested (do they make sense?), the constructs used (are they different from each other?) and whether the arguments are coherent (what are they really saying?). Furthermore, being critical may also highlight some fundamental flaws in a discipline if we start to ask about an author's underlying assumptions (such as whether people really have a consistent personality or whether what people say they think is what they really think), or what a discipline chooses to focus on and chooses to ignore (why do psychologists focus on behaviour while sociologists focus on society-level variables such as social class, education, social capital, economic stability, etc.?). And finally, being critical involves learning to trust the feeling that something 'isn't quite right' or 'doesn't quite make sense' or 'is so obvious that it's not interesting'. This section describes how to think critically of health psychology in terms of theory, methods, measurement and the discipline itself.

BEING CRITICAL OF THEORY

Health psychology uses theories such as the stages of change model (SOC), the theory of planned behaviour (TPB) or the COM-B. It also uses constructs such as self-efficacy, behavioural intentions, illness cognitions and coping. Some theories are based on stages and see their components as leading from one to the other in a linear progression. The SOC model is one such model. Other theories are more dynamic and describe their components as being interrelated. Examples of these are the TPB and the COM-B. Being critical of theory involves learning to ask questions about constructs and theories such as the ones described below. Additional ways to think critically about the SOC, TPB and COM-B can be found at the end of Chapters 2 and 7.

Constructs

Health psychology uses a wide range of constructs such as coping, illness beliefs, perceived control, quality of life depression and anxiety. We need to ask whether these constructs are meaningful and discrete. For example:

- Is 'I feel depressed' an emotion or a cognition?
- Can depression cause poor quality of life or is it part of quality of life?
- Can poor health status lead to poor quality of life or is health status part of quality of life?
- Is the illness belief 'my illness won't last a long time' an illness belief or a coping mechanism?
- Are different personality types mutually exclusive to each other: can I be extrovert and introvert?

Stage Models

Health psychology uses a number of stage models such as the SOC. We need to ask:

- Are the different stages qualitatively separate from each other?
- Are stages real or a product of statistics? (That is, if I ask if people across stages are different, will I then find that they are different, because I am imposing difference on the data?)
- Are stages an artefact of labelling them as such?

Finding Associations in our Theories

Many of our theories argue that different constructs are associated with each other (e.g. self-efficacy predicts behavioural intentions; control-related illness cognitions predict coping). We need to ask:

- Are these associations true by definition (e.g. control cognitions relate to coping *only* because control cognitions are part of the definition of coping)?
- Are the associations true by observation (e.g. smoking actually does cause cancer AND smoking is defined and measured as separate to the ways in which cancer is define and measured)?

Finding Differences in our Theories

Many theories also look for differences between populations (e.g. men versus women; old versus young; doctor versus patient). We need to ask:

- Are these differences artefacts of the statistics we use (e.g. if we ask a differences-based question we can find a difference, but if we ask an association-based question we can find an association)? A good example of this is that daughters have higher body dissatisfaction than their mothers (i.e. they are different) *but* daughter body dissatisfaction is correlated with their mothers (i.e. they are associated). The answer depends on the question asked and the statistical test used.
- Are the variables that we use to explore differences (men versus women; old versus young) really dichotomous variables or artificially created as binary variables? (What about all the people who fall somewhere in between?)

Can Theories Be Tested?

Much research in health psychology aims to test a theory. We need to ask:

- Can the theory ever be rejected? (E.g. it didn't work but it was the fault of the sample/measures/confounding variables – let's keep the theory.)
- Can the theory ever be accepted? (Statistics are based on probabilities; our results are never true all the time but true within an accepted level of probability.)

We can therefore learn to be more critical of theories in terms of the constructs we use and the ways in which we explore whether or not these constructs are related to each other.

BEING CRITICAL OF METHOD

In health psychology we use both qualitative and quantitative methods and a range of research designs including cross-sectional studies, experiments and cohort studies. Being critical involves asking questions about all aspects of methodology.

Quantitative Studies

Quantitative studies are the mainstay of more traditional forms of empirical research and involve collecting numerical data through questionnaires, experiments (or trials) or computer tasks. Such quantitative data is often assumed to be more objective and controlled than qualitative data. But being critical involves asking questions such as:

- Is quantitative data really objective and value-free? The researcher chooses what questions to ask, how the data should be coded, what sample to select, what variables to analyse, what tests to use and what story to tell in the final paper. All these processes involve subjective judgements which are value-laden.

Qualitative Studies

Health psychology uses a range of qualitative methods such as focus groups and interviews and applies different data analysis approaches, such as thematic analysis, interpretative phenomenological analysis (IPA) or narrative analysis. Qualitative researchers are clear about the subjective nature of their data and argue that their findings are neither generalizable nor representative. But we need to ask the following questions:

- If the data analysis is open to subjective interpretation by the researcher, how much of the analysis reflects only what the researcher wants to see and is any of the analysis reflective of what went on in the interview? Is qualitative analysis purely a product of what is in the mind of the researcher?
- Although qualitative findings are not supposed to be generalizable, are we in fact interested to see if they can tell us about people other than those few (maybe just ten people) who took part in the study?

The Sample

Quantitative research requires larger samples that are representative so that the results can be generalized. Qualitative studies involve much smaller samples as generalization is not the aim. But . . .

- Can a sample ever be representative and if so of whom? Samples may well be selected from a school, or a clinic, or even a city or country but can the data ever be representative of all schools, clinics, cities or countries? Yet we assume that data on people with diabetes who took part in the trial can tell us about people with diabetes in general even though the trial population were all under 65 and living in London.
- Qualitative studies use small samples but can a study on seven people really tell us much apart from about those seven people? Are people so consistent that what seven people tell us can inform what we know about other people with a similar condition, illness or behaviour? And if it can't, then why do we only study seven people?

Research Designs

We have a number of research designs all of which have their strengths and weaknesses. We need to ask:

- How can the authors describe 'cause' or predict anything when a cross-sectional design was used?
- How can the results be generalized when the data were collected in an artificial laboratory setting?
- How can the results be trusted when they were collected in a natural setting with so many uncontrolled potentially confounding variables?

Health psychology uses a range of methods, all of which have their problems. Being critical of methodology involves understanding these problems and making sure that the conclusions from any study are justified. Central to all research is the assumption that data can be collected about the world and that data is separate to the tool that is collecting it. This raises the problem of whether research collects or creates the very things it is trying to measure.

BEING CRITICAL OF MEASUREMENT

Research within health psychology involves using a wide range of measurement tools including subjective questionnaires to detect 'caseness' or variables on a continuum, interview schedules, computer tasks and objective measures of factors such as adherence (blood levels of the drug), smoking (blood levels of nicotine) or stress (measured cortisol). These all have their problems and the following questions can be asked.

Subjective Measures

It is acknowledged that self-report measures such as questionnaires and interviews are subjective. This raises problems such as:

- Are participants just saying what they believe the researcher wants them to say?
- Does the participant have the language and insight to express what they really feel?
- Can people really differentiate their feelings, beliefs or behaviours into the level of detail expected by numerical scales with 5 or 7 or even 100 options?

Objective Measures

Some measures are more objective but these also have their problems:

- Most measures still involve the possibility of human error or bias through coding, choosing what to measure and when, and deciding how the data should be analysed.
- An objective measure of a psychological construct may miss the important part of that construct. (E.g. is cortisol really a reflection of stress or just one component of it?)

A Leap of Faith

Throughout the different areas of health psychology, researchers develop research tools to assess quality of life, pain, stress, beliefs and behaviours. These tools are then used by the researchers to examine how the subjects in the research feel/think/behave. However, this process involves an enormous leap of faith – that our measurement tool actually measures something *out there*. How do we know this? Perhaps what the tool measures is simply what the tool measures. A depression scale may not assess 'depression' but only the score on the scale. Likewise, a quality of life scale may not assess quality of life but simply how someone completes the questionnaire.

BEING CRITICAL OF A DISCIPLINE

Finally, being critical also involves analysing and criticizing the discipline of health psychology itself in terms of its key perspective and core assumptions. Health psychology positions itself as a discrete discipline separate to other related disciplines such as medicine and medical sociology. It has some core underlying approaches which were outlined earlier in this chapter as emphasizing a biopsychosocial approach and highlighting a more holistic understanding of health and illness. Furthermore, it is founded on the belief that research will help us to understand health and illness and that the more we research our beliefs and behaviour, the better our understanding will be. These are explored here in terms of the mind–body split, how the individual is integrated into their social context and the notion of progression.

The Mind–Body Split

Health psychology sets out to provide an integrated model of the individual by establishing a holistic approach to health. Therefore it challenges the traditional medical model of the mind–body split and provides theories and research to support the notion of a mind and body that are one. For example, it suggests that beliefs influence behaviour, which in turn influences health; that stress can cause illness and that pain is a perception rather than a sensation. In addition, it argues that illness cognitions relate to recovery from illness and coping relates to longevity. However, does this approach really represent an integrated individual? Although all these perspectives and the research that has been carried out in their support indicate that the mind and the body interact, they are still defined as separate. The mind reflects the individual's psychological states (i.e. their beliefs, cognitions, perceptions), which influence but are *separate from* their bodies (i.e. the illness, the body, the body's systems).

Integrating the Individual with their Social Context

Psychology is traditionally the study of the individual. Sociology is traditionally the study of the social context. Recently, however, health psychologists have made moves to integrate this individual with their social world. To do this they have turned to social epidemiology (i.e. the exploration of class, gender and ethnicity), social psychology (i.e. subjective norms) or social constructionism (i.e. qualitative methods). Therefore health psychologists access either the individual's location within their social world via their demographic factors or ask individuals for their beliefs about the social world. However, does this really integrate the individual with the social world? A belief about the social context is still an individual's belief. Can psychology really succeed with this integration? Would it still be psychology if it did?

The Problem of Progression

Health psychology uses a number of theories, methods and measurement tools. Being critical involves developing the confidence to evaluate and assess any paper (or book) in terms of all of these dimensions and learning to question whether a conclusion is justified, whether a theory makes sense or whether the underlying assumptions which form the basis of any piece of work are clear and transparent.

BOX 1.1
Critical Approaches to Health Psychology

Over the past few years a subsection of health psychology has developed which has become known as 'critical health psychology'. Researchers within this area emphasize the qualitative, critical and alternative approaches to understanding health and illness. Further, they highlight the role of the social context and the political dimensions to health. Some of the assumptions addressed in this chapter are also addressed within the domain of critical health psychology. Over recent years this approach has started to address some of the concerns emerging about the focus of our discipline, the samples we use, the questions we ask and the conclusions we draw. These will be considered through this book but include:

- **WEIRD samples:** Much research in psychology draws upon White, Educated participants from Industrialized, Rich and Democratic countries. This is very much the case when research draws upon university students, particularly psychology students, for its studies. In health psychology we are actually less likely to be guilty of this than other areas of psychology, as many of our studies include patient populations. Yet it remains the case that our research certainly does not access the breadth of diversity that it could.

- **Gender differences:** Much research within psychology explores gender differences with a focus on men versus women. Within health psychology we have a literature on how men and women differ on factors such as coping styles, body dissatisfaction, responses to stress, pain thresholds, health-related behaviour such as diet, smoking and exercise and help seeking. While such research can help to inform our understanding of how people make sense and manage their health, it tends to focus on a binary notion of gender and does not sit comfortably with a world in which gender is becoming more fluid. Asking research questions that focus on gender differences not only, however, finds differences by gender but also reifies the notion that there are only two genders and that these are fixed. This is a problem for how health psychology sits in the modern world.

- **Sexuality:** In line with gender, research also classifies participants according to their sexuality and research and looks for differences between heterosexual and homosexual individuals. For example, we have a body of literature of sexuality differences in attitudes to sex, sexual behaviours, help-seeking behaviours and health behaviours both related to sex and not such as smoking, diet and exercise. This is problematic in many ways. First, it assumes that these classifications are fixed and that a person's sexuality is stable. Second, it assumes that there are a limited number of key classifications. Third, it assumes that classifying people in this way to look for individuals differences is useful. Health Psychology therefore needs to grasp a more diverse and flexible approach to sexuality as it moves through the twenty-first century.

- **The individual vs the social vs the political:** as a discipline we focus on the individual. Our history comes from 'the psyche', our research methods study individuals through experiments, questionnaires or interviews and our constructs such as 'cognitions', 'emotions', 'behaviours' belong to the individual. This approach can be criticized for neglecting our place within the broader world such as the family, the friendship group, the community, culture, religion, ethnicity and the broader world. It can also be criticized for being 'apolitical'. Some of these issues will be considered throughout the book.

- **The mind vs the body:** Psychology is the study of the mind and emphasizes this rather than the body. Health psychology emphasizes the interaction between the mind and the body and attempts to challenge a dualist approach. Throughout this book I explore the extent to which this challenge is successful.

6 WORKING IN HEALTH PSYCHOLOGY

Health psychology is an expanding discipline in the UK, across Europe, in Australia and New Zealand, and in the USA. For many students this involves taking a health psychology course as part of their psychology degree. For some students, health psychology plays a part of their studies for other allied disciplines, such as medicine, nursing, health studies and dentistry. However, in addition to studying health psychology at this preliminary level, an increasing number of students carry out higher degrees in health psychology as a means to develop their careers within this field. This has resulted in discussions about the possible roles for a health psychologist. Health psychologists may teach, carry out research, do consultancy or work with patients as practitioners. To date there are four possible career pathways for those in health psychology, which are not always mutually exclusive. These are: the clinical health psychologist, the health psychology practitioner, the community health psychologist and the academic health psychologist.

THE CLINICAL HEALTH PSYCHOLOGIST

A clinical health psychologist has been defined as someone who merges 'clinical psychology with its focus on the assessment and treatment of individuals in distress . . . and the content field of health psychology' (Belar and Deardorff 1995). In order to practise as a clinical health psychologist, it is generally accepted that someone would first gain training as a clinical psychologist and then later acquire an expertise in health psychology, which would involve an understanding of the theories and methods of health psychology and their application to the health care setting. A trained clinical health psychologist would tend to work within the field of physical health, including stress and pain management, rehabilitation for patients with chronic illnesses (e.g. cancer, HIV or cardiovascular disease) or the development of interventions for problems such as spinal cord injury and disfiguring surgery. A clinical health psychologist could work with people face to face or see people through group work. They could work in a hospital setting (e.g. seeing out-patients), in the community (e.g. in primary care) or through their own private practice seeing people either online or face to face in a designated therapy room. All clinical health psychologists should have regular supervision to support them with their clinical workload.

Case Study: A Clinical Health Psychologist

Devon is a Clinical Health Psychologist. He completed his undergraduate degree in psychology and then spent some time as a psychology assistant, working as part of a clinical team and seeing patients with a range of mental health issues such as depression, anxiety and eating disorders. He then secured a place on a Clinical Psychology Doctorate Programme which took 3 years and gave him a broad range of clinical skills such as CBT, person-centred therapy and family therapy, which enabled him to work clinically with patients either one-to-one or in a group. Devon then graduated and got a job as a Clinical

Psychologist in a pain clinic. Over the past 10 years he has gained experience in a number of health care settings but still mostly works with patients in the pain clinic where he draws upon his clinical skills to help patients manage their pain and encourages them towards acceptance.

THE HEALTH PSYCHOLOGY PRACTITIONER

A health psychology practitioner is someone who is trained to an acceptable standard in health psychology and works as a health psychologist. Within the UK, the term 'health psychologist' is now used and is managed by the Health Care Professions Council. Across Europe, Australasia and the USA, the term 'professional health psychologist' or simply 'health psychologist' is used. At the present time it is generally agreed that a health psychology practitioner should have competence in five areas: ethical practice, research, teaching, interventions and consultancy. In addition, they should be able to show a suitable knowledge base of academic health psychology, normally by completing a higher degree in health psychology. Having demonstrated that they meet the required standards, a health psychology practitioner could work within the health promotion setting, within schools or industry, and/or within the health service. If they have a PhD they could also work as an academic within the university sector. Their work could include research, teaching, the development and evaluation of interventions to reduce risk-related behaviour or working with charities or with government bodies to develop, implement and evaluate health-related policy.

Case Study: A Health Psychology Practitioner

Eleni is a Health Psychology Practitioner. She initially completed her undergraduate degree in psychology and then her master's in health psychology. After a few years working in a hospital as a health care worker, Eleni decided to complete her Stage 2 training in health psychology. She discussed this with various course leaders and decided that rather than taking the PhD route she would do the professional doctorate. She therefore worked alongside the doctorate in a number of health psychology roles including a smoking cessation clinic, a stress management clinic and in cardiac rehabilitation while completing her portfolio of competencies and carrying out a research study. Since qualification Eleni has worked in Public Health where she designs and evaluates interventions. She also feeds into policy making and sometimes advises government bodies.

THE COMMUNITY HEALTH PSYCHOLOGIST

Much psychology and health psychology focuses on the individual in terms of the individual's beliefs and behaviours and how these can be changed or supported. In contrast, the focus of a community health psychologist is on the community as a means to understand the role of the social context in facilitating or undermining health. Likewise, the key outcome for this approach is concerned with reducing health inequalities across communities rather than just changing the health status of the individual. From this perspective, poor health and health inequalities are seen as a result of aspects of the social world such as the environment, political choices, industry, access to education, funding or access to health care (Campbell and Murray 2004). A community health psychologist could therefore work in a public health setting to develop and/or evaluate public health interventions. They could also work as a researcher based in a University to synthesize existing evidence for the effectiveness of public interventions or they could work alongside a service provider to provide a theoretical/evidence-based input into the development of a public health intervention. Examples of community health psychology interventions could include working with local church communities to increase uptake of vaccines during the COVID pandemic, encouraging local councils to provide better street lighting and cycle paths to facilitate increased activity, or working with local charities to support those with chronic conditions such as dementia or cancer. To make things more complicated, community health psychologists may also be known as public health psychologists!

Case study: A Community Health Psychologist

Ravi is a community health psychologist. He completed his undergraduate degree which included a final year module in health psychology that he really enjoyed. He then completed the MSc in Health Psychology which gave him his stage 1 qualification. During this time he realized he was interested in making a difference and helping as many people as possible and so felt that a public health route would be best for him. After the MSc he then secured a post with a local public health department where he was linked in with the obesity and COVID teams. His role involved working with local councils to improve public areas for exercise, setting up social media networks to support those trying to lose weight, helping the local hospital get its COVID messaging right for its staff and working with local care homes to encourage staff to be vaccinated. During this time he decided to further his training and found himself a mentor who was able to support him through the stage 2 health psychology training. After several years of working and completing his portfolio he qualified as a Health Psychologist and continued to work in a public health setting.

THE ACADEMIC HEALTH PSYCHOLOGIST

An academic health psychologist usually has a first degree in psychology and then completes a master's in health psychology and a PhD in a health psychology-related area. For example, they may focus their PhD on obesity, stress, coronary heart disease or behaviour change. They will then enter the pathway for an academic health psychologist by getting a postdoctoral position or a lectureship at a university. The pathway in the UK involves the progression from lecturer, to senior lecturer, to reader and then professor (although in many countries the terms 'assistant professor', 'associate professor' and 'full professor' are used). The career of an academic involves teaching at all levels (undergraduate and postgraduate), project supervision for students, carrying out research, writing books and research articles in peer review journals and presenting work at conferences. Most academics also have an administrative role, such as managing the examination process or directing the teaching programmes for undergraduate or postgraduate students.

Case Study: An Academic Health Psychologist

Jane is an Academic Health Psychologist. She did her undergraduate degree in neurobiology (which was recognized by the British Psychological Society). She then completed her PhD in the area of eating behaviour. Her first job was as a lecturer where she set up a undergraduate module in Health Psychology. She decided to turn this into a textbook on health psychology. Her next job was in a medical school where she taught psychology to medical students and GPs. She was promoted to Senior Lecturer and Reader while she was there. She then moved jobs to take up the role of Professor in Health Psychology at the University of Surrey. Jane teaches health psychology to psychology, veterinary, nutrition, dietician and medical students. She carries out research, mostly on eating behaviour and obesity, publishes research papers and books, often does consultancy and works with the media. She also manages the PhD programme and supervises many BSc, MSc and PhD students.

7 THE AIMS OF THIS BOOK

Health psychology is an expanding area in terms of teaching, research and practice. Health psychology *teaching* occurs at both the undergraduate and postgraduate level and is delivered to both mainstream psychology students and those studying other health-related subjects. Health psychology *research* also takes many forms. Undergraduates are often expected to produce research projects as part of their assessment, and academic staff and research teams carry out research to develop and test theories and to explore new areas. Such research often feeds directly into *practice*, with intervention programmes aiming to change the factors identified by research. This book aims to provide a comprehensive introduction to the main topics of health psychology. The book will focus on psychological theory supported by research. In addition, how these theories can be turned into practice will also be described. The book is now supported by a comprehensive website which includes teaching aids such as lectures and assessments.

A COMPLETE COURSE IN HEALTH PSYCHOLOGY

This book takes the format of a complete course in health psychology. Each chapter could be used as the basis for a lecture and/or reading for a lecture and consists of the following features:

- Seven learning objectives for each chapter which map directly onto the structure the chapter.
- A case study for each chapter to illustrate how the theories and research are relevant to everyday life.
- A set of questions for seminar discussions or essay titles.
- Recommendations for further reading.
- Diagrams to illustrate the models and theories discussed within the text.
- A 'thinking critically about. . .' section which describes some of the main methodological and conceptual problems for each area of research.
- A 'being critical of health psychology' section to generate discussions about some of the bigger issues in our discipline to reflect a changing world.

In addition, there is a glossary at the end of the book, which describes terms within health psychology relating to methodology.

ONLINE/HYBRID LEARNING

Since the start of the COVID pandemic in 2019, teaching has changed. While some universities were known for their online courses, most had to adjust to the limitations imposed by COVID and lecturers (like me!) had to quickly get to grips with recording videos, teaching through Zoom, organizing break-out rooms, trying to engage a sea of blank screens and maintaining our energy and enthusiasm while sitting in a stuffy room back home and not seeing our colleagues. Then once we went back to the lecture theatre we needed to master the art of hybrid teaching and suffer fails in technology as we attempted to interact both with the real room and the virtual one. Now, even though the end of COVID seems in sight and we are all pretty much back in the lecture theatre (at the time of writing this), online and/or hybrid teaching seems here to stay. And at times it even feels like a bonus that can work well (and save the planet). Here are some ways this book could be used for online/hybrid teaching.

Pre-recorded Videos

The PowerPoint slides on the website could be used to create online videos to provide students with a concise overview of the key theories and research.

Figures and Images

There are many figures and images throughout this book used to illustrate theories or the ways in which psychology can be used to understand specific health issues. These could be used as a forum for generating discussion.

Essay Questions

The questions at the end of each chapter could be used for homework before each lecture to generate debate in the lecture. They could also be used to assess learning throughout the semester and provide formative feedback.

Break-out Groups

When working online, break-out groups are a good way to encourage discussion and get people speaking. I tend to put people either into pairs or groups of about five, set a specific task, give them about 15 minutes to discuss the task and then ask one member to be responsible for feeding back from each group. If you want to discuss a slide or figure, remember this disappears when they go into groups so I ask them to photograph it on their phones! Some ideas are below:

Why health is clearly psychological: Get into break-out groups of two people and think about the last time you went to the doctor. What factors, other than medical factors, can you think of that influenced why you felt ill and why you decided to go to the doctor? (Only share a health problem you are happy to share with others!) Then re-join the main group and see if these factors fit in with the focus of health psychology.

Why people do not always behave as they should: Get into groups of five and consider why people continue to smoke even when they know it is not good for them. What other factors are involved? (Think about beliefs, childhood, emotions, expectations, etc. NOT addiction!)

Why do people go to the doctor for trivial reasons? Some people go to the doctor for just a cold. Get into groups of five and consider what psychological reasons might influence their decision to seek help.

Why do people not go to the doctor for serious problems? Some people delay seeking help even when they have a very worrying lump. Get into groups of five and think why this might be.

Why do people differ in their responses to illness? Two people might have a sore throat but whereas one stays in bed the other is determined to carry on. What psychological factors could explain this difference.

Mind–body relationships: I strongly believe that the mind and body are intertwined and that how we think and feel affects our bodies. Get into pairs and think about the ways in which your own thoughts and feelings have effected changes in your body.

Psychology and health outcomes: Two people can have the same illness but whereas one person recovers quickly the other goes to bed and gets worse. Get into groups of five and think through all the psychological factors that could contribute to this difference in health outcomes.

Hybrid Discussions

Sometimes we have people in the classroom and people at home. When this happens I put the people in the class into groups but sometimes let the people at home just chat in the chat! This can work well and writing can feel less stressful than talking.

A NOTE ON REFERENCING

This is now the seventh edition of this book and I am now 56. For me, 'recent research' means about 1990, but I am aware that many of the students reading this book were not born then. This edition has therefore been revised and updated throughout. I have not, however, removed *all* earlier references in favour of more recent ones for two reasons. Firstly, some of the key theories used in health psychology were developed in the 1980s and 1990s. I have retained these original references throughout. Secondly, many of the studies testing these theories were carried out in the 1990s. Therefore, I have also retained some of these as, although many more studies may have been done in recent years, testing the same theories using the same populations and methods, it feels unjust to use the more recent less original papers rather than the earlier original ones.

A NOTE ON COVID

Since the last edition, the COVID pandemic has happened. This has had two key implications for updating this book. First, a wealth of research has been published about COVID relevant to health psychology, exploring areas such as mask wearing, hand washing, vaccination uptake, help seeking and changes in health-related behaviours such as exercise, healthy eating, smoking and drinking. I have included some of this research where relevant throughout with a particular focus on exercise changes (Chapter 5) and health inequalities (Chapter 14). I have also, however, been wary of including too much COVID research for fear of saturation with future students being bored with reading about it! Furthermore, much of the research published by the time of writing this (2022) was collected quite early in the pandemic and may well not reflect what happened as the pandemic progressed. Second, COVID had a massive impact on all health behaviours and all diagnoses of all illnesses. Throughout this book I draw upon large-scale surveys to describe the prevalence of behaviours such as smoking, alcohol use, exercise and healthy eating and similarly describe conditions such as HIV, cancer and CHD. This relies upon regular surveys being conducted by organizations such as the ONS and WHO. During COVID some of these studies were stopped so the data is not available. For those that were carried out, the data is not representative of a 'normal year' and cannot be taken as showing an increase or decrease compared to previous years if COVID had not happened. For this reason, some of my more epidemiological figures may seem a bit dated but at times this is because either there is no more up-to-date data OR that the up to date data is 'odd' due to COVID.

TO CONCLUDE

Health psychology explores how a number of psychological factors impact upon health and illness and emphasizes four frameworks: a biopsychosocial perspective, health and illness as being on a continuum, the direct and indirect pathways between psychology and health, and the problem of variability. This book covers the breadth of health psychology and can be used as the basis for a complete course for students at both undergraduate and postgraduate levels and for those both within psychology and in other allied disciplines such as nutritionists, nurses, doctors and dieticians.

QUESTIONS

1 To what extent does health psychology challenge the assumptions of the biomedical model of health and illness?
2 Why do health psychologists consider health and illness to be on a continuum?
3 Is the biopsychosocial model a useful perspective?
4 What problems are there with dividing up the pathways between health and illness into indirect and direct pathways?
5 What factors could explain variability between people in terms of their behaviour and health outcomes?
6 To what extent does health psychology enable the whole person to be studied?
7 Can you design a research study to illustrate the impact of the bio, psycho and social processes in an illness of your choice?

FOR DISCUSSION

Consider the last time you were ill (e.g. flu, headache, cold, etc.). Discuss the extent to which factors other than biological ones may have contributed to your illness.

FURTHER READING

Kaptein, A. and Weinman, J. (eds) (2010) *Health Psychology*, 2nd edn. Oxford: BPS Blackwell. This edited collection provides further detailed description and analysis of a range of areas central to health psychology.

Michie, S. & Abraham, C. (eds) (2004) *Health Psychology in Practice*. Oxford: Blackwell. This edited collection provides a detailed account of the competencies and skills required to be a chartered health psychologist in the UK. However, the information is also relevant internationally to anyone interested in pursuing a career in health psychology.

Ogden, J. (2007). *Essential Readings in Health Psychology*. Maidenhead: Open University Press. This is my reader which consists of 29 papers I have selected as good illustrations of theory, research, methodology or debate. The book also contains a discussion of each paper and a justification for its inclusion.

RESEARCH METHODS

Bowling, A. (2023) *Research Methods in Health: Investigating Health and Health Services,* 5th edn. Maidenhead: McGraw-Hill Education.
This provides an excellent overview of research methods including systematic reviews, surveys, questionnaire design, modelling and trials. Its focus is on health research.

Lyons, E. and Coyle, A. (eds.) (2007) *Analyzing Qualitative Data in Psychology*. London: Sage.
This book provides an excellent overview of four different qualitative approaches (IPA, grounded theory, narrative analysis, discourse analysis) and then explores how they can be used and the extent to which they produce different or similar accounts of the data.

Ogden, J. (2019) *Thinking Critically about Research: A Step-by-step Approach*. London: Routledge.
This is my new critical thinking book. The first half describes the basics of research (sampling, research questions, variables), research design, measures, data analysis and theory. The second half then takes a step-by-step approach to critically analysing each component of research and addresses the questions 'What evidence is there?' and 'How is it presented?' using a critical tool kit. It is full of worked examples, tasks to be used in class and illustrations.

Smith, J. A. (2015) *Qualitative Psychology: A Practical Guide to Research Methods.* London: Sage.

This offers a very clear hands-on guide to the different qualitative approaches and is extremely good at showing how to carry out qualitative research in practice.

Willig, C. (2012) *Qualitative Interpretation and Analysis in Psychology.* Maidenhead: McGraw-Hill Education.

An extremely well-written and clear guide to the different qualitative approaches, which offers an accessible overview of their similarities and differences in terms of epistemology and method.

CRITICAL HEALTH PSYCHOLOGY

Below are some of my own papers that have attempted to take a more critical stance on health psychology. Read if you are interested!

Ogden, J. (1995) Changing the subject of health psychology, *Psychology and Health,* **10:** 257–65.
This paper addresses some of the assumptions in health psychology and discusses the interrelationship between theory, methodology and the psychological individual.

Ogden, J. (1995) Psychosocial theory and the creation of the risky self, *Social Science and Medicine,* **40:** 409–15.
This paper examines the changes in psychological theory during the twentieth century and relates them to discussions about risk and responsibility for health and illness.

Ogden, J. (1997) The rhetoric and reality of psychosocial theories: a challenge to biomedicine? *Journal of Health Psychology,* **2:** 21–9.
This paper explores health psychology's apparent challenge to biomedicine.

Ogden, J. (2002) *Health and the construction of the individual.* London: Routledge.
This book explores how both psychological and sociological theories construct the individual through an exploration of methodology, measurement, theory and the construction of boundaries.

Ogden, J. (2003) Some problems with social cognition models: a pragmatic and conceptual analysis, *Health Psychology,* **22:** 424–8.
This paper provides a critique of social cognition models but is also of relevance to other theoretical perspectives used in health psychology. In particular, it questions whether measuring beliefs accesses them or changes (or even creates) them and whether our theories are tautological.

Ogden, J. and Lo, J. (2012) How meaningful is data from Likert scales? An evaluation of how ratings are made and the role of the response shift in the socially disadvantaged. *International Journal of Health Psychology,* **12:** 350–61.
This paper explores some of the fundamental problems with using quantitative measures to explore between-group differences and questions why quantitative and qualitative methods can often produce very contradictory results.

Ogden, J. (2016) Celebrating variability and a call to end a systematising approach to research: the example of the Behaviour Change Taxonomy and the Behaviour Change Wheel. *Health Psychology Review* (with 5 commentaries), **10** (3): 245–50.

This paper presents a critique of the behaviour change wheel and COM-B models of behaviour change and was published as part of a special issue with discussions with other authors. It is a useful start for seminars and tutorial discussions.

Ogden, J. (2019) Do no harm: balancing the costs and benefits of patient outcomes in health psychology research and practice. *Journal of Health Psychology,* **24**; 25-37. doi: 10.1177/1359105316648760

This paper presents a critical analysis of the ways in which health psychology may inadvertently do harm by encouraging people to seek help unnecessarily or over-use health care services.

Other useful texts on critical health psychology include the following:

Crossley, M. (2000) *Rethinking Health Psychology.* Maidenhead: Open University Press.

This book argues that 'mainstream' health psychology neglects some of the contextual factors that impact upon health and is over-reliant upon quantitative methodologies.

Hardey, M. (1998) *The Social Context of Health.* Maidenhead: Open University Press.

This book explores the role of a range of social factors that contribute both to our understanding of health and to the decisions we make about how to behave.

PART TWO

Staying Well: Health Beliefs, Behaviour and Behaviour Change

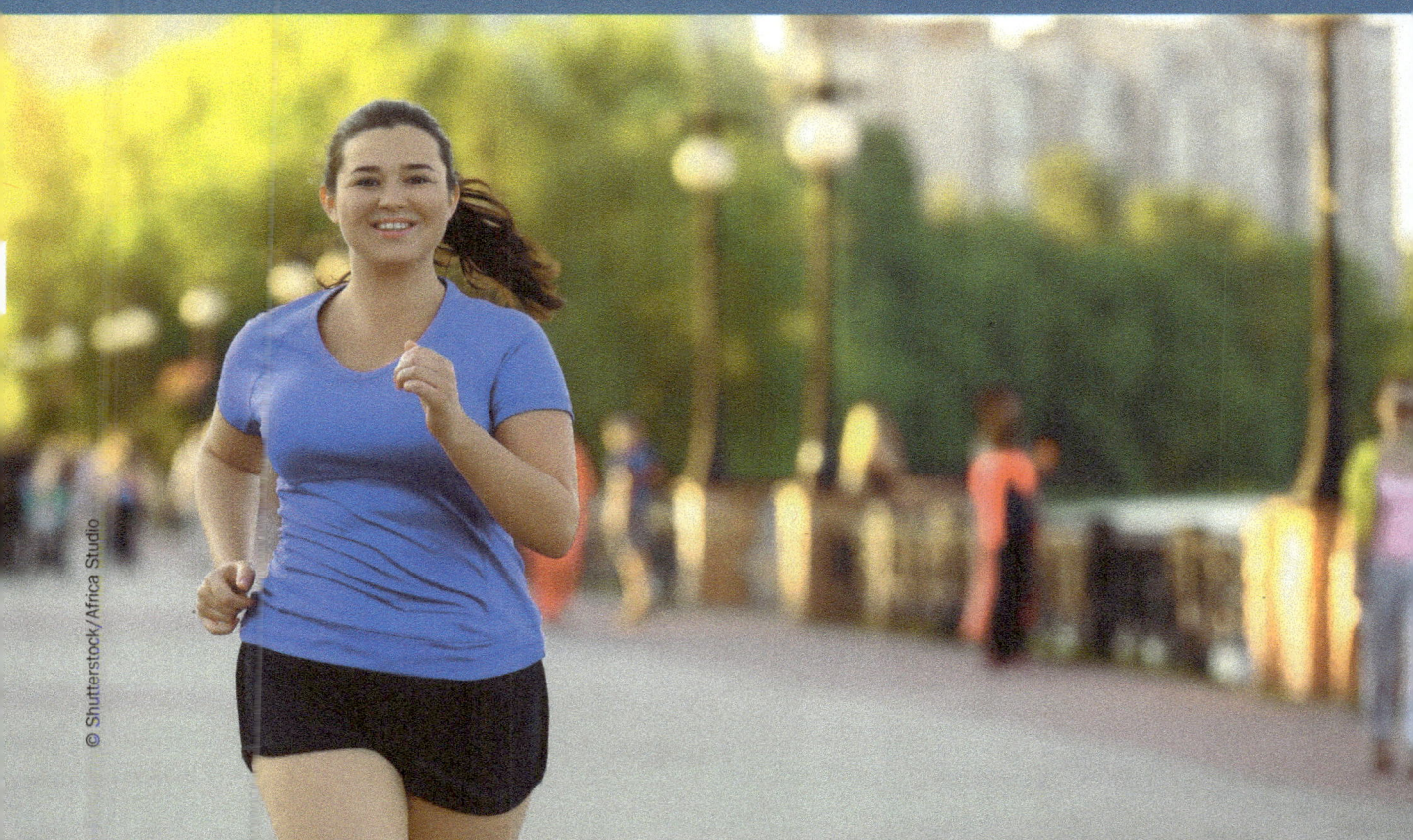

© Shutterstock/Africa Studio

Part Two

Staying Well: Health Beliefs, Behaviour and Behaviour Change

2
Health Beliefs

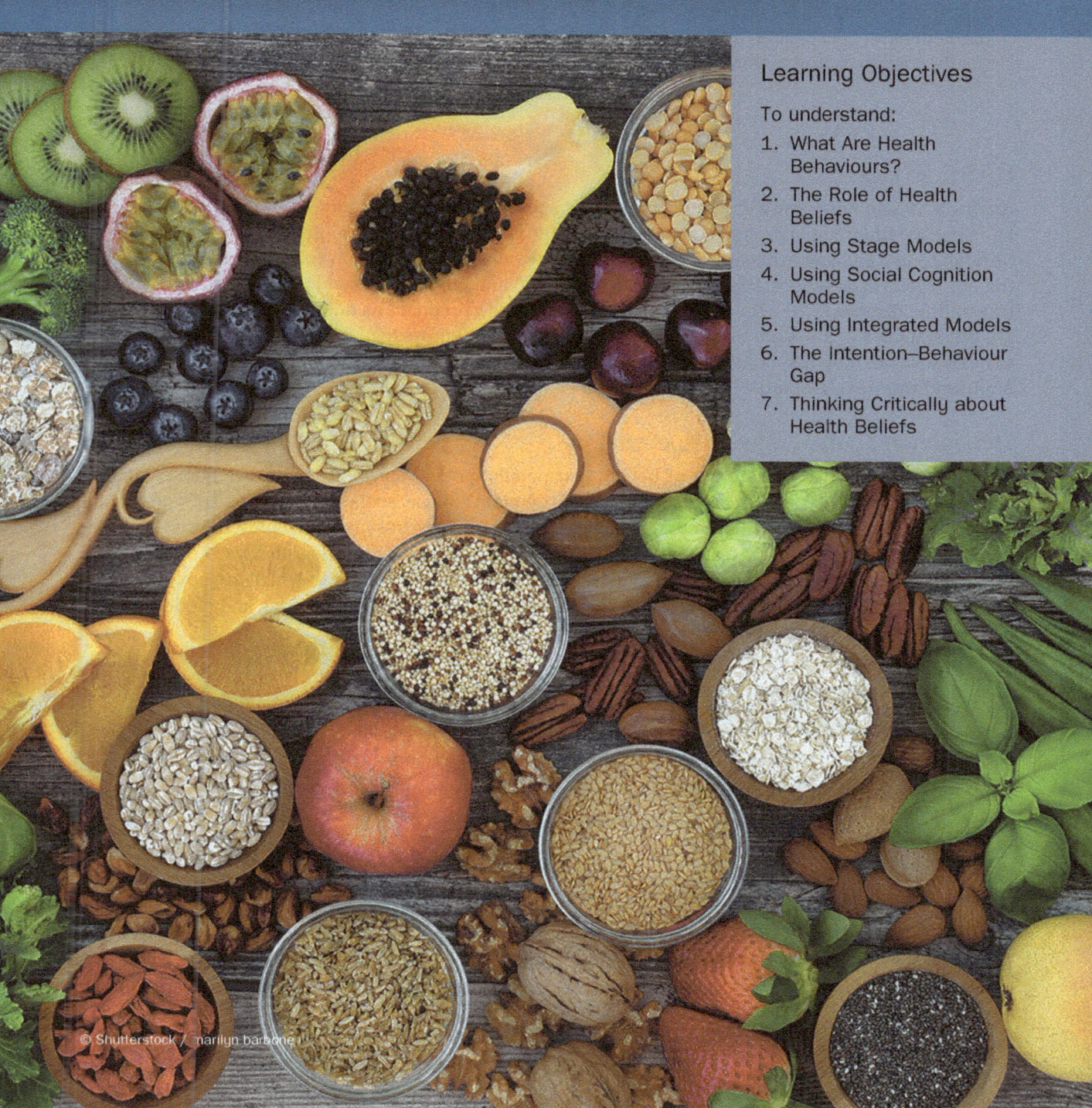

© Shutterstock / marilyn barbone

Learning Objectives

To understand:
1. What Are Health Behaviours?
2. The Role of Health Beliefs
3. Using Stage Models
4. Using Social Cognition Models
5. Using Integrated Models
6. The Intention–Behaviour Gap
7. Thinking Critically about Health Beliefs

CHAPTER OVERVIEW

Chapter 1 introduced the discipline of health psychology and highlighted a key role for health-related behaviours such as diet, exercise and smoking. For example, the aim of health psychology was described as being to predict and change health behaviours and the focus of health psychology illustrated a role for behaviour in the development of health conditions such as coronary heart disease (CHD), obesity, cancers and HIV. This chapter explores what health behaviours are and the extent to which they can be predicted by health beliefs, with a focus on attributions, risk perception, motivation and self-efficacy. The chapter then describes a number of key stage models, social cognition models and integrated models which are often used to predict health behaviours. It then explores the problem of the intention–behaviour gap and finally describes how to think critically about research on health beliefs.

CASE STUDY

Amara is 19 and has been with her boyfriend for about 6 months. They have decided to have sex and have had a rather embarrassing conversation about contraception. Her boyfriend thinks condoms are difficult to use and embarrassing to buy and Amara would rather be in control so has decided to go on the pill. The doctor suggests that she uses both the pill and condoms to avoid pregnancy and sexually transmitted disease (STD). Amara is very scared of getting pregnant as one of her friends from school got pregnant at 17. She is not that worried about STDs as she knows her boyfriend well and only intends to have sex with him. Six months later she starts to have an unpleasant discharge and finds out that her boyfriend was also sleeping with a girl from his college. She is very angry.

Through the Eyes of Health Psychology. . .

Amara's story illustrates a number of beliefs that people have about their health behaviours such as the costs (embarrassing) and benefits (not getting pregnant) of use, social norms (friend got pregnant), self-efficacy (condoms are difficult to use) and perceptions of control (using the pill). It also illustrates the role of emotions such as fear and embarrassment. These beliefs and emotions are relevant to a range of health behaviours such as eating, exercise, smoking and alcohol use which are covered in the next few chapters. This chapter focuses on the beliefs themselves and the theories and models used in health psychology to study how people think about what they do.

1 WHAT ARE HEALTH BEHAVIOURS?

Kasl and Cobb (1966) defined three types of health-related behaviour:

- A *health behaviour* aims to prevent disease (e.g. eating a healthy diet).
- An *illness behaviour* aims to seek remedy (e.g. going to the doctor).
- A *sick role behaviour* aims at getting well (e.g. taking prescribed medication, resting).

Health behaviours were further defined by Matarazzo (1984) as either:

- *Health-impairing habits,* which he called 'behavioural pathogens' (e.g. smoking, eating a high fat diet), or
- *Health protective behaviours,* which he defined as 'behavioural immunogens' (e.g. attending a health check).

In health psychology, health behaviours are generally regarded as any behaviour that is related to the health status of the individual.

WHY STUDY HEALTH BEHAVIOURS?

McKeown (1979) examined health and illness throughout the twentieth century and argued that contemporary illness is caused by 'influences . . . which the individual determines by his own behaviour (smoking, eating, exercise, and the like)' (p. 118). More recent data support this emphasis on behaviour and their links with chronic illnesses. For example, in 2008 Allender et al. published data on the most common causes of death across Europe (including the UK) and concluded that cardiovascular diseases and cancer account for 64 per cent of male and 71 per cent of female deaths (Allender et al. 2008a, 2008b). Similar figures are also found in the USA where cardiovascular diseases and cancer accounted for 56 per cent of deaths in men and 55 per cent of deaths in women (National Center for Health Statistics 2009).

BEHAVIOUR AND LONGEVITY

The role of behaviour has also been highlighted by the work of Belloc and Breslow and their colleagues (Belloc and Breslow 1972; Breslow and Enstrom 1980) who examined the relationship between mortality rates and behaviour among 7,000 people as part of the Alameda County study in the USA, which began in 1965. They concluded from their original correlational analysis that seven behaviours were related to positive health status. These behaviours were:

1   Sleeping 7–8 hours a day.
2   Having breakfast every day.
3   Not smoking.
4   Rarely eating between meals.
5   Being near or at prescribed weight.
6   Having moderate or no use of alcohol.
7   Taking regular exercise.

Their large sample was followed up over 5.5 years and 10 years in a prospective study and the authors reported that these seven behaviours were related to mortality. In addition, they suggested for people aged over 75 who carried out all of these health behaviours, health was comparable to those aged 35–44 who followed less than three.

BEHAVIOUR AND MORTALITY

In 2016, data from the Global Burden of Disease protocol shows that behavioural risk factors account for more deaths than metabolic or environmental risk factors. Specifically, dietary risk factors accounted for 20 per cent, smoking accounted for about 14 per cent, with behaviour in general accounting for about 50 per cent. This data is shown in Figure 2.1.

Lung cancer, which is the most common form of cancer, accounts for 36 per cent of all cancer deaths in men and 15 per cent in women in the UK. It has been calculated that 90 per cent of all lung cancer mortality is attributable to cigarette smoking, which is also linked to other illnesses such as cancers of the bladder, pancreas, mouth, larynx and oesophagus and CHD. The impact of smoking on mortality was shown by McKeown when he examined changes in life expectancies in males from 1838 to 1970. His data are shown in Figure 2.2 which indicates that the increase in life expectancy shown in non-smokers is much reduced in smokers.

In 2004, Mokdad et al. also explored the role of health behaviour in illness and mortality. Their analysis was based upon studies which had identified a link between risk behaviours such as smoking,

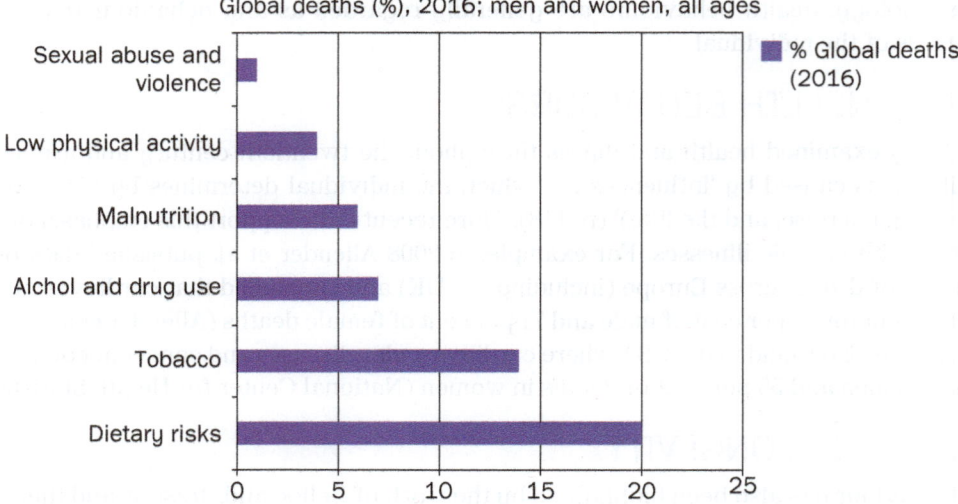

Figure 2.1 Global deaths from behaviour, 2016, men and women, all ages

SOURCE: Global Burden of Disease (2016)

diet, activity, alcohol consumption, car crashes and sexual behaviour and the deaths of 2.4 million people who had died in the year 2000 in the USA. The results from this analysis showed that the percentage of deaths caused by behaviours were as follows: tobacco: 18.1 per cent; diet and inactivity: 16.6 per cent; alcohol: 3.5 per cent; motor vehicle: 1.8 per cent; firearms: 1.2 per cent; sexual behaviour: 0.8 per cent; illicit drug use: 0.7 per cent. In 2008, data from a study in England also illustrated the impact of behaviour on mortality. Khaw et al. (2008) carried out a longitudinal study over 11 years of 20,244 men and women and concluded that death from all causes, cancer and cardiovascular disease was related to four health behaviours: smoking, not being physically active, drinking more than moderate amounts of alcohol and not eating five or more portions of fruit and vegetables per day. This study therefore again supported the link between behaviour and mortality. In addition, it supports the role of a healthy lifestyle as mortality was predicted by the combined impact of these four behaviours, not just individual behaviours.

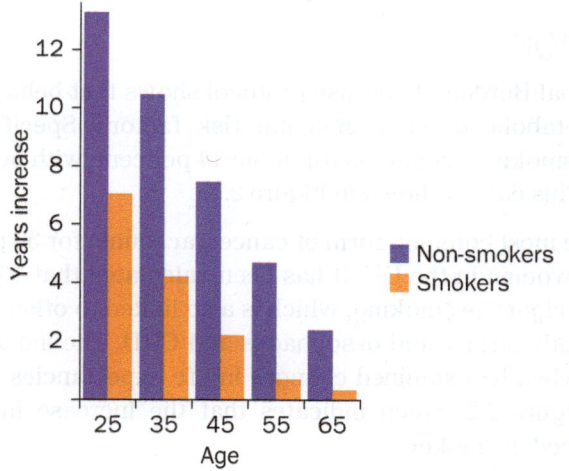

Figure 2.2 The effect of smoking on increase in expectation of life: males, 1838–1970

SOURCE: Adapted from McKeown (1979)

The relationship between behaviour and mortality can also be illustrated by the longevity of people in different countries. For example, in the USA and the UK, only 3 people out of every 100,000 live to be over 100. However, in Georgia, among the Abkhazians, 400 out of every 100,000 live to be over 100, and the oldest recorded Abkhazian was 170 (although this is obviously problematic in terms of the validity of any written records in the early 1800s). Weg (1983) examined the longevity of the Abkhazians and suggested that, relative to that in other countries, it is due to a combination of biological, lifestyle and social factors including:

- genetics
- maintaining vigorous work roles and habits
- a diet low in saturated fat and meat and high in fruit and vegetables
- no alcohol or nicotine
- high levels of social support
- low reported stress levels.

Analysis of this group of people suggests that health behaviours may be related to longevity and are therefore worthy of study. However, such cross-sectional studies are problematic to interpret, particularly in terms of the direction of causality: does the lifestyle of the Abkhazians cause their longevity or is it a product of it?

Research therefore points to a role for behaviour in explaining health, illness and mortality, particularly in the developed world where the most common problems are chronic illness such as cancer, CHD, obesity and diabetes, which have strong links to behaviour.

2 | THE ROLE OF HEALTH BELIEFS

Health promotion and health education perspectives tend to emphasize the role of knowledge and aim to change behaviour by improving what people know. This is the basis of campaigns which state 'smoking kills', 'eat more fruit and vegetables', 'wear a condom' and 'exercise is good for you'. In line with this, some studies indicate that knowledge does play a role in how we behave (Rimer et al. 1991; Lashley 1987; Champion 1990; O'Brien and Lee 1990). Within health psychology it is now generally accepted that knowledge is not enough and that what people believe is more important. Most research has therefore emphasized health beliefs as the key predictors of behaviour. This chapter describes the role of individual beliefs, stage models, social cognition models and integrated models as the four key approaches to health beliefs.

INDIVIDUAL BELIEFS

There are a number of different health beliefs that relate to health behaviours. This section will focus on attribution theory, risk perception, motivation and self-efficacy.

Attribution Theory

The origins of attribution theory can be found in the work of Heider (1958), who argued that individuals are motivated to see their social world as predictable and controllable – that is, there is a need to understand causality. Kelley (1971) developed these original ideas and proposed a clearly defined attribution theory suggesting that attributions about causality were structured according to causal schemata made up of the following criteria:

- *Distinctiveness:* the attribution about the cause of a behaviour is specific to the individual carrying out the behaviour.
- *Consensus:* the attribution about the cause of a behaviour would be shared by others.

- *Consistency over time:* the same attribution about causality would be made at any other time.
- *Consistency over modality:* the same attribution would be made in a different situation.

Kelley argued that attributions are made according to these different criteria and that the type of attribution made (e.g. high distinctiveness, low consensus, low consistency over time, low consistency over modality) determines the extent to which the cause of a behaviour is regarded as a product of a characteristic internal to the individual or external to them (i.e. the environment or situation).

Since its original formulation, attribution theory has been developed extensively and differentiations have been made between self-attributions (i.e. attributions about one's own behaviour) and other attributions (i.e. attributions made about the behaviour of others). In addition, the dimensions of attribution have been redefined as follows:

- *Internal versus external* (e.g. my failure to get a job is due to my poor performance in the interview versus the interviewer's prejudice).
- *Stable versus unstable* (e.g. the cause of my failure to get a job will always be around versus was specific to that one event).
- *Global versus specific* (e.g. the cause of my failure to get a job influences other areas of my life versus only influenced this specific job interview).
- *Controllable versus uncontrollable* (e.g. the cause of my failure to get a job was controllable by me versus was uncontrollable by me).

Attribution theory has been applied to the study of health and health-related behaviour. Herzlich (1973) interviewed 80 people about the general causes of health and illness and found that health is regarded as internal to the individual and illness is seen as something that comes into the body from the external world. Recently, attribution theory has been used to explore reactions to the COVID pandemic. For example, Yao and Siegel (2021) used an experimental design and manipulated perceived intentionality and controllability using a Chinese sample (n=271) in the context of a passenger spreading COVID-19 on an airplane. The results showed that stronger perceptions of intentionality and controllability of the passenger resulted in increased perceptions of responsibility, anger, and the desire to punish. Higher perceptions of controllability also decreased sympathy toward those who transmitted the virus. Further, there was an interaction between perceived intentionality and controllability: perceived controllability increased anger only when perceived intentionality was low; however, when intentionality was high, participants were angered regardless of perceived controllability. This indicates that beliefs about intentionality and controllability change attributions of responsibility together with feelings of anger and the desire to punish.

The internal versus external dimension of attribution theory has also been specifically applied to health in terms of the concept of a *health locus of control.* Individuals differ as to whether they tend to regard events as controllable by them (an internal locus of control) or uncontrollable by them (an external locus of control). Wallston and Wallston (1982) developed a measure of the health locus of control which evaluates whether an individual regards their health as controllable by them (e.g. 'I am directly responsible for my health'), whether they believe their health is not controllable by them and in the hands of fate (e.g. 'whether I am well or not is a matter of luck'), or whether they regard their health as under the control of powerful others (e.g. 'I can only do what my doctor tells me to do'). Researchers have also assessed parent's health locus of control for their children and Tremolada et al. (2020) showed that that parents of children with leukaemia were more likely to have an external locus of control than an internal one. Health locus of control has been shown to be related to whether an individual changes their behaviour (e.g. gives up smoking) or adheres to recommendations made by their doctor (see Norman and Bennett 1995 for a review). In addition, it has also been shown to relate to the kind of communication style people require from health professionals. For example, if a doctor encourages an individual who is generally *external* to change their lifestyle, the individual is unlikely to comply as they do not deem themselves responsible for their health (see e.g. Weiss and Larson 1990). Further, in a study of young people with diabetes, whereas an internal locus of control related to seeing the benefits of adhering to a self-care regimen for diabetes as outweighing the costs, a belief in powerful others was associated with a lower perception of the risks associated with the disease (Gillibrand and Stevenson 2006). Likewise, Muschetto and Siegel (2019) explored the impact of perceived controllability of depression on responses to individuals with the illness and found that perceiving depression as controllable generated more anger and less sympathy, which in turn increased a desire for social distance from the person with depression. Research also indicates that health locus of control can be changed. For example, Zhu et al. (2022) carried out an intervention study and randomly allocated half of the participants with Type 2 diabetes mellitus (n = 60) to receive a health locus of control-based education programme on self-management. Following the intervention, participants had significantly higher scores on internal health locus of control together with higher levels of self-management, dietary management, foot care, medication management and lower glycated haemoglobin level than the control group.

Risk Perception

One key health belief that people hold relates to their perception of risk and their sense of whether or not they are susceptible to any given health problem. For example, people may believe that because their grandmother smoked all her life and didn't die until she was 85, they are not at risk from lung cancer if they smoke. In contrast, others may overestimate their risk of illness, believing that obesity runs in their family and that there is little they can do to prevent themselves from becoming overweight. Perceptions of risk have been studied within two frameworks: unrealistic optimism and risk compensation.

Unrealistic Optimism

Weinstein (1983) suggested that one of the reasons that people continue to practise unhealthy behaviours is due to inaccurate perceptions of risk and susceptibility – their *unrealistic optimism*. He asked subjects to examine a list of health problems and to state 'compared to other people of your age and sex, what are your chances of getting [the problem] – greater than, about the same, or less than theirs?' The results of the study showed that most subjects believed that they were less likely to get the health problem. Weinstein called this phenomenon unrealistic optimism as he argued that not everyone can be less likely to contract an illness. Weinstein described four cognitive factors that contribute to unrealistic optimism: (1) lack of personal experience with the problem; (2) the belief that the problem is preventable by individual action; (3) the belief that if the problem has not yet appeared, it will not appear in the future; and (4) the belief that the problem is infrequent. These factors suggest that perception of own risk is not a rational process. Rouyard et al. (2017) carried out a systematic review on 18 studies reporting lay perceptions of risks of developing complications in Type 2 diabetes. They found substantial evidence for the existence of optimistic bias and low risk awareness, particularly from those from ethnic minority groups.

In an attempt to explain why individuals' assessment of their risk may go wrong, and why people are unrealistically optimistic, Weinstein argued that individuals show *selective focus*. He claimed that individuals ignore their own risk-increasing behaviour ('I may not always practise safe sex but that's not important') and focus primarily on their risk-reducing behaviour ('but at least I don't inject drugs'). He also argues that this selectivity is compounded by egocentrism: individuals tend to ignore others' risk-decreasing behaviour ('my friends all practise safe sex but that's irrelevant'). Therefore an individual may be unrealistically optimistic if they focus on the times they use condoms when assessing their own risk and ignore the times they do not and, in addition, focus on the times that others around them do not practise safe sex and ignore the times that they do.

In one study, subjects were required to focus on either their risk-increasing ('unsafe sex') or their risk-decreasing ('safe sex') behaviour. The effect of this on their unrealistic optimism for risk of HIV was examined (Hoppe and Ogden 1996). Heterosexual subjects were asked to complete a questionnaire concerning their beliefs about HIV and their sexual behaviour. Subjects were allocated to either the risk-increasing or risk-decreasing condition. Subjects in the risk-increasing condition were asked to complete questions such as 'since being sexually active how often have you asked about your partners' HIV status?' It was assumed that only a few subjects would be able to answer that they had done this frequently, thus making them feel more at risk. Subjects in the risk-decreasing condition were asked questions such as 'since being sexually active how often have you tried to select your partners carefully?' It was believed that most subjects would answer that they did this, making them feel less at risk. The results showed that focusing on risk-decreasing factors increased optimism by increasing perceptions of others' risk. Therefore, by encouraging the subjects to focus on their own healthy behaviour ('I select my partners carefully'), they felt more unrealistically optimistic and rated themselves as less at risk compared with those whom they perceived as being more at risk.

Risk Compensation

Risk perception has also been understood within the framework of risk compensation. People are exposed to often competing desires and motivations. For example, they may like eating cake but want to be thin. Some individuals opt for an extremely healthy approach to life and ensure that all their behaviours are protective and that the only desires they give in to are the healthy ones. Many, however, show risk compensation and believe that 'I can smoke because I go to the gym at the weekend' or 'I can eat chocolate because I play tennis'. From this perspective people believe that one set of risky behaviours can be neutralized or compensated for by another.

Such beliefs have been studied by Rabiau et al. (2006) who developed the compensatory health beliefs model and argued that such beliefs may explain why people don't always adhere to dietary or exercise programmes. Similarly, Radtke et al. (2010) developed a scale to assess compensatory beliefs in the context of adolescent smoking and concluded that more compensatory health beliefs about smoking predicted a lower readiness to stop smoking. They argued that smokers are often in a state of cognitive dissonance (e.g. 'I want to be healthy' *but* 'I know smoking is unhealthy') and that compensatory health beliefs may be a mechanism for them to resolve this dissonance. During the COVID pandemic much was written about risk compensation and researchers argued whether or not mask wearing would generate risk compensation and encourage people to take more risks such as mixing in public areas. For example, Trogen and Caplan (2021) argued that risk compensation would prolong the pandemic and in 2020 the WHO (2020) were quoted as saying 'Masks can also create a false sense of security, leading people to neglect measures such as hand hygiene and physical distancing.' While there are a few studies indicating that people may have taken more risks when wearing a mask such as not complying with social distancing rules (Aranguren 2022) or spending less time at home and more time in restaurants (Yan et al. 2021) most public health experts argued that the benefits of mask wearing outweighed the costs and some also stated that concerns about risk compensation were delaying the introduction of public health measures (Mantzari et al. 2020).

Motivation and Self-Determination Theory

The motivation to carry out a behaviour is a core construct in a lot of research exploring health behaviour and it is widely accepted that an individual needs to be motivated to either start a new behaviour or change an existing one. The notion of motivation can be found either implicitly or explicitly in most models of health behaviour but plays a central role in self-determination theory (SDT) (Deci and Ryan 1985, 2000). SDT focuses on the reasons or motives that regulate behaviour and distinguishes between two kinds of motivation. First it describes autonomous motivations which relate to engaging in behaviours that fulfil personally relevant goals such as eating nice food or talking to friends. This is also referred to as *intrinsic motivation* and tends to make the person feel satisfied or rewarded. Deci and Ryan (1985, 2000) argue that such autonomous motivations satisfy three basic needs:

autonomy ('I can manage my own behaviour'), competence ('I can master my environment') and relatedness ('I can develop close relationships with others'). Autonomous motivations tend to be associated with a sense of well-being and the persistence of health-related behaviours. Second it describes *controlled motivations* which are driven by external factors such as the need to please friends, and are also referred to as *extrinsic motivations*. These controlled motivations tend to make the person feel less personally satisfied and are linked with the avoidance of health behaviours.

Self-Efficacy

The notion of self-efficacy was first developed by Bandura in 1977 and then expanded as part of his social learning theory which has been used extensively to explain a range of behaviours from aggression and parenting to eating and exercise. Self-efficacy is 'the belief in one's capabilities to organize and execute the sources of action required to manage prospective situations' (Bandura 1986) and is very closely related to feeling confident in one's ability to engage in any given behaviour. Therefore stopping smoking would be related by the belief 'I am confident I can stop smoking' and eating more vegetables would be predicted by 'I can eat more vegetables in the future'. In 2020, Martinez-Calderon et al. carried out a systematic review of 11 studies assessing the role of self-efficacy in health outcomes in people with rheumatoid arthritis. The results suggest an association between higher self-efficacy and greater goal achievement, positive affect, acceptance of illness, problem-solving coping, physical function, physical activity and quality of life. Similarly, Jiang et al.'s (2019) systematic review and meta-analysis of the effectiveness of self-efficacy-focused education on health outcomes in patients with diabetes concluded that improved self efficacy was related to an increased ability to regulate self-management behaviours.

In Summary

In summary, there are four sets of individual beliefs that relate to health behaviours: attributions, risk perception, motivation and self-efficacy. These different beliefs have been used to study and change all types of health behaviours including diet, exercise, smoking, medication taking, screening uptake and safer sex. They have also been incorporated into models of health beliefs and behaviour. This chapter will now describe stage models, social cognition models and integrated models.

3 USING STAGE MODELS

Some models of health beliefs and health behaviour consider individuals to be at different ordered *stages* and describe how they move through these stages as they change their behaviour. A stage model is deemed to have four basic properties (Weinstein et al. 1998):

1 *A classification system to define the different stages:* each stage is therefore labelled and defined.

2 *Ordering of stages:* people pass through each stage in a predictable order, although they may not all reach the end-point, and some may pass backwards through the stages.

3 *People within the same stage face similar barriers:* in particular each stage is characterized by a similar set of barriers that prevent people from moving to the next stage.

4 *People from different stages face different barriers:* this means that each stage comes with a different set of barriers.

Stage models of behaviour can be found across a number of areas within psychology including models of child development, stages of grief and bereavement and the stages of adjustment to a serious illness or accident. The two-stage models most relevant to health psychology are the *stages of change model* (SOC) and the *health action process approach* (HAPA).

THE STAGES OF CHANGE MODEL (SOC)

The transtheoretical model of behaviour change was originally developed by Prochaska and DiClemente (1982) as a synthesis of 18 therapies describing the processes involved in eliciting and maintaining change. It is now more commonly known as the stages of change model (SOC).

Components of the SOC

The stages of change model is based upon the following stages:

1 *Pre-contemplation:* not intending to make any changes.

2 *Contemplation:* considering a change.

3 *Preparation:* making small changes.

4 *Action:* actively engaging in a new behaviour.

5 *Maintenance:* sustaining the change over time.

These stages, however, do not always occur in a linear fashion (simply moving from 1 to 5), and the theory describes behaviour change as dynamic and not 'all or nothing'. For example, an individual may move to the preparation stage and then back to the contemplation stage several times before progressing to the action stage. Furthermore, even when an individual has reached the maintenance stage, they may slip back to the contemplation stage over time.

The model also examines how the individual weighs up the costs and benefits of a particular behaviour, which is referred to as *decisional balance*. In particular, its authors argue that individuals at different stages of change will differentially focus on either the costs of a behaviour (e.g. 'stopping smoking will make me anxious in company') or the benefits of the behaviour (e.g. 'stopping smoking will improve my health'). For example, a smoker at the action stage ('I have stopped smoking') and the maintenance stage ('for four months') tends to focus on the favourable and positive feature of their behaviour ('I feel healthier because I have stopped smoking'), whereas smokers in the pre-contemplation stage tend to focus on the negative features of the behaviour ('it will make me anxious'). Central to any stage model is the position that the stages are qualitatively different to each other. For the SOC this means that the decisional balance of a person at the preparation change (for example) would be different to the decisional balance of someone at the action stage.

Using the SOC

If applied to smoking cessation, the model would suggest the following set of beliefs and behaviours at the different stages:

1 *Pre-contemplation:* 'I am happy being a smoker and intend to continue smoking'.

2 *Contemplation:* 'I have been coughing a lot recently, perhaps I should think about stopping smoking'.

3 *Preparation:* 'I will stop going to the pub and will buy lower tar cigarettes'.

4 *Action:* 'I have stopped smoking'.

5 *Maintenance:* 'I have stopped smoking for four months now'.

This individual, however, may well move back at times to believing that they will continue to smoke and may relapse (known as the *revolving door schema*).

Evidence for the SOC

The SOC has been applied to several health-related behaviours, such as smoking, alcohol use, exercise and screening behaviour (e.g. DiClemente et al. 1991; Cox et al. 2003; Armitage 2009a).

It is also increasingly used as a basis to develop interventions that are tailored to the particular stage of the specific person concerned. For example, a smoker who has been identified as being at the preparation stage would receive a different intervention to one who was at the contemplation stage. Gourlan et al. (2016) conducted a meta-analysis on the effects of theory-based interventions on the promotion of physical activity and concluded that those based on the SOC had an overall significant effect. Marshall and Biddle (2001) and Rosen (2000) have carried out meta-analyses on the use of the model to understand a range of health-related behaviours. In general, their conclusions indicate that the SOC can be used in research to explore changes in health behaviours and that some differences in decisional balance appear to exist between people classified as being at different stages. However, their analyses also revealed many inconsistencies in the data and the SOC has been subjected to many criticisms.

THE HEALTH ACTION PROCESS APPROACH (HAPA)

The HAPA (see Figure 2.3) is another stage model of health beliefs and health behaviour and was developed by Schwarzer (1992) following his review of the literature, which highlighted the need to include a *temporal* element in the understanding of beliefs and behaviour. In addition, it emphasized the importance of self-efficacy as a determinant of both behavioural intentions and self-reports of behaviour. The HAPA includes several individual beliefs (see earlier) and several elements from the social cognition models (see next section) and attempts to predict both behavioural intentions and actual behaviour.

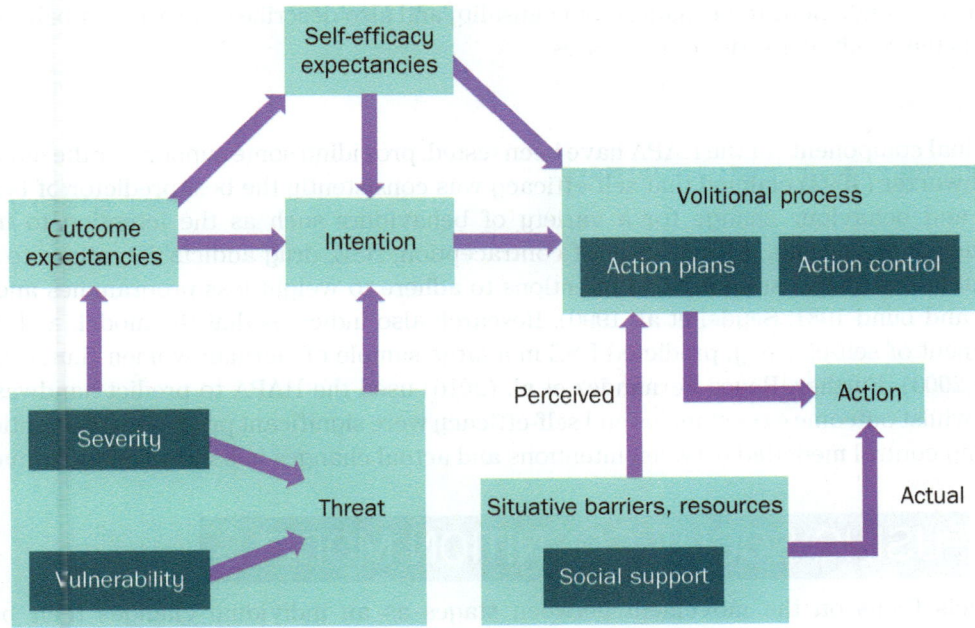

Figure 2.3 The health action process approach (HAPA)

Components of the HAPA

The main novel component of the HAPA is the distinction between a decision-making/motivational stage and an action/maintenance stage. Therefore the model adds a temporal and process factor to understanding the relationship between beliefs and behaviour and suggests that individuals initially decide whether or not to carry out a behaviour (the *motivation* stage), and then make plans to initiate and maintain this behaviour (the *action* phase).

According to the HAPA, the motivation stage is made up of the following components:

- *Self-efficacy* (e.g. 'I am confident that I can stop smoking').
- *Outcome expectancies* (e.g. 'stopping smoking will improve my health'), which has a subset of *social outcome expectancies* (e.g. 'other people want me to stop smoking and if I stop smoking I will gain their approval').
- *Threat appraisal*, which is composed of beliefs about the severity of an illness and perceptions of individual vulnerability.

According to the HAPA the end result of the process is an intention to act.

The action stage is composed of cognitive (volitional), situational and behavioural factors. The integration of these factors determines the extent to which a behaviour is initiated and maintained via these self-regulatory processes. The cognitive factor is made up of action plans (e.g. 'if offered a cigarette when I am trying not to smoke I will imagine what the tar would do to my lungs') and action control (e.g. 'I can survive being offered a cigarette by reminding myself that I am a non-smoker'). These two cognitive factors determine the individual's determination of will. The situational factor consists of social support (e.g. the existence of friends who encourage non-smoking) and the absence of situational barriers (e.g. financial support to join an exercise club).

Schwarzer (1992) argued that the HAPA bridges the gap between intentions and behaviour and emphasizes self-efficacy, both in terms of developing the intention to act and also implicitly in terms of the cognitive stage of the action stage, whereby self-efficacy promotes and maintains action plans and action control, therefore contributing to the maintenance of the action. He maintained that the HAPA enables specific predictions to be made about causality and also describes a process of beliefs whereby behaviour is the result of a series of processes.

Evidence for the HAPA

The individual components of the HAPA have been tested, providing some support for the model. In particular, Schwarzer (1992) claimed that self-efficacy was consistently the best predictor of behavioural intentions and behaviour change for a variety of behaviours such as the intention to use dental floss, frequency of flossing, effective use of contraception, BSE, drug addicts' intentions to use clean needles, intentions to quit smoking and intentions to adhere to weight loss programmes and exercise (e.g. Beck and Lund 1981; Seydel et al. 1990). Research also indicates that the model, and in particular the element of self-efficacy, predicted BSE in a large sample of German women (Luszczynska and Schwarzer 2003). Further, Reyes Fernández et al. (2016) used the HAPA to predict handwashing and found that whilst outcome expectancies and self-efficacy were significant predictors of intention, action and planning control mediated between intentions and actual changes in hand washing frequency.

4 | USING SOCIAL COGNITION MODELS

Stage models focus on the movement between stages as an individual changes their behaviour. Social cognition models examine the predictors and precursors to health behaviours and take a continuum approach to behaviour and behaviour change. They draw upon subjective expected utility theory (SEU) (Edwards 1954), which suggests that behaviour results from weighing up the costs and benefits of any given action and emphasizes how individuals are rational information processors. Social cognition models are also based upon social cognition theory which was developed by Bandura (1977, 1986) and suggests that behaviour is governed by expectancies, incentives and social cognitions. Expectancies include:

- *Situation outcome expectancies:* the expectancy that a behaviour may be dangerous (e.g. 'smoking can cause lung cancer').

- *Outcome expectancies:* the expectancy that a behaviour can reduce the harm to health (e.g. 'stopping smoking can reduce the chances of lung cancer').
- *Self-efficacy expectancies:* the expectancy that the individual is capable of carrying out the desired behaviour (e.g. 'I can stop smoking if I want to').

The concept of *incentives* suggests that a behaviour is governed by its consequences. For example, smoking behaviour may be reinforced by the experience of reduced anxiety, having a cervical smear may be reinforced by a feeling of reassurance after a negative result.

Social cognitions are a central component of social cognition models and reflect the *individual's representations of their social world.* Accordingly, social cognition models attempt to place the individual within the context both of other people and the broader social world, although the extent to which this is achieved varies between models. The main models currently in use within health psychology are the health belief model (HBM), protection motivation theory (PMT) and the theory of planned behaviour (TPB).

THE HEALTH BELIEF MODEL

The HBM (see Figure 2.4) was developed initially by Rosenstock (1966) and further by Becker and colleagues throughout the 1970s and 1980s in order to predict preventive health behaviours and also the behavioural response to treatment in acutely and chronically ill patients. However, over recent years, the HBM has been used to predict a wide variety of health-related behaviours.

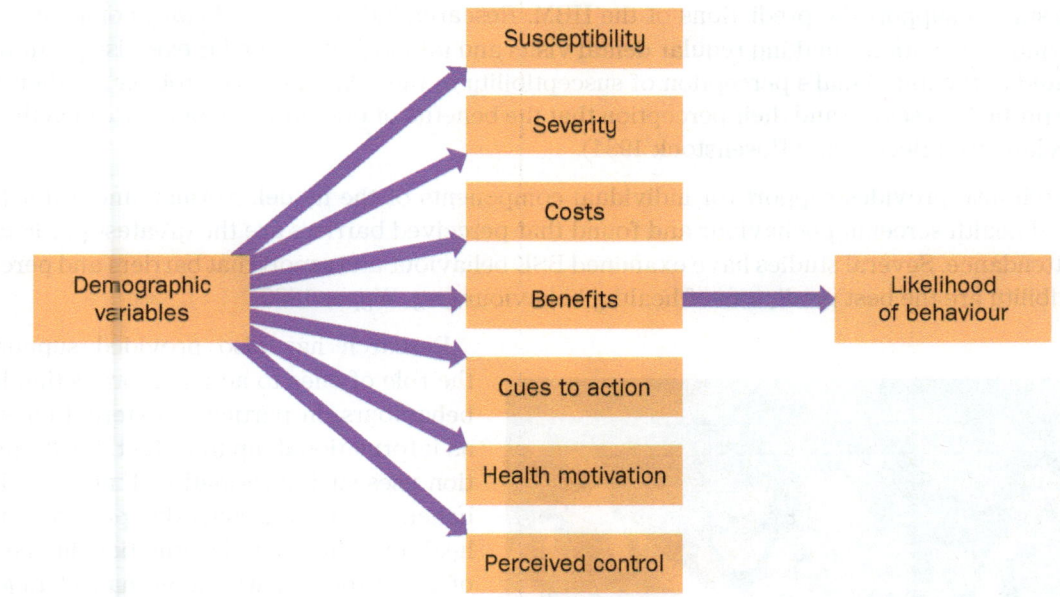

Figure 2.4 Basics of the health belief model

Components of the HBM

The HBM predicts that behaviour is a result of a set of core beliefs, which have been redefined over the years. The original core beliefs are the individual's perception of:

- Susceptibility to illness (e.g. 'my chances of getting lung cancer are high').
- The severity of the illness (e.g. 'lung cancer is a serious illness').
- The costs involved in carrying out the behaviour (e.g. 'stopping smoking will make me irritable').

- The benefits involved in carrying out the behaviour (e.g. 'stopping smoking will save me money'; 'smoking is cool').
- Cues to action, which may be internal (e.g. the symptom of breathlessness), or external (e.g. information in the form of health education leaflets).

The HBM suggests that these core beliefs should be used to predict *the likelihood that a behaviour will occur*. In response to criticisms the HBM has been revised to add the construct 'health motivation' to reflect an individual's readiness to be concerned about health matters (e.g. 'I am concerned that smoking might damage my health'). Becker and Rosenstock (1987) also suggested that perceived control (e.g. 'I am confident that I can stop smoking') should be added to the model.

Using the HBM

If applied to a health-related behaviour such as screening for cervical cancer, the HBM predicts regular screening if an individual perceives that she is highly susceptible to cancer of the cervix, that cervical cancer is a severe health threat, that the benefits of regular screening are high, and that the costs of such action are comparatively low. This will also be true if she is subjected to cues to action that are external, such as a leaflet in the doctor's waiting room, or internal, such as a symptom perceived to be related to cervical cancer (whether correct or not), such as pain or irritation. When using the new amended HBM, the model would also predict that a woman would attend for screening if she is confident that she can do so and if she is motivated to maintain her health.

Evidence for the HBM

Several studies support the predictions of the HBM. Research indicates that dietary compliance, safe sex, having vaccinations, making regular dental visits and taking part in regular exercise programmes are related to the individual's perception of susceptibility to the related health problem, to their belief that the problem is severe and their perception that the benefits of preventive action outweigh the costs (e.g. Becker 1974; Becker and Rosenstock 1984).

Research also provides support for individual components of the model. Norman and Fitter (1989) examined health screening behaviour and found that perceived barriers are the greatest predictors of clinic attendance. Several studies have examined BSE behaviour and report that barriers and perceived susceptibility are the best predictors of healthy behaviour (e.g. Wyper 1990).

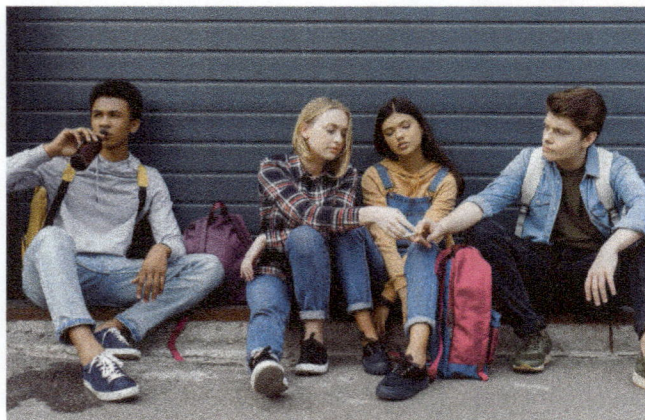

People weigh up the costs and benefits of a health behaviour: 'smoking is cool' may be a perceived benefit

SOURCE: © LightField Studios Inc./Alamy Stock Photo

Research has also provided support for the role of cues to action in predicting health behaviours, in particular external cues such as informational input. In fact, health promotion uses such informational input to change beliefs and consequently promote future healthy behaviour. Information in the form of fear-arousing warnings may change attitudes and health behaviour in such areas as dental health, safe driving and smoking (e.g. Sutton and Hallett 1989). General information regarding the negative consequences of a behaviour is also used both in the prevention and cessation of smoking behaviour (e.g. Flay 1985). To date, reviews of the HBM show support for some but not all of its components and at times the links between beliefs and behaviour within the model have been very small (see Abraham and Sheeran 2005 for an analysis of HBM data). Further, Jones et al. (2014) carried out a systematic review to assess the effectiveness of HBM interventions to promote adherence and concluded that 78 per cent of studies reported significant improvements in adherence although only six studies utilized the full version of the HBM.

Although there is much contradiction in the literature surrounding the HBM, research has used aspects of this model to predict screening for hypertension, screening for cervical cancer, genetic screening, exercise behaviour, decreased alcohol use, changes in diet and smoking cessation.

PROTECTION MOTIVATION THEORY (PMT)

Rogers (1975, 1985) developed the PMT (see Figure 2.5), which expanded the HBM to include additional factors. The main contribution of PMT over the HBM was the addition of fear and an attempt to include an emotional component into the understanding of health behaviours.

Components of PMT

PMT describes health behaviours as a product of five components:

1 Severity (e.g. 'bowel cancer is a serious illness').
2 Susceptibility (e.g. 'my chances of getting bowel cancer are high').
3 Response effectiveness (e.g. 'changing my diet would improve my health').
4 Self-efficacy (e.g. 'I am confident that I can change my diet').
5 Fear (e.g. an emotional response: 'I am scared of getting cancer').

These components predict *behavioural intentions* (e.g. 'I intend to change my behaviour'), which are related to behaviour. PMT describes severity, susceptibility and fear as relating to *threat appraisal* (i.e. appraising to outside threat) and response effectiveness and self-efficacy as relating to *coping appraisal* (i.e. appraising the individual themselves). According to PMT, there are two types of sources of information – environmental (e.g. verbal persuasion, observational learning) and intrapersonal (e.g. prior experience). This information influences the five components of PMT (self-efficacy, response effectiveness, severity, susceptibility, fear), which then elicit either an 'adaptive' coping response (i.e. behavioural intention) or a 'maladaptive' coping response (e.g. avoidance, denial).

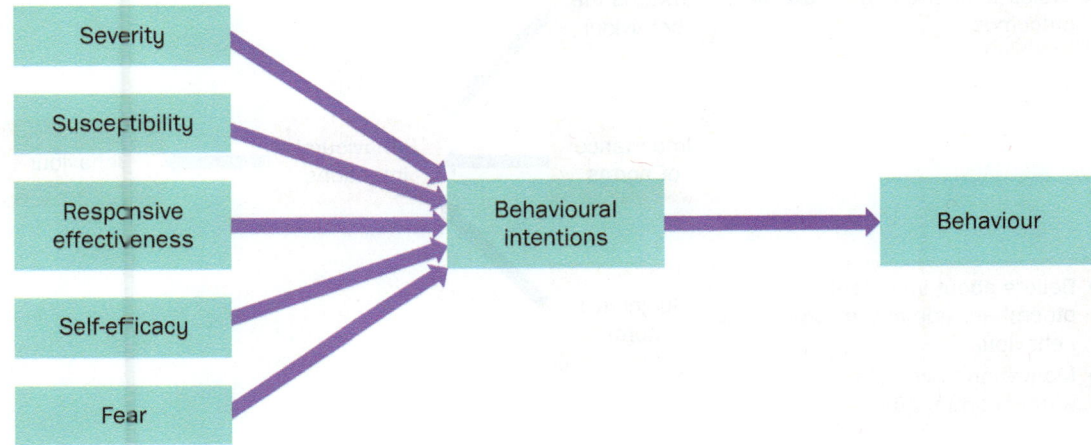

Figure 2.5 Basics of protection motivation theory

Using the PMT

If applied to dietary change, PMT would make the following predictions: information about the role of a high fat diet in CHD would increase fear, increase the individual's perception of how serious CHD is (perceived severity) and increase their belief that they are likely to have a heart attack (perceived susceptibility/susceptibility). If the individual also felt confident that they could change their diet (self-efficacy) and that this change would have beneficial consequences (response effectiveness), they would report high intentions to change their behaviour (behavioural intentions). This would be seen as an adaptive coping response to the information.

Evidence for the PMT

Norman et al. (2003) used the PMT to predict children's adherence to wearing an eye patch. Parents of children diagnosed with eye problems completed a baseline questionnaire concerning their beliefs and a follow-up questionnaire after two months describing the child's level of adherence. The results showed that perceived susceptibility and response costs were significant predictors of adherence. Similarly, Plotnikoff et al. (2010) used PMT to predict physical activity in adults with type 1 diabetes and reported that self-efficacy and severity were good predictors of intention, although perceived vulnerability was not. Furthermore, similar results were found for predicting activity in a large sample of healthy adults (Plotnikoff et al. 2009). Bui et al. (2013) conducted a systematic review of 20 studies investigating the effectiveness of PMT in physical activity and concluded that self-efficacy was generally the most effective predictor.

THEORIES OF REASONED ACTION AND PLANNED BEHAVIOUR (TRA AND TPB)

The theory of reasoned action (TRA) (see Figure 2.6) has been extensively used to examine predictors of behaviours and was central to the debate within social psychology concerning the relationship between attitudes and behaviour (Fishbein 1967; Fishbein and Ajzen 1975). The TRA emphasized a central role for social cognitions in the form of subjective norms (the individual's beliefs about their social world) and included both beliefs and evaluations of these beliefs (both factors constituting the individual's attitudes).

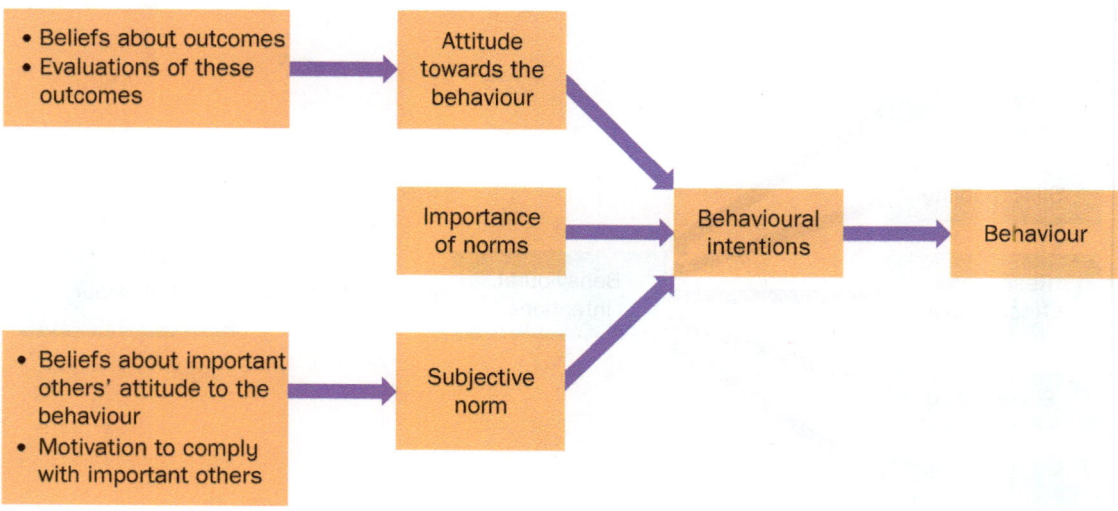

Figure 2.6 Basics of the theory of reasoned action

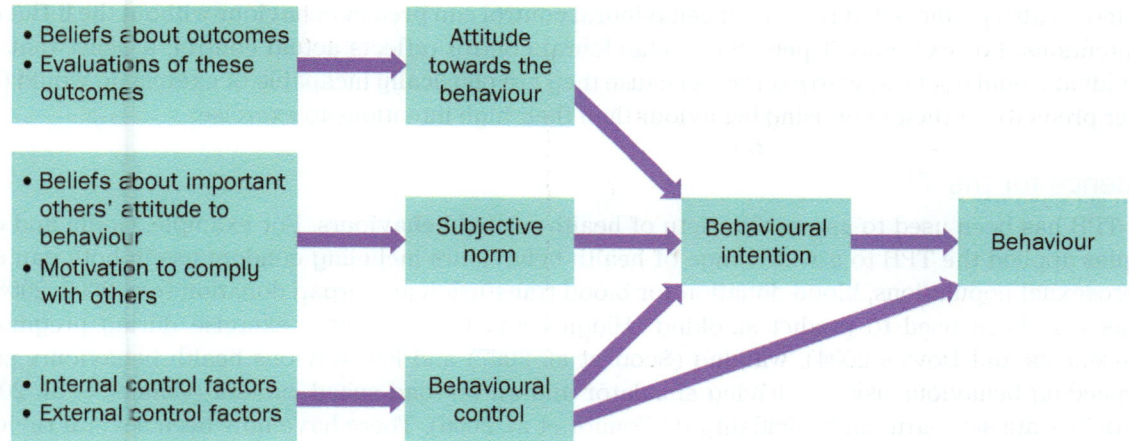

Figure 2.7 Basics of the theory of planned behaviour

The TRA was therefore an important model as it placed the individual within the social context and in addition suggested a role for *value,* which was in contrast to the traditional more rational approach to behaviour. The theory of planned behaviour (TPB) (see Figure 2.7) was developed by Ajzen and colleagues (Ajzen and Madden 1986; Ajzen 1988) and represented a progression from the TRA. Where the TRA had added subjective norms to previous models, the TPB added both subjective norms and a measure of *behavioural control.* Both models also emphasize behavioural intentions as an important precursor to actual behaviour.

Components of the TPB

The TPB emphasizes *behavioural intentions* as the outcome of a combination of several beliefs. The theory proposes that intentions should be conceptualized as 'plans of action in pursuit of behavioural goals' (Ajzen and Madden 1986) and are a result of the following beliefs:

- *Attitude towards a behaviour,* which is composed of either a positive or negative evaluation of a particular behaviour and beliefs about the outcome of the behaviour (e.g. 'exercising is fun and will improve my health').
- *Subjective norm,* which is composed of the perception of social norms and pressures to perform a behaviour, and an evaluation of whether the individual is motivated to comply with this pressure (e.g. 'people who are important to me will approve if I lose weight and I want their approval').
- *Perceived behavioural control,* which is composed of a belief that the individual can carry out a particular behaviour based upon a consideration of internal control factors (e.g. skills, abilities, information) and external control factors (e.g. obstacles, opportunities), both of which relate to past behaviour.

According to the TPB, these three factors predict behavioural intentions, which are then linked to behaviour. The TPB also states that perceived behavioural control can have a direct effect on behaviour without the mediating effect of behavioural intentions.

Using the TPB

If applied to alcohol consumption, the TPB would make the following predictions: if an individual believed that reducing their alcohol intake would make their life more productive and be beneficial to their health (attitude to the behaviour), and believed that the important people in their life wanted them to cut down (subjective norm), and in addition believed that they were capable of drinking less alcohol due to their past behaviour and evaluation of internal and external control factors (high behavioural control), then this would predict high intentions to reduce alcohol intake (behavioural intentions).

The model also predicts that perceived behavioural control can predict behaviour without the influence of intentions. For example, if perceived behavioural control reflects actual control, a belief that the individual would not be able to exercise because they are physically incapable of exercising would be a better predictor of their exercising behaviour than their high intentions to exercise.

Evidence for the TPB

The TPB has been used to assess a variety of health-related behaviours. For example, Godin and colleagues applied the TPB to a wide range of health behaviours including condom use in both gay and heterosexual populations, blood donation for blood transfusion and organ donation (e.g. 2007, 2008a). It has also been used to predict smoking (Higgins and Conner 2003), exercise during pregnancy (Hausenblas and Downs 2004), walking (Scott et al. 2007) and less obvious health behaviours such as speeding behaviour using a driving simulator and an on-road speed camera (Conner et al. 2006) and deliberate self-harm and suicidality (O'Connor et al. 2006). There have now been several reviews and meta-analyses of the TPB which describe the extent to which this model can predict a range of health behaviours (e.g. Armitage and Conner 2001; Trafimow et al. 2002). For example, Sutton and White (2016) conducted a systematic review and meta-analysis of 38 studies using the TPB to predict sun-protective intentions and reported significant effects for perceived behavioural control, subjective norms and attitudes, with attitudes having the strongest relationship with behavioural intentions.

5 | USING INTEGRATED MODELS

Over recent years there has been a call to integrate models to form one definitive model that consists of the most useful cognitions and can be used to predict (and change) most health behaviours. One integrated model has been called the 'major theorist's model' as it emerged out of a workshop attended by many of the most prominent researchers within psychology (e.g. Becker, Fishbein, Bandura and Kanfer). Through discussion they identified eight key variables which they believed should account for most of the variance in any given (deliberative) behaviour (Fishbein et al. 2001). These were divided into those that directly impact upon behaviour (e.g. environmental constraints, intention, skills) and those that relate to the intention (e.g. self-discrepancy, advantages/disadvantages, social pressure, self-efficacy, emotional reaction). Research has also tested the effectiveness of integrating models in other ways. For example, Lippke and Plotnikoff (2009) integrated PMT with the SOC as a means to predict exercise and concluded that PMT variables functioned differently at the different stages of the SOC and that this was a useful way to examine behaviour. Further, Jacobs et al. (2011) explored the usefulness of integrating the TPB with STD in the context of diet and physical activity. In 2009 Hagger and Chatzisarantis carried out a meta-analysis of the integration of these two perspectives and concluded that this was a partially (but not totally) useful way forward.

THE COM-B

An integrated model which has probably been used the most over recent years is the COM-B developed by Michie and colleagues (e.g. Michie et al. 2011; Michie et al. 2014; Michie and Wood 2015; see Figure 2.8). The COM-B was derived from carrying out an analysis of 83 theories and 1659 constructs by a cross disciplinary team of researchers in terms of three dimensions: comprehensiveness, coherence and a clear link to an overarching model of behaviour. The core components of this new model are *Capability* (derived from the individual's psychological or physical ability to enact the behaviour), *Opportunity* (reflecting the physical and social environment that enables the behaviour) and *Motivation* (describing the reflective and automatic mechanisms that activate or inhibit the behaviour. These in turn predict *behaviour*. The COM-B finds reflection in the models used in a number of domains such as criminology (the opportunity, motive, capability triad) and workplace and environmental interventions (Motivations, opportunities, ability model, MOA) and has been applied beyond health psychology to many other areas of research.

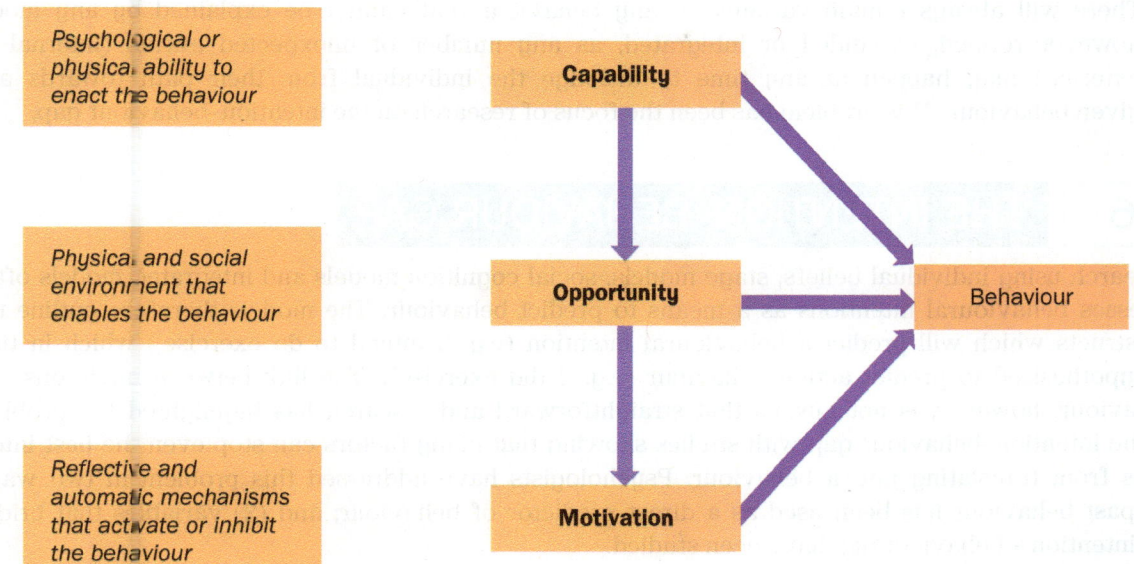

Figure 2.8 The COM-B

SOURCE: Michie et al. (2011)

Using the COM-B

Using the COM-B to predict a behaviour such as cooking would indicate the following: people cook because they are capable of cooking (i.e. have cooking skills), because they are motivated to cook (i.e. want to cook and believe that it is the right thing to do) and because they have the opportunity to cook (i.e. have food and a cooker).

Evidence for the COM-B

Since its development the COM-B has been used in a multitude of studies to predict a wide range of behaviours such as physical activity, weight loss, hand hygiene, dental hygiene, diet, smoking, medication adherence, prescribing behaviours, condom use and female genital mutilation (e.g. Jackson et al. 2014; Brown et al. 2015; Bailey et al. 2015; Chadwick and Benelam 2013; Asimakopoulou and Newton 2015; Heneghan et al. 2020; Willmott et al. 2021; see Michie and Wood 2015; Atkins et al. 2015 and Michie et al. 2014 for reviews). It has also been used to frame a number of qualitative studies and as the basis for interventions. For example, Bentley et al. (2019) use the COM-B as a theoretical lens to explore the qualitative accounts of sports nutritionists, Timlin et al. (2021) used the COM-B model to identify ways to modify dietary patterns of 40–55-year-olds living in the UK as a means to reduce the risk of cognitive decline in later life and O'Donovan et al. (2021) carried out a qualitative study of women aged 25–65 years to investigate factors that either promote or inhibit cervical screening uptake.

Although the idea of integrating models makes common sense as there is substantial overlap between the different approaches, there are some problems:

- Models which are small and focused can be tested in research and used to develop interventions *but* may miss important other variables.
- Larger models that are more inclusive may miss out less but are more unwieldy to use in both research and practice.

- Theories and models are often the work of individuals who have invested a large part of their career in their development. They may be reluctant to have their model subsumed within someone else's model.
- There will always remain variance in any behaviour that cannot be explained by any model however refined, expanded or integrated, as any number of unexpected events (internal or external) may happen at any time to dislodge the individual from their path towards any given behaviour. This problem has been the focus of research on the intention–behaviour gap.

6 THE INTENTION–BEHAVIOUR GAP

Research using individual beliefs, stage models, social cognition models and integrated models often assesses behavioural intentions as a means to predict behaviour. The models therefore outline the constructs which will predict a behavioural intention (e.g. 'I intend to do exercise') which in turn is hypothesized to predict actual behaviour (e.g. 'I did exercise'). The link between intentions and behaviour, however, is not always that straightforward and research has highlighted the problem of the intention–behaviour gap with studies showing that many factors can stop even the best intentions from translating into a behaviour. Psychologists have addressed this problem in two ways: (1) past behaviour has been used as a direct predictor of behaviour; and (2) variables that bridge the intention – behaviour gap have been studied.

THE ROLE OF PAST BEHAVIOUR AND HABIT

Most research assumes that cognitions predict behavioural intentions, which in turn predict behaviour. This is in line with the shift from 'I think, therefore I intend to do, therefore I do'. It is possible, however, that behaviour is not predicted by cognitions but by behaviour. From this perspective, individuals are more likely to eat healthily tomorrow if they ate healthily today. They are also more likely to go to the doctor for a cervical smear if they have done so in the past. Research suggests that such past behaviour can account for about 13 per cent of future behaviour (Conner and Armitage 1998) and predicts behaviours such as cycle helmet use (Quine et al. 1998), breast self examination (Hodgkins and Orbell 1998), bringing up condom use (Yzer et al. 2001), wearing an eye patch (Norman et al. 2003), attendance at health checks (Norman and Conner 1993) and breakfast consumption (Wong and Mullan 2009). In addition, past behaviour may itself predict cognitions that then predict behaviour (Gerrard et al. 1996).

SO HOW DOES PAST BEHAVIOUR INFLUENCE FUTURE BEHAVIOUR?

Ouellette and Wood (1998) identified two possible routes for the link between past behaviour and future behaviour. First, they argued that past behaviour may influence future behaviour indirectly through a conscious change in cognitions – for example, 'I had breakfast yesterday and it made me realize that I had more energy so I will have breakfast again today'. Such a route is more common for behaviours which are infrequent as they offer a new experience. Secondly, they argued for a role of habit with future behaviour occurring after past behaviour in a more automatic way, with very little effort or conscious processing. This route is more likely to be taken for frequently occurring behaviours which offer no new experience. In line with this second route, Verplanken and colleagues (e.g. Verplanken et al. 1994; Verplanken and Aarts 1999) have explored ways to measure habit strength, and research indicates a role for habit in explaining a number of behaviours such as travel mode (Verplanken et al. 1994), condom use (Trafimow 2000), people's use of information (Aarts et al. 1998) and health care professionals' behaviour (Potthoff et al. 2019). This has resulted in a theory of habit and its impact upon behaviour (eg. see Gardner et al. 2019; Gardner et al. 2020; Phillips and Mullan 2022 for reviews). To date, from these reviews it seems clear that habit plays a key role in behaviour change and sustaining behaviours over time and that habit formation offers an acceptable, easily understood intervention strategy to promote behaviour change. It is also argued, however, that it is important to identify the 'facilitating conditions' that may determine the relative influence of habit and intention on behaviour. One of these factors may be self control and Gardner et al. (2020) suggest that when self-control is diminished, people act habitually regardless of intention direction or strength. Yet when people possess self-control, habits can help people to act on favourable but weakened intentions, but intentions that oppose habitual tendencies can override habitual influence. Another key factor in habit change may be a break in context such as moving home or coming back from holiday. This can disrupt the association between familiar contexts and behaviours and opens up a 'window of opportunity' during which people are amenable to changing their behaviour and new habits can be established (Verplanken et al. 2008). Interestingly, even when old habits are broken, the desire to perform the old behaviour doesn't just go away but fades over a long period. This suggests that there is a window of time when people will be vulnerable to relapsing back into old habits if their usual environment reappears (Walker et al. 2015).

Therefore, even when a habit has been formed, some conscious motivation may be required to sustain behaviours over time. This suggests that even though past behaviour predicts future behaviour this may still need some cognitive effort. Further, even though habits can be broken by a 'window of opportunity' there is also a window following this when they can be formed again.

BRIDGING THE INTENTION–BEHAVIOUR GAP

The second approach to address the limited way in which research has predicted behaviour has been to suggest variables that may bridge the gap between intentions to behave and actual behaviour. Some research has emphasised the role of habit and perceived behavioural control in bridging the intention–behaviour gap (e.g. Verplanken et al. 1994; Verplanken and Aarts 1999) although recently the strength of this association has been questioned and may attributed to methodological and/or statistical artefacts (Rebar et al. 2019). Other research has highlighted the role of plans for action, health goals commitment, action control and trying as a means to tap into the kinds of cognitions that may be responsible for the translation of intentions into behaviour (Schwarzer 1992; Bagozzi 1993; Luszczynska and Schwarzer 2003; Sniehotta et al. 2005). Most research, however, has focused on Gollwitzer's (1993) notion of implementation intentions, which are a simple form of action plans. According to Gollwitzer, carrying out an intention involves the development of specific plans as to what an individual will do given a specific set of environmental factors. Therefore, implementation intentions describe the 'what' and the 'when' of a particular behaviour. For example, the intention 'I intend to stop smoking' will be more likely to be translated into 'I have stopped smoking' if the individual makes the implementation intention 'I intend to stop smoking tomorrow at 12.00 when I have finished my last packet'. Further, 'I intend to eat healthily' is more likely to be translated into 'I am eating healthily' if the implementation intention 'I will start to eat healthily by having an apple tomorrow lunchtime' is made. Some experimental research has shown that encouraging individuals to make implementation intentions can actually increase the correlation between intentions and behaviour for behaviours such as adolescent smoking (Conner and Higgins 2010), fruit consumption (Armitage 2007a), exercise (Brickell et al. 2006), taking a vitamin C pill (Sheeran and Orbell 1998), reducing dietary fat (Armitage 2004) and reducing binge drinking in university students (Norman and Wrona-Clarke 2016). Gollwitzer and Sheeran (2006) carried out a meta-analysis of 94 independent tests of the impact of implementation intentions on a range of behavioural goals including eating a low fat diet, using public transport, exercise and a range of personal goals. The results from this analysis indicated that implementation intentions had a medium to large effect on goal attainment and the analysis provides some insights into the processes involved in this approach. The use of implementation intentions is also supported by the goal-setting approach of cognitive behavioural therapy (CBT). Therefore, by tapping into variables such as implementation intentions it is argued that the models may become better predictors of actual behaviour.

BOX 2.1
Critical Approaches to Health Psychology

Research exploring health beliefs and their role in predicting health behaviour highlights some of the bigger issues in research in health psychology:

WEIRD samples: A lot of research exploring beliefs and behaviours has been carried out on WEIRD samples often drawing upon University students and sometimes even psychology students. And as we know students (particularly psychology students!) are not always like everyone else. So which beliefs they have and which beliefs predict which behaviour may be different for them than for other people.

A focus on the individual: Research in this area focuses on the individual and explores individual beliefs and individual behaviours. This conceptualizes the individual as separate to their social and political world. Attempts are (kind of) made to capture some of this broader context with 'boxes' in models such as 'social norms', 'opportunity' or 'social context' but this can't capture the richness of a person's culture, religion or ethnicity or family influences.

A snapshot in time: Research assessing beliefs captures these at a specific time and treats this as if it is a stable variable. However, beliefs are complex and ever changing so what one person thinks when they are asked may not reflect what they think a few minutes (or even seconds) later. It is hard to generalize from what has been measured to what someone thinks and know whether this is what they still think by the time you measure their next belief or their behaviour.

Behaviours are complex too: We describe health behaviours such as eating, drinking, smoking, exercise as if they are simple boundaried behaviours. But in fact they are complex and multi faceted. For example, exercise might mean running 5km. But it also might mean walking up the stairs rather than using the lift, putting the kettle on, fidgeting on a seat or, in my case, bouncing on a ball (!). And it might mean running fast, slow, being out of breath or just about moving faster than walking (again in my case!). It is therefore hard to know if our simple measures of behaviour actually capture what people are doing.

7	THINKING CRITICALLY ABOUT HEALTH BELIEFS

This chapter has outlined a number of different approaches to understanding the role of beliefs in predicting behaviour with a focus on individual beliefs, stage models, social cognition models and integrated models. Thinking critically about health beliefs involves challenging the ways the models have been developed and constructed, understanding problems with research in this area and recognizing the problems with any models trying to predict (and therefore change) behaviours as variable as diet, exercise, safer sex and smoking. This final section will outline ways to think critically about these different approaches to understanding health beliefs and their role in predicting health behaviours.

SOME CRITICAL QUESTIONS

When reading or thinking about the theories and research relating to health beliefs, ask yourself the following questions:

- How important are our beliefs compared to our emotions?
- Can we really measure what someone believes without changing it through our questions?
- To what extent are our beliefs captured by those described in our models?

- What factors might influence why people don't always behave as they intend to?
- Why are some of our models too simple?
- Why are some of our models too complex?

SOME PROBLEMS WITH . . .

Below are some specific problems with research in this area.

Problems with Stage Models

Stage models such as the stages of change model (SOC) and the HAPA have been used to underpin research and to develop behaviour change interventions. The SOC has recently been criticized for the following reasons (Weinstein et al. 1998; Sutton 2000, 2002a, 2005; West 2006). These criticisms are also relevant to most other stage theories:

- It is difficult to determine whether behaviour change occurs according to stages or along a continuum. Researchers describe the difference between linear patterns between stages which are not consistent with a stage model and discontinuity patterns which are consistent.
- The absence of qualitative differences between stages could either be due to the absence of stages or because the stages have not been correctly assessed and identified.
- Changes between stages may happen so quickly as to make the stages unimportant.
- Most studies based on the SOC use cross-sectional designs to examine differences between different people at different stages of change. Such designs do not allow conclusions to be drawn about the role of different causal factors at the different stages (i.e. people at the preparation stage are driven forward by different factors than those at the contemplation stage). Experimental and longitudinal studies are needed for any conclusions about causality to be valid.
- The concept of a 'stage' is not a simple one as it includes many variables: current behaviour, quit attempts, intention to change and time since quitting. Perhaps these variables should be measured separately.
- The model focuses on conscious decision-making and planning processes. Further, it assumes that people make coherent and stable plans.
- Using the model may be no better than simply asking people, 'Do you have any plans to try to . . . ?' or 'Do you want to . . . ?'.

Problems with Social Cognition Models

Social cognition models provide a structured approach to understanding health beliefs and the prediction of health behaviours and offer a framework for designing questionnaires and developing interventions. Over recent years, however, several papers have been published criticizing these models (Sutton 2002a; Smedslund 2000; Ogden 2003, 2015; Sniehotta et al. 2014). These problems can be categorized as conceptual, methodological and predictive.

Conceptual Problems

Some researchers have pointed to some conceptual problems with the models in terms of their variables and their ability to inform us about the world. These problems are as follows:

- Each model is made up of different concepts such as perceived behavioural control, behavioural intentions, perceived vulnerability and attitudes. Norman and Conner (1996) have argued that there is some overlap between these variables and Armitage and Conner (2000) have argued for a 'consensus' approach to studying health behaviour, whereby key constructs are integrated across models (see integrated models).

- The models describe associations between variables which assume causality. For example, the TPB describes attitude as causing behavioural intention. Sutton (2002a) argues that these associations are causally ambiguous and cannot be concluded unless experimental methods are used. Similarly, Smedslund (2000) criticized the models for their logical construction and said that assumptions about association are flawed.

- A theory should enable the collection of data which can either lead to that theory being supported or rejected. Ogden (2003) carried out an analysis of studies using the HBM, TRA, PMT and TPB over a 4-year period and concluded that the models cannot be rejected as caveats can always be offered to perpetuate the belief that the model has been supported.

- Research should generate truths which are true by observation and require an empirical test (e.g. smoking causes heart disease) rather than by definition (i.e. heart disease causes narrowing of the arteries). Ogden (2003) concluded from her analysis than much research using the models produces statements that are true by definition (i.e. 'I am certain that I will use a condom therefore I intend to use a condom'). She argues that the findings are therefore tautological.

- Research should inform us about the world rather than create the world. Ogden (2003) argues that questionnaires that ask people questions such as 'Do you think the female condom decreases sexual pleasure for a man?' may change the way in which people think rather than get them to just describe their thoughts. This is similar to changes in mood following mood checklists, and the ability of diaries to change behaviour. Much research has now explored this possibility within the framework of the 'mere measurement effect' and 'measurement reactivity' and illustrates that the simple process of measuring can change cognitions, emotion and behaviour across a number of areas including blood donation and cervical screening attendance (e.g. Godin et al. 2008b, 2010; French and Sutton 2010).

Methodological Problems

Research using models such as the TPB, TRA and HBM often uses cross-sectional designs involving questionnaires which are analysed using multiple regression analysis or structural equation modelling. Researchers have highlighted some problems with this approach.

- Cross-sectional research can only show associations rather than causality. To solve this, prospective studies are used which separate the independent and dependent variables by time. Sutton (2002a) argues that both these designs are problematic and do not allow inferences about causality to be made. He suggests that randomized experimental designs are the best solution to this problem.

- Hankins et al. (2000) provide some detailed guidelines on how data using the TRA and TPB should be analysed and state that much research uses inappropriate analysis. They point out that if multiple regression analysis is used, adjusted R^2 should be the measure of explained variance, that residuals should be assessed and that semi-partial correlations should be used to assess the unique contribution of each variable. They also state that 'structural equation modelling' might be a better approach as this makes explicit the assumptions of the models.

- Darker and French (2009) carried out a think-aloud study of a questionnaire based upon the TPB to explore how people made sense of the different items. On average the results showed around 16 problems with the 52 questions, indicating that research participants may not always interpret questions in the ways intended by the researchers.

Predictive Problems

Models such as the TRA, TPB, HBM and PMT are designed to predict behavioural intentions and actual behaviour. However, two main observations have been made.

- First, it has been suggested that these models are not that successful at predicting behavioural intentions. For example, Sutton (1998a) argued that studies using social cognition models only manage to predict between 40 and 50 per cent of the variance in behavioural intentions. Therefore, up to 50 per cent of the variance remains unexplained.

• Secondly, it has been observed that such models are even less effective at predicting actual behaviour. Sutton (1998a) also argued that studies using these models only predict 19–38 per cent of the variance in behaviour. Some of this failure to predict behaviour may be due to the behaviour being beyond the control of the individual concerned. For example, 'I intend to study at university' may not be translated into 'I am studying at university' due to economic or educational factors. Further, 'I intend to eat healthily' may not be translated into 'I am eating healthily' due to the absence of healthy food.

Problems with Integrated Models

Although integrated models such as the COM-B are a relatively new approach to understanding health related behaviour, these too have their problems and have been criticized in the following ways (Ogden 2016a, 2016b).

The Problem of Variability

The COM-B is an integrated model designed to reduce variability in research (so one model is used rather than many), in practice (so practitioners use a systematic approach rather than many) and between patients (so we can predict as much of the variance as possible of any one person's health behaviour). This aim is worthy if the goal is to produce research studies which can be compared and synthesized through systematic reviews or meta-analyses as all studies would be using the same approach. It also comes with problems. First, such a systematized approach can limit research and reduce creativity if everyone is encouraged to use the same approach in their research. Second, it rules out the 'art' of practitioner work and can reduce professionals to technicians who follow rules and guidelines leaving no space for responding to the needs of the client or the dynamic with the professional. And finally, there are so many variables that predict what we do and when, it seems naive to believe that one model could possibly ever explain all behaviours carried out by all people for all the time. So it might not be desirable to rule out variability. Nor might it be feasible.

The Tension between Inclusivity and Specificity

Some models include a multitude of different constructs and cover every possible idea from every possible angle. These inclusive models can never be criticized for missing anything out but are unwieldy and difficult to operationalize and test. In contrast, some models are very narrow and focused. These are much easier to test as they have fewer constructs and can be turned into measures. However, such specific models can also be criticized as 'but surely its more complex than that?', 'what about. . .?' and they seem to oversimplify the world we live in. Integrated models illustrate this tension between inclusivity and specificity as they are either too complex or too simple.

The Tension between Now and When

Research into health beliefs and their role in predicting health behaviours has been around since about the 1960s. Now would therefore seem the right time to consolidate what we know, build a simple and integrated model and synthesize the research we have, to come up with a solution. But although health psychologists have been on the task for a while the evidence we have is very often weak, flawed and often absent. Therefore, although the impatient response is to integrate and synthesize now, perhaps it is too early and we need to wait a while longer until our evidence base is stronger.

The Tension between Who We Are Speaking To

Academics are trained with 'Research suggests that. . .', 'It could be argued that. . .', 'It is complex', and 'More research is needed'. As a result, our models are often complex and inclusive and our conclusions are tentative. This is appropriate if our audience are fellow academics who see the world through academic eyes. But for policy makers and practitioners this is pretty useless if they want to know what to say or do next. In contrast, simplified, integrated and common-sense models are useful when talking to policy makers and practitioners who just want a simple answer to what they see as a simple question. There is therefore a tension between using a language for researchers and a language for those out there in the real world. Integrated models reflect this tension as some can be too complex (useless but truthful) or too simple (useful but not reflecting the complexity of the situation).

Problems with All Models

Health psychology emphasizes the role of health beliefs in predicting health behaviours. Underpinning this approach is the assumption that human beings are rational information processors governed by cognitions. Much of what we do, however, is also governed by less rational factors such as our social context and emotions. For example, we might eat just because it is there or because we feel sad, guilty or lonely. These less rational factors are not fully included in our models.

In summary, thinking critically about health beliefs involves a consideration of a wide range of problems relating to the conceptualization of models, the methodologies used in research and the assumptions behind this area of research. These problems are apparent in all the models we use in health psychology. This does not undermine the value of our discipline. It just means that it should be seen with a critical eye within an understanding of what is feasible in research when you are researching something as complicated as the human being (Ogden 2019).

TO CONCLUDE

Behaviour plays an increasingly important role in health, illness and longevity. This chapter has described the key role of health beliefs in predicting health behaviours with a focus on individual beliefs such as attribution, risk perception, motivation and self-efficacy. It has then described models of beliefs in terms of stage models (SOC, HAPA), social cognition models (HBM, PMT, TPB) and integrated models (COM-B). The chapter has then addressed the problem of the intention–behaviour gap and methods to close this gap such as past behaviour, habit, goals, planning and implementation intentions. Finally, the chapter has described some of the many issues with research in this area such as conceptual, methodological and predictive problems.

QUESTIONS

1 Why is it important to explain and predict health-related behaviours?
2 Discuss the contribution of attribution theory to understanding health behaviours.
3 Health beliefs predict health behaviours. Discuss with reference to two models.
4 Discuss some of the problems with the stage models of health behaviour.
5 Discuss some of the problems with the social cognition models of health behaviour.
6 What are some of the problems with integrated models of health behaviours such as the COM-B?
7 How might the problem of the intention–behaviour gap be solved?
8 Describe the ways in which researchers have tried to improve models of health behaviour.
9 Most of our models describe human beings as rational processors of information. Discuss some of the less rational factors that might influence how we behave.

FOR DISCUSSION

Consider one of your regular health-related behaviours (e.g. smoking, what you eat for breakfast, how much you sleep, any recent check-ups you have had). Discuss how your health beliefs relate to this behaviour and whether other factors are involved.

FURTHER READING

Conner, M. and Norman, P. (eds)(2015) *Predicting Health Behaviour,* 3rd edn. Maidenhead: Open University Press.
This book provides an excellent overview of the different models, the studies that have been carried out using them and the new developments in this area. Each chapter is written by an expert in each model, yet the book still has a clear narrative that is often missing from edited books.

Verplanken, B. (2018) (ed) *The Psychology of Habit.* Berlin: Springer.
This is a great book which describes the role of habit in behaviour and behaviour change and is relevant to understanding any health behaviour.

Webb, T.L. and Sheeran, P. (2006) Does changing behavioural intentions engender behaviour change? A meta-analysis of the experimental evidence, *Psychological Bulletin,* **132:** 249–68.
This paper presents a meta-analysis of the research exploring the links between intentions and behaviour. It is useful in itself but also provides an excellent source of references.

Woodcock, A., Stenner, K. and Ingham, R. (1992) Young people talking about HIV and AIDS: interpretations of personal risk of infection, *Health Education Research: Theory and Practice,* **7:** 229–47.
This paper is now getting quite old but I have always used it to illustrate a qualitative approach to health beliefs and it is a good example of how to present qualitative data.

3

Addictive Behaviours

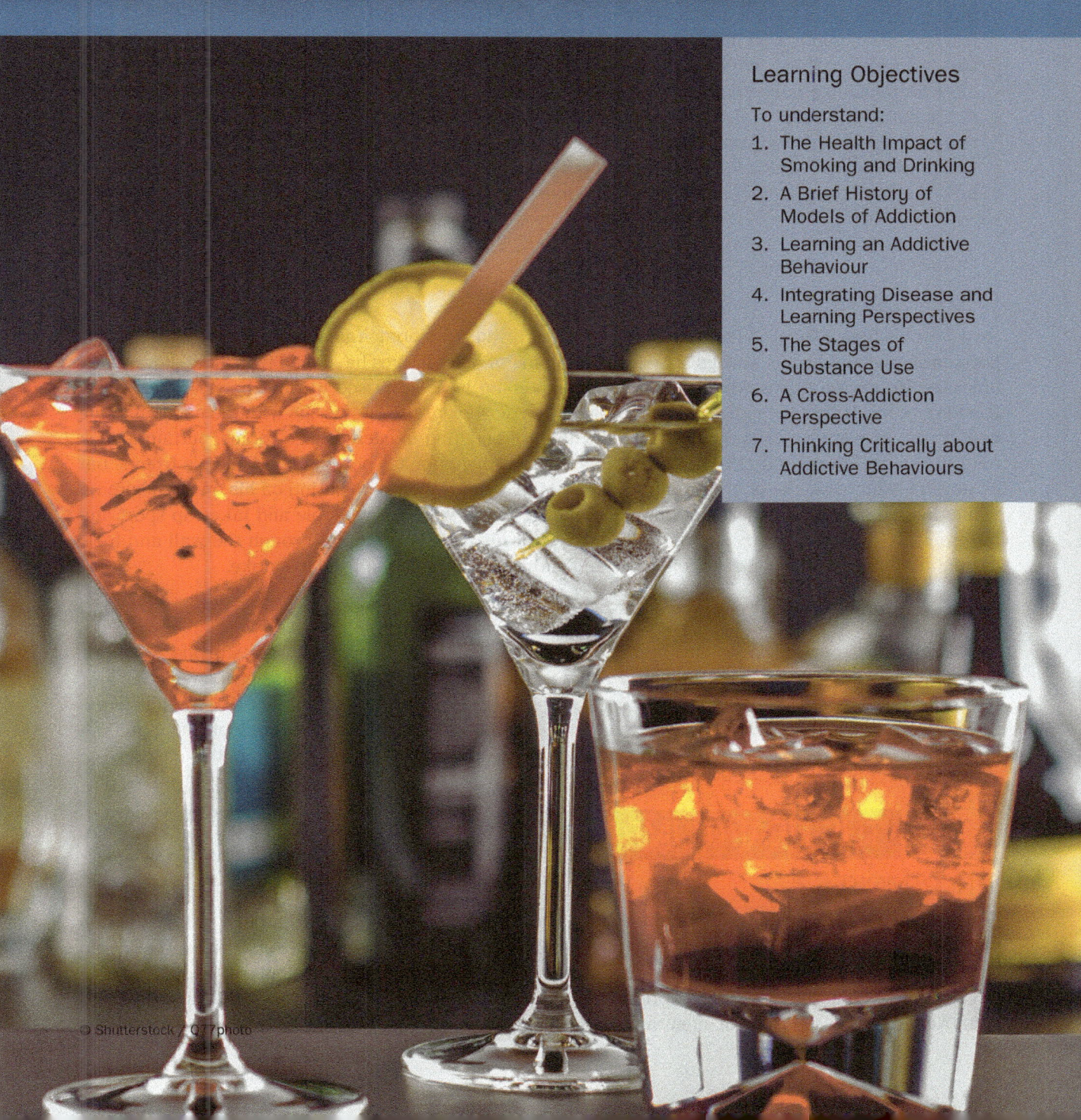

CHAPTER OVERVIEW

Within health psychology, smoking and alcohol use tend to be studied using the models described in Chapter 2 while interventions tend to be based upon the theories described in Chapter 7. This chapter presents research and theories that are specific to more 'addictive' types of behaviour and should be read alongside the chapters on health behaviours in general (Chapters 4, 5, 6). This chapter examines the prevalence of smoking and alcohol consumption and evaluates the health consequences of these behaviours. A brief history of models of addiction is then described, highlighting the shift from a disease model to the social learning theory perspective. Details are then given to describe how an addictive behaviour can be learned. The chapter next illustrates the disease and social learning perspectives through two examples: caffeine, which is the most commonly used drug across all societies, and exercise dependence, showing how a healthy behaviour can become excessive and potentially detrimental. The chapter also examines the four stages of substance use from initiation and maintenance to cessation and relapse. It then describes two models – excessive appetites theory and prime theory – which take a cross-addictive perspective. Finally, it concludes by outlining how to think critically about addictive behaviours.

CASE STUDY

Sam is in his first year of university and has moved away from home for the first time. Neither of his parents smoke and he has always been told that many of his relatives have died from smoking related illnesses. He knows that smoking kills. But at university he is surprised to find that lots of his new friends smoke. At first they all sit out on the steps having a cigarette and he sits with them enjoying the banter. But as winter comes they get into the habit of smoking in each other's rooms, putting a sock over the smoke alarm and closing the windows so that they aren't reported. Sam likes his friends but he doesn't want to smoke or sit in smoky rooms. After a time he ends up sitting on his own in his room while they all smoke together next door. He tries to join in with other people and takes up sport and different societies which are fun but he can still hear his friends laughing through the wall and feels left out. Eventually, he decides to join them and within weeks he has started to smoke.

Through the Eyes of Health Psychology. . .

Nowadays most people know that smoking is harmful and yet people are still starting smoking. Sam's story illustrates some of the many reasons why people smoke, including peer pressure (new friends smoke), social benefits (sitting on steps) and a desire to fit in (banter). It also illustrates how key transitional stages, such as leaving home, can be trigger points for behaviour change both good and bad. The factors which lead to smoking uptake and cessation are covered in this chapter.

1 | THE HEALTH IMPACT OF SMOKING AND DRINKING

WHO SMOKES?

Worldwide data in 2014 showed that about 20 per cent of the world population smoked (about 1 billion people). Of these, about 800 million were men and 200 million were women. In countries in the Global North, smoking rates have levelled off or declined over recent years, particularly in men, but in developing nations tobacco consumption continues to rise. Worldwide data show that in developed countries about 35 per cent of men and 22 per cent of women smoke, whereas in countries in the

Global South about 50 per cent of men and 9 per cent of women smoke. For example, in China, Cuba, Albania, Armenia, Thailand, Indonesia, Korea and the Congo about 50 per cent of the population smoke, whereas in New Zealand, Iceland, Canada, Sweden, the UK and Australia less than 20 per cent of the population smoke (WHO 2017). China has the highest percentage of male smokers at about 300 million. This is equivalent to the entire US population. In the UK the overall prevalence of smoking has decreased in men from 52 per cent in 1974, to 30 per cent in 1990, to 26 per cent in 2004, to 18.7 per cent in 2017 and down to 14.1 per cent in 2019 (Office for National Statistics 2019). In women it has decreased from 41 per cent in 1970, to 29 per cent in 1990, to 23 per cent in 2004, to 15 per cent in 2017 and down to 12.5 per cent in 2019 (Office for National Statistics 2019). This decrease in smoking behaviour follows a trend for an overall decline, as shown in Figure 3.1.

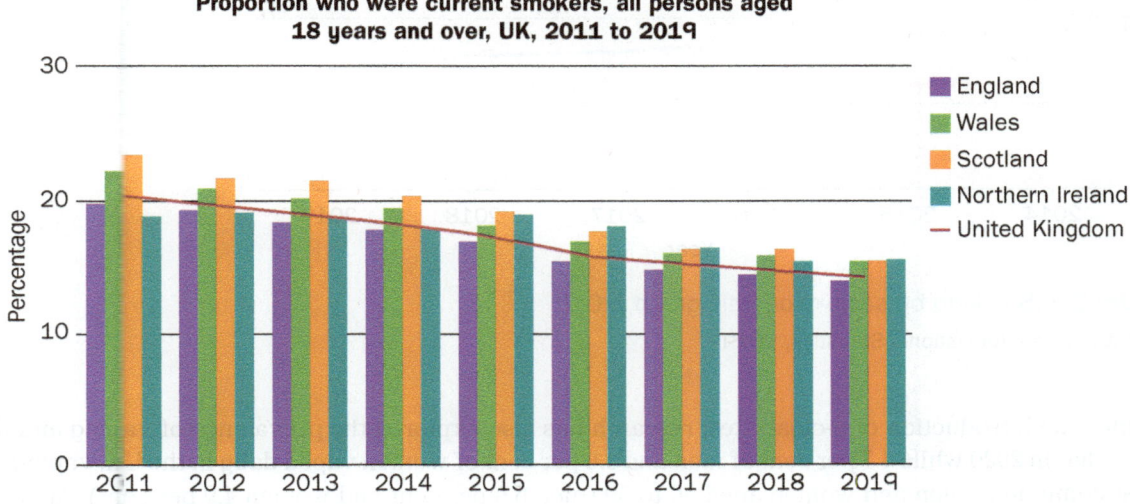

Figure 3.1 Changes in smoking, 2011–2019

SOURCE: Adapted from Office for National Statistics (2019)

Despite this overall decline in smoking the highest prevalence of smoking is in those aged between 25 and 34 whereas the biggest decrease is in those aged 18 to 24 years. These data are shown in Figure 3.2.

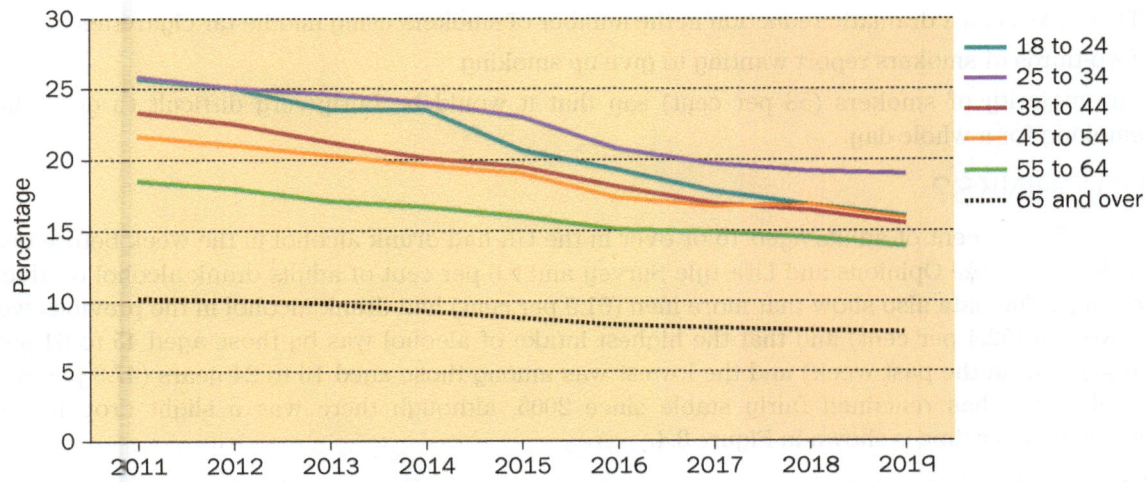

Figure 3.2 Percentage of people who smoke by age 2011–2019

SOURCE: Office for National Statistics (2019)

Smoking also varies by socio-economic status group. In 2019, the number of people who smoked in the lowest group was more than twice the number of people who smoked in the highest group. These data are shown in Figure 3.3.

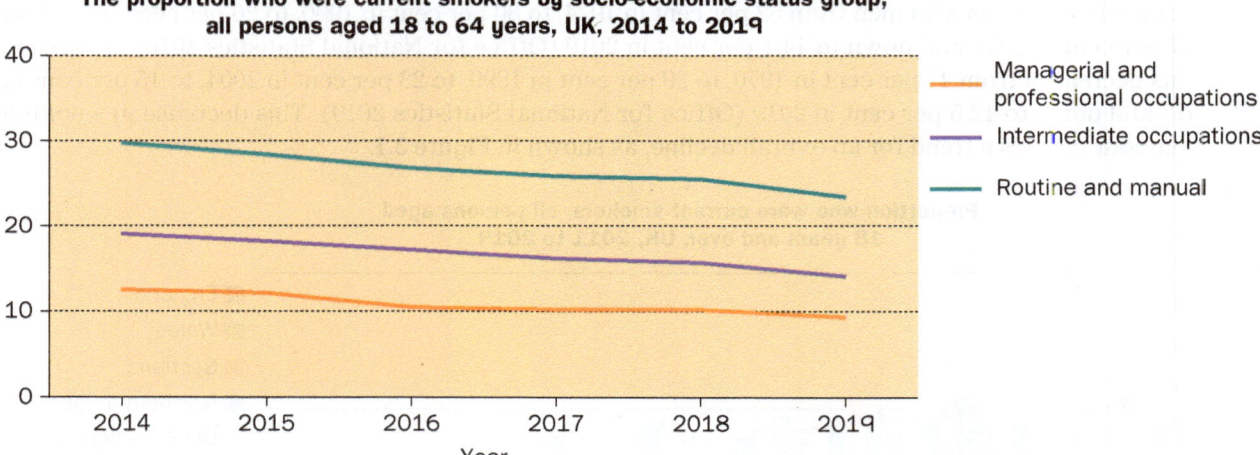

Figure 3.3 Smoking by socio-economic group, 2019
SOURCE: Office for National Statistics, 2019

Since the introduction of e-cigarettes, research has also explored the prevalence of vaping and indicates that in 2020 while 4.7 per cent of men and 3.0 per cent of women vaped daily in the UK, vaping was most common in men and women aged 50 to 59 (men 6.6 per cent and women 4.9 per cent). Although, of those aged 25 to 34, 4.6 per cent of men and 4.4 per cent of women also vaped daily (ONS 2020).

In general, data about smoking behaviour suggest the following about smokers:

- Smoking behaviour is on the decline, but this decrease is greater in men than in women.
- Smokers tend to be in the unskilled manual group.
- Smokers tend to earn less than non-smokers.
- There has been a dramatic reduction in the number of smokers using middle-tar cigarettes.
- Two-thirds of smokers report wanting to give up smoking.
- The majority of smokers (58 per cent) say that it would be fairly/very difficult to go without smoking for a whole day.

WHO DRINKS?

In 2017, 57.0 per cent of adults aged 16 or over in the UK had drunk alcohol in the week before being interviewed for the Opinions and Lifestyle Survey and 9.6 per cent of adults drank alcohol on five or more days. The data also show that more men (61.9 per cent) had drunk alcohol in the previous week than women (52.4 per cent) and that the highest intake of alcohol was by those aged 45 to 64 years (64.6 per cent in the past week) and the lowest was among those aged 16 to 24 years (47.9 per cent). Alcohol intake has remained fairly stable since 2005, although there was a slight drop in 2017. This change over time is shown in Figure 3.4.

Research also shows that alcohol intake varies by income. For example, those from the highest income groups were more likely to drink alcohol compared to those with lower incomes (see Office for National Statistics 2019; Figure 3.5).

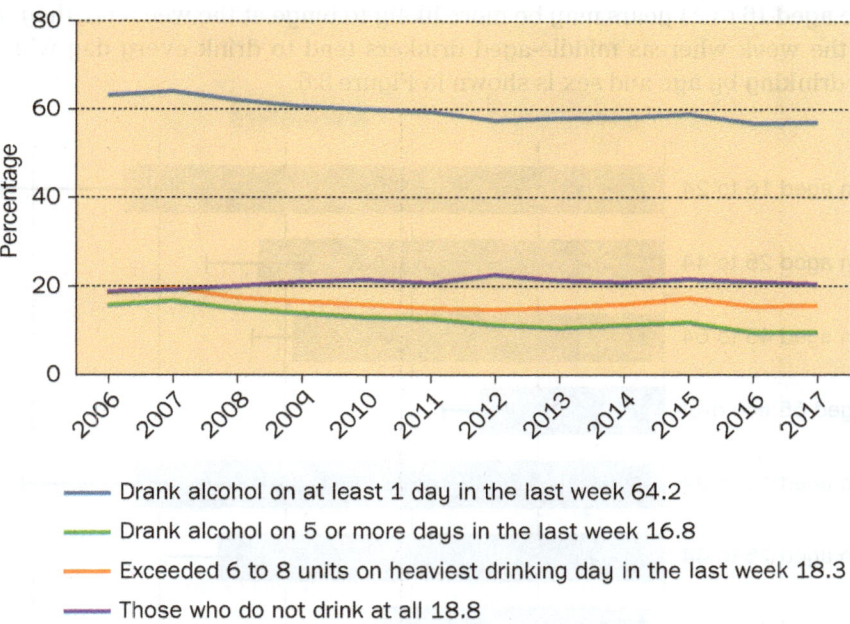

Drank alcohol on at least 1 day in the last week 64.2
Drank alcohol on 5 or more days in the last week 16.8
Exceeded 6 to 8 units on heaviest drinking day in the last week 18.3
Those who do not drink at all 18.8

Figure 3.4 Self reported changes in alcohol consumption 2005–2017
SOURCE: Office for National Statistics, 2018

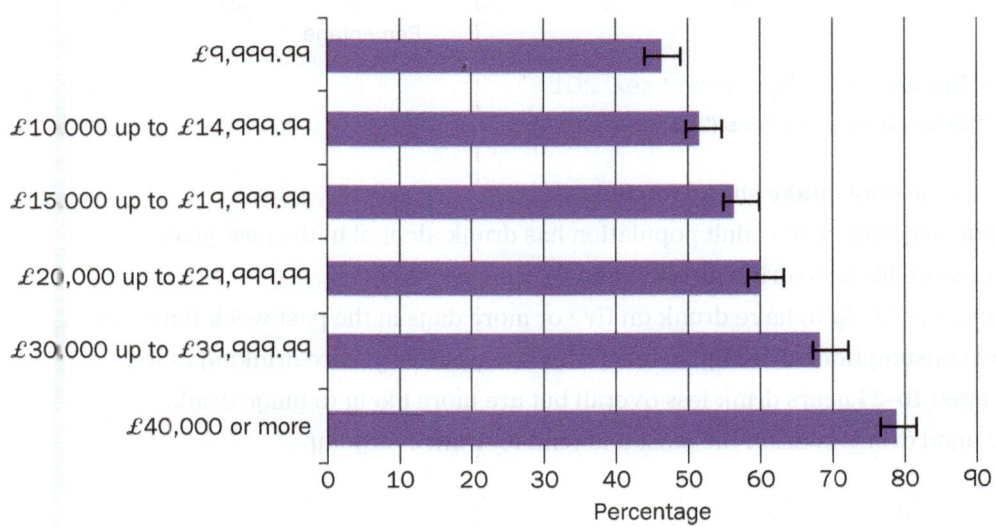

Figure 3.5 Income differences for drinking alcohol
SOURCE: Office for National Statistics (2017)

Research has also explored the prevalence of binge drinking defined as more than twice the recommended amount on any given day (>8 units for men and >6 units for women). The data indicate that 28.7 per cent of men and 25.6 per cent of women binged alcohol on their heaviest drinking day and that although those aged 16 to 24 years were the least likely to say they drank in the past week, when they did drink both men and women in this age group were the most likely to binge on alcohol. Those aged 65 years and over were the least likely to binge although men in this age group were twice as likely to binge (14.7 per cent) compared to women of the same age (7.6 per cent). Data also indicates that while those aged 16 to 24 years may be more likely to binge at the weekend, they tend not to drink for the rest of the week whereas middle-aged drinkers tend to drink every day which may be more harmful. Binge drinking by age and sex is shown in Figure 3.6.

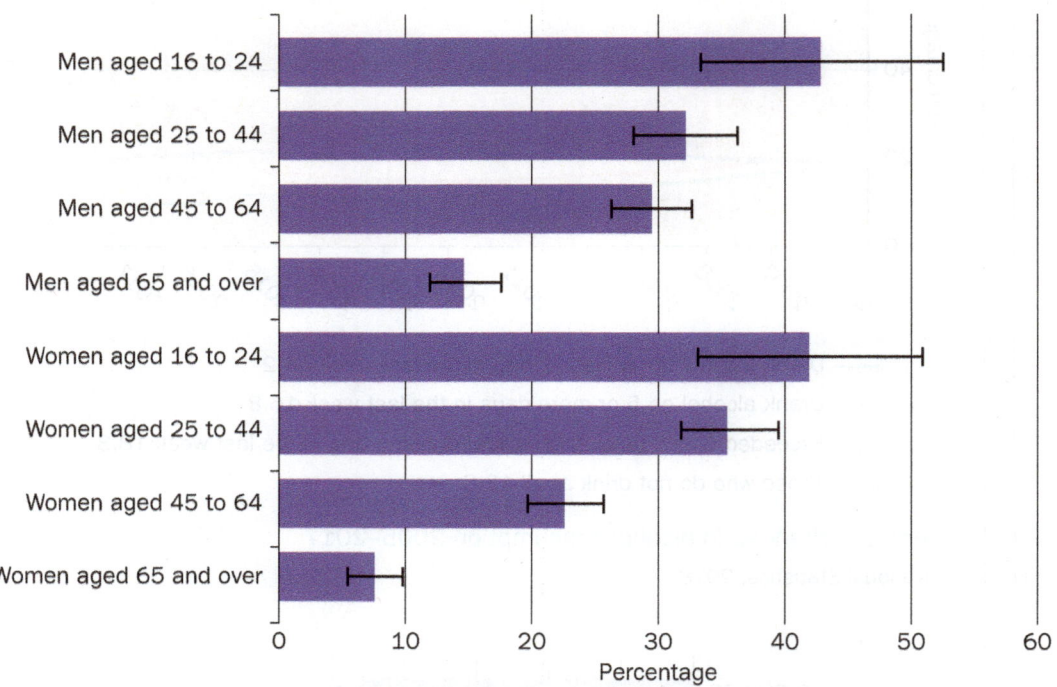

Figure 3.6 Binge drinking by age and sex, 2017

SOURCE: Office for National Statistics (2017)

The data on alcohol intake shows the following:

- The large majority of the adult population has drunk alcohol in the past year.
- Men are more likely to drink alcohol than women.
- Men are more likely to have drunk on five or more days in the past week than women.
- Alcohol consumption varies by income, with those earning more drinking more.
- Those aged 16–24 years drink less overall but are more likely to binge drink.
- Middle-aged drinkers drink the most and tend to drink everyday.

SMOKING AND HEALTH

In 1954 Doll and Hill reported that smoking cigarettes was related to lung cancer. Since then, smoking has also been implicated in coronary heart disease (CHD) and a multitude of other cancers such as throat, stomach and bowel. In addition, the increase in life expectancy over the past 150 years is considerably less for smokers than for non-smokers. The risks of smoking were made explicit in a book by Peto et al. (1994), who stated that of 1,000 20-year-olds in the UK who smoke cigarettes regularly, about 1 will be murdered, 6 will die from traffic accidents, 250 will die from cigarettes in middle age (35–69) and another 250 will die from smoking in old age (70 and over). In industrialized countries smoking is the leading cause of loss of healthy life years. The average smoker dies 8 years early and starts to suffer disability 12 years early, while a quarter of smokers who fail to stop die an average of 23 years early (West and Shiffman 2004). Worldwide it is estimated that 4 million deaths per year are attributable to smoking. In the USA, an estimated 443,000 people die each year from smoking-related diseases (Center for Disease Control 2008). In 2016, it was estimated that 77,900 deaths in England were attributable to smoking, representing 16 per cent of all deaths. This is a decrease by 2 per cent on the previous year (2015) and a decrease of 7 per cent from 2006 (Office for National Statistics 2016). The number of deaths by smoking in the USA compared to other common causes of deaths is shown in Figure 3.7.

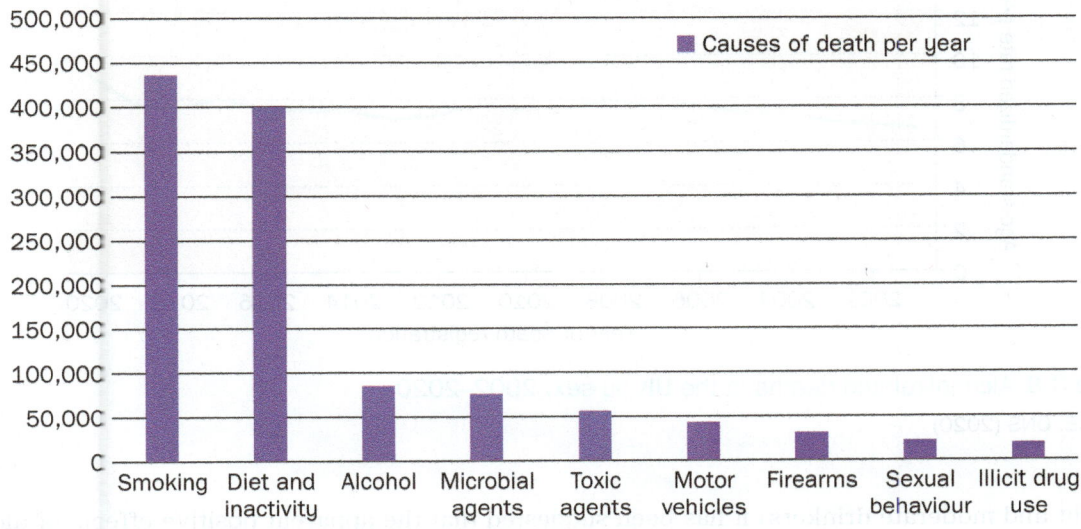

Figure 3.7 Deaths attributable to smoking in the USA in 2000

SOURCE: Adapted from Mokdad et al. (2004)

Smoking in adolescence has also been found to have more immediate effects and is linked with shortness of breath, asthma, higher blood pressure and an increased number of respiratory tract infections (American Lung Association 2002a, 2002b). There has also been an interest in passive smoking and research suggests an association between passive smoking and lung cancer in adults, and respiratory ill health in children (US Environmental Protection Agency 1992).

ALCOHOL AND HEALTH

Alcohol consumption also has many negative effects on health. For example, alcoholism increases the chance of disorders such as liver cirrhosis, cancers (e.g. pancreas and liver), hypertension and memory deficits (White et al. 2002). Alcohol also increases the chances of harm through car accidents, non-traffic accidents, accidental falls, violence and unsafe sex (e.g. Corbin and Fromme 2002). In terms of the impact of alcohol on mortality, rates of alcohol-related deaths in the UK increased from 9.1 per 100,000 in 1994 to 10.6 in 2001 and to 14.3 in 2014 but then remained fairly stable. In 2020, however, the rates were 14 per 100,000 which was statistically significantly higher than 2019 and any other year since 2001. Data also shows that death rates are higher for men than for women and that this gap has widened over recent years. Change in alcohol-related deaths by sex is shown in Figure 3.8.

Some research has also pointed to the positive effects of alcohol on health. For example, Friedman and Kimball (1986) reported that light and moderate drinkers had lower morbidity and mortality rates than both non-drinkers and heavy drinkers. They argued that alcohol consumption reduces CHD via the following mechanisms: (1) a reduction in the production of catecholamines when stressed; (2) the protection of blood vessels from cholesterol; (3) a reduction in blood pressure; (4) self-therapy; and (5) a short-term coping strategy. The results from the *General Household Survey* (OPCS 1992) also showed some benefits of alcohol consumption with the reported prevalence of ill health being higher among non-drinkers than among drinkers. Although these data have been well received (particularly

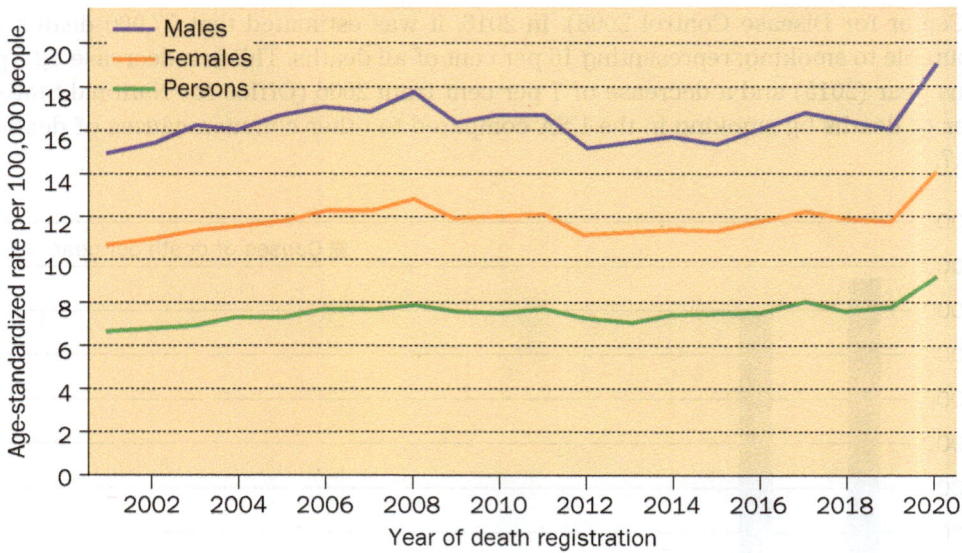

Figure 3.8 Alcohol-related deaths in the UK by sex, 2002–2020

SOURCE: ONS (2020)

by light and moderate drinkers) it has been suggested that the apparent positive effects of alcohol on health may be an artefact of poor health in the non-drinkers who have stopped drinking due to health problems.

In an attempt to understand why people smoke and drink, much health psychology research has drawn upon the social cognition models described in Chapter 2. However, there is a vast addiction literature which has also been applied to smoking and drinking. These models are also relevant to all other potentially addictive behaviours such as caffeine drinking, drug-taking, gambling, food addiction and even sex addiction (see Orford 2002 for an excellent cross-addictive behaviour perspective). Addiction theories will now be explored. Exercise dependence and caffeine drinking are covered in detail later.

2 | A BRIEF HISTORY OF MODELS OF ADDICTION

WHAT IS AN ADDICTION?

Many theories have been developed to explain addictions and addictive behaviours, including moral models which regard an addiction as the result of weakness and a lack of moral fibre; biomedical models which see an addiction as a disease; and social learning theories which regard addictive behaviours as behaviours that are learned according to the rules of learning theory. The multitude of terms that exist, and are used with respect to behaviours such as smoking and alcohol, are indicative of these different theoretical perspectives and in addition illustrate the tautological nature of the definitions. For example:

- *An addict:* someone who 'has no control over their behaviour', 'lacks moral fibre', 'uses a maladaptive coping mechanism', 'has an addictive behaviour'.
- *An addiction:* 'a need for a drug', 'the use of a substance that is psychologically and physiologically addictive', 'showing tolerance and withdrawal'.

- *Dependency:* 'showing psychological and physiological withdrawal'.
- *Drug:* 'an addictive substance', 'a substance that causes dependency', 'any medical substance'.

These different definitions indicate the relationship between language and theory. For example, concepts of 'control', 'withdrawal' and 'tolerance' are indicative of a biomedical view of addictions. Concepts such as 'lacking moral fibre' suggest a moral model of addictions, and 'maladaptive coping mechanism' suggests a social learning perspective. In addition, the terms illustrate how difficult it is to use one term without using another, with the risk that the definitions become tautologies.

Many questions have been asked about different addictive behaviours, including the following:

- What causes someone to start smoking?
- What causes drinking behaviour to become a problem?
- Why can some people just smoke socially while others need to smoke first thing in the morning?
- Is it possible for an alcoholic to return to normal drinking?
- Do addictions run in families?

Questions about the causes of an addiction can be answered according to the different theoretical perspectives that have been developed over the past 300 years to explain and predict addictions, including the moral model, the first disease concept, the second disease concept and social learning theory. These different theories, their development and how they relate to attitudes to different substances will now be examined.

THE SEVENTEENTH CENTURY AND THE MORAL MODEL OF ADDICTIONS

During the seventeenth century, alcohol was generally held in high esteem by society. It was regarded as safer than water, nutritious and the innkeeper was valued as a central figure in the community. In addition, at this time humans were considered to be separate from nature, in terms of possessing a soul and a will and being responsible for their own behaviour. Animals' behaviour was seen as resulting from biological drives, whereas the behaviour of humans was thought to be a result of their own free choice. Accordingly, alcohol consumption was considered an acceptable behaviour, but excessive alcohol use was regarded as a result of free choice and personal responsibility. Alcoholism was therefore seen as a behaviour that deserved punishment, not treatment; alcoholics were regarded as choosing to behave excessively. This model of addiction was called the *moral model*. This perspective is similar to the arguments espoused by Thomas Szasz in the 1960s concerning the treatment versus punishment of mentally ill individuals and his distinction between being 'mad' or 'bad'. Szasz (1961) suggested that to label someone 'mad', and to treat them, removed the central facet of humanity, namely personal responsibility. He proposed that holding individuals responsible for their behaviour gave them back their sense of responsibility even if this resulted in them being seen as 'bad'. Similarly, the moral model of addictions considered alcoholics to have chosen to behave excessively and therefore be deserving of punishment (acknowledging their responsibility), not treatment (denying their responsibility). In effect, contemporary social attitudes were reflected in contemporary theory.

THE NINETEENTH CENTURY AND THE FIRST DISEASE CONCEPT

During the nineteenth century, attitudes towards addictions, and in particular alcohol, changed. The temperance movement was developed and spread the word about the evils of drink. Alcohol was regarded as a powerful and destructive substance and alcoholics were seen as its victims. This perspective is also reflected in prohibition and the banning of alcohol consumption in the USA. During this time, the *first disease concept* of addiction was developed. This was the earliest form of a biomedical approach to addiction and regarded alcoholism as an illness. Within this model, the focus for the illness was the substance. Alcohol was seen as an addictive substance, and alcoholics were viewed as passively succumbing to its influence. The first disease concept regarded the substance as the problem and called for the treatment of excessive drinkers. Again, social attitudes to addiction were reflected in the development of theory.

THE TWENTIETH CENTURY AND THE SECOND DISEASE CONCEPT

Attitudes towards addiction changed again at the beginning of the twentieth century. The USA learned quickly that banning alcohol consumption was more problematic than expected, and governments across the western world realized that they could financially benefit from alcohol sales. In parallel, attitudes towards human behaviour were changing and a more liberal, laissez-faire attitude became dominant. Likewise, theories of addiction reflected these shifts. The *second disease concept* of addiction was developed, which no longer saw the substance as the problem but pointed the finger at those individuals who became addicted. In this perspective, the small minority of those who consumed alcohol to excess were seen as having a problem, but for the rest of society alcohol consumption returned to a position of an acceptable social habit. This perspective legitimized the sale of alcohol, recognized the resulting government benefits and emphasized the treatment of addicted individuals. Alcoholism was regarded as an illness developed by certain people who therefore needed support and treatment. In the second disease perspective there are three different arguments: (1) pre-existing physical abnormalities; (2) pre-existing psychological abnormalities; and (3) acquired dependency theory. All of these have a similar model of addiction in that they:

- Regard addictions as discrete entities (you are either an addict or not an addict).
- Regard an addiction as an illness.
- Focus on the individual as the problem.
- Regard the addiction as irreversible.
- Emphasize treatment.
- Emphasize treatment through total abstinence.

Problems with a Disease Model of Addiction

Although many researchers still emphasize a disease model of addiction, there are several problems with this perspective:

- The disease model encourages treatment through lifelong abstinence. However, lifelong abstinence is very rare and may be difficult to achieve.
- The model does not incorporate relapse into its concept of treatment. However, this 'all or nothing' perspective may actually promote relapse through encouraging individuals to set unreasonable targets of abstinence and by establishing the self-fulfilling prophecy of 'once a drunk, always a drunk'.
- The description of controlled drinking, which suggested that alcoholics can return to 'normal drinking' patterns (Davies 1962; Sobel and Sobel 1978), challenged the central ideas of the disease model. The phenomenon of controlled drinking indicated that perhaps an addiction was not irreversible and that abstinence might not be the only treatment goal.

THE 1970S AND ONWARDS: SOCIAL LEARNING THEORY

In the latter part of the twentieth century, attitudes towards addictions changed again. With the development of behaviourism, learning theory and a belief that behaviour was shaped by an interaction with both the environment and other individuals, the belief that excessive behaviour and addictions were illnesses began to be challenged. Since the 1970s, behaviours such as smoking, drinking and drug-taking have been increasingly described within the context of all other behaviours. In the same way that theories of aggression shifted from a biological cause (aggression as an instinct) to social causes (aggression as a response to the environment/upbringing), addictions were also seen as learned behaviours. In this perspective, the term 'addictive behaviour' replaced 'addictions' and such behaviours were regarded as a consequence of learning processes. This shift challenged the concepts of addictions, addict, illness and disease; however, the theories still emphasized treatment. The social learning perspective differs from the disease model of addiction in several ways:

- Addictive behaviours are seen as acquired habits, which are learned according to the rules of social learning theory.
- Addictive behaviours can be unlearned; they are not irreversible.
- Addictive behaviours lie along a continuum; they are not discrete entities.
- Addictive behaviours are no different from other behaviours.
- Treatment approaches involve either total abstinence or relearning 'normal' behaviour patterns.

3   LEARNING AN ADDICTIVE BEHAVIOUR

From a social learning perspective, addictive behaviours are learned according to the following processes: (1) classical conditioning; (2) operant conditioning; (3) observational learning; and (4) cognitive processes.

CLASSICAL CONDITIONING

The rules of classical conditioning state that behaviours are acquired through the processes of associative learning. For example, an unconditioned stimulus (US; e.g. going to the pub) may elicit an unconditioned response (UR; e.g. feeling relaxed). If the unconditioned stimulus is associated with a conditioned stimulus (CS; e.g. a drink), then eventually this will elicit the conditioned response (CR; e.g. feeling relaxed). Classical conditioning may also result in two addictive behaviours such as smoking and drinking being linked together. This process of classical conditioning can happen as follows:

The unconditioned stimulus and the unconditioned response:

- going to the pub + feeling relaxed
- (US) + (UR)

Pairing the unconditioned stimulus and the conditioned stimulus:

- going to the pub + a drink
- (US) + (CS)

The conditioned stimulus and the conditioned response:

- a drink + feeling relaxed
- (CS) + (CR)

Therefore the conditioned stimulus now elicits the conditioned response.

What Factors Can Pair with the Conditioned Stimulus?

Two types of factor can pair with the conditioned stimulus: *external* (e.g. the pub) and *internal* (e.g. mood) cues. In terms of a potentially addictive behaviour, smoking

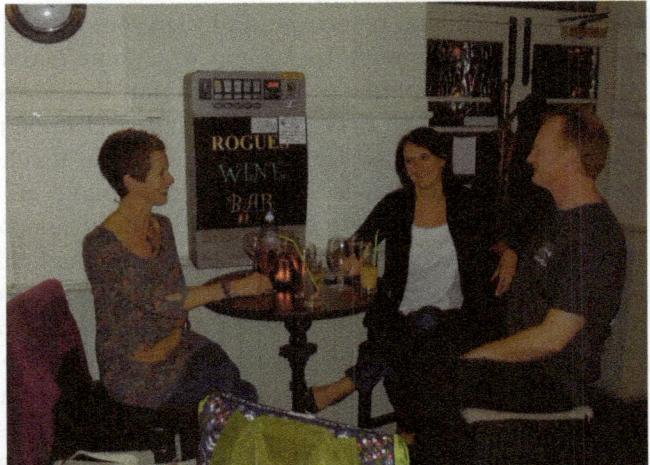

Smoking and drinking alcohol can become associated with each other through classical conditioning

cigarettes may be associated with external cues (e.g. seeing someone else smoking, being with particular friends), or with internal cues (e.g. anxiety, depression or happiness). It has been argued that a pairing with an internal cue is more problematic because these cues cannot be avoided. In addition, internal cues also raise the problem of *generalization*. Generalization occurs when the withdrawal symptoms from a period of abstinence from an addictive behaviour act as cues for further behaviour. For example, if an individual has paired feeling anxious with smoking, their withdrawal symptoms may be interpreted as anxiety and therefore elicit further smoking behaviour; the behaviour provides relief from its own withdrawal symptoms.

OPERANT CONDITIONING

The rules of operant conditioning state that the probability of behaviour occurring is increased if it is either *positively reinforced* by the presence of a positive event, or *negatively reinforced* by the absence or removal of a negative event. In terms of an addictive behaviour such as smoking, the probability of smoking will be increased by feelings of social acceptance, confidence and control (the positive reinforcer) and removal of withdrawal symptoms (the negative reinforcer).

OBSERVATIONAL LEARNING/MODELLING

Behaviours are also learned by observing significant others carrying them out. For example, parental smoking, an association between smoking and attractiveness/thinness, and the observation of alcohol consumption as a risk-taking behaviour may contribute to the acquisition of the behaviour.

COGNITIVE FACTORS

Factors such as self-image, problem-solving behaviour, coping mechanisms and attributions also contribute to the acquisition of an addictive behaviour.

4 INTEGRATING DISEASE AND LEARNING PERSPECTIVES

Researchers often polarize a disease and a social learning perspective of addiction. For example, while some researchers argue that smoking is entirely due to the addictive properties of nicotine, others argue that it is a learned behaviour. However, implicit within each approach is the alternative explanation. For example, while a disease model may emphasize acquired tolerance following smoking or drinking behaviour and therefore draws upon a disease perspective, it implicitly uses a social learning approach to explain why some people start smoking/drinking in the first place and why only some continue to the extent that they develop acquired tolerance. People need exposure and reinforcement to make the smoking or drinking enough to develop tolerance. The concept of tolerance may be a disease model concept but it relies upon some degree of social learning theory for it to operate. Likewise, people might smoke an increasing number of cigarettes because they have learned that smoking relieves withdrawal symptoms. However, while this form of association is derived from a social learning perspective, it implicitly uses a disease perspective in that it requires the existence of physical withdrawal symptoms. Therefore most researchers draw upon both disease and social learning perspectives. Sometimes this interaction between the two forms of model is made explicit and the researchers acknowledge that they believe both sources of influence are important. However, at times this interaction is only implicit. The role of a disease model and a social learning model is explored here with two case studies. The first is on caffeine (see Box 3.1), which highlights the addictive nature of a common drug and its impact upon health, and the second is on exercise dependence (see Box 3.2), which reflects the addictive nature of a behaviour.

BOX 3.1
Caffeine: The Most Widely Consumed Psychoactive Substance in History

(This information is synthesized from the work of Jack James, who is the world expert in this field. Please see references such as James 2004, 2010; James and Rogers 2005; James and Keane 2007 for more detail.)

Caffeine is a psychoactive substance that causes physical changes in the body. It is also central to much social behaviour, and coffee and tea form the basis for many interactions with friends and family as well as offering a means to punctuate a busy working day.

Caffeine illustrates the ways in which a substance can be harmful and is in line with other forms of drug addiction. It also illustrates how all addictive behaviours have some form of learning processes implicit in them. This case study will describe what caffeine is and how it affects our bodies. It will then describe the impact of caffeine on performance and mood and physical health.

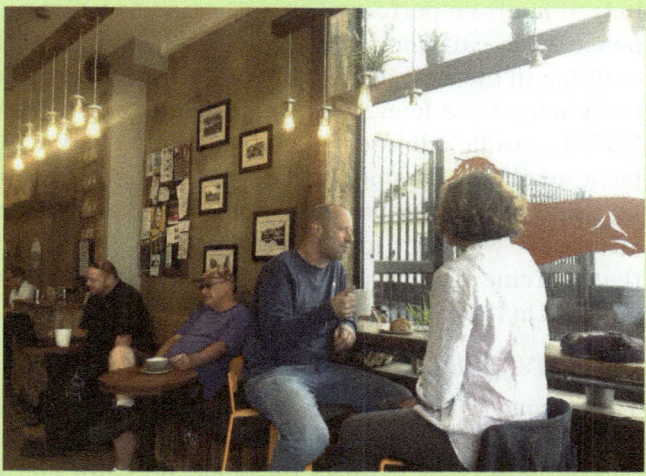

Coffee drinking is central to many social interactions

CAFFEINE AND ITS USE

Caffeine, otherwise known as 1,3,7-trimethylxanthine, first became widely available after European colonization in the seventeenth and eighteenth centuries. It is mostly consumed through tea, coffee, soft drinks or energy drinks, but is also present in chocolate and some painkillers. For most people, their first exposure occurs while still in the womb as caffeine can cross the placenta. Use continues in childhood through the intake of soft drinks and then consolidates in adolescents and early adulthood. After this time, patterns of intake tend to stabilize and continue throughout life. Worldwide, more than 80 per cent of people consume caffeine daily and its use is universal regardless of age, gender, geography and culture, far outweighing any other drug including nicotine, alcohol, cannabis or cocaine. Caffeine has a strong social role in that it forms the rationale and centrepiece for many social interactions. It is also a psychoactive drug that affects how we function. Once ingested, caffeine is quickly distributed around the body and is cleared from the stomach within about 20 minutes, reaching peak blood levels within 40–60 minutes. It has a half-life of about five hours in adults, which means that a daily intake of three or four cups will stay at active levels for most of a person's waking day. Caffeine is addictive in that repeated use results in physical dependence leading to behavioural, physiological and subjective withdrawal symptoms such as sleepiness, lethargy, headaches and reduction in psychomotor performance, including concentration and reaction time. Caffeine use has two important implications for health. First, people are motivated to use caffeine through expected benefits to performance and mood. Second, research highlights many detrimental effects on physical health.

PERFORMANCE AND MOOD

Those who consume caffeine tend to hold two key expectancies of how the drug will affect them. First, they believe that caffeine enhances their mood, and second they believe it increases their performance, particularly by keeping them awake. Research has explored these expected effects to see if they are real. Some studies have compared consumers vs non-consumers and pre- and post-consumption, but such approaches have methodological problems. James and colleagues (James and Rogers 2005; James et al. 2005) have employed more power-ful experimental designs with double-blinding and a placebo control. The results from these studies offer substantial support for the withdrawal reversal hypothesis: that caffeine does indeed improve performance and mood *but* only in relation to the impact of overnight absti-nence from caffeine which has caused an initial deficit. Accordingly, if people didn't drink caffeine in the first place, then there would be no deficit to rectify by drinking more. In fact, in a study of academic achievement, James et al. (2010) explored the impact of caffeine use in 7,377 Icelandic adolescents and concluded that achievement deficits that would usually have been attributed to smoking and alcohol use were in fact accounted for by caffeine intake. In addition, the results indicated that this might be because caffeine also causes daytime sleepiness which in turn affects academic achievement. From this evidence it would seem that caffeine is not a psychostimulant as is often believed and only has cognitive and mood benefits in those experiencing withdrawal.

CARDIOVASCULAR DISEASE AND BLOOD PRESSURE

The second main area of research relates to the impact of caffeine on physical health, particularly in relation to cardiovascular disease. Evidence for this comes from the acute and chronic effects of caffeine on blood pressure and epidemiological data on caffeine use and cardiovascular disease. Blood pressure has direct implications for cardiovascular disease, stroke and heart attacks and research conclusively shows that caffeine increases blood pressure acutely in both men and women of all ages with either no prior health problems or hypertension (James 1997). Increases tend to be between 5 to 15mm Hg systolic and 5 to 10mm Hg diastolic for an average daily intake. In addition, this increase adds to that caused by other factors such as smoking and stress. Research also indicates that, over time, rather than developing tolerance to caffeine, the acute effects of caffeine on blood pressure persist. There also appear to be chronic effects of caffeine on blood pressure although evidence for this is less conclusive.

EPIDEMIOLOGICAL DATA

More than 100 large epidemiological studies have also explored links between caffeine and health at a population rather than an individual level and generally the conclusion is that caffeine is bad for cardiovascular function. There are, however, some problems with these studies, including the measurement of caffeine use which has resulted in some conflicting findings. Some authors have argued that these conflicts indicate that caffeine is not harmful, whereas others argue that this is due to measurement error and that the effects on health may be even larger than found in the research literature (James 2011). Similarly, epidemiological studies have also explored links between caffeine and population blood pressure levels. Again there are inconsistencies in the literature. However, it seems clear that people do not show tolerance to caffeine and there-fore repeated use results in repeated episodes of raised blood pressure which, overall, causes population increases in blood pressure which in turn impacts negatively upon health.

OTHER ASPECTS OF HEALTH

Generally there are mixed results for the impact of caffeine on a range of cancers, although in the laboratory setting it has been shown to be carcinogenic under some conditions. More convincing evidence relates caffeine use to miscarriage, lower birth weight and some adverse reactions with some medicines.

CAFFEINE DRINKING AS AN ADDICTIVE BEHAVIOUR

Caffeine clearly has psychoactive properties and acts as a drug on our bodies. People are motivated to use caffeine for its effects on their performance and mood, but research indicates that these benefits are in fact just compensating for the negative effects of withdrawal symptoms. However, caffeine drinking is also a learned behaviour as people associate coffee with social interactions, as an excuse for conversation ('going out for coffee') or with the end of a meal. They also hold positive outcome expectancies on the basis of their previous experiences. Caffeine drinking is therefore learned in all the ways that other behaviours are learned: through associative learning, reinforcement and modelling. Caffeine is a good example of an addictive drug that also involves a strong social learning component in its maintenance and cessation.

BOX 3.2
Exercise Dependence: When Is There Too Much of a Good Thing?

Smoking and alcohol use (and caffeine, heroine, cannabis, etc.) illustrate addictive behaviours which involve a combination of physical responses to a drug (e.g. nicotine) and the consequences of a learned behaviour (e.g. social drinking with friends). Over recent years researchers have also recognized that people can become 'addicted' to behaviours which do not involve the intake of any external drug. For example, there are now literatures on shopping addiction ('shopaholics'), gambling addiction, sex addiction, food addiction and exercise dependence (see Orford 2002 for an excellent overview). A disease model of such addictions would argue that the behaviours become addictive because they generate endorphins which create a sense of arousal and pleasure. From a social learning perspective, however, it would be argued that these behaviours become excessive because they are reinforced by factors such as mood, social interaction, changes in body shape and financial gain, and are paired with cues such as friends, the pub, stress and relief from stress, which become triggers for subsequent behaviour. There is an alternative perspective which says they are not addictive behaviours at all, but this purely depends upon the definition of addiction being used (see pp. 72–3). This case study will focus on exercise dependence as an example of a behaviourally triggered addiction which has consequences for an individual's well-being. Exercise dependence is described in terms of its definition, possible causes and impact on the individual.

DEFINING EXERCISE DEPENDENCE

Early articles examined the concept of 'exercise addiction', discussed positive versus negative exercise addiction and deliberated over whether excessive exercise was harmful. The term 'exercise addiction' was later replaced by others such as 'obligatory running' (Coen and Ogles 1993), 'compulsive running' (Nash 1987), 'morbid exercising' (Chalmers et al. 1985) and 'exercise dependence' (Veale 1987). Several measures have been developed in an attempt to assess this behaviour, with some being specific to certain forms of exercise, including the 'Feelings About Running Scale' (Carmack and Martens 1979) and the 'Running Addiction Scale' (Chapman and de Castro 1990), and others being more generic, such as the Obligatory Exercise Questionnaire (Pasman and Thompson 1988) and the Exercise Dependence Questionnaire (Ogden et al. 1997).

In general, exercise dependence relates to the disease perspective:

- **Tolerance:** 'I need to do more and more to get the same effects'.
- **Withdrawal symptoms:** 'If I don't exercise I feel dreadful'.

And to the social learning perspective:

- **Feeling out of control:** 'I live to exercise'; 'I have to exercise'.
- **Interference with social life:** 'I cancel seeing my friends so I can exercise'.
- **Interference with family life:** 'My family complain I exercise too much'.
- **Interference with work:** 'My exercise makes me tired at work'.
- **Stereotypical behaviour:** 'I must not miss an exercise session'.
- **Excessive behaviour:** 'I exercise more than most people I know'.

Hence, exercise dependence (or whichever term is used) describes excessive exercise which impacts upon a person's life and reflects a feeling of being out of control. As with all definitions of addictive behaviours this is problematic as it assumes that there *is* a normal life (i.e. work, family, friends) and that a behaviour that interferes with this is harmful. Furthermore, it is quite possible that a person who exercises excessively feels perfectly in control of their behaviour as long as their life enables them to exercise to the level that they need. The definition of 'excessive' is also flawed because it depends upon social norms and a model of how we *should* distribute our time.

CAUSES OF EXERCISE DEPENDENCE

There are several possible explanations as to why people can become addicted to exercise which can be understood in terms of the disease and social learning perspectives.

Disease Model
- **Tolerance:** people become tolerant to their level of exercise and therefore need to exercise more to achieve the same benefits.
- **Withdrawal symptoms:** exercise improves mood and generates a sense of arousal. After a period of time, however, this state deteriorates and the individual experiences a sense of withdrawal. They therefore exercise to reverse the withdrawal process (similar to caffeine, see Box 3.1).
- **Endorphins:** exercise generates endorphins in the brain which create a sense of euphoria ('joggers' high') but endorphins then decay, leaving the person wanting that feeling again.

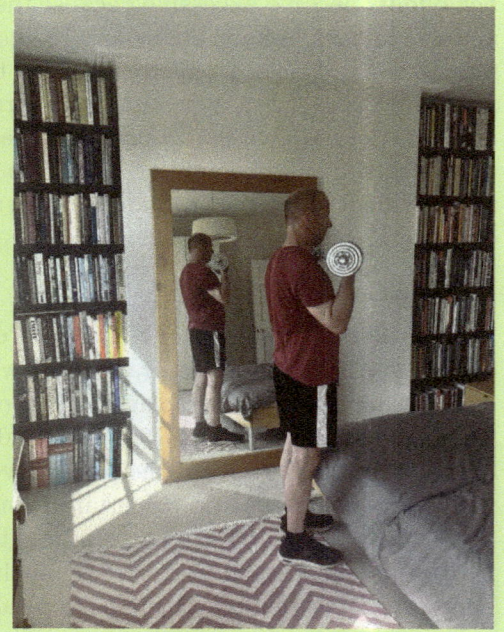

Social learning model
- **Feeling out of control:** exercise can make people feel more in control of their lives and similarities have often been drawn with eating disorders. For example, if a person feels out of control of their relationships or their career, they may find satisfaction in being able to control how much they exercise.
- **Reinforcement:** exercise has many positive consequences (some of which are fairly immediate)

Exercise can become addictive if it starts to interfere with work and social life

Social Learning Model

such as improved mood, stress reduction, improved body shape and body image, and increased energy. These can become reinforcing for the behaviour with the individual exercising more as a means to experience these benefits. Changes in body shape are also frequently reinforced through the compliments of others.

- **Modelling:** social learning may also encourage excessive exercise if people start to socialize in groups of other excessive exercisers (e.g. body-building clubs, jogging clubs, rowing clubs, etc.).

- **Associative learning:** excessive exercise can be learned through association with a range of cues such as social groups (e.g. jogging clubs, gyms), being in the fresh air, feeling stressed, feeling unattractive and feeling fat. These internal and external factors can become cues for further exercise behaviour.

CONSEQUENCES OF EXERCISE DEPENDENCE

Regular exercise may result in physiological and psychological benefits and is recommended for both the prevention and treatment of physical disorders such as CHD, hypertension and obesity, and psychological problems such as depression and anxiety (see Chapters 5, 13). When taken to excess, however, exercise may be harmful. For example, people with exercise dependence often have physical injuries associated with their behaviour (e.g. problems with knees, ankles, feet and back) and rather than rest to allow these injuries to recover may continue to exercise, thereby exacerbating their problems. Excessive exercise may also have negative effects on interpersonal relationships – for example, becoming an absent parent or neglecting family/partner responsibilities. Finally, although exercise improves mood for most people, excessive exercise may be detrimental to depression and anxiety in the longer term if a person becomes overly dependent on exercise to manage their well-being (Orford 2002).

Exercise dependence is an example of how a behaviour can become excessive and therefore 'addictive'. It also shows how even a behaviourally generated addiction can be explained through both disease and social learning perspectives. Parallel processes may well be involved for other problem behaviours such as shopping, gambling and sex addiction.

5 THE STAGES OF SUBSTANCE USE

Research into addictive behaviours has defined four stages of substance use: (1) initiation; (2) maintenance; (3) cessation; and (4) relapse. These four stages will now be examined in detail for smoking and alcohol use and are illustrated in Figure 3.9.

STAGES 1 AND 2: INITIATING AND MAINTAINING AN ADDICTIVE BEHAVIOUR

Smoking Initiation and Maintenance

Many children and adolescents try a puff of a cigarette. It is therefore difficult to distinguish between actual initiation and maintenance of smoking behaviour. Accordingly, these stages will be considered together. In an attempt to understand initiation and maintenance, researchers have searched for the psychological and social processes that may promote smoking behaviour with a focus on cognitions and social norms.

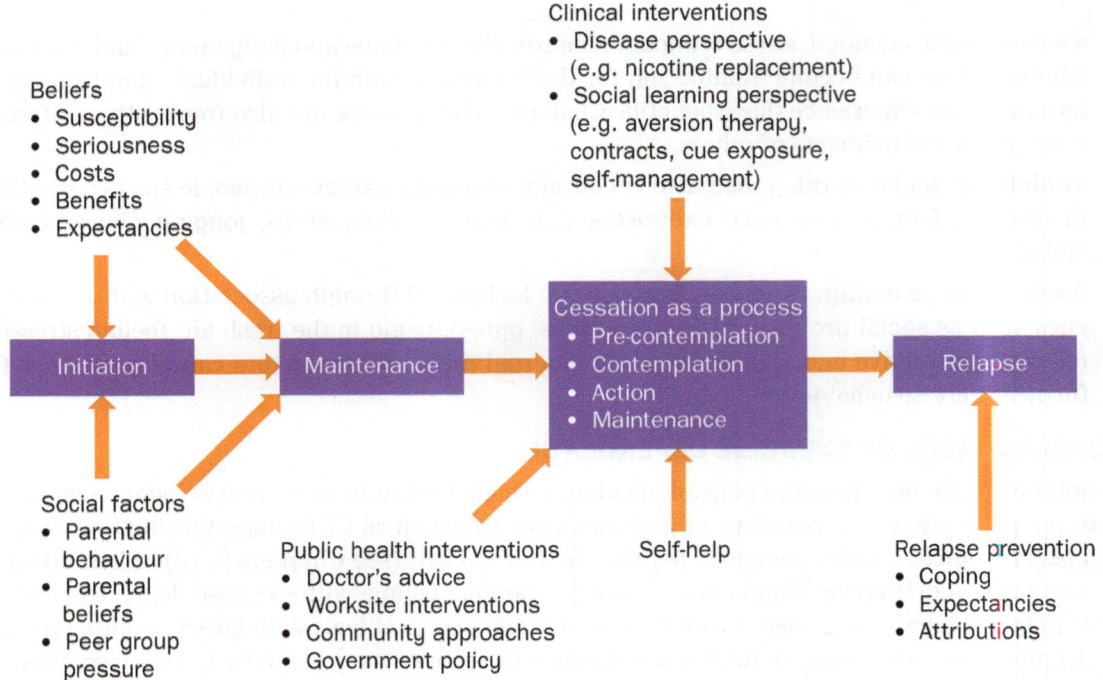

Figure 3.9 The stages of substance use

Cognitions

Models of health behaviour such as the health belief model (HBM), protection motivation theory (PMT), the theory of reasoned action (TRA) and the health action process approach (HAPA) (see Chapter 2) have been used to examine the cognitive factors that contribute to smoking initiation (e.g. Wilkinson and Abraham 2004; Connor et al. 2006; Reisi et al. 2014). Additional cognitions that predict smoking behaviour include associating smoking with fun and pleasure, smoking as a means of calming nerves and smoking as being sociable and building confidence, all of which have been reported by young smokers (Charlton 1984; Charlton and Blair 1989; see also Chapter 10 for a discussion of smoking and stress reduction). Research also highlights a role for self-esteem and perceived ease of smoking (Wilkinson and Abraham 2004). Conner et al. (2006) explored the role of theory of planned behaviour (TPB) variables (see Chapter 2) as well as anticipated regret and intention stability in predicting smoking initiation in adolescents aged between 11 and 12. Non-smoking adolescents (n = 675) completed measures at baseline and then were followed up after nine months to see if they had tried smoking, which was assessed using a carbon monoxide breath monitor. The results showed that smoking initiation was predicted by baseline intentions. This association between intentions and behaviour was only present, however, in those who did not express regret about starting smoking at baseline and who showed stable intentions. In terms of maintenance of smoking, Lawton et al. (2009) explored the relative role of cognitive attitudes (e.g. 'smoking is harmful') and affective attitudes (e.g. 'smoking is enjoyable') in predicting smoking at one month follow-up and concluded that affective attitudes had a direct impact upon behaviour (regardless of intentions), and that this might be a useful variable to target in interventions. Research also explored smoking during the COVID pandemic and has described how people used smoking as a coping strategy. For example, Shepherd et al. (2021) carried out a cross-sectional study and concluded that increased worry about COVID-19 was related to using smoking to cope with the pandemic and increased ratings of the barriers and negative consequences of giving up smoking.

Social Norms

Much research focuses on the individual and takes them out of their social context. Interactions with the social world help to create and develop a child's beliefs and behaviour. In Britain, there have been five longitudinal studies that have identified elements of the child's social world that are predictive of smoking behaviour (Murray et al. 1984; McNeil et al. 1988; Charlton and Blair 1989; Gillies and Galt 1990; Goddard 1990). The main factor that predicts smoking is parental smoking, with reports that children are twice as likely to smoke if their parents smoke (Lader and Matheson 1991). In addition, parents' attitudes to smoking also influence their offspring's behaviour. For example, if a child perceives the parents as being strongly against smoking, he or she is up to seven times less likely to be a smoker (Murray et al. 1984). The next most important influence on smoking is peer group pressure. Mercken et al. (2011) explored the beliefs and behaviours of 1,475 Dutch adolescents and concluded that their smoking behaviour was predicted by parental, sibling and friend smoking. In addition, even those people that they would like to be friends with in the future influenced whether or not they smoked in the present. Liu et al. (2017) conducted a meta-analysis of 75 studies across 16 countries which showed that having peers who smoke, doubled the odds of adolescents beginning or continuing to smoke. Research also shows an impact of an individual's wider social context. For example, a Cancer Research Campaign study in 1991 found that smoking prevalence was lower in schools that had a 'no smoking' policy, particularly if this policy included staff as well as students. Further, Helweg-Larsen et al. (2010) carried out a qualitative study of smokers from Denmark (where smoking is accepted) and the USA (where it is not) as a means to explore the role of an individual's cultural background. The results showed that although all smokers were aware of the risks of their behaviour, the Danes were more likely to minimize these risks. In addition, although all smokers also said that they had been the target for moralized attitudes from others, the Danes were more rejecting of these views.

Alcohol Initiation and Maintenance

Most people try alcohol at some time in their lives, with about 90 per cent of all adults having drunk alcohol in the past year. Some do describe themselves as lifelong abstainers (OPCS 1994) and the most common reasons for never drinking alcohol are religion and not liking it. Therefore, rather than examining predictors of drinking 'ever' or 'occasionally', this section examines which factors predict developing a problem with drinking. Research has focused on cognitive factors, affect and social factors.

Cognition and Affect

The tension-reduction hypothesis (Cappell and Greeley 1987) suggests that individuals may develop a drink problem because alcohol reduces tension and anxiety. Tension creates a heightened state of arousal and alcohol reduces this state, which perpetuates further drinking behaviour. However, it has been suggested that it is not the *actual* effects of alcohol use that promote drinking but the *expected* effects (George and Marlatt 1983). Therefore, because a small amount of alcohol may have positive effects, people assume that these positive effects will continue with increased use. During the COVID pandemic, alcohol drinking increased with more people drinking more at home than before. Avery et al. (2020) carried a large-scale study of adult twins (n = 3971) during the COVID pandemic and reported that about 14 per cent of the respondents reported an increase in alcohol use. Further, while there was no significant difference in stress or anxiety levels between non-drinkers and those who reported no change in alcohol use, in drinkers, increased stress and anxiety was related to increased alcohol consumption. Studies have also focused on cognitions using social cognition models (see Chapter 2). For example, Norman and Conner (2006) used the TPB to predict binge drinking in undergraduate students and included a measure of past binge drinking as a means to measure habit. The results showed that the best predictors of intentions to binge drink at one week follow-up were attitude, self-efficacy and lower perceived control, and that intentions and self-efficacy in turn predicted actual behaviour.

Furthermore, past behaviour also predicted both intentions and behaviour, showing an important role for habit in alcohol use.

Social Factors

Many of the social factors that relate to smoking behaviour are also predictive of alcohol consumption. For example, parental drinking is predictive of problem drinking in children. According to a disease model of addictions, it could be argued that this reflects the genetic predisposition to develop an addictive behaviour. However, parental drinking may be influential through 'social hereditary factors', with children being exposed to drinking behaviour and learning this behaviour from their parents (Orford and Velleman 1991).

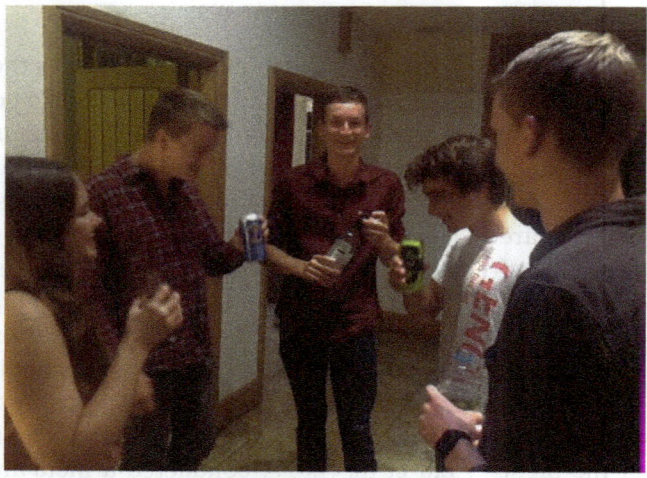

Social factors have a strong role to play in drinking behaviour

For example, Homel and Warren (2019) carried out a longitudinal study with 2,800 teenagers aged 14–15 years (48.9 per cent female) living in two-parent households from the Longitudinal Study of Australian Children to assess the relationship between mother's and father's heavy binge drinking and adolescent drinking. The results showed that parent heavy binge drinking predicted adolescent drinking, even after controlling for potential confounding variables, and that girls in early adolescence were more influenced by their parents' drinking than boys. Furthermore, a large study in the Netherlands of children aged 6 to 8 years and 12 to 15 years explored the relationship between their expectancies of the consequences of alcohol and their parents' drinking (Smit et al. 2019). The results concluded that while there was an association between parental drinking and children's expectancies about the effects of alcohol, it was how much they *saw* their father drink rather than how much he actually drank that was the best predictor of their alcohol expectancies. Likewise, peer group alcohol use and abuse also predict drinking behaviour, as does being someone who is sensation-seeking, with a tendency to be aggressive and having a history of getting into trouble with authority. Johnston and White (2003) used the TPB to predict binge drinking in students. However, given the social nature of binge drinking, they focused on the role of norms. Using a longitudinal design, 289 undergraduate students completed a questionnaire concerning their beliefs with follow-up collected about reported binge drinking. The results showed an important role for norms, particularly if the norms were of a behaviourally relevant reference group with which the student strongly identified.

STAGE 3: CEASING AN ADDICTIVE BEHAVIOUR

Because of the potential health consequences of both smoking and alcohol consumption, research has examined different means to help smokers and drinkers quit their behaviour. (Much of this research can be understood in terms of the strategies for behaviour change described in Chapter 7.)

The Process of Cessation

Most research to date has conceptualized cessation as the result of a slow process of cognitive shifts. In contrast, recent research has emphasized a more unplanned approach to cessation. These two approaches will now be considered.

Cessation as a Slow Process

Much research emphasizes the 'drip, drip' approach to cessation and the development of behavioural intentions or plans (see Chapters 2, 7). Such approaches include the use of health behaviour models, implementation intentions, a stages of change approach and in recent years has drawn upon text messaging and social media.

Health behaviour models: Research has used models such as TPB, HBM and the COM-B (see Chapter 2) to examine the predictors of both intentions to stop smoking and successful smoking cessation. For example, Norman et al. (1999) examined the usefulness of the TPB at predicting intention to quit smoking and making a quit attempt in a group of smokers attending health promotion clinics in primary care. The results showed that the best predictors of intentions to quit were perceived behavioural control and perceived susceptibility. At follow-up, the best predictors of making a quit attempt were intentions at baseline and the number of previous quit attempts. Other similar studies report a role for individual cognitions such as perceptions of susceptibility, past cessation attempts and perceived behavioural control as predictors of smoking behaviour (Giannetti et al. 1985; Godin et al. 1992). Further, an extended TPB including descriptive norms and affective attitudes has been shown to be a good predictor of cessation (Rise et al. 2008). The HBM has also been used as a framework for understanding smoking cessation, and Battle et al. (2015) found evidence from their focus group discussions with 71 participants for the HBM components in smoking cessation. Some research has also focused on the impact of social norms which is a component of the TPB. For example, Blok et al. (2017) carried out a longitudinal study on 4,623 adults. They reported that social networks, especially among household members and friends, were strongly linked to smoking cessation and relapse and that those who had a higher number of smokers in their social networks were less likely to quit smoking, and more likely to relapse. Some research has also used the COM-B to explore successful changes to both smoking and alcohol behaviours (eg. Kwah et al. 2019; Minian et al. 2020; Rosário et al. 2021). For example, Minian et al. (2020) carried out a rapid realist review of the literature and concluded that the best predictor of smoking cessation was through increasing opportunities (i.e. factors that lie outside the individual that prompt the behaviour or make it possible) so that people can engage in healthier behaviours leading to smoking cessation success. Similarly, Rosário et al. (2021) carried out a systematic review of 84 studies to explore the aim to conduct a theory-informed review of the factors influencing general practitioners' and primary care nurses' routine delivery of alcohol screening and brief interventions (SBI) to adults. The authors concluded that increasing all aspects of capability, opportunity and motivation may be needed to successfully implement alcohol SBI in primary health care.

Implementation intention research highlights the development of plans (Gollwitzer 1993) and has been used to promote changes in both smoking and alcohol use. For example, Conner and Higgins (2010) randomly allocated adolescents (aged 11–12) to receive either an implementation intention intervention (i.e. planning how, where and when they could refuse to smoke) or a self-efficacy intervention (i.e. planning how to refuse to smoke in increasingly difficult situations). They were then followed up for up to 24 months. The results showed that the implementation intention intervention was most effective at reducing adolescent smoking by two years. Similarly, Armitage (2008, 2009a) concluded from his experimental studies that implementation intentions could also reduce both smoking and alcohol intake by one month.

The stages of change model (SOC) focuses on the gradual progression through a series of stages (Prochaska and DiClemente 1982). In particular, Prochaska and DiClemente (1984) adapted their SOC to examine cessation of addictive behaviours. This model highlighted the processes involved in the transition from a smoker to a non-smoker and from a drinker to a non-drinker. They argued that cessation involves a shift across five basic stages:

1 *Pre-contemplation:* defined as not seriously considering quitting.

2 *Contemplation:* having some thoughts about quitting.

3 *Preparation:* seriously considering quitting.

4 *Action:* initial behaviour change.

5 *Maintenance:* maintaining behaviour change for a period of time.

Prochaska and DiClemente maintain that individuals do not progress through these stages in a straightforward and linear fashion but may switch backwards and forwards (e.g. from pre-contemplation to contemplation and back to pre-contemplation again). They call this 'the revolving door' schema and emphasize the dynamic nature of cessation. This model of change has been tested to provide evidence for the different stages for smokers and outpatient alcoholics (DiClemente and Prochaska 1982, 1985; DiClemente and Hughes 1990), and for the relationship between stage of change for smoking cessation and self-efficacy. In addition, it has formed the basis of several interventions to promote smoking cessation. In a very early study by the model's authors, DiClemente et al. (1991) examined the relationship between stage of change and attempts to quit smoking and actual cessation at one- and six-month follow-ups. The authors categorized smokers into either pre-contemplators or contemplators and examined their smoking behaviour at follow-up. They further classified the contemplators into either contemplators (those who were smoking, seriously considering quitting within the next six months, but not within the next 30 days) or those in the preparation stage (those who were seriously considering quitting smoking within the next 30 days). The results showed that those in the preparation stage of change were more likely to have made a quit attempt at both one and six months, that they had made more quit attempts and were more likely to be not smoking at the follow-ups. Aveyard et al. (2006) also used the SOC to promote smoking cessation in pregnant women and concluded that a stage-matched intervention was more effective at moving women forward a stage than a non-stage-matched intervention. Further, Caponnetto et al. (2017) concluded that training pharmacists to use the SOC along with motivational interviewing improved their effectiveness at promoting smoking cessation in their patients.

Text messaging, MHealth platforms and social media are increasingly used to deliver smoking cessation and alcohol reduction interventions. Over recent years a number of systematic reviews and meta analyses have been carried out to assess their effectiveness. Some of the conclusions are as follows:

- Villanti et al. (2020) carried out a systematic review of 32 studies of smoking-cessation interventions for young adults (aged 18–24 years) in the US. They concluded that three new approaches could be effective additions to existing approaches to promote smoking cessation. These were: text message interventions, sustained quit-and-win contests, and multiple behaviour interventions.

- Luo et al. (2021) carried out a systematic review of 16 studies and concluded that due to the low cost and widespread use of social media, smoking cessation interventions should be embedded within popular social media platforms.

- Song et al. (2019) carried out a systematic review of 19 studies to synthesize evidence about the efficacy of MHealth interventions for unhealthy alcohol use. They concluded that most studies showed that MHealth interventions improved self control for unhealthy alcohol use, especially those delivered by short message service and interactive voice response systems.

- Bendtsen et al. (2021) carried out a systematic review and meta-analysis of 10 studies and concluded that text messaging interventions may reduce alcohol consumption among risky drinkers when compared with no or basic health information.

Text messaging, social media and MHealth platforms may therefore offer a low cost and easily accessible way to deliver smoking cessation and alcohol reduction interventions.

Cessation as Unplanned

In contrast to this 'drip, drip' approach to cessation West (2006; West and Sohal 2006) has argued that sometimes cessation of an addictive behaviour can be unplanned. In a large-scale cross-sectional survey of smokers who had made at least one quit attempt (n = 918) and ex-smokers (n = 996) the researchers asked participants to describe whether they had made a serious quit attempt ('By serious attempt I mean you decided that you would try to make sure you never smoked another cigarette').

Those who had tried were then asked to describe the extent to which their attempt had been planned (ranging from 'I did not plan the quit attempt in advance' to 'I planned the quit attempt a few months beforehand') (West and Sohal 2006). The results showed that almost half (48.6 per cent) of the attempts had been made *without* planning. In addition, the results showed that unplanned attempts were more likely to last for at least six months (65.4 per cent) compared to planned attempts (42.3 per cent). These results remained even when age, sex and social class were controlled for. These findings are in contrast to much of the research described earlier which emphasizes the role of plans and stages.

STAGE 4: RELAPSE

Although many people are successful at initially stopping smoking and changing their drinking behaviour, relapse rates are high. For example, nearly half of those smokers who make a quit attempt return to smoking within the year (National Statistics 2005). Interestingly, the pattern for relapse is consistent across a number of different addictive behaviours, with high rates initially tapering off over a year. This relapse pattern is shown in Figure 3.10.

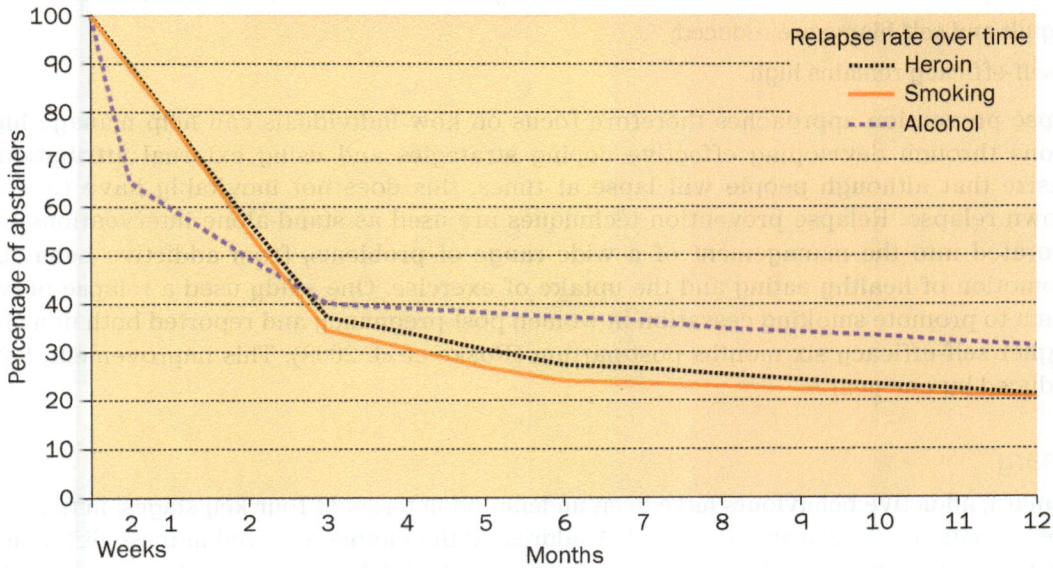

Figure 3.10 Relapse curves for individuals treated for heroin, smoking and alcohol addiction

SOURCE: Hunt and Bespalec (1974)

In 1985, Marlatt and Gordon developed a relapse prevention model of addictions to address the processes involved in successful and unsuccessful cessation of any given addictive behaviour. This approach challenged some of the aspects of a disease model of addictions by emphasizing how addictive behaviours could be unlearned and arguing that believing in an abstinence-only model and that 'one drink = a drunk' is a self-fulfilling prophecy. This model is described in detail in Chapter 7. The key novel component is the focus on the transition from a lapse, which entails a minor slip (e.g. a cigarette, a couple of drinks), and a relapse, which entails a return to former behaviour (e.g. smoking 20 cigarettes, getting drunk). Marlatt and Gordon examined the processes involved in the progression from abstinence to lapse to relapse and called this the abstinence violation effect (AVE). The AVE occurs as follows:

- *Abstinence:* the individual sets abstinence as their target behaviour.
- *High-risk situation:* lowered mood, being in a drinking environment, being offered a cigarette, are all high-risk situations.

- *Coping behaviour:* if they can cope effectively, then abstinence will be maintained. If not, then the person will lapse.
- *Positive outcome expectancies:* Successful coping is helped by negative outcome expectancies (e.g. getting drunk will make me feel sick) but hindered by positive outcome expectancies (e.g. smoking will make me feel less anxious).
- *Self-efficacy:* successful coping is also helped by high levels of self-efficacy.
- *Lapse:* the initial lapse happens.
- *Full-blown relapse:* the lapse is then turned into a full-blown relapse (smoking a packet of cigarettes, getting drunk) if the following happens:
  - the lapse is attributed to the self (e.g. 'I am useless, it's my fault');
  - feeling guilt and self-blame;
  - this internal attribution lowers self-efficacy.
- *Abstinence returns:* the lapse returns to abstinence if the following happens:
  - the lapse is attributed to the external world (e.g. the situation, the presence of others);
  - guilt and self-blame are reduced;
  - self-efficacy remains high.

Relapse prevention approaches therefore focus on how individuals can help manage high-risk situations through developing effective coping strategies and using external attributions, and emphasize that although people will lapse at times, this does not inevitably have to lead to a full-blown relapse. Relapse prevention techniques are used as stand-alone interventions but also incorporated into the management of a wide range of problems, from addictive behaviours to the promotion of healthy eating and the uptake of exercise. One study used a relapse prevention approach to promote smoking cessation in women post-pregnancy and reported both non-smoking and higher self-efficacy six months post-partum (Roske et al. 2008). This improvement, however, had reduced by one year.

Summary

In summary, addictive behaviours have been understood in terms of four key stages: initiation, maintenance, cessation and relapse. Research has addressed the factors involved in these different stages from both a disease and social learning perspective and highlights a role for pharmacological action on the body as well as conditioning, cognitions, mood and motivations. Nowadays, most attempts to change addictive behaviours incorporate both these perspectives and the evidence seems to point to a role for multiple approaches, with much social support and longer-term follow-ups as being predictive of better cessation in the longer term.

6   A CROSS-ADDICTION PERSPECTIVE

According to the disease models of addiction, each behaviour is examined separately. Therefore an addiction to cigarettes is seen as separate and different from an addiction to alcohol as they are based upon a different substance with different effects on the body. From a social learning perspective, however, it is possible to examine similarities between behaviours and throughout this chapter many commonalities can be seen in terms of initiation, maintenance, cessation and relapse, and the role of conditioning, cognitions, mood and motivation. Furthermore, these factors are not only relevant to smoking, alcohol and caffeine use but also to other addictions such as exercise, sex, gambling and eating. Such an approach reflects a cross-addictive behaviours perspective and two models using this are now described.

EXCESSIVE APPETITES THEORY

Orford's (2002) book, *Excessive Appetites,* describes the ways in which any appetitive behaviour, such as gambling, eating, sex or exercise can become so excessive as to ruin people's lives. His complex model, called *excessive appetites theory,* was then further refined in terms of the ways in which some core addictions can emerge out of behaviours which are often ordinary and unproblematic. The following is a simplified version of his model.

- *Appetitive consumption:* appetitive behaviours are those which feel good, and Orford identifies core addictions as drinking, gambling, drug-taking, eating, exercise and sex. The model uses the term *appetitive consumption* rather than addiction.

- *Behaviour as rewarding:* all appetitive behaviours cause emotional rewards such as pleasure, fun or arousal or have positive consequences such as feeling relaxed, less stressed and more socially at ease. This reinforces the behaviour whether it be a drug-based pleasure or the consequences of a behaviour, and can engender feelings of necessity and lack of control.

- *Deterrents and restraints:* the model argues that although they are rewarding, most appetitive behaviours are limited by a set of barriers. For example, excessive alcohol use causes headaches, sickness, inability to get to work and a sense of being drunk that some people don't like. These deterrents and restraints would usually limit a behaviour. When these are reduced, however, the behaviour spills over like a river flooding its banks.

- *Methods of escalation:* Orford proposes two ways in which casual behaviour escalates into an excessive behaviour:
  - *low proportionate effect:* this reflects the notions of choice and self-control and describes how a behaviour will escalate if the incentives are perceived as great and the restraints to stop are perceived as weak;
  - *strong attachments:* the individual develops a strong attachment to the behaviour through reinforcements and this is exacerbated by increasing generalized anxiety and a reduction in the normal restrictions that limit the behaviour.

- *Social norms:* people are more likely to show excessive behaviour if their peer group also does the same. As people develop excessive behaviours, they also change peer groups to be with similar people with similar levels of behaviour.

- *AVE:* in line with relapse prevention (see below) Orford argues that escalation is also exacerbated by the AVE and feelings of guilt, self-blame and internal attributions for lapses.

- *Social response to addiction:* once behaviours become excessive they have social consequences such as frustration and upset from others, breakdown of relationships, loss of employment, loss of property, loss of money (gambling) and secrecy. This gives rise to a secondary form of emotional cycles as the individual tries to compensate for these social consequences (e.g. gambling more to regain lost money; becoming more isolated and secretive to hide behaviour).

- *Conflict:* the strong attachment to the behaviour, due to high incentives and reinforcements and low deterrents and restraints in the context of the negative social response to addiction, causes conflict. This conflict may be a motivation to change. Orford calls this 'motivation for self-liberation'. It may, however, exacerbate feelings of anxiety which heighten the individual's attachment to the appetitive behaviour even more.

This model is relevant to a wide range of potential addictive behaviours whether they be drug- or behaviourally based. It draws upon social learning perspectives on addictive behaviours with its emphasis on reinforcements, social norms, AVE and restraints, but it also allows for a disease element in terms of drug effects. The model is complex, however, and it is therefore difficult to operationalize and test. But it is hard to think of examples of addictive behaviour that cannot be accounted for by this approach.

PRIME THEORY

West (2006) developed an alternative model of addictive behaviours that could also be applied to all drug-based and behaviourally based addictions. This was called PRIME theory and was based upon a motivational model that could capture both conscious choice processes and non-conscious motivational systems, as well as classical and operant conditioning processes. The model is illustrated in Figure 3.11.

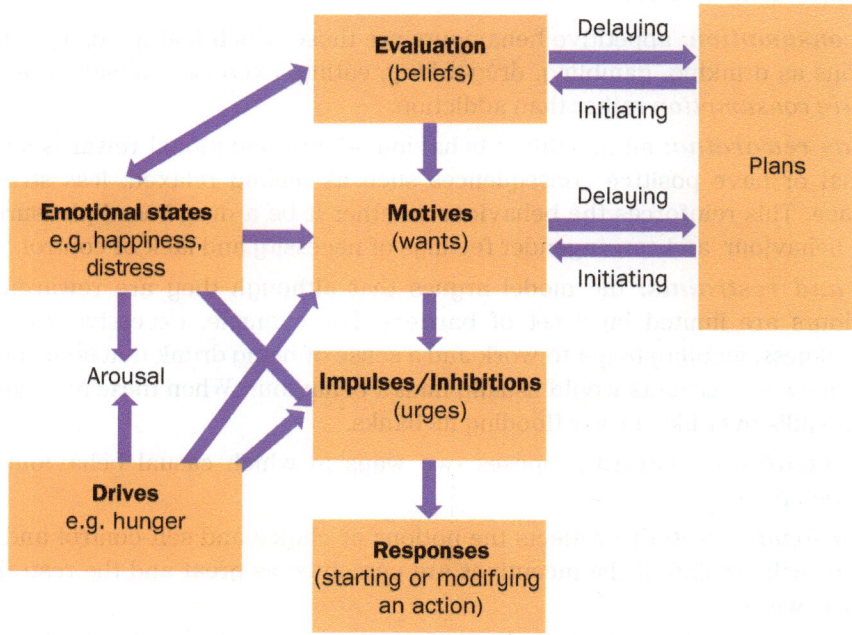

Figure 3.11 PRIME theory of addiction

SOURCE: Adapted from West (2006)

PRIME stands for the following aspects of the model:

P – plans (conscious mental representations of future actions plus commitment).

R – responses (starting, stopping or modifying actions)

I – impulses/inhibitory forces (can be experienced as urges)

M – motives (can be experienced as desires)

E – evaluations (evaluative beliefs)

These aspects influence addictive behaviours in the following ways. In terms of alcohol dependence, an individual who is emotionally vulnerable, who feels relief when drinking and lives within a social context where it is normal to drink heavily, will be more likely to drink to excess. Even if they do not respond well to the negative effects of alcohol, their problem will continue because, in terms of PRIME theory, this drinking behaviour will then be maintained through their impulses ('I need a drink'), emotional states ('I am anxious'), motives ('I want a drink') and evaluations ('drinking will make me feel better') which in turn make it unlikely they will make plans to change or stop their behaviour.

West's PRIME theory focuses more on the maintenance of an addictive behaviour rather than its uptake. It also highlights ways in which therapy could intervene by reducing impulses (e.g. NRT, alcohol reduction medication, methodone); changing evaluations (e.g. focusing on the negative consequences of a behaviour); changing emotional states (e.g. cognitive behavioural therapy – CBT – relaxation, counselling) or challenging motives (e.g. reframing the craving for a drink as the need for something more healthy – exercise, social support, etc.).

Although most research focuses on specific behaviours such as smoking *or* alcohol use *or* drug-taking, there are many similarities across behaviours in terms of factors relating to initiation, maintenance, cessation and relapse. These two cross-addiction behaviour models explore some of these similarities and also highlight how individuals may show excessive behaviours for both drug-based and behaviourally based addictions.

BOX 3.3
Critical Approaches to Health Psychology

Research exploring addictive behaviours highlights some of the bigger issues with research in health psychology:

Gender differences: Much research in this area explores differences between men and women in terms of smoking uptake or cessation or drinking behaviour. This imposes a simple dichotomous model, assumes that people belong to one of these two groups and that these two groups tell us about the people within these groups. Is gender as simple as this? How much do we really find out about a person by knowing they are a man or a woman? Is it time to deprioritize gender and find other more useful ways to classify people?

The individual vs the social vs the political: Smoking, alcohol drinking, coffee drinking, exercise, gambling, shopping and all the other behaviours that become addictive are clearly products of an individual's social and political world. In our models we capture this as 'social norms' or 'opportunity' but this doesn't in any way reflect the complexity of an abusive family driving their teenager to gamble online, a culture that normalises excessive alcohol drinking in middle aged women or a culture that has been so annihilated through invasion, history and neglect that they find comfort in smoking and drinking too much. Yet in health psychology our focus on the individual through our theories, constructs and methods neglects the bigger picture.

The problem of choice: In health psychology we have a dilemma. We focus on the individual and explore the role of their beliefs in predicting behaviour. Then to change behaviour we try to change these beliefs. This is considered empowering as the individual can 'choose' to change. But if they are behaving in a certain way because of their social or political world, this focus on them takes the responsibility for change away from the world around them and places it onto them. So if work stress makes someone smoke, do we change their beliefs about the stress or ask their manager to reduce their workload?

---

7 | THINKING CRITICALLY ABOUT ADDICTIVE BEHAVIOURS

There are several problems with the research and theories of addictive behaviours including the key constructs, the language and the methodologies used in research.

SOME CRITICAL QUESTIONS

When thinking about research and theories relating to addictive behaviours ask yourself the following questions:

- Is the divide between psychological and disease approaches useful?
- Why is it so difficult to measure behaviours such as smoking and drinking?
- How does the history of addictive behaviours influence the words we use to describe them?
- Are addictive behaviours really different to other behaviours?

SOME PROBLEMS WITH . . .

Thinking critically about addictive behaviours involves an understanding of some of these problems as follows:

Polarized theories: There are very different theoretical perspectives on addictive behaviours which colour research in terms of theory, methods and interpretation. For example, those from a medical perspective emphasize the addictive nature of the drug while those from a behavioural perspective emphasize the behaviour. At times these two perspectives contradict each other but mostly the two camps publish in different journals and do not really communicate. This can lead to polarizing our understanding of these behaviours.

Measurement issues: Most measures of smoking and alcohol are self-reported. This can be problematic as people may under-report their behaviour in order to seem healthier than they are. There are some more objective measures available such as cotinine levels. However, these involve more commitment by both the researcher and the subject. In addition, measuring these behaviours may change them as any form of measurement can make people more aware of their behaviour.

The problem of language: The language used when talking about addiction is problematic as every term is embedded with meaning from a specific theoretical perspective. For example, the terms 'addiction', 'addict' and 'drug' tend to reflect a disease perspective emphasizing how the problem lies with the substance or the personal. Likewise 'withdrawal' and 'tolerance' highlight the medical impact of a 'drug' on the body. In contrast using words such as 'dependency' or even 'habit' encourages a more learning perspective and suggests a notion of choice or control. These terms are core to how we talk about the onset, maintenance and management of an addictive behaviour and therefore influence our beliefs about what an 'addiction' is and how it should be treated.

Complex vs simple models: The factors that explain smoking and alcohol use are many and complex. Related theories are therefore complex and often difficult to operationalize. Simpler theories are easier to operationalize but may miss many of the variables that predict these behaviours. Therefore a trade-off is always needed between comprehensiveness and usefulness.

TO CONCLUDE

Addictive behaviours such as smoking and alcohol use both have negative effects on health and yet are common. There are many different theories to explain why people smoke or drink and how they can be encouraged to adopt healthier behaviours. This chapter presented a brief history of models of addiction with a focus on the moral model, first and second disease models and the social learning perspective. It then examined the mechanisms involved in learning an addictive behaviour and the ways in which the different models can be integrated with a focus on caffeine use and exercise dependence. The chapter then described the stages of substance use from initiation and maintenance to cessation and relapse. The chapter also examined a cross-addiction perspective with a focus on two approaches which highlight similarities between behaviours and the ways in which many ordinary and unproblematic behaviours can become excessive if the conditions are right. Finally, the chapter explored some of the problems with research in this area.

QUESTIONS

1 Could we become addicted to anything?
2 Discuss the role of learning in the initiation and maintenance of an addictive behaviour.
3 Smoking is an addiction to nicotine. Discuss.
4 Discuss the role of health beliefs in the initiation of smoking behaviour.
5 Discuss the role of withdrawal reversal effects in the maintenance of an addictive behaviour.
6 It is the government's responsibility to prevent smoking. Discuss.
7 Lung cancer from smoking is a self-inflicted disease. Discuss.
8 To what extent are addictions governed by similar processes?
9 We have known for a half a century that smoking causes lung cancer. Why do people still continue to smoke?

FOR DISCUSSION

Have you ever tried a puff of a cigarette? If so, consider the reasons that you did or did not become a smoker. If you have never even tried a cigarette, discuss the possible reasons for this.

FURTHER READING

Marlatt, G.A. and Gordon, J.R. (1985) *Relapse Prevention*. New York: Guilford Press.
Provides a detailed analysis and background to relapse prevention and applies this approach to a variety of addictive behaviours. Chapter 1 is a particularly useful overview.

Orford, J. (2002) *Excessive Appetites: A Psychological View of Addictions,* 2nd edn. Chichester: John Wiley.
Illustrates the extent to which different addictive behaviours share common variables in both their initiation and maintenance and discusses the interrelationship between physiological and psychological factors.

Svanberg, J. (2018) *The Psychology of Addiction*. London: Routledge.
This is a great little book that covers the theories research around addiction in an accessible way.

West, R. and Brown, J. (2013) *Theory of Addiction*. 2nd edn. Oxford: Blackwell.
An interesting and comprehensive book which describes existing theories of addiction and offers a new synthetic model of addiction which combines a range of psychological processes.

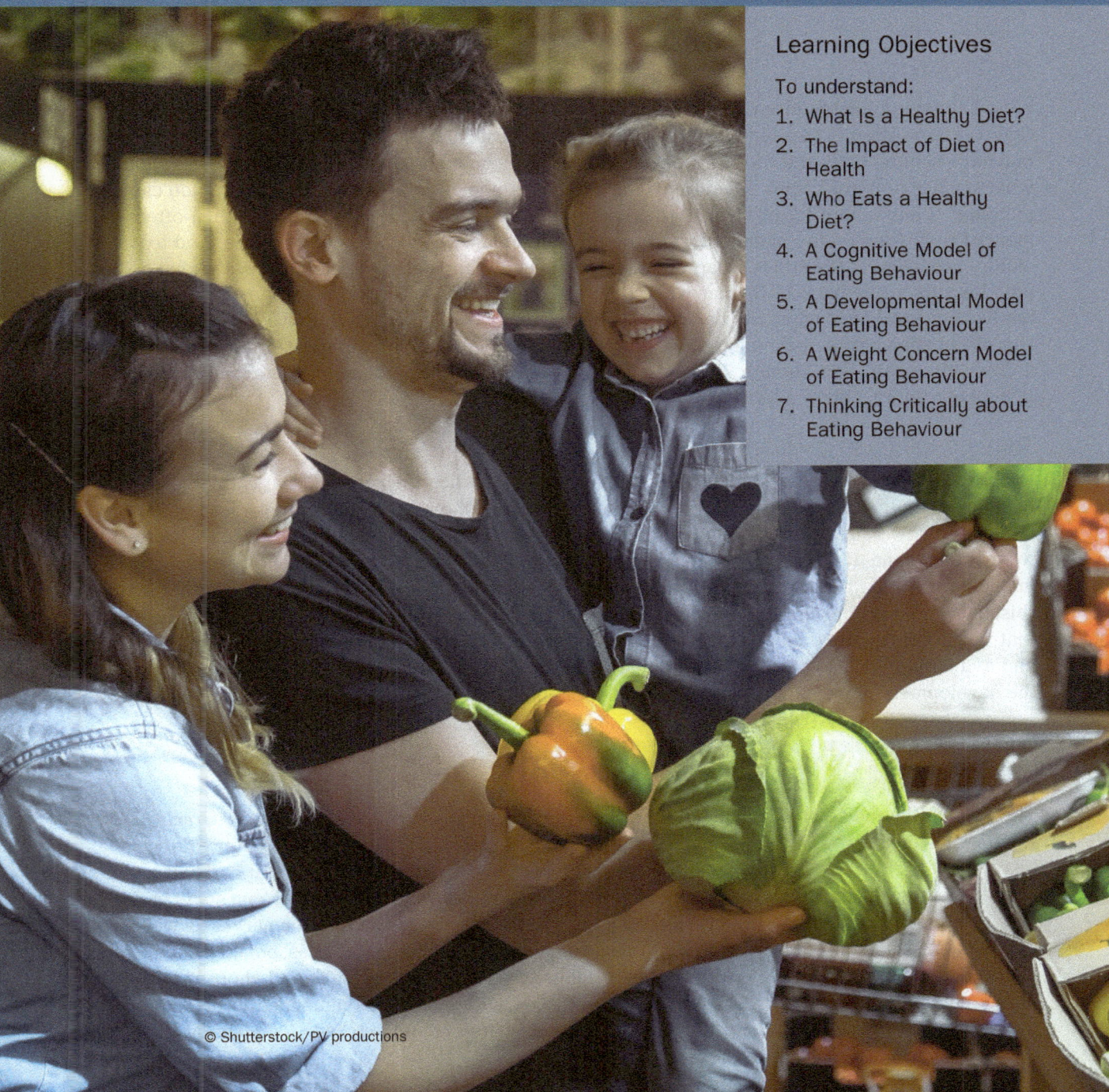

4
Eating Behaviour

Learning Objectives

To understand:

1. What Is a Healthy Diet?
2. The Impact of Diet on Health
3. Who Eats a Healthy Diet?
4. A Cognitive Model of Eating Behaviour
5. A Developmental Model of Eating Behaviour
6. A Weight Concern Model of Eating Behaviour
7. Thinking Critically about Eating Behaviour

© Shutterstock/PV productions

CHAPTER OVERVIEW

This chapter examines what constitutes a healthy diet, the links between diet and health and who does and does not eat healthily. Three main psychological models of eating behaviour are then described. First, the chapter describes the cognitive model with its emphasis on social cognition and the role of cognition in predicting food intake. Then it focuses on the developmental model of eating behaviour and the role of exposure, social learning and associative learning. Third, it explores the weight concern model and the role of body dissatisfaction and restrained eating. Finally, the chapter concludes with a summary of how to think critically about eating behaviour.

CASE STUDY

Sona has two young children aged 6 and 4. She has a busy job, has been working from home since COVID and is often exhausted when the children's tea-time comes. She wants the children to eat well and have healthy diets and tries to cook as much as she can but is often frustrated when they don't eat what she has prepared. Sona encourages them to eat saying 'if you eat your vegetables you can have pudding', 'I have put a lot of effort into cooking this' and 'eat this it is healthy' but they often leave most of their food on the plate and want to go off and play. She also sometimes uses food to get the children to behave, finds that a bag of crisps will keep them quiet while she makes a phone call and puts biscuits in the back of the car when they are on long car journeys. Sona doesn't eat with them but has her meal later when her partner gets home from work, by which time the children are in bed. Her eldest seems to be becoming quite fussy about food and often announces 'I don't like pasta' or 'I don't like peas' even though he has eaten them before and the youngest is starting to copy him. It is all becoming a bit of a battle.

Through the Eyes of Health Psychology. . .

People often think they eat when they are hungry and stop when they are full. But eating behaviour is far more complex than just a response to biology. From the moment we are born we learn what foods to like and how much to eat through our interactions with others, which in turn influences how we eat when we become adults. Sona's story illustrates many of the factors that influence eating behaviour including modelling (not eating with the children, siblings copying each other), associative learning (biscuits and car journeys), reinforcement (food to get the children to behave), parental control (eat vegetables and you can have pudding) and the impact of situational factors such as time, money and availability of healthy food. These factors are covered in this chapter. They are also relevant to the development of obesity, which is covered in Chapter 12.

1   WHAT IS A HEALTHY DIET?

The nature of a good diet has changed dramatically over the years. In 1824 *The Family Oracle of Good Health* published in the UK recommended that young ladies should eat the following at breakfast: 'plain biscuit (not bread), broiled beef steaks or mutton chops, under done without any fat and half a pint of bottled ale, the genuine Scots ale is the best', or if this was too strong it suggested 'one small breakfast cup . . . of good strong tea or of coffee – weak tea or coffee is always bad for the nerves as well as the complexion'. Dinner is later described as similar to breakfast with 'no vegetables, boiled meat, no made dishes being permitted much less fruit, sweet things or pastry . . . the steaks and chops must always be the chief part of your food'. Similarly in the 1840s Dr Kitchener recommended in his diet book a lunch of 'a bit of roasted poultry, a basin of good beef tea, eggs poached . . . a sandwich – stale bread – and half a pint of good home brewed beer' (cited in Burnett 1989: 69). Nowadays, there is, however, a consensus among nutritionists as to what constitutes a healthy diet (Public Health England 2016). Descriptions of healthy eating tend to describe food in terms of broader food groups and make recommendations as to the relative consumption of each of these groups. Current recommendations are as follows and illustrated in Figure 4.1.

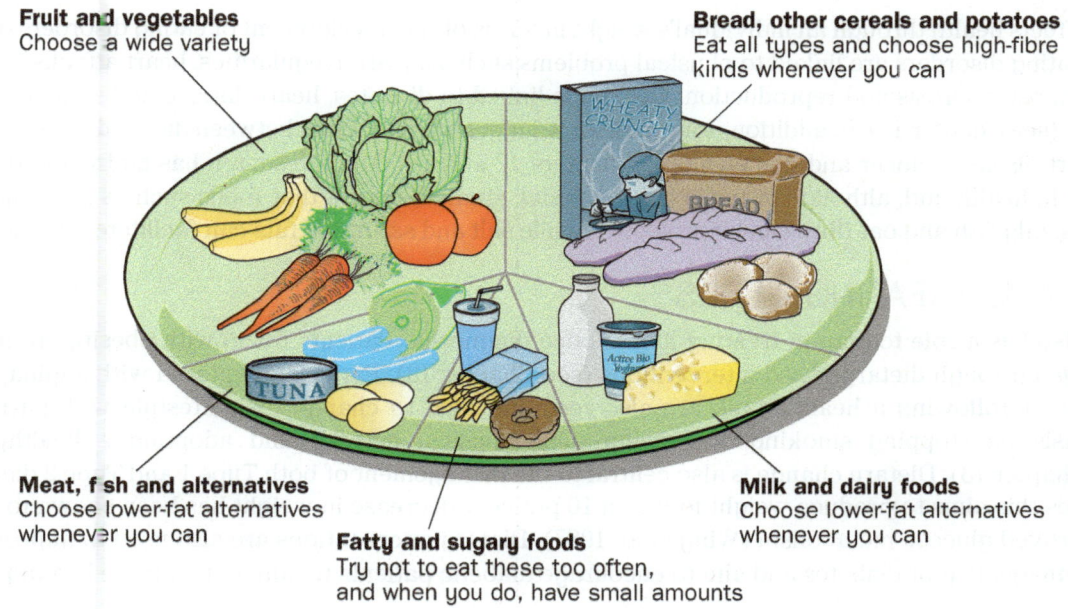

Fruit and vegetables
Choose a wide variety

Bread, other cereals and potatoes
Eat all types and choose high-fibre kinds whenever you can

Meat, fish and alternatives
Choose lower-fat alternatives whenever you can

Fatty and sugary foods
Try not to eat these too often, and when you do, have small amounts

Milk and dairy foods
Choose lower-fat alternatives whenever you can

Figure 4.1 The balance of good health

- *Fruit and vegetables:* a wide variety of fruit and vegetables should be eaten and preferably five or more servings should be eaten per day.
- *Bread, pasta, other cereals and potatoes:* plenty of complex carbohydrate foods should be eaten, preferably those high in fibre.
- *Meat, fish and alternatives:* moderate amounts of meat, fish and alternatives should be eaten and it is recommended that the low-fat varieties are chosen. Ideally two portions of fish should be eaten each week, one of which should be oily.
- *Milk and dairy products:* these should be eaten in moderation and the low-fat alternatives should be chosen where possible.
- *Fatty and sugary foods:* food such as crisps, sweets and sugary drinks should only be eaten infrequently and in small amounts and lower sugar ones should be chosen where possible.

Other recommendations for a healthy diet include eating more beans and pulses, less red and processed meat, and fruit juices and smoothies should be limited to 150 ml a day. Women should take in a total of 2,000 kcal and men should take in a total of 2,500 kcal (including food and drink), a moderate intake of alcohol (a maximum of 3–4 units per day for men and 2–3 units per day for women), the consumption of fluoridated water where possible, a limited salt intake of 6 g per day, eating unsaturated fats from olive oil and oily fish rather than saturated fats from butter and margarine, and consuming complex carbohydrates (e.g. bread and pasta) rather than simple carbohydrates (e.g. sugar). It is also recommended that men aged between 19 and 59 require 2,550 calories per day and that similarly aged women require 1,920 calories per day although this depends upon body size and degree of physical activity (DH 1995).

2   THE IMPACT OF DIET ON HEALTH

Diet is linked to health in two ways: by influencing the onset of illness and as part of treatment and management once illness has been diagnosed.

DIET AND ILLNESS ONSET

Diet affects health through an individual's weight in terms of the development of eating disorders or obesity. Eating disorders are linked to physical problems such as heart irregularities, heart attacks, stunted growth, osteoporosis and reproduction. Obesity is linked to diabetes, heart disease and some forms of cancer (see Chapter 13). In addition, some research suggests a direct link between diet and illnesses such as heart disease, cancer and diabetes (see Chapters 12 and 13). Much research has addressed the role of diet in health and, although at times controversial, studies suggest that foods such as fruit and vegetables, oily fish and oat fibre can be protective while salt and saturated fats can facilitate poor health.

DIET AND TREATING ILLNESS

Diet also has a role to play in treating illness once diagnosed. Patients living with obesity are mainly managed through dietary-based interventions (see Chapter 13). Patients diagnosed with angina, heart disease or following a heart attack are also recommended to change their lifestyle with particular emphasis on stopping smoking, increasing their physical activity and adopting a healthy diet (see Chapter 13). Dietary change is also central to the management of both Type 1 and Type 2 diabetes. At times this aims to produce weight loss as a 10 per cent decrease in weight has been shown to result in improved glucose metabolism (Wing et al. 1987). Dietary interventions are also used to improve the self-management of diabetes and aim to encourage diabetic patients to adhere to a more healthy diet.

3   WHO EATS A HEALTHY DIET?

A healthy diet should be high in fruit and vegetables, high in complex carbohydrates and low in fat and sugary foods and links have been found between diet and both the onset of illnesses and their effective management. However, research indicates that many people across the world do not eat according to these recommendations. Research has explored the diets of children, adults and the elderly.

- *Children:* data on children's diets in the Global North do not match the recommendations for a healthy diet, and children have been shown to eat too much fat and too few fruit and vegetables (USDA 1999). Therefore dietary recommendations aimed at the western world in the main emphasize a reduction in food intake and the avoidance of becoming overweight. For the majority of the Global South, however, undereating remains a problem, resulting in physical and cognitive problems and poor resistance to illness due to lowered intakes of both energy and micronutrients. The World Health Organization (WHO) indicates that 174 million children under the age of 5 in the Global South are malnourished and show low weight for age and that 230 million are stunted in their growth. Further, the WHO estimates that 54 per cent of childhood mortality is caused by malnutrition, particularly related to a deficit of protein and energy consumption. Such malnutrition is the highest in South Asia which is estimated to be five times higher than in the western hemisphere, followed by Africa, then Latin America.

- *Adults:* research has also explored the diets of young adults. One large-scale study carried out between 1989–90 and 1991–2 examined the eating behaviour of 16,000 male and female students aged between 18 and 24 from 21 European countries (Wardle et al. 1997). The results suggest that the prevalence of these fairly basic healthy eating practices was low in this large sample of young adults. In terms of gender differences, the results showed that the women in this sample reported more healthy eating practices than the men. The results also provided insights into the different dietary practices across the different European countries. Overall, there was most variability between countries in terms of eating fibre, red meat, fruit and salt. Fat consumption seemed to vary the least. Countries such as Sweden, Norway, the Netherlands and Denmark ate the most fibre, while Italy, Hungary, Poland and Belgium ate the least. Mediterranean countries such as Italy, Portugal and Spain ate the most fruit and England and Scotland ate the least. Further, Belgium and Portugal made least attempts to limit red meat while Greece, Austria, Norway and Iceland made more attempts. Finally, salt consumption was highest in Poland and Portugal and lowest in Sweden, Finland and Iceland.

- *The elderly:* research exploring the diets of the elderly indicates that although many younger and non-institutionalized members of this group have satisfactory diets, many elderly people, particularly the older elderly, report diets that are deficient in vitamins, too low in energy and have poor nutrient content.

The *National Diet and Nutrition Survey* coordinated by Public Health England profiles the types and quantities of foods consumed by a nationally representative sample of people of all ages in the UK. Data collected between August and October 2020 showed that consumption of fruit and vegetables was below the '5 a day' recommendation in all age groups; that red and processed meat consumption met the maximum recommendation for adults but was over for children; that oily fish consumption was well below the recommendation for all age groups; that intakes of saturated fat and free sugars exceeded maximum recommendations in all age groups; that fibre intake was below recommendations in all age groups; that mean intakes of folate, iron and calcium met recommended levels in all age groups.

In the UK a large-scale survey explored the consumption of fruit and vegetables and the types of fruit and vegetables by age and sex. The results showed that overall the average daily intake of fruit and vegetables was higher in women, with age differences showing lower intakes in the youngest and oldest groups (see Figure 4.2).

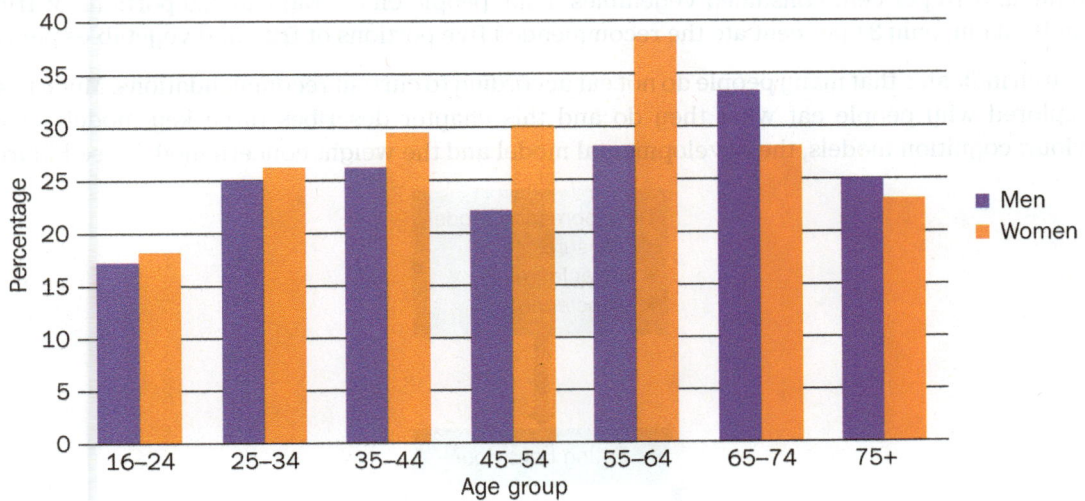

Figure 4.2 Daily intakes of five or more portions of fruit and vegetables by age and sex

SOURCE: Copyright © 2011, Health and Social Care Information Centre annual report 2011 to 2012, Reproduced under the Open Government Licence v3.0.
https://www.nationalarchives.gov.uk/doc/open-government-licence/version/3/

The survey also explored fruit and vegetable intake by social class as measured by household income and showed a linear relationship between income and fruit and vegetable intake, with intake being the highest in the highest income quartile and lowest in the lowest income quartile. This pattern was fairly similar for men and women (see Figure 4.3).

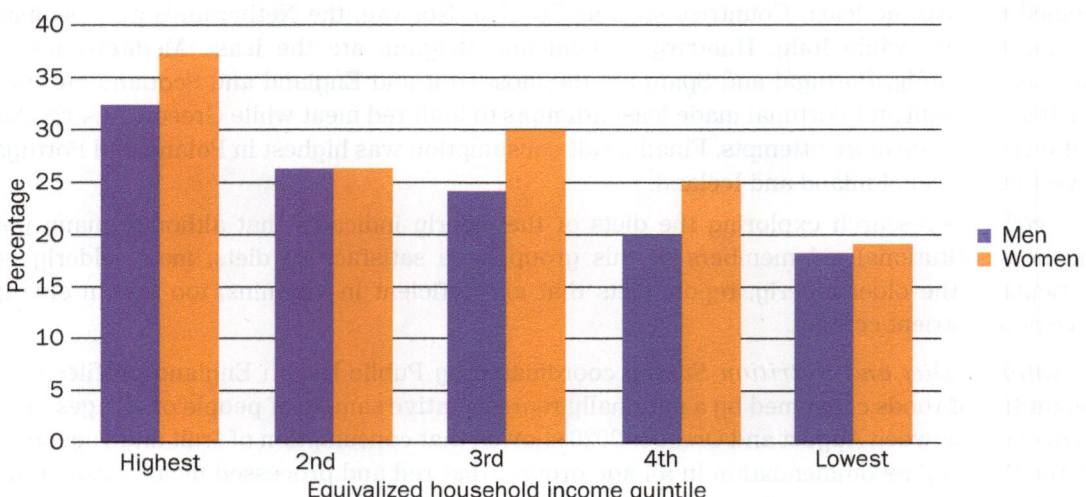

Figure 4.3 Daily intake of five or more portions of fruit and vegetables by sex and household income

SOURCE: Copyright © 2011, Health and Social Care Information Centre annual report 2011 to 2012, Reproduced under the Open Government Licence v3.0

https://www.nationalarchives.gov.uk/doc/open-government-licence/version/3/

In Ireland, a large scale survey (n=7545) in 2021 also showed that most people were not eating in line with guidelines. For example, 36 per cent reported consuming two or more unhealthy snack foods daily; 29 per cent consumed sugar sweetened drinks weekly and 8 per cent drank these daily; 65 per cent ate fruit daily and 75 per cent consumed vegetables daily; people on average ate 2.9 portions of fruit and vegetables daily; only 34 per cent ate the recommended five portions of fruit and vegetables per day.

Research indicates that many people do not eat according to current recommendations. Much research has explored why people eat what they do and this chapter describes three key models of eating behaviour: cognition models, the developmental model and the weight concern model (see Figure 4.4).

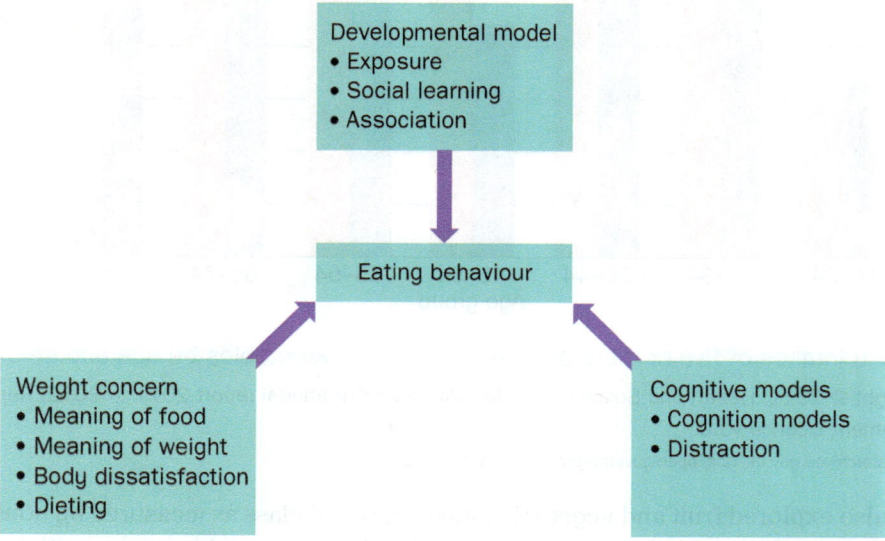

Figure 4.4 The cognitive, developmental and weight concern models of eating behaviour

4 A COGNITIVE MODEL OF EATING BEHAVIOUR

A cognitive model of eating behaviour focuses on an individual's cognitions and has explored the extent to which cognitions predict and explain behaviour. Most research using a cognitive model has drawn upon health behaviour models such as the theory of reasoned action (TRA), the theory of planned behaviour (TPB) and the COM-B (see Chapter 2 for details). Some research has also addressed the broader impact of cognitions with a focus on distraction, memory and language.

USING HEALTH BEHAVIOUR MODELS

Some research using social cognition models has explored the role of specific cognitions in predicting intentions to consume specific foods. For example, research has explored the extent to which cognitions relate to the intentions to eat biscuits and wholemeal bread (Sparks et al. 1992), skimmed milk (Raats et al. 1995), organic food (Arvola et al. 2008) and fish (Verbeke and Vackier 2005). Much research suggests that behavioural intentions are not particularly good predictors of behaviour per se, which has generated work exploring the intention–behaviour gap (Gollwitzer 1993; Sutton 1998a). Therefore, studies have also used the TRA and TPB to explore the cognitive predictors of actual behaviour. For example, Shepherd and Stockley (1985) used the TRA to predict fat intake and reported that attitude was a better predictor than subjective norms. Similarly, attitudes have also been found to be the best predictor of table salt use (Shepherd and Farleigh 1986), eating in fast-food restaurants (Axelson et al. 1983), the frequency of consuming low-fat milk (Shepherd 1988) and healthy eating conceptualized as high levels of fibre, fruit and vegetables and low levels of fat (Povey et al. 2000). Research has also pointed to the role of perceived behavioural control in predicting behaviour particularly in relation to healthy eating (Povey et al. 2000). In addition, studies highlight the importance of past behaviour and habit in predicting a number of different aspects of eating including seafood consumption, having breakfast and the intake of sweetened drinks (e.g. Wong and Mullan 2009). The social norms component of these models has consistently failed to predict eating behaviour. Riebl et al. (2015) conducted a meta-analysis on 34 studies using TPB to predict eating behaviour in adolescents. The authors concluded that attitudes were the best predictor of intentions and that intentions were the best predictor of actual behaviour. Research has also used the COM-B to explore food intake. For example, Timlin et al. (2021) carried out a qualitative study to identify which components of the COM-B influenced the dietary patterns in 40–55-year-olds living in the UK in order to influence the risk of cognitive decline in later life (the Mediterranean-DASH Intervention for Neurodegenerative delay (MIND). The results indicated that the main barriers to uptake of the MIND diet were time, work environment, taste preference and convenience whereas the facilitators were improved health, memory, planning and organization, and access to good quality food. Similarly, Rockliffe et al. (2022) carried out a cohort study to compare the utility of the COM-B versus a Teachable Moments model to explain changes in eating behaviour during pregnancy (n = 516). The authors concluded that neither model provided a satisfactory explanation of eating behaviour during pregnancy and that motivation in particular may not play a key role in what women eat when pregnant.

Research from a cognitive perspective has also developed a number of interventions to change and improve diet. For example, Jacobs et al. (2011) used the TPB and self-determination theory, Gratton et al. (2007) used the TPB together with a motivational intervention and implementation intentions, and Armitage (2007a) and Keller and Abraham (2005) used an implementation intention intervention. The results generally show that such interventions can change dietary behaviour in the short term but that these changes may not always persist in the longer term (see Chapter 7 for a description of behaviour change interventions).

THE BROADER IMPACT OF COGNITION

In terms of the broader impact of cognition, several studies indicate a role for distraction. For example, research indicates that watching television increases food intake in both the current meal (Bellissimo et al. 2007; Ogden et al. 2013b) and subsequent meal (Higgs and Woodward 2009). Further, this impact persists even when participants have comparable levels of hunger (Blass et al. 2006) with estimates of food intake being less accurate when eating when watching television (Moray et al. 2007). Research also indicates increased food intake due to other forms of distraction such as listening to a story (Bellisle and Dalix 2001; Long et al. 2011), listening to music (Stroebele and de Castro 2006), playing a computer game (Oldham-Cooper et al. 2011), engaging in a word counting task (Boon et al. 2002), eating on the go (Ogden et al. 2015) and social interaction (Hetherington et al. 2006). In addition, research indicates that attention to food cues through either chopping food (to make a wrap) or watching someone else chop food (to make a wrap) can increase both food intake and the desire to eat compared to attention away from food cues (Ogden et al. 2021).

It has been suggested that distraction may disrupt the link between food intake and subsequent reductions in desire to eat (Ogden et al. 2013b). Research also highlights a role for memory and it has been argued that distraction interrupts episodic memory formation and prevents the encoding of a meal (Oldham-Cooper et al. 2011; Robinson et al. 2013). This is supported by research indicating decreased food intake when the amount consumed is made more salient by leaving sweet wrappers nearby (Polivy et al. 1986). Research also indicates that reminding participants of recent meals makes the memories of these meals more apparent which in turn suppresses subsequent food intake (Higgs 2002, 2005, 2008; Higgs et al. 2008a). Further, studies show that lacking a memory of meals or having impaired memory such as amnesia can increase food intake (Higgs et al. 2008b). Higgs and Spetter (2018) carried out a review of the recent literature on the role of memory in eating behaviours

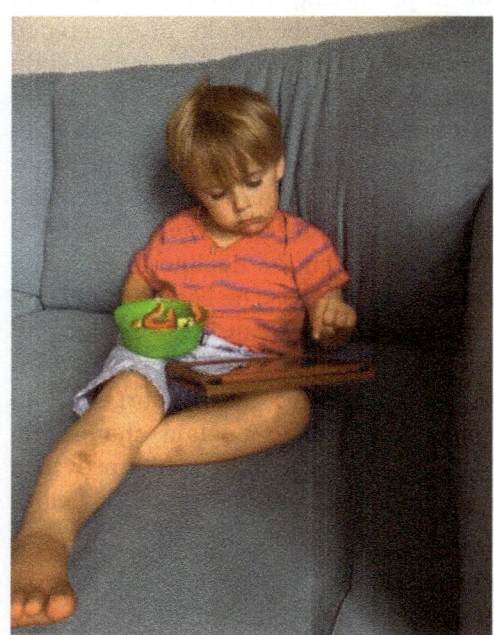

The environment can distract people from what they are eating. This is sometimes called mindless eating. It is a useful way to get children to eat vegetables but not helpful if the food is less healthy

and concluded that both working memory and episodic memory are critical for food-related decision-making, and that disrupting these processes can cause problems with appetite control and weight gain. They also argued that weight loss programmes might be improved by the addition of cognitive training which has been supported by Yang et al.'s (2019) systematic review and meta-analysis. This review concluded that whereas eating behaviour was influenced by inhibition training, attention bias modification training and episodic future thinking training, approach/avoidance training had no effect.

Studies have also explored the ways in which the food environment can trigger overeating by making it harder to monitor how much is being consumed. For example, research illustrates how overeating can be triggered by the ambience of the room, container size, plate size, variety of food and perceived time of day (DiSantis et al. 2013; Stroebele & de Castro, 2004; Wansink et al. 2006a; Wansink et al. 2006b). In addition, research indicates that notions of a 'normal' portion size vary according to exposure to larger or smaller portions, suggesting that changes in the food environment may influence what is considered a 'normal meal' (Robinson et al. 2016). Findings also suggest that not only does the food environment encourage automatic decisions to eat without any conscious processing, but that people deny that the environment has an impact on their food intake (Wansink 2009; Wansink and Sobal 2007). This process has been termed 'mindless eating' and can be contrasted with 'mindful' eating when people are encouraged to self monitor and process what they eat (Wansink and Sobal, 2007).

Some research has also highlighted a role for language on food intake and in the main this has explored the impact of food labels. For example, Provencher et al. (2009) reported that participants consumed 35 per cent more cookies when they were described as containing 'healthy' ingredients compared to 'unhealthy' ingredients. Likewise, Irmak et al. (2011) indicated that restrained eaters consumed significantly more sweets when given the healthier label 'fruit chews' compared to the less healthy label 'candy chews'. Some research has also explored the broader impact of language using a preload/taste test design and indicates that food intake in a subsequent taste test is influenced by what people are told about their preload rather than its actual calorific content. For example, Ogden and Wardle (1990b) found that restrained eaters showed changes in hunger reflecting the stated (rather than actual) content of the preload.

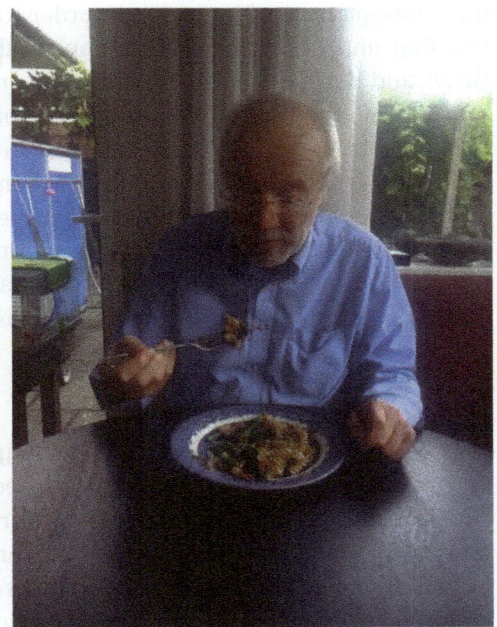

Eating at a table as a 'meal' may help people to eat less later on

Similarly, Crum et al. (2011) showed changes in satiety and ghrelin levels consistent with what the participant believed they had consumed rather than what they had actually consumed. Ogden et al. (2018) further tested the impact of language together with where food is consumed. For this experimental study participants were asked to eat a pasta pot which was labelled either 'snack' or 'meal' and eaten either as a 'snack' (standing up with a plastic fork from the pot) or as a 'meal' (at a table, sitting down with a ceramic plate and metal fork).

All participants then took part in a taste test to assess their subsequent eating. The results showed that those who were told the pasta pot was a 'snack' ate more than those told it was a 'meal' and those who ate it as a 'snack' ate more than those who ate it as a 'meal'. Those who ate the most had been told it was a 'snack' and ate it as a 'snack'.

Eating behaviour is therefore influenced by cognitions in the broader sense and research has highlighted a role for distraction, memory and language.

5 A DEVELOPMENTAL MODEL OF EATING BEHAVIOUR

A developmental model of eating behaviour emphasizes the importance of learning and experience and focuses on the development of food preferences in childhood. An early pioneer of this research was Davis (1928), who carried out studies of infants and young children living in a paediatrics ward in the USA for several months. The results from this study generated a theory of 'the wisdom of the body' that emphasized the body's innate food preferences and Davis concluded that children have an innate regulatory mechanism and are able to select a healthy diet. She also, however, emphasized that they could only do so as long as healthy food was available and argued that the children's food preferences changed over time and were modified by experience. Birch (1989), who has extensively studied the developmental aspects of eating behaviour, interpreted Davis's data to suggest that what was innate was the 'ability to learn about the consequences of eating [and] to learn to associate food cues with the consequences of ingestion in order to control food intake'. Birch therefore emphasized the role of learning and described a developmental systems perspective (e.g. Birch 1999; Anzman et al. 2010; Birch and Anzman 2010). In a recent qualitative think-aloud study (Ogden and Roy Stanley 2020), 27 children aged 9–10 were asked to voice their thoughts while making different meals and snacks using pictures of food. The results indicated how children of this age are transitioning from a passive child whose decisions were made for them to an active child with autonomy and agency. This involved a number of processes including: i) drivers of food decisions (hunger, health, liking, emotions, availability); ii) sources of these drivers (parents, peers, routine); iii) polarized reasoning whereby food was often dichotomized as good or bad. This illustrates the factors involved in the development of food preferences which can be understood in terms of exposure, social learning and associative learning.

EXPOSURE

Human beings need to consume a variety of foods in order to have a balanced diet and yet show fear and avoidance of novel foodstuffs called *neophobia*. This has been called the 'omnivore's paradox' (Rozin 1976). Young children will therefore show neophobic responses to food but must come to accept and eat foods that may originally appear as threatening. Research has shown that mere exposure to novel foods can change children's preferences. For example, Birch and Marlin (1982) gave 2-year-old children novel foods over a six-week period. One food was presented 20 times, one 10 times, one 5 times while one remained novel. The results showed a direct relationship between exposure and food preference and indicated that a minimum of about 8 to 10 exposures was necessary before preferences began to shift significantly. Wardle et al. (2003) carried out a trial which involved identifying a least preferred vegetable in children aged 2–6 years and then assigning them to one of three groups: exposure, information or control. The results showed that after 14 days those in the exposure group, involving daily exposure to the vegetable, ate more of the vegetable in a taste test and reported higher ratings of liking and ranking compared to the other two groups. Likewise, Dazeley and Houston-Price (2015) designed an intervention to improve children's willingness to try fruits and vegetables and examined its effectiveness on 92 children aged between 12 and 36 months old. The children took part in activities which involved looking at, touching, smelling and listening to unusual fruits and vegetables every day for 4 weeks. In a subsequent taste test, the children touched and tasted more of the fruits and vegetables that they had become familiar with, compared to the unfamiliar foods. Research also indicates that the impact of exposure to new foods is accumulative: if more and more new foods are added to a diet, they take fewer exposures before they become acceptable (Williams et al. 2008).

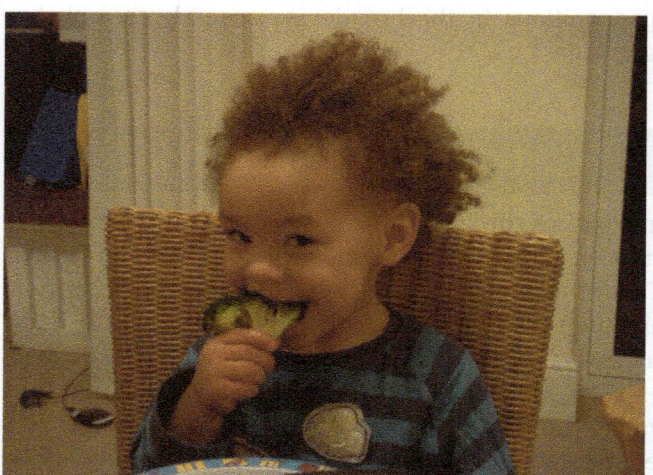

Further, children can identify and are willing to taste vegetables if their parents buy them (Busick et al. 2008). Simple exposure can therefore change intake and preference.

Neophobia has been shown to be greater in males than females (both adults and children), to run in families (Hursti and Sjoden 1997), to be minimal in infants who are being weaned onto solid foods but greater in toddlers, preschool children and adults (Birch et al. 1998). Neophobia is sometimes called being a 'picky eater' or a 'fussy eater' and can be measured using a questionnaire (MacNicol et al. 2003).

Simple exposure can help children prefer healthy foods

One hypothesized explanation for the impact of exposure is the 'learned safety' view (Kalat and Rozin 1973) which suggests that preference increases because eating the food has not resulted in any negative consequences. This suggestion has been supported by studies that exposed children either to just the sight of food or to both the sight and taste of food. The results showed that looking at novel foods was not sufficient to increase preference and that tasting was necessary (Birch et al. 1987). It would seem, however, that these negative consequences must occur within a short period of time after tasting the food as telling children that a novel food is 'good for you' has no impact on neophobia whereas telling them that it will *taste* good does (Pliner and Loewen 1997). The exposure hypothesis is also supported by evidence indicating that neophobia reduces with age (Birch 1989).

SOCIAL LEARNING

Social learning describes the impact of observing other people's behaviour on one's own behaviour and is sometimes referred to as 'modelling' or 'observational learning'. This has been explored in terms of peers, parents and the media.

Peers

An early study explored the impact of 'social suggestion' on children's eating behaviours and arranged to have children observe a series of role models engaging in eating behaviours different from their own (Duncker 1938). The models chosen were other children, an unknown adult and a fictional hero. The results showed a greater change in the child's food preference if the model was an older child, a friend or the

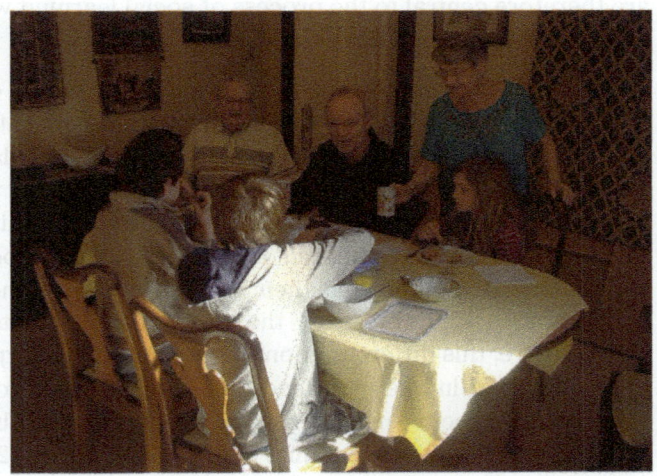

Social eating: food preferences can change as a result of watching others eat

fictional hero. The unknown adult had no impact on food preferences. In another study, peer modelling was used to change children's preference for vegetables (Birch 1980). The target children were placed at lunch for four consecutive days next to other children who preferred a different vegetable to themselves (peas versus carrots). By the end of the study the children showed a shift in their vegetable preference which persisted at a follow-up assessment several weeks later. Similarly, Salvy et al. (2008) asked children to play a sorting task while exposed to cookies either on their own, with an unfamiliar peer or a sibling, and reported that the consumption of cookies was highest in those who sat with their sibling. Furthermore, overweight girls have been found to eat more when sitting with another overweight girl than with one of normal weight (Salvy et al. 2007). The impact of social learning has also been shown in an intervention study designed to change children's eating behaviour using video-based peer modelling (Lowe et al. 1998). This series of studies used video material of 'food dudes' who were older children enthusiastically consuming refused food, which was shown to children with a history of food refusal. The results showed that exposure to the 'food dudes' significantly changed the children's food preferences and specifically increased their consumption of fruit and vegetables. The Food Dudes programme is now used in parts of England and Ireland and is based upon the three 'Rs': role modelling, repeated tasting and rewards. Following their evaluation of the programme, Marcano-Olivier et al. (2021) reported an increase in children's intake of fruit, vegetables, vitamin C and E and a decrease in their total energy consumption, fat, saturated fat, and sodium intake in the intervention school but not in the control school. Food preferences therefore change through watching others eat.

Parents

Parental attitudes to food and eating behaviours are also central to the process of social learning. For example, research indicates that adolescents are more likely to eat breakfast if their parents do (Pearson et al. 2009) and that emotional eating is concordant between adolescents and their parents (Snoek et al. 2007). Klesges et al. (1991) showed that children selected different foods when they were being watched by their parents compared to when they were not, and Olivera et al. (1992) reported a correlation between mothers' and children's food intakes for most nutrients in preschool children, and suggested targeting parents to try to improve children's diets. Likewise, Contento et al. (1993) found a relationship between mothers' health motivation and the quality of children's diets, and Brown and Ogden (2004) reported consistent correlations between parents and their children in terms of snack food intake, eating motivations and body dissatisfaction. Parental behaviour and attitudes are therefore central to the process of social learning with research highlighting a positive association between parents' and children's diets.

There is, however, some evidence that mothers and children are not always in line with each other. For example, Wardle (1995) reported that mothers rated health as more important for their children than for themselves. Alderson and Ogden (1999) similarly reported that whereas mothers were more motivated by calories, cost, time and availability for themselves, they rated nutrition and long-term health as more important for their children. In addition, mothers may also differentiate between themselves and their children in their choices of food. For example, Alderson and Ogden (1999) indicated that mothers fed their children more of the less healthy dairy products, breads, cereals and potatoes and fewer of the healthy equivalents to these foods than they ate themselves. Furthermore, this differentiation was greater in dieting mothers, suggesting that mothers who restrain their own food intake may feed their children more of the foods that they are denying themselves. A relationship between maternal dieting and eating behaviour is also supported by a study of 197 families with pre-pubescent girls by Birch and Fisher (2000). This study concluded that the best predictors of the daughter's eating behaviour were the mother's level of dietary restraint and the mother's perceptions of the risk of her daughter becoming overweight. In summary, parental behaviours and attitudes may influence those of their children through the mechanisms of social learning. This association, however, may not always be straightforward with parents differentiating between themselves and their children both in terms of food-related motivations and eating behaviour.

The Media

Radnitz et al. (2009) analysed the nutritional content of food on television aimed at children under 5 years and showed that unhealthy foods were given almost twice as much air time and were shown as valued significantly more than healthy foods. The role of social learning is also shown by the impact of television and food advertising. Halford et al. (2004) used an experimental design to evaluate the impact of exposure to food-related adverts. Lean, overweight and obese children were shown a series of food and non-food-related adverts and their snack food intake was then measured in a controlled environment. The results showed that overall the obese children recognized more of the food adverts than the other children and that the degree of recognition correlated with the amount of food consumed. Furthermore, all children ate more after exposure to the food adverts than the non-food adverts. Similarly, King and Hill (2008) showed children adverts for healthy or less healthy foods and measured their hunger, food choice and product recall. No effects were found for hunger or food choice but children could remember more of the less healthy than the healthy foods. Likewise, Zhou et al. (2017) reported that participants ate more food if they had watched a movie clip where a character continued to eat rather than had finished eating.

In summary, social learning factors are central to choices about food. In fact a recent review by Cruwys et al. (2015) concluded that food intake is largely determined by social influence, particularly modelling, and reported near universal support for the norms provided by others. This process of modelling includes peers, parents and the media, which offer new information, present role models and illustrate behaviour and attitudes that can be observed and incorporated into the individual's own behavioural repertoire.

ASSOCIATIVE LEARNING

Associative learning refers to the impact of contingent factors on behaviour. For example, food can be paired with specific places, times of day, people or other foods or drinks which can change what and when people eat (e.g. Van den Akker et al. 2017; Cornwell and McAlister 2013). At times, these contingent factors can be considered reinforcers in line with operant conditioning. In particular, food has been paired with a reward, used as the reward and paired with physiological consequences. Research has also explored the relationship between control and food.

Rewarding Eating Behaviour

Some research has examined the effect of rewarding eating behaviour as in 'if you eat your vegetables I will be pleased with you'. For example, Birch et al. (1980) gave children food in association with positive adult attention compared with more neutral situations. This was shown to increase food preference. Similarly an intervention study using videos to change eating behaviour reported that rewarding vegetable consumption increased that behaviour (Lowe et al. 1998). Further, an intervention introduced a 'kids' choice' school lunch programme whereby children were given tokens for eating fruit or vegetables which could be later traded in for prizes. The results showed that preference and consumption increased at two weeks after the programme (Hendy et al. 2005). However, by seven months, when the programme had finished, levels had returned to baseline. One recent experimental study explored the impact of pairing images of snack foods with potential negative health consequences such as obesity or an unhealthy heart (Hollands et al. 2011). The results showed that not only did the pairing result in more negative implicit attitudes to the snacks but it also reduced intake in a behavioural choice task which offered snacks or fruit. Rewarding food choice can therefore encourage healthy eating either by positively reinforcing healthy foods or negatively reinforcing unhealthy ones.

Food as the Reward

Other research has explored the impact of using food as a reward. For these studies gaining access to the food is contingent upon another behaviour, as in 'if you are well behaved you can have a biscuit'. Birch et al. (1980) presented children with foods either as a reward, as a snack or in a non-social situation (the control). The results showed that food acceptance increased if the foods were presented as a reward but that the more neutral conditions had no effect. This suggests that using food as a reward increases the preference for that food.

The relationship between food and rewards, however, appears to be more complicated than this. In one study, children were offered their preferred fruit juice as a means to be allowed to play in an attractive play area (Birch et al. 1982). The results showed that using the juice as a means to get the reward reduced the preference for the juice. Similarly, Lepper et al. (1982) told children stories about children eating imaginary foods called 'hupe' and 'hule' in which the child in the story could only eat one if he or she had finished the other. The results showed that the food that was used as the reward became the most preferred one, which has been supported by similar studies (see Birch 1999). These examples are analogous to saying, 'if you eat your vegetables you can eat your pudding'. Although parents use this approach to encourage their children to eat vegetables, the evidence indicates that this may be increasing their children's preference for pudding even further as pairing two foods results in the 'reward' food being seen as more positive than the 'access' food. As concluded by

Birch, 'although these practices can induce children to eat more vegetables in the short run, evidence from our research suggests that in the long run parental control attempts may have negative effects on the quality of children's diets by reducing their preferences for those foods' (1999: 10).

Food and Control

The associations between food and rewards highlight a role for parental control over eating behaviour. Some research has addressed the impact of control as studies indicate that parents often believe that restricting access to food and forbidding children to eat food are good strategies to improve food preferences (Casey and Rozin 1989). Birch (1999) reviewed the evidence for the impact of imposing any form of parental control over food intake and argued that it is not only the use of foods as rewards that can have a negative effect on children's food preferences but also attempts to limit a child's access to foods. She concluded from her review that 'child feeding strategies that restrict children's access to snack foods actually make the restricted foods more attractive' (1999: 11). For example, when food is made freely available, children will choose more of the restricted than the unrestricted foods, particularly when the mother is not present (Fisher and Birch 1999; Fisher et al. 2000). From this perspective parental control would seem to have a detrimental impact upon a child's eating behaviour. In contrast, however, some studies suggest that parental control may actually reduce weight and improve eating behaviour. For example, Wardle et al. (2002: 453) suggested that 'lack of control of food intake [rather than higher control] might contribute to the emergence of differences in weight'. Similarly, Brown and Ogden (2004) reported that greater parental control was associated with higher intakes of healthy snack foods. Ogden et al. (2006b) argued that these conflicting results are due to parental control being more complex than acknowledged by existing measures and examined the impact of differentiating between 'overt control' which can be detected by the child (e.g. being firm about how much your child should eat) and 'covert control' which cannot be detected by the child (e.g. not buying unhealthy foods and bringing them into the house). The results showed that these different forms of control differently predicted snack food intake and that, while higher covert control was related to decreased intake of unhealthy snacks, higher overt control predicted an increased intake of healthy snacks. Similar results were also found in another sample of parents with small children (Brown et al. 2008), indicating that while some forms of control may well be detrimental to a child's diet, others may be beneficial. Further, in a longitudinal study Jarman et al. (2015) reported that increased covert control by parents over a 2-year period predicted healthier children's diets by follow-up whereas an increase in overt control was associated with increased neophobia. It would therefore seem that controlling the child's environment in terms of what food is brought into the house, or which cafes and restaurants they visit, may encourage healthy eating without having the rebound effect of more obvious forms of control to overeat.

There is a consistent problem, however, with much of the research exploring parental control; it uses cross-sectional designs which limit conclusion about causality. For example, it may well be that increased parental control *causes* a child to eat more. But it may also be that parents use more parental control *because* their child already overeats. To address this problem Ogden et al. (2013a) carried out two experimental studies to explore the impact of imposing parental control versus no control on a child's eating behaviour. The authors chose two naturally occurring times when children are bought chocolate: Easter eggs and chocolate coins at Christmas. For both studies, parents were randomly allocated to either the control condition (limit the chocolate to set times and amounts) or no control condition (allow the child to have whatever they like) and rated their child's preoccupation with the target food and other sweet foods at the start and end of the interventions. The results showed that children ate less chocolate in the control conditions. But by the end of both interventions children who had had their intake controlled showed greater preoccupation with the food that had been controlled. This study provides experimental evidence for the causal link between parental control and a child's food intake. But it could not differentiate between covert and overt control as all parents needed to allow the chocolate into the house in order for the study to take place.

FOOD AND PHYSIOLOGICAL CONSEQUENCES

Studies have also explored the association between food cues and physiological responses to food intake. There is a wealth of literature illustrating the acquisition of food aversions following negative gastrointestinal consequences (e.g. Garcia et al. 1974). For example, an aversion to shellfish can be triggered after one case of stomach upset following the consumption of mussels. Research has also explored pairing food cues with the sense of satiety which follows their consumption. One early study of infants showed that by about 40 days of age infants adjusted their consumption of milk depending upon the calorific density of the drink they were given (Formon 1974). Similarly, children can adjust their food intake according to the flavour of foods if certain flavours have been consistently paired with a given calorific density (Birch and Deysher 1986).

6 — A WEIGHT CONCERN MODEL OF EATING BEHAVIOUR

THE MEANING OF FOOD AND WEIGHT

So far this chapter has explored cognitive and developmental models of eating behaviour. Cognitive models emphasize the role of attitudes and beliefs whereas developmental models emphasize the role of learning and association. Food, however, is associated with many meanings such as a treat, a celebration, the forbidden fruit, a family get-together, being a good mother and being a good child (Ogden et al. 2012). Furthermore, once eaten, food can change the body's weight and shape, which is also associated with meanings such as attractiveness, control and success (Ogden 2010, 2018). As a result of these meanings, many women, in particular, show weight concern in the form of body dissatisfaction, which often results in dieting. This in turn changes eating behaviour.

BODY DISSATISFACTION

Body dissatisfaction comes in many forms (see Grogan 2016 for a review of the literature on body dissatisfaction). It has been described as follows.

Distorted Body Size Estimation

Some research has conceptualized body dissatisfaction in terms of a *distorted body size estimation* and a perception that the body is larger than it really is. This can be measured by asking people to adjust the distance between two light beams to match the width of different aspects of their body (Slade and Russell 1973), by asking participants to mark either ends of a life-size piece of paper (Gleghorn et al. 1987), to adjust the horizontal dimensions on either a television or video image of themselves (Freeman et al. 1984), or to change the dimensions on a distorting mirror (Brodie et al. 1989). This research has consistently shown that individuals with clinically defined eating disorders show greater perceptual distortion than non-clinical subjects. However, the research has also shown that the vast majority of women, with or without an eating disorder, think that they are fatter than they actually are.

Discrepancy between Ideal versus Perceived Reality

Some research has emphasized a discrepancy between *perceptions of reality versus those of an ideal*, without a comparison to the individual's actual size as objectively measured by the researcher. This research has tended to use whole-body silhouette pictures of varying sizes whereby the subject is asked to state which one is closest to how they look now and which one best illustrates how they would like to look. It has consistently been shown that most girls and women would like to be thinner than they are and most males would like to be either the same or larger (see Figure 4.5).

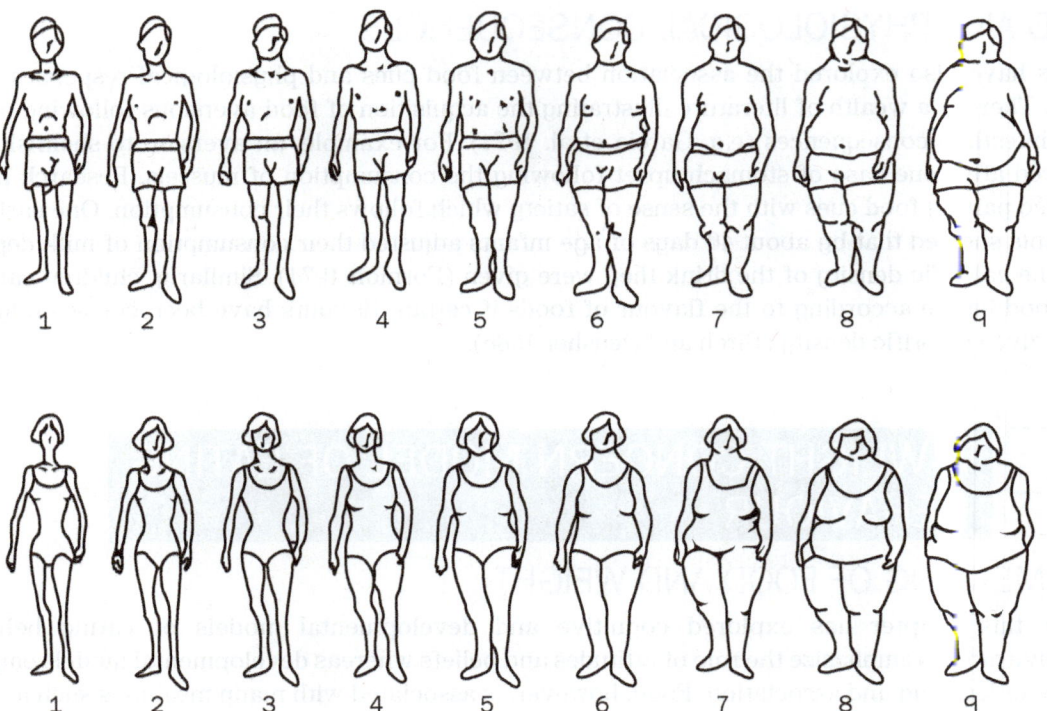

Figure 4.5 Measuring body dissatisfaction – which one would you prefer to be?

SOURCE: Cheung et al. (2011); Adapted from: Stunkard et al. (1983)

Negative Feelings about the Body

The final and most frequent way in which body dissatisfaction is understood is simply in terms of *negative feelings* and cognitions towards the body. This has been assessed using questionnaires such as the Body Shape Questionnaire (Cooper et al. 1987), the Body Areas Satisfaction Scale (Brown et al. 1990) and the body dissatisfaction subscale of the Eating Disorders Inventory (Garner 1991). These questionnaires ask questions such as 'Do you worry about parts of your body being too big?', 'Do you worry about your thighs spreading out when you sit down?' and 'Does being with thin women make you feel conscious of your weight?'

Body dissatisfaction can be conceptualized as either a discrepancy between individuals' perception of their body size and their real body size, a discrepancy between their perception of their actual size and their ideal size, or simply as feelings of discontent with the body's size and shape.

The prevalence of body dissatisfaction has been explored in terms of a wide range of demographics including sexuality, gender, age, ethnic group and cultural differences (see Grogan 2016 for a review). Overall, research indicates that body dissatisfaction is common. In general, individuals with eating disorders show greater body dissatisfaction than those without, dieters show greater body dissatisfaction than non-dieters and women in general show greater body dissatisfaction than men, although men still show dissatisfaction with the way they look. So what causes this problem?

Causes of Body Dissatisfaction

Much research has looked at the role of the media and the family.

The Media

The most commonly held belief in both the lay and academic communities is that body dissatisfaction for women is a response to representations of thin women in the media. Magazines, newspapers, television, films and even novels predominantly use images of thin women. These women may be advertising body-size related items such as food and clothes or neutral items such as vacuum cleaners and wallpaper, but they are always thin. Alternatively, they may be characters in a story or simply passers-by to illustrate the real world, but this real world is always represented by thinness. Whatever their role and wherever their existence, women used by the media are generally thin, and we are therefore led to believe that thinness is not only the desired norm but also *the* norm. When, on those rare occasions, a fatter woman appears, she is usually there making a statement about being fat (fat comedians make jokes about chocolate cake and fat actresses are either evil or unhappy), not simply as a normal woman. Research has addressed whether these representations make women dissatisfied with their bodies, how the process works and whether interventions can make people less influenced by what they see in the media.

Some empirical research has directly explored the association between media presentations of women and experiences of body dissatisfaction. For example, using correlational designs research shows an association between the frequency of reading popular magazines and the importance placed on the images used in such magazines, and factors such as body dissatisfaction, drive for thinness and pathological eating (e.g. Harrison and Cantor 1997; Tiggemann and McGill 2004). Similarly, McCabe and Ricciardelli (2001) reported that greater exposure to television and magazines had a greater impact upon adolescent girls, and Field et al. (1999) concluded from their survey of young girls that the majority stated that magazine images of women influenced their idea of the perfect shape and that nearly a half wanted to lose weight because of the images they saw in magazines.

Other research has used experimental designs and has explored the impact of showing women magazine images of the 'ideal body shape'. Using this approach research suggests that acute exposure to media images for only a few minutes increases body size distortion in those with anorexia, bulimia and pregnant women compared to neutral images (Waller et al. 1992; Hamilton and Waller 1993). Such exposure can also make women report a significant increase in their body dissatisfaction (see Figure 4.6) (Ogden and Mundray 1996; Halliwell and Dittmar 2004; see Groesz et al. 2002 for a review). In contrast, exposure to more diverse images of attractiveness, even for a short period of time can have positive results on women's body image (Ogden et al. 2020; Stewart and Ogden 2021).

Social comparison theory provides an explanation for why media images may cause body dissatisfaction (Martin and Kennedy 1993). Upward social comparisons occur when an individual compares themselves to someone perceived to be socially better than them. If a discrepancy is perceived between the individual and the comparison figure, the individual will be motivated to make personal alterations in order to progress towards the comparison standard. Models in the media signify the societal ideal, so are subsequently used as comparison figures. Upward social comparisons reveal a discrepancy between their self and the media causing a self-discrepancy, which in turn may increase body dissatisfaction (Posavac and Posavac 2002). Not all women exposed to such media images however, show body dissatisfaction and research also highlights *internalization* (Stice et al. 1994; Stormer and Thompson 1996). Body dissatisfaction may therefore be exacerbated by media images of the 'perfect woman' if a woman internalizes these ideals and makes favourable upward comparisons to these images. Accordingly, if internalization and upward comparisons could be prevented, body dissatisfaction may then not transpire. Interventions have been designed for this purpose.

Body dissatisfaction is therefore common particularly among women, and the media would seem to have a major role in both its development and perpetuation. Some researchers have argued that women could be taught to be more critical of the methods used by the media as a means to minimize its impact (Oliver 2001). In line with this, Stormer and Thompson (1996) developed an educational intervention concerning the methods used by the media to manipulate images, making them more 'ideal', and reported improvements in young women's body image and decreased internalization of the ideal image.

Please now study the following photographs and rate on a scale of 1–10, in the boxes below, how attractive you think the person is : 1 = not at all, 10 = very attractive.

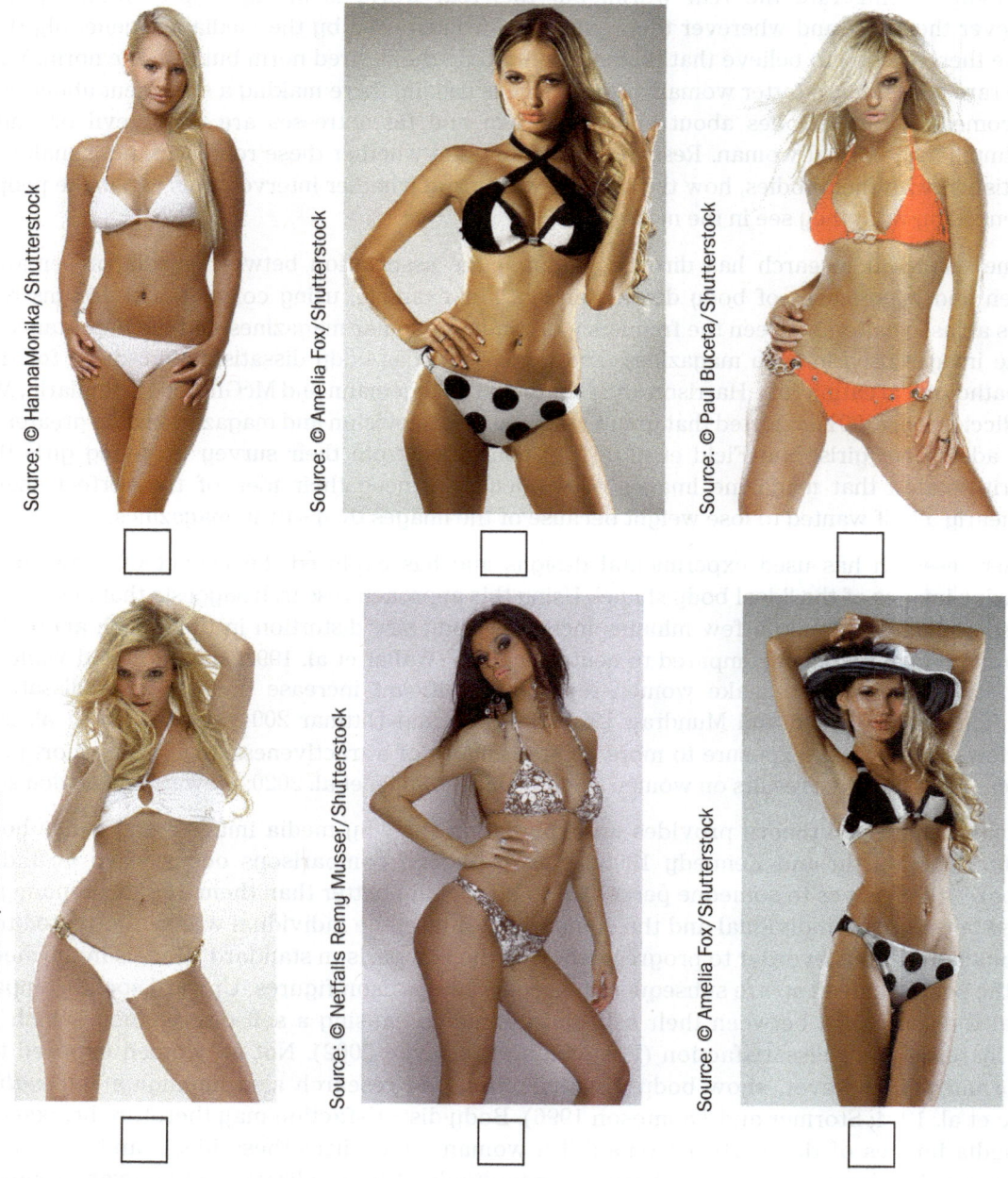

Figure 4.6 Acute exposure to thin images

Similarly, Thompson and Heinberg (1999) developed an intervention to show how images of beauty are created using techniques such as airbrushing and computer-generated images and reported decreases in weight-related anxiety. Ogden and Sherwood (2008) and Ogden et al. (2011) explored whether the impact of exposure to media images of thin or fatter women could be minimized if participants were shown the extent to which airbrushing, photoshopping or makeup can change how women look.

(see Figure 4.7). The results showed that in line with previous research, seeing the thin images made women more critical of their bodies. However, this effect was much reduced if they had been taught about the power of the media to manipulate the images used. Therefore, although women may be influenced by the media, they can also be taught to be more critical of the images it provides.

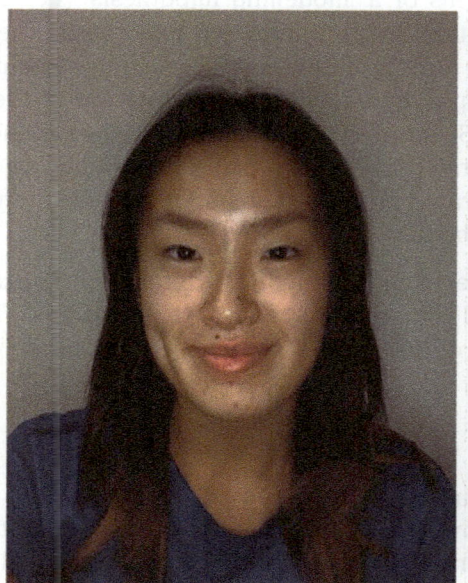 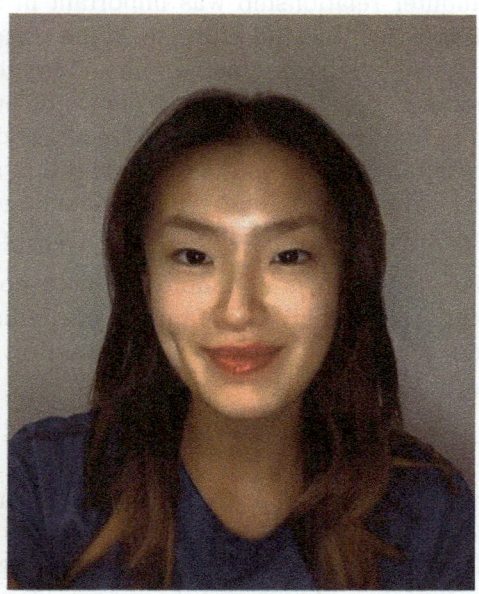

Figure 4.7 The power of airbrushing (before and after)

SOURCE: Photo by Symone Allijohn (subject: Bobo)

The Family

Research has also focused on the impact of the family on predicting body dissatisfaction in terms of associations between mothers' and daughters' body dissatisfaction and the mother–daughter relationship. Studies have highlighted a role for the mother and suggested that mothers who are dissatisfied with their own bodies communicate this to their daughters, which results in the daughters' own body dissatisfaction. For example, Hall and Brown (1982) reported that mothers of girls with anorexia show greater body dissatisfaction than mothers of non-disordered girls. Likewise, Steiger et al. (1994) found a direct correspondence between mothers' and daughters' levels of weight concern, and Hill et al. (1990) reported a link between mothers' and daughters' degree of dietary restraint. However, research examining concordance between mothers and daughters has not always produced consistent results. For example, Attie and Brooks-Gunn (1989) reported that mothers' levels of compulsive eating and body image could not predict these factors in their daughters. Likewise, Ogden and Elder (1998) reported discordance between mothers' and daughters' weight concern in both Asian and white families.

Some research has also explored the nature of the mother–daughter relationship. For example, Crisp et al. (1980) argued that undefined boundaries within the family and the existence of an enmeshed relationship between mother and daughter may be important factors. Likewise, Smith et al. (1995) suggested that a close relationship between mother and daughter may result in an enmeshed relationship and problems with separation in adolescence. Further, Minuchin et al. (1978) argued that although optimum autonomy does not mean breaking all bonds between mother and daughter, mother–daughter relationships that permit poor autonomy for both parties may be predictive of future psychopathology. Further, Bruch (1974) argued that anorexia may be a result of a child's struggle to develop her own self-identity within a mother–daughter dynamic that limits the daughter's autonomy. Some authors have also examined the relationship between autonomy, enmeshment and intimacy. For example, Smith et al. (1995) argued that an increased recognition of autonomy within the mother–daughter relationship corresponds with a decrease in enmeshment and a resulting increase in intimacy. Further, it is suggested that such intimacy may be reflected in a reduction in conflict and subsequent psychological problems (Smith et al. 1995). One study directly explored whether the mother–daughter relationship was important in terms of a 'modelling hypothesis' (i.e. the mother is body dissatisfied and therefore so is the daughter) or an 'interactive hypothesis' (i.e. it is the relationship itself between mother and daughter that is important). The study examined both the mothers' and the daughters' own levels of body dissatisfaction and the nature of the relationship between mother and daughter (Ogden and Steward 2000). The results showed no support for the modelling hypothesis but suggested that a relationship in which mothers did not believe in either their own or their daughter's autonomy and rated projection as important was more likely to result in daughters who were dissatisfied with their bodies.

Body dissatisfaction is common and may come from the media through internalization and social comparisons and the family, particularly mother–daughter relationships. The most common consequences of body dissatisfaction are dieting and an attempt to change body size through eating less.

DIETING

The weight concern model of eating behaviour includes a role for body dissatisfaction as described above. Research indicates that feeling critical of how you look consistently relates to dieting which in turn influences eating behaviour. The term 'restrained eating' has become increasingly synonymous with dieting, and restraint theory was developed as a framework to explore this behaviour. Restrained eating is measured using scales such as the Restraint Scale (Heatherton et al. 1988), the restrained eating section of the Dutch Eating Behaviour Questionnaire (van Strien et al. 1986) and the dietary restraint section of the Three Factor Eating Questionnaire (Stunkard and Messick 1985). These self-report measures ask questions such as 'How often are you dieting?', 'How conscious are you of what you are eating?', 'Do you try to eat less at mealtimes than you would like to eat?', and 'Do you take your weight into account with what you eat?' Restraint theory (e.g. Herman and Mack 1975; Herman and Polivy 1984) was developed to evaluate the causes and consequences of dieting (referred to as restrained eating) and suggests that dieters show signs of both undereating and overeating.

Dieting and Undereating

Restrained eating aims to reduce food intake and several studies have found that at times this aim is successful. Thompson et al. (1988) used a preload/taste test methodology to examine restrained eaters' eating behaviour. This experimental method involves giving subjects either a high calorie preload (e.g. a high calorie milk shake, a chocolate bar) or a low calorie preload (e.g. a cracker). After eating/drinking the preload, subjects are asked to take part in a taste test. This involves asking subjects to rate a series of different foods (e.g. biscuits, snacks, ice cream) for a variety of different qualities, including saltiness, preference and sweetness. The subjects are left alone for a set amount of time to rate the foods and then the amount they have eaten is weighed (the subjects do not know that this will happen). The aim of the preload/taste test method is to measure food intake in a controlled environment (the laboratory) and to examine the effect of preloading on participants' eating behaviour. Thompson and colleagues reported that in this experimental situation the restrained eaters consumed fewer calories than the unrestrained eaters after both the low and high preloads. Some studies also show that dieters eat the same as unrestrained eaters (e.g. Sysko et al. 2007). Restrained eaters aim to eat less and are sometimes successful. At other times these attempts may be ineffective but at least they do not do harm (see Chapter 13 for a discussion of dieting and obesity management).

Dieting and Overeating

Several studies have suggested that higher levels of restrained eating are also related to increased food intake. For example, the original study by Herman and Mack (1975) used a preload/ taste test paradigm, and involved giving groups of dieters and non-dieters either a high calorie preload or a low calorie preload. The results are illustrated in Figure 4.8 and indicated that, whereas the non-dieters showed compensatory regulatory behaviour, and ate less at the taste test after the high calorie preload, the dieters consumed more in the taste test if they had had the high calorie preload than if they had had the low calorie preload. This has been called 'disinhibition', 'counter regulation' or the 'what the hell effect' and has been identified as characteristic of overeating in restrained eaters (Herman and Mack 1975).

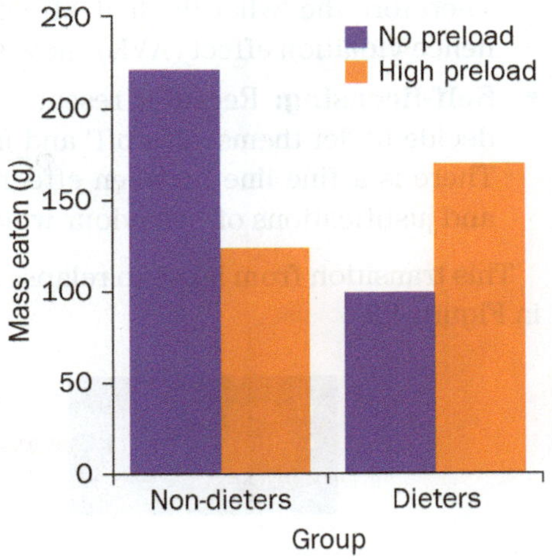

Figure 4.8 Overeating in dieters in the laboratory

SOURCE: Adapted from Herman and Mack (1975)

This form of disinhibition or the 'what the hell' effect illustrates overeating in response to a high calorie preload. Disinhibition in general has been defined as 'eating more as a result of the loosening of restraints in response to emotional distress, intoxication or preloading' (Herman and Polivy 1988: 342) and its definition paved the way for a wealth of research examining the role of restraint in predicting overeating behaviour.

Causes of Overeating

Dieters therefore show episodes of overeating. Research indicates that overeating can be triggered by the following factors:

- **Giving in:** overeating is sometimes triggered by a 'motivational collapse' and a cognitive shift towards a passive state of 'giving in' to the overpowering drives to eat (Polivy and Herman 1983; Ogden and Wardle 1991).

- **Rebellion:** in contrast, some episodes of overeating reflect a more active state of mind characterized by cognitions such as 'rebellious', 'challenging' and 'defiant' and thoughts such as 'I don't care now, I'm just going to stuff my face' (Ogden and Wardle 1991; Ogden and Greville 1993).

- **Mood modification:** Some researchers have argued that overeating enables the individual to mask their negative mood with the temporary heightened mood caused by eating. This has been called the 'masking hypothesis' (Polivy and Herman 1999) and explains why dieters overeat when feeling miserable.

- **Denial:** Cognitive research illustrates that thought suppression can have the paradoxical effect of making the thoughts that the individual is trying to suppress more salient (Wenzlaff and Wegner 2000). This has been called the 'theory of ironic processes of mental control' (Wegner 1994). For example, in an early study participants were asked to try not to think of a white bear but to ring a bell if they did (Wegner et al. 1987). The results showed that those who were trying not to think about the bear thought about the bear more frequently than those who were told to think about it. A decision not to eat specific foods or to eat less is central to the dieter's cognitive set. Therefore, as soon as food is denied it simultaneously becomes forbidden which translates into eating which undermines any attempts at weight loss. Boon et al. (2002) and Soetens et al. (2006) directly applied the theory of ironic processes of thought control to dieting and overeating. Their studies provide some support that trying not to think about food can make people think about food more.

- **Relapse:** Parallels exist between the overeating of the dieter and the bingeing of the relapsing smoker or alcoholic as all tend to have an 'all or nothing' approach to their behaviours.

Therefore the 'what the hell' effect characterized by disinhibition in dieters is similar to the abstinence violation effect (AVE) shown by alcoholics when they relapse (described in Chapters 3 and 7).

- **Self-licensing:** Recently researchers have also explored the role of self-licensing when people decide to 'let themselves off' and indulge in moments of lowered self-control (Prinsen et al. 2016). There is a fine line between effective self-compassion and self-licensing which may be beneficial and justifications of behaviour which may not be.

This transition from lapse to relapse and the associated changes in mood and cognitions is illustrated in Figure 4.9.

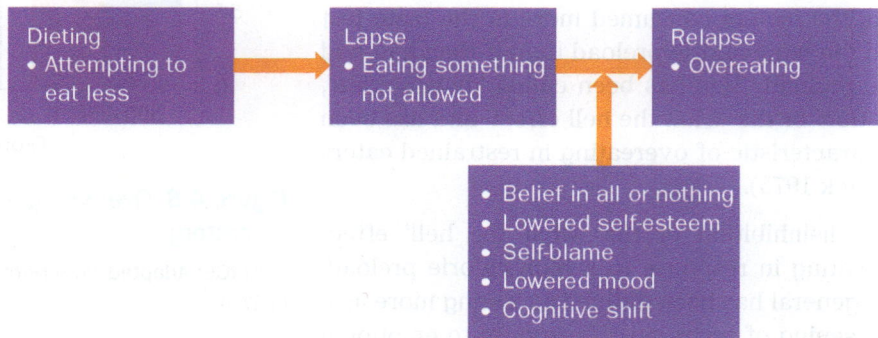

Figure 4.9 The 'what the hell' effect as a form of relapse

These parallels have been supported by research suggesting that both excessive eating and alcohol use can be triggered by high-risk situations and low mood (Brownell et al. 1986b). In addition, the transition from lapse to relapse in both alcohol and eating behaviour has been found to be related to the internal attributions (e.g. 'I am to blame') for the original lapse (e.g. Ogden and Wardle 1990a).

The Role of Control

Dieting is linked to overeating and many different mechanisms have been described to explain this process. Central to these is the role of control. For example, control is challenged by a high-risk situation, undermined by lowered mood or cognitive shifts and problems with control are exacerbated by internal attributions – a rebound effect against denial. These processes are illustrated in Figure 4.10.

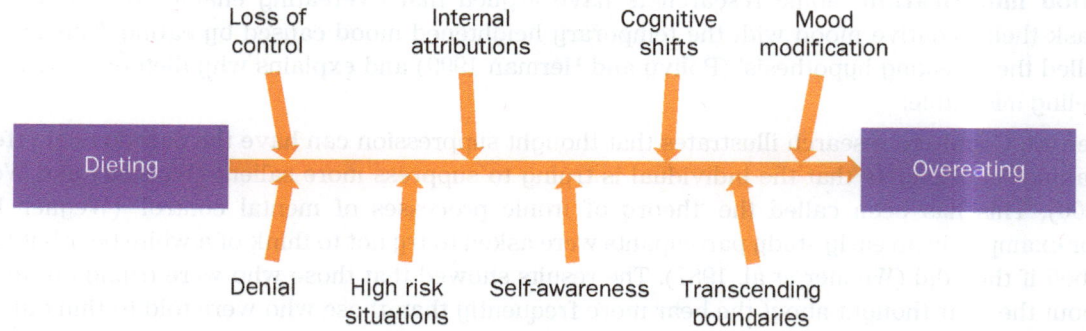

Figure 4.10 From dieting to overeating

Dieting and Weight Loss

A classic study by Keys et al. (1950) suggested that overeating is not the only possible consequence of restricting food intake. The study involved 36 healthy non-dieting men who were conscientious objectors from the Korean War. They received a carefully controlled daily food intake of approximately half their normal intake for a period of 12 weeks, and consequently lost 25 per cent of their original body weight. Keys stated that they developed a preoccupation with food, often resulting in hoarding or stealing it. They showed an inability to concentrate and mood changes, with depression and apathy being common. At the end of the period of dieting, the men were allowed to eat freely. They often ate continuously and reported loss of control over their eating behaviour, sometimes resulting in binge eating. The authors concluded that these effects were probably due to the restriction of their diet. To examine the effects of dieting without extreme weight loss, Warren and Cooper (1988) carried out a controlled study for a two-week period and found that food restriction resulted in increased preoccupation with food. In a further study, Ogden (1995) monitored the effects of self-imposed dieting over a six-week period and reported increased depression and preoccupation with food. These results suggest that dieting can have several negative consequences and that these changes are possibly involved in causing overeating.

Restraint theory therefore suggests that:

- Dieters aim to eat less as a means to lose weight and change their body shape. At times this aim is achieved and they successfully manage to restrict their food intake. Dieters therefore sometimes show undereating. Sometimes they eat the same as non-dieters.

- Dieters, however, also show episodes of overeating, particularly in response to triggers such as high calorie preloads, anxiety or smoking abstinence.

- This overeating can be understood in terms of shifts in cognitive set, mood modification, a response to denial, a lapse or changes in self-control. Increasing or promoting dieting can result in an increased preoccupation with food, increased depression and, paradoxically, increased eating behaviour.

The dieter's aim to eat less and consequently to lose weight is rarely achieved and this failure may be a product of changes that occur as a direct response to imposing a cognitive structure upon eating behaviour. Dieting is also related to changes in weight in terms of weight variability, the development of eating disorders and the onset and progression of obesity (see Chapter 13 for the links between dieting and obesity).

BOX 4.1
Critical Approaches to Health Psychology

Research exploring eating behaviour highlights some of the bigger issues with research in health psychology:

Gender differences: Much research focusing on eating behaviour, particularly that also concerned with body dissatisfaction focuses on women. This is often based upon the assumption that only women have problems with food and body image. It is also dichotomizes gender in a ways that undermines the complexity of this variable.

WEIRD samples: Work exploring eating behaviour is often carried out on university students due to convenience. Often they are also psychology students. This limits the generalizability of the data to other samples. Some research on body dissatisfaction is also carried out on female psychology students. This is also convenient. But it seems more reasonable if the focus is on those who are known to have concerns about body image, as this problem is common among psychology students.

The individual vs social vs political: Food is a political and social issue and the way we eat is very much a product of our culture, our economic situation and the politics of our country. Our individualistic models cannot capture this, they can only capture our thoughts or feelings about food which have been shaped by these outside influences.

7 THINKING CRITICALLY ABOUT EATING BEHAVIOUR

Thinking critically about eating behaviour involves considering the theories used and how they are constructed, the methods used in eating research and the ways in which eating behaviour is measured.

SOME CRITICAL QUESTIONS

When thinking about this area ask yourself the following questions.

- Why is measuring eating behaviour so difficult?
- What problems are there with carrying out laboratory research in this area?
- Much research is carried out in the west. What are the problems of this for understanding eating behaviour?
- The different models emphasize different predictors of eating behaviour. Are these predictors really that different?

SOME PROBLEMS WITH . . .

The problems with each specific model will now be considered, followed by some of the general problems with research in this area.

Problems with a Cognitive Model

A cognitive model of eating behaviour highlights the role of cognitions and provides a useful framework for studying these cognitions and their impact upon behaviour. However, there are some problems with this approach.

- Most research carried out within a cognitive perspective uses quantitative methods and devises questionnaires based upon existing models. This approach means that the cognitions being examined are chosen by the researcher rather than offered by the person being researched. It is possible that many important cognitions that are central to understanding eating behaviour are missed.
- Although focusing on cognitions, those incorporated by the models are limited and ignore the wealth of meanings associated with food and body size.
- Research from a cognitive perspective assumes that behaviour is a consequence of rational thought and ignores the role of affect. Emotions such as fear (of weight gain, of illness), pleasure (over a success which deserves a treat) and guilt (about overeating) might contribute towards eating behaviour.
- Some cognitive models incorporate the views of others in the form of the construct 'subjective norm'. This does not adequately address the central role that others play in a behaviour as social as eating.
- At times the cognitive models appear tautological in that the independent variables do not seem conceptually separate from the dependent variables they are being used to predict. For example, is the cognition 'I am confident I can eat fruit and vegetables' really distinct from the cognition 'I intend to eat fruit and vegetables'?
- Although the social cognition models have been applied extensively to behaviour, their ability to predict actual behaviour remains poor, leaving a large amount of variance to be explained by undefined factors.

Problems with a Developmental Model

A developmental approach to eating behaviour provides detailed evidence on how food preferences are learned in childhood. This perspective emphasizes the role of learning and places the individual within an environment that is rich in cues and reinforcers. However, there are some problems with this perspective as follows.

- Much of the research carried out within this perspective has taken place within the laboratory as a means to provide a controlled environment. Although this methodology enables alternative explanations to be excluded, the extent to which the results would generalize to a more naturalistic setting remains unclear.

- A developmental model explores the meaning of food in terms of food as a reward, food as a means to gain a reward, food as status, food as pleasant and food as aversive. However, food has a much more diverse set of meanings which are not incorporated into this model. For example, food can mean power, sexuality, religion and culture.

- Once eaten, food is incorporated into the body and can change body size. This is also loaded with a complex set of meanings such as attractiveness, control, lethargy and success. A developmental model does not address the meanings of the body.

- A developmental model includes a role for cognitions because some of the meanings of food, including reward and aversion, are considered to motivate behaviour. These cognitions remain implicit, however, and are not explicitly described.

Problems with a Weight Concern Model

Although a weight concern model of eating has generated a wealth of research and provided an insight into overeating behaviour, there are also several problems with this approach:

- Restraint theory relies on a belief in the association between food restriction and overeating. Although dieters, bulimics and bingeing anorexics report episodes of overeating, restricting anorexics cannot be accounted for by restraint theory. If attempting not to eat results in overeating, how do anorexics manage to starve themselves?

- If attempting not to eat something results in eating it, how do vegetarians manage never to eat meat?

- Weight concern is derived from body dissatisfaction which in turns leads to dieting. Not all those with body dissatisfaction go on diets. Some turn to exercise and some live with their body dissatisfaction.

Some General Problems with Eating Research

- Measuring behaviour is always difficult. Measuring eating behaviour is particularly difficult as it is made up of many different components, happens at many different times and in different places. Further, measuring it either by self-report, observation or in the laboratory can both be inaccurate and can actually change the ways in which people eat.

- Much research uses healthy eating as the outcome variable by trying to predict healthy eating or promote a better diet. However, trying to define what is a healthy diet and what foods are either 'good' or 'bad' is very problematic.

- There are very different models and theories of eating behaviour which take different perspectives and emphasize different variables. How these fit together or can be integrated is unclear.

TO CONCLUDE

Diet is related to health in terms of promoting good health and managing illness. Yet many people do not follow the guidelines for a healthy diet. This chapter has explored three models which have been used to understand eating behaviour. The first was a cognitive model with the use of social cognition models and an emphasis on the role of distraction, memory and language. The second was the developmental model which emphasizes the importance of exposure, social learning and associative learning and highlights the impact of parental control on what children eat. The third was the weight concern model which illustrates how the meaning of food and weight can lead to body dissatisfaction and in turn dieting which can cause overeating rather than under-eating. Finally, the chapter described some of the problems with each of the three models and with research generally in this area.

QUESTIONS

1 Why should people try to eat a healthy diet?
2 How do our beliefs influence what we eat?
3 How might parents influence their children's eating behaviour?
4 To what extent are food preferences learned?
5 How could a parent limit their child's intake of unhealthy foods without making those foods 'forbidden fruit'?
6 What are the problems with the developmental and cognitive models of eating behaviour?
7 What factors contribute towards body dissatisfaction?
8 Dieting causes overeating. Discuss.
9 To what extent is our food intake governed by hunger?
10 What are some of the methodological problems with research in this area?

FOR DISCUSSION

Think of someone you know who has successfully changed their eating behaviour (e.g. become a vegetarian or vegan, eaten less, cut out chocolate). What factors contributed towards their success?

FURTHER READING

Apologies – but this is my research area so I am unashamedly putting my own books into the reading list!

Grogan, S. (2016) *Body Image: Understanding Body Dissatisfaction in Men, Women and Children*, 3rd edn. London: Routledge.
An accessible and comprehensive book that reviews the vast literature on body image in a useful and interesting way.

Ogden, J. (2020) *The Good Parenting Food Guide: Managing what Children Eat without Making Food a Problem.* This book is now free and open access https://openresearch.surrey.ac.uk/esploro/outputs/book/The-Good-Parenting-Food-Guide/99604423802346?institution=44SUR_INST

This book is based upon extensive research on children's eating behaviour and how parents can bring up their children to have a good relationship with food. It is written for parents and offers a step-by-step guide. I wrote this as a mum and a researcher.

Ogden, J. (2018) *The Psychology of Dieting.* London: Routledge.

This is my little yellow book which explores the psychology of dieting in terms of why diets fail and how they can be made more successful. It is written for those who want to help others lose weight or those who want to lose weight themselves.

Rumsey, N. and Harcourt, D. (2005) *The Psychology of Appearance.* Maidenhead: Open University Press.

This is an excellent book that reviews issues of body image and appearance concerns. Some of this relates to eating and weight-related issues but it also presents research on disfigurement following injury or illness or the experiences of those born with a visible difference. It therefore takes a much broader perspective on body image than the current chapter in a clearly written way.

5
Exercise

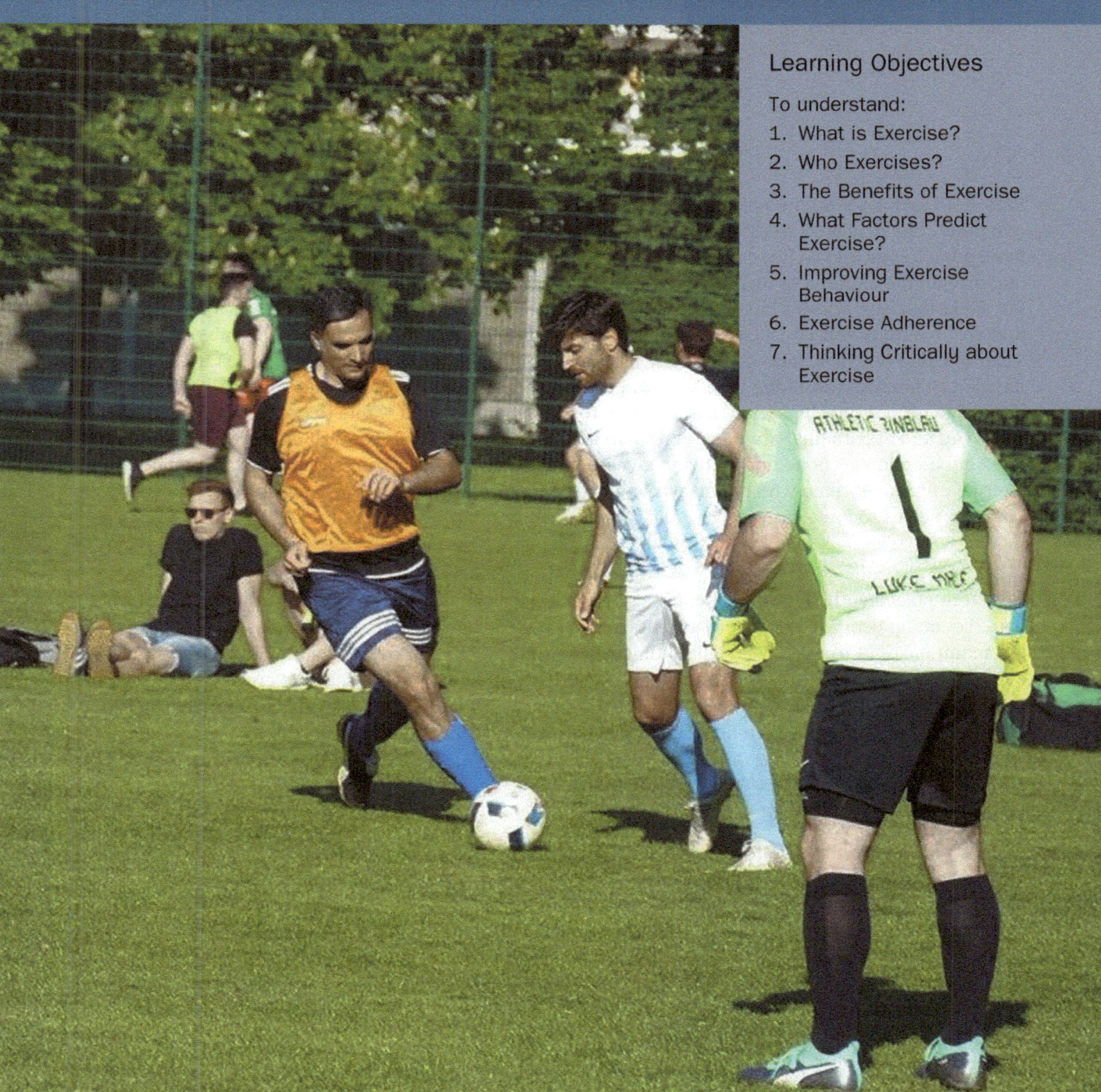

Learning Objectives

To understand:
1. What is Exercise?
2. Who Exercises?
3. The Benefits of Exercise
4. What Factors Predict Exercise?
5. Improving Exercise Behaviour
6. Exercise Adherence
7. Thinking Critically about Exercise

CHAPTER OVERVIEW

Over the past few decades, there has been an increasing interest in the role of exercise in promoting health. This chapter examines the development of the contemporary interest in exercise and describes definitions of exercise, physical activity and fitness. The chapter next examines who exercises and then describes the physical and psychological benefits of exercise and the harms associated with a sedentary lifestyle. It next describes the predictors of exercise behaviour with a focus on demographics, social, cognitive and emotional factors. The chapter then describes how these factors can be used to promote exercise uptake and adherence for the longer term, using interventions which work at both the social/political and individual level. Finally, the chapter outlines how to think critically about research in this area.

CASE STUDY

Safa is 45 and moderately overweight. She works in an office and spends most of her day sitting at a computer. She drives to work and back and is too tired to do much in the evenings after the children have gone to bed and so lies on the sofa watching TV. At the weekends she is busy doing the shopping and driving the children to their different clubs and activities. Safa knows she should do more exercise but feels that she doesn't have the time. She feels too unfit to join a gym or go to a keep fit class and she is sure it will be embarrassing as she will get red and sweaty and won't be able to keep up. Then one day her firm announces a new initiative to improve the well-being of their staff. They have decided to introduce walking meetings and offer a special deal for those who want to cycle to work. They also offer a new lunchtime Zumba class for free. Safa's friend wants to go but needs a friend for company and eventually Safa decides to give it a try. She finds she loves it. It is great fun, everyone is equally bad and everyone goes red and sweaty. Safa then decides to run with the local running group every Saturday morning who lap the park and go for coffee afterwards. She soon starts to like feeling a bit fitter, seems to have more energy and without really trying loses a bit of weight.

Through the Eyes of Health Psychology . . .

Research consistently shows the benefits of exercise for physical and mental health in every possible way. Yet many people remain very sedentary due to the demands of modern life. Safa's case illustrates the many barriers to exercise such as time (a busy life), beliefs (feels too unfit) and embarrassment (of being red and sweaty). It also illustrates the factors which can increase exercise such as social norms (friends), fun (all together) and accessibility (at work). This chapter will describe the benefits of exercise and the factors which limit or increase the amount of exercise people do.

1   WHAT IS EXERCISE?

At first glance the notion of 'exercise' might seem a simple one. But people do 'exercise' in many different ways. Some exercise is a discrete activity and takes time, such as running a marathon, going to the gym and playing team sports. In contrast, exercise can also just be part of daily life such as walking to work, mowing the lawn or doing housework. Further, while some exercise is strenuous and generates a sweat and change in heart rate – such as playing tennis – other forms of exercise are less noticeable – for example, going upstairs to get a jumper or even getting off the sofa to change the lighting. These different aspects of exercise have been defined in different ways according to intention, outcome and location.

1 *Intention.* Some researchers have differentiated between different types of behaviour in terms of the individual's intentions. For example, Caspersen et al. (1985) distinguished between physical activity and exercise. *Physical activity* has been defined as 'any bodily movement produced by skeletal muscles which results in energy expenditure'. This perspective emphasizes the physical and biological changes that happen both automatically and through intention. *Exercise* has been defined as 'planned, structured and repetitive bodily movement done to improve or maintain one or more components of physical fitness'. This perspective emphasizes the physical and biological changes that happen as a result of intentional movements.

2 *Outcome.* Distinctions have also been made in terms of the outcome of the behaviour. For example, Blair et al. (1992) differentiated between physical exercise that improves fitness and physical exercise that improves health. This distinction illustrates a shift in emphasis from intensive exercise resulting in cardiovascular fitness to moderate exercise resulting in mild changes in health status. It also illustrates a shift towards using a definition of health that includes both biological and psychological changes.

3 *Location.* Distinctions have been made in terms of location. For example, Paffenbarger and Hale (1975) differentiated between *occupational activity*, which was performed as part of an individual's daily work, and *leisure activity*, which was carried out in the individual's leisure time.

These definitions are not mutually exclusive and illustrate the different ways that exercise has been conceptualized. Most research nowadays uses the term 'exercise' to reflect discrete episodes of activity (e.g. running, going to the gym, playing sport) and 'physical activity' to describe all levels of non-sedentary behaviour.

DEVELOPING THE CONTEMPORARY CONCERN WITH EXERCISE BEHAVIOUR

Until the 1960s exercise was generally done by the young and talented and the emphasis was on excellence. The Olympics, Wimbledon tennis and football leagues were for those individuals who were the best at their game and who strove to win. At this time, the focus was on high levels of physical fitness for the elite. However, at the beginning of the 1960s there was a shift in perspective. The 'Sport for All' initiative developed by the Council of Europe, the creation of a Minister for Sport and the launching of the Sports Council suggested a move towards exercise for everyone. Local councils were encouraged to build swimming pools, sports centres and golf courses. Although these initiatives included everyone, however, the emphasis was still on high levels of fitness and the recommended levels of exercise were intensive. The 'no pain, no gain' philosophy abounded. More recently, however, there has been an additional shift. Exercise is no longer for the elite, nor does it have to be at intensive and often impossible levels. Government initiatives such as 'Look After Yourself', 'Feeling Great' and 'Fun Runs' encourage everyone to be involved at a manageable level. In addition, the emphasis is no longer on fitness, but on both physical and psychological health. Contemporary messages promote moderate exercise for everyone to improve general (physical and psychological) well-being. There is also an increasing recognition that exercise that can be included in a person's daily life may be the way to create maximum health benefits. The most sedentary members of the population are more likely to make and sustain smaller changes in lifestyle such as walking, cycling and stair use rather than the more dramatic changes required by the uptake of rigorous exercise programmes. Interventions are therefore designed to make people more active and do more exercise. In addition, the emphasis is now also on making people less sedentary.

MEASURING EXERCISE

As with all health-related behaviour, measuring exercise is not simple as all methods have their strengths and limitations. Subjective self-report measures ask people to record how much exercise they do using either retrospective questionnaires (e.g. 'over the past week', 'in an average week') or daily diaries. They ask about specific activities ('climbing stairs', 'walking', 'playing sport') or target a specific intensity of exercise ('exercise to raise your heart rate' or 'until you feel breathless'). They may also ask about the location of exercise ('at your work' or 'in your leisure time'). Such subjective measures are useful for large-scale surveys but are liable to error due to problems with recall bias, social desirability and individual variability in the interpretation of the terms (e.g. 'feeling breathless'). Other studies therefore use more objective measures of exercise such as pedometers and heart rate monitors. These produce more detailed physiological data and are good for small-scale studies. However, they are not feasible for large-scale surveys. In addition, they may well change exercise behaviour as participants are aware that they are being monitored. Finally, some studies involve laboratory measures of exercise by bringing people into the laboratory to use exercise bikes or treadmills. These obviously produce reliable objective data but cannot be used on a large scale and also have limited ecological validity as the laboratory setting is controlled but unlike real life. As an alternative solution, some studies measure sedentary behaviour as a means to measure the converse to exercise. This can be done through questions about TV viewing, computer use or car use and is very useful for larger-scale studies, particularly with children. But again, this approach is problematic because a very active person (lots of exercise in the evenings) could also be very sedentary during the day.

CURRENT RECOMMENDATIONS

Recommendations for exercise have changed over time and vary between countries depending upon how sedentary a culture is and what is deemed to be a reasonable, yet beneficial, level. It is therefore no use recommending that a sedentary population do one hour per day of heart-rate raising exercise as this will simply make people give up. However, recommending too little will have no health benefits. The current UK Department of Health (DH 2011) recommends the following:

- *Adults:* should engage in a minimum of 150 minutes of moderate exercise spread across the week in bouts of 10 minutes or more OR 75 minutes of vigorous intensity activity spread across the week OR a combination of moderate and vigorous intensity activity. Adults should also undertake physical activity to improve muscle strength on at least two days a week and should minimize the time spent being sedentary for extended periods.
- *Children:* every day should include at least 60 minutes of at least moderate intensity physical activity with at least two sessions including activities to improve bone health, muscle strength and flexibility.

Another simple target that has been used, particularly in Australia, followed on from the increased availability of pedometers and recommended 10,000 steps per day. This is a clear target, which can be clearly assessed and some evidence indicates that just wearing a pedometer and/or getting feedback from a pedometer can increase walking (Rooney et al. 2003; Stovitz et al. 2005). Nowadays steps can also be monitored by smartphones, which may make people more aware of how active (or inactive) they are being.

2   WHO EXERCISES?

The Healthy People 2000 programmes in the USA show that only 23 per cent of adults engage in light to moderate physical activity five times per week and up to a third remain completely sedentary across all industrialized countries. A survey in England in 2017 asked men and women about their exercise behaviour over the past 12 months (Sport Participation in England 2017). The results were analysed in terms of broad physical activity types (see Figure 5.1) and specific sporting activities (see Figure 5.2). The results show that the most common broad activity types were sporting activities (23 per cent) and walking for leisure (22 per cent) and that the most common sports were running (15 per cent), taking fitness classes (14 per cent), a gym session (12 per cent) and swimming (11 per cent).

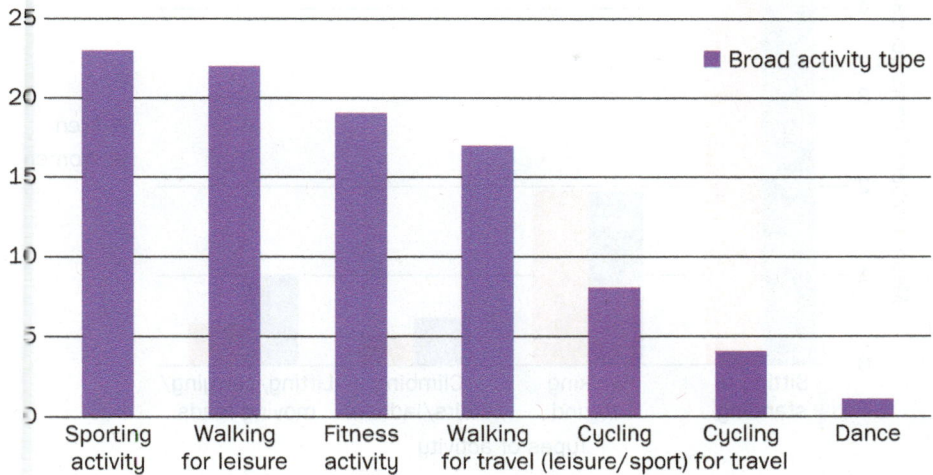

Figure 5.1 Percentage participation in exercise by broad activity types in the past 12 months (150+ minutes a week, England, 2017)

SOURCE: Sport England, Active Lives Survey data, cited in *Sport participation in England,* Commons Library Briefing Paper 8181, 14 December 2017.

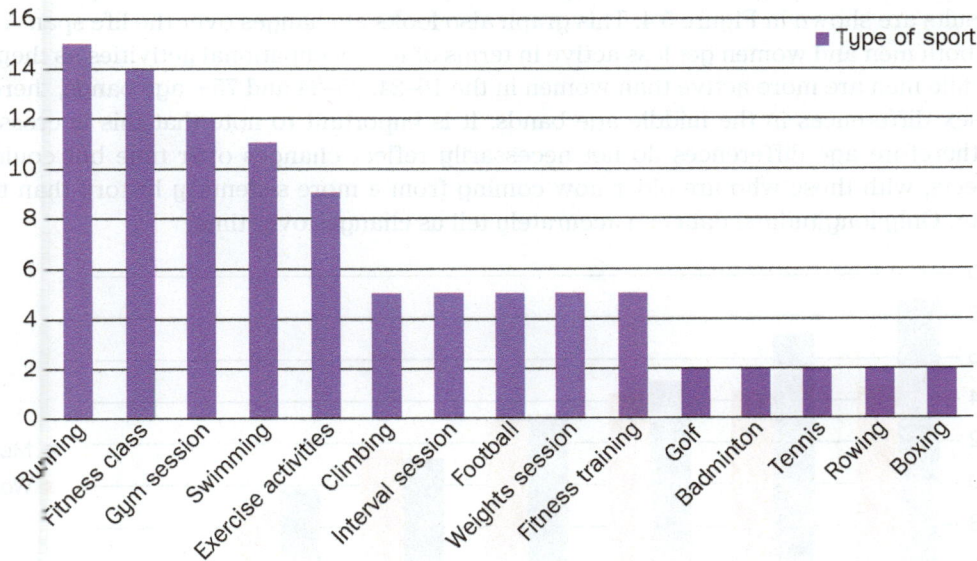

Figure 5.2 Percentage participation in type of sport (England, 2017)

SOURCE: Sport England, Active Lives Survey data, cited in *Sport participation in England,* Commons Library Briefing Paper 8181, 14 December 2017.

A large survey in the UK in 2010 also asked about exercise but this time the data were explored in terms of occupational activities (i.e. sitting or standing, walking around, climbing stairs or ladders, lifting or carrying loads) or non-occupational activities (i.e. heavy housework or walking). The results for men and women for occupational activities are shown in Figure 5.3 and demonstrate that the most common activity was sitting or standing and the least common was lifting or carrying loads. The only main difference between men and women was that men spent more time carrying loads than women.

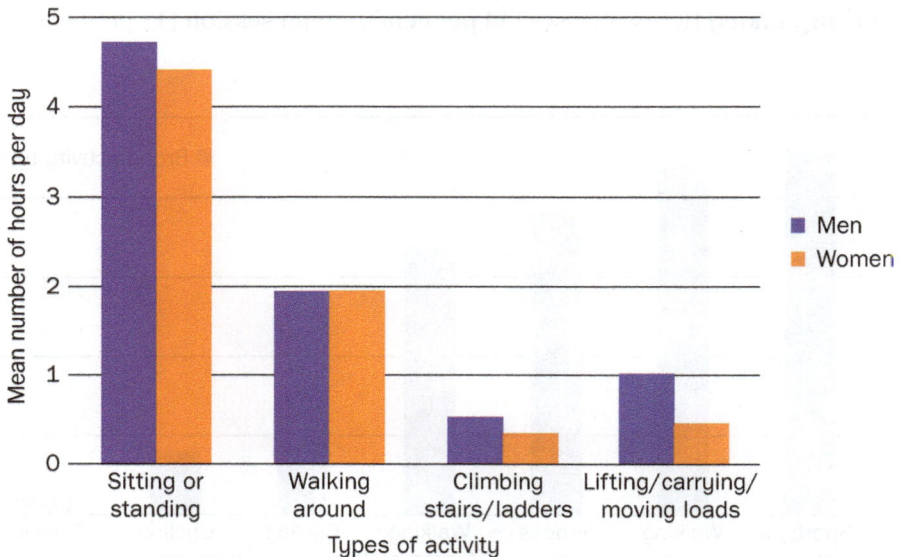

Figure 5.3 Occupational activities by sex

SOURCE: Copyright © 2011, Health and Social Care Information Centre annual report 2011 to 2012, Reproduced under the Open Government Licence v3.0.

https://www.nationalarchives.gov.uk/doc/open-government-licence/version/3/

The data from this survey were also analysed to explore differences in non-occupational activities and the results are shown in Figure 5.4. This graph also looks at changes over the life span. The results show that both men and women get less active in terms of non-occupational activities as they get older and that while men are more active than women in the 16–24, 25–34 and 75+ age bands, there are only marginal sex differences in the middle age bands. It is important to note that this is cross-sectional data and therefore age differences do not necessarily reflect changes over time but could indicate cohort effects, with those who are older now coming from a more sedentary history than those who are younger. Only longitudinal data can accurately tell us changes over time.

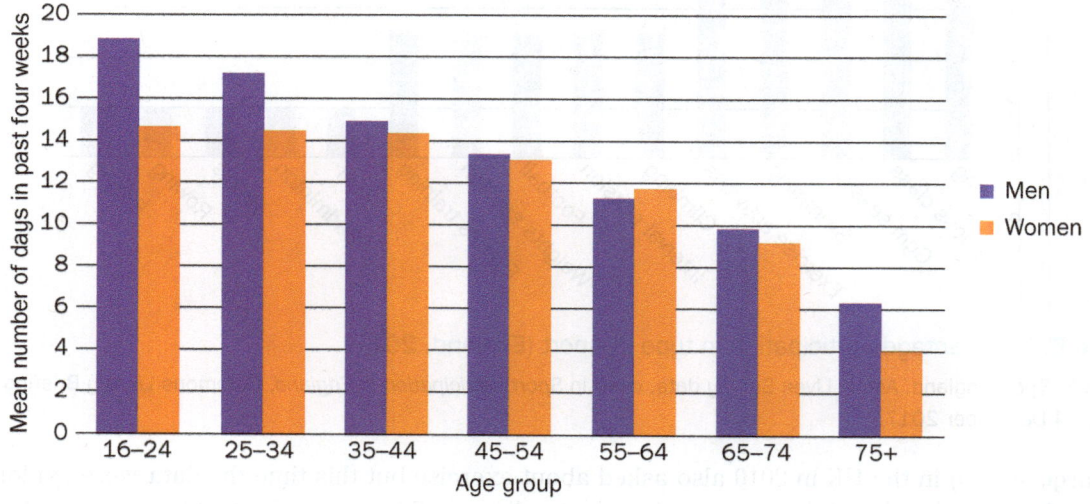

Figure 5.4 Non-occupational activity by sex and age

SOURCE: Copyright © 2011, Health and Social Care Information Centre annual report 2011 to 2012, Reproduced under the Open Government Licence v3.0.

https://www.nationalarchives.gov.uk/doc/open-government-licence/version/3/

In the UK, it is estimated that 29 per cent of adults do not achieve even 30 minutes of moderate-intensity exercise each week (Sport England, 2013). Research has also explored whether or not people reach the target of 150 minutes of moderate intensity activity per week set by the DH. Globally, about 40 per cent of people around the world with coronary heart disease (CHD), cancer and diabetes do not reach this target (Hallal et al. 2012). This rises to about 70 per cent in high income countries in Europe and North America and if objective measures are used, such as accelerometers, then it seems that about 95 per cent of adults in the general population can be classified as inactive (Troiano et al. 2008; NHS Information Centre 2009). Data for the UK for meeting the target by sex are shown in Figure 5.5. The results show that more men reach the target than women and that about 40 per cent of the population report low levels of activity.

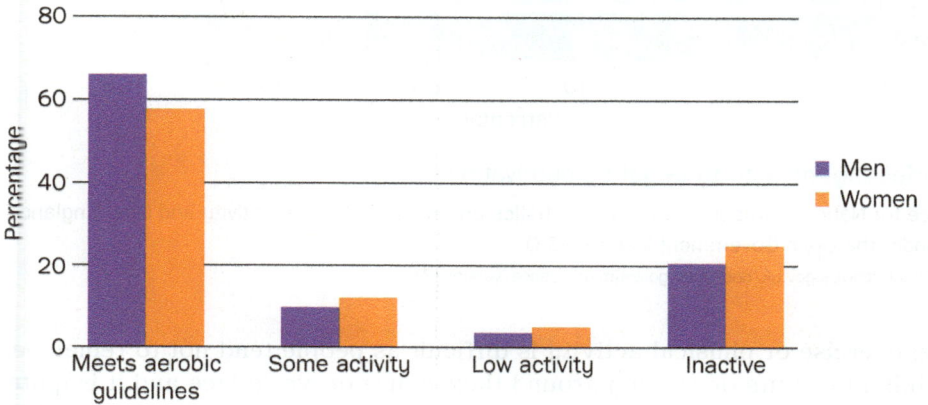

Figure 5.5 Meeting the recommended activity target by sex

SOURCE: Office for National Statistics (2017c), Statistics on Obesity, Physical Activity and Diet, England 2017, Reproduced under the Open Government Licence v3.0.
https://www.nationalarchives.gov.uk/doc/open-government-licence/version/3/

The data were also analysed by age and are shown in Figure 5.6. The results show that younger people are more likely to meet the activity target than older people and that the highest rates for meeting the target are for those aged 25–34.

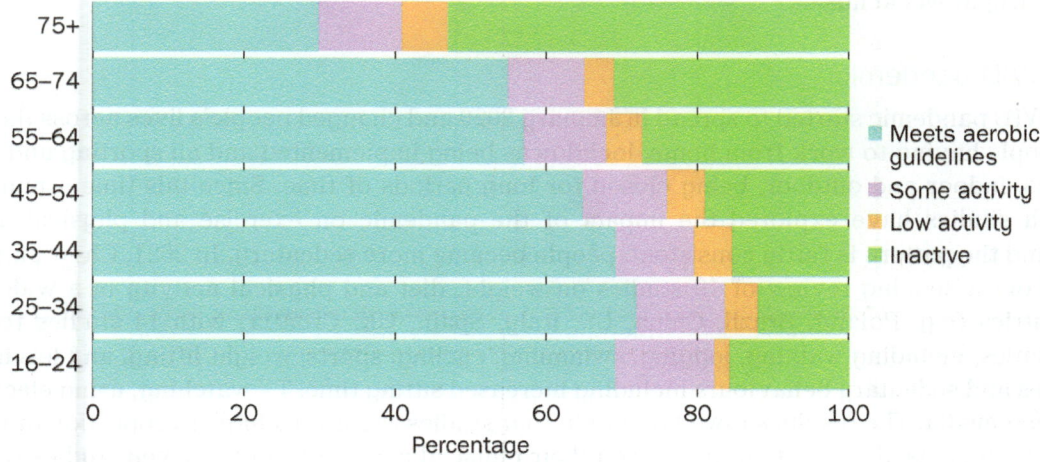

Figure 5.6 Meeting the recommended activity target by age

SOURCE: Office for National Statistics (2017c), Statistics on Obesity, Physical Activity and Diet, England 2017, Reproduced under the Open Government Licence v3.0.
https://www.nationalarchives.gov.uk/doc/open-government-licence/version/3/

Differences in meeting the target were also analysed by deprivation score and are shown in Figure 5.7. This analysis indicates that those who are most deprived are less active and less likely to meet the activity target.

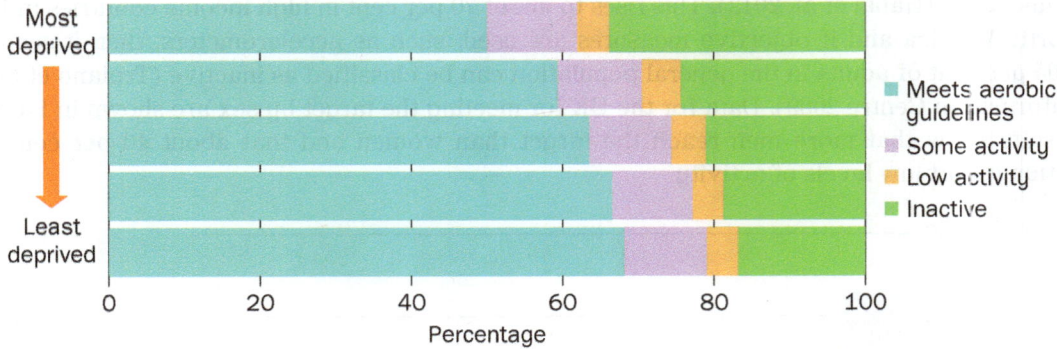

Figure 5.7 Meeting the activity target by deprivation

SOURCE: Office for National Statistics (2017c), Statistics on Obesity, Physical Activity and Diet, England 2017, Reproduced under the Open Government Licence v3.0.

https://www.nationalarchives.gov.uk/doc/open-government-licence/version/3/

Measuring exercise or physical activity is difficult as people tend not to remember small tasks such as walking up stairs or moving around their house or workplace and it is quite possible for two people to spend the same amount of time on any given activity but for one to use up much more energy than the other. An alternative approach is to ask people how sedentary they are and in the UK this was done in terms of watching TV and being sedentary in general. Figure 5.8 shows the data for men and women across the life span on weekdays and at weekends. The results from this analysis show a U-shaped curve with people being most sedentary in the youngest age band (16–24) and the oldest age bands (65–74, 75+). The results show only minimal sex differences for weekday activity but men tended to be more sedentary at the weekend. In terms of TV watching, these data are shown in Figure 5.9. The results show a more linear relationship between age and TV watching with men in the middle bands (35–44, 45–54, 55–64) watching more TV than women, particularly at weekends.

The COVID pandemic

The COVID pandemic started to spread in January 2020 and changed people's lives across the world with people having to work from home, lockdowns being implemented and all sporting and leisure facilities, indoor and outdoor, being closed for long periods of time. Since this time a number of research studies have explored the impact of the pandemic on exercise and physical activity levels and the pattern is fairly consistent: people became more sedentary. In 2021, Chew and Lopez carried out a scoping review of 19 studies on weight, diet and physical activity in a wide range of countries (e.g. Poland, Brazil, China, US, Italy, Spain, UK, Croatia) with 14 studies focusing on activities, including walking, jogging, swimming, cycling, sports, weight lifting, and leisure-time activities and sedentary behaviours including increased sitting time, TV watching, using electronics and social media. The results showed that only four studies reported a higher proportion of respondents who increased rather than decreased their physical activity whereas seven studies reported

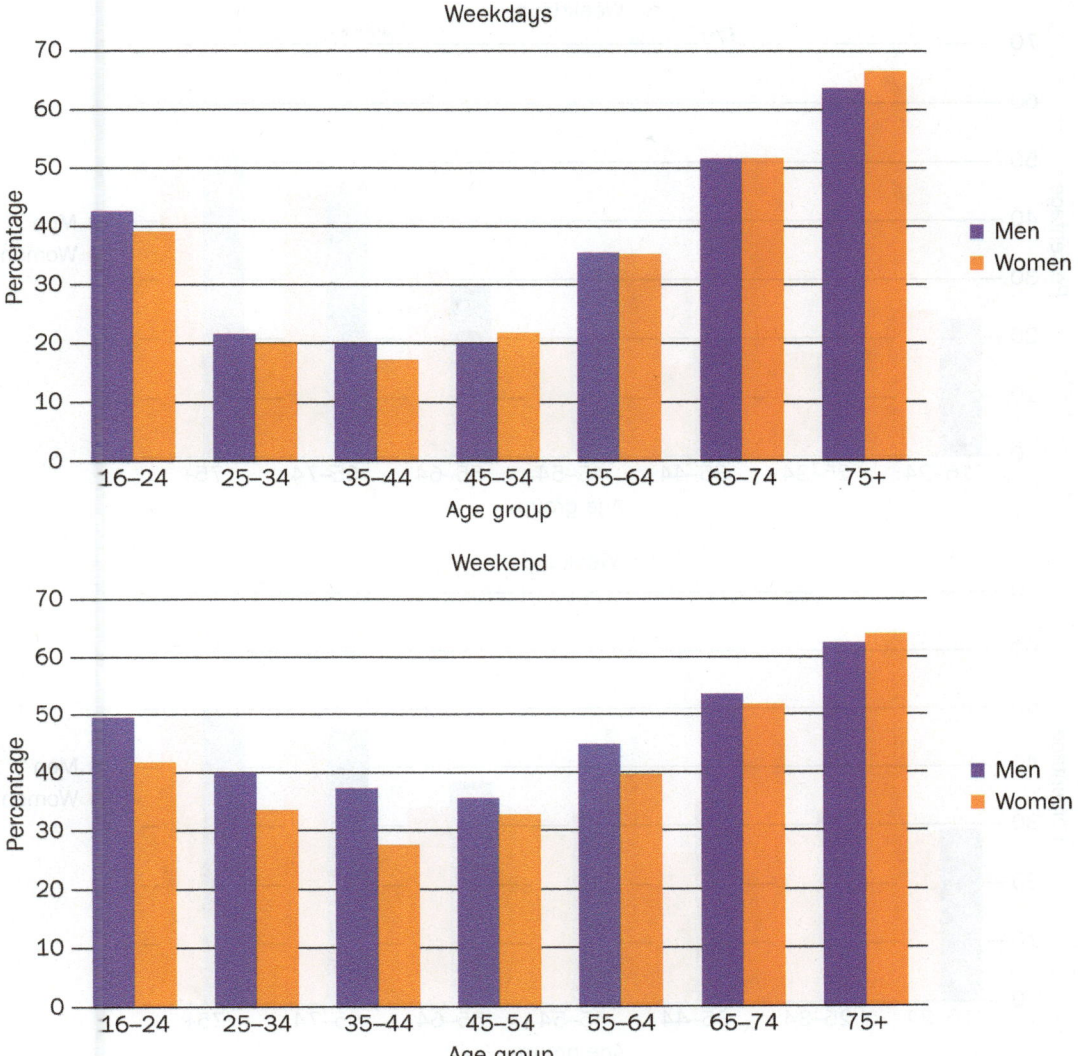

Figure 5.8 Being sedentary by age and sex on weekdays and at the weekend

SOURCE: Copyright © 2011, Health and Social Care Information Centre annual report 2011 to 2012, Reproduced under the Open Government Licence v3.0.

https://www.nationalarchives.gov.uk/doc/open-government-licence/version/3/

the majority decreasing their activity levels. Further, four studies reported a significant increase in sedentary behaviours.

Overall, data seem to indicate that the majority of people do not meet the recommended targets for activity, that generally people get more sedentary and less active as they get older and that men are more active than women, particularly when young, but watch more TV than women as they get older. Further, across the world, people became less active and more sedentary during the COVID pandemic.

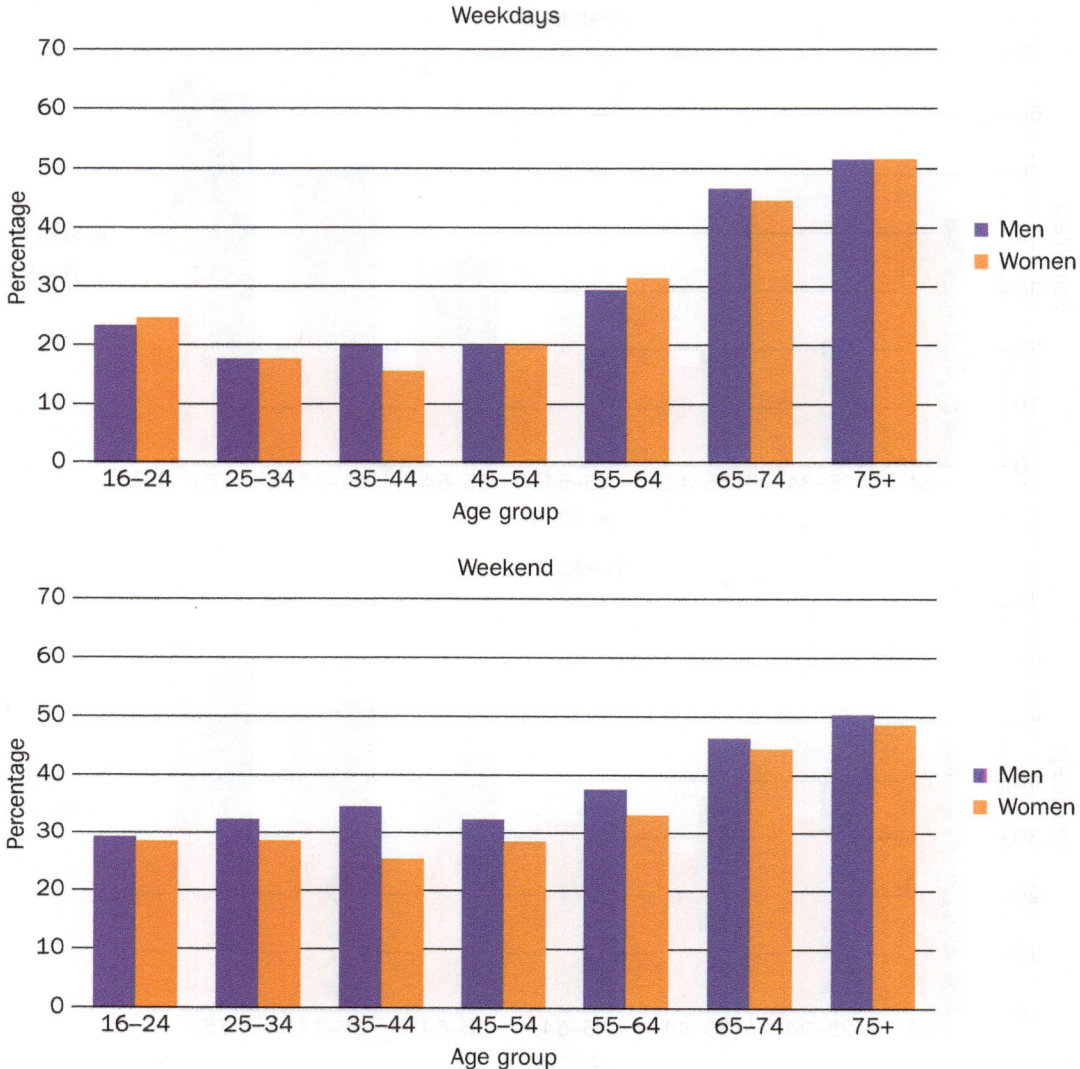

Figure 5.9 Watching TV on weekdays and at the weekend by age and sex

SOURCE: Copyright © 2011, Health and Social Care Information Centre annual report 2011 to 2012, Reproduced under the Open Government Licence v3.0.

https://www.nationalarchives.gov.uk/doc/open-government-licence/version/3/

3 THE BENEFITS OF EXERCISE

Research has examined the physical and psychological benefits of exercise.

THE PHYSICAL BENEFITS

Physical activity has been shown to improve health in terms of longevity and a number of chronic illnesses, particularly through a reduction in cardiovascular disease. It also improves subjective health status and recent evidence indicates that it is an effective treatment approach for chronic fatigue syndrome (CFS).

Longevity

Paffenbarger et al. (1986) examined the relationship between weekly energy expenditure and longevity for a group of 16,936 Harvard alumni aged 35 to 70 years. They reported the results from a longitudinal study which suggested that individuals with a weekly energy expenditure of more than 2,000 kcal on exercise reported as walking, stair climbing and sports lived for 2.5 years longer on average than those with an energy expenditure of less than 500 kcal per week on these activities. Further, data from the Global Burden of Disease protocol shows that physical inactivity is one of the leading behavioural risk factors of deaths (see Figure 2.1 in Chapter 2). In addition, Jefferis et al. (2018) carried out a cohort study over 30 years in the UK and reported that light physical activity was protective against all-cause mortality in older men. Similarly, Wen et al. (2011) carried out a cohort study in Taiwan over 10 years and reported that even 15 minutes a day or 90 minutes a week of moderate-intensity exercise was protective against all-cause mortality.

Over recent years there has also been evidence to illustrate the impact of sedentary lifestyles, indicating that prolonged sitting is related to reduced life expectancy (Buckley et al. 2015). This has been quantified by Lee et al. (2012) who concluded from their analysis that inactivity causes 6 per cent of the burden of disease from coronary heart disease, 7 per cent of Type 2 diabetes, 10 per cent of breast cancer, 10 per cent of colon cancer and 9 per cent of premature mortality, which is the equivalent of more than 5.3 million of the 57 million deaths that occurred worldwide in 2008. Further, Chau et al. (2013) carried out a meta analysis and concluded that adults who sat for more than 10 hours per day had a 34 per cent higher mortality risk, even when physical activity was accounted for and estimated that daily sitting time accounted for 5.9 per cent of all-cause mortality.

Being sedentary also affects children, with research indicating that watching more than 2 hours of TV per day is associated with unfavourable body composition, decreased fitness, lowered scores for self-esteem and pro-social behaviour and decreased academic achievement in those aged 5 to 17 years old (Tremblay et al. 2011). Ekelund et al. (2016) conducted a meta-analysis of data from 16 studies including over one million men and women and found high levels of moderate intensity physical activity (60–75 minutes a day) could eliminate the increased risk of death associated with prolonged sitting.

Blair has also carried out much research in this area and has argued that increases in fitness and physical activity can result in significant reductions in the relative risk of disease and mortality (see e.g. Blair et al. 1989, 1996). Blair et al. (1989) examined the role of generalized physical fitness and health status in 10,224 men and 3,120 women for eight years and reported that physical fitness was related to a decrease in both mortality rates (all cause) and coronary heart disease (CHD). Blair has also explored the relationship between fatness and fitness and the data from one study are shown in Figure 5.10. This study indicated that overweight men and women who showed low fitness scores had a high risk of all-cause mortality. Those overweight individuals, however, who showed either medium fitness scores or high fitness scores showed a substantial reduction in this risk. Fitness was therefore protective against the effects of fatness. This finding has been supported by a recent review of the evidence of the impact of body weight on CHD and mortality (Ortega et al. 2018). This showed that metabolically healthy patients with obesity had a lower risk of CHD than metabolically unhealthy patients with obesity, which was mostly explained by their levels of fitness. The review also showed, however, that regardless of fitness levels (and cholesterol and blood pressure) body weight per se was an independent predictor of CHD (see Chapter 13 for details of risks for CHD).

Chronic Illness

In 2004 the Department of Health completed a report exploring the evidence for physical activity as a cause or prevention for physical health problems (DH 2004). The conclusions are summarized in

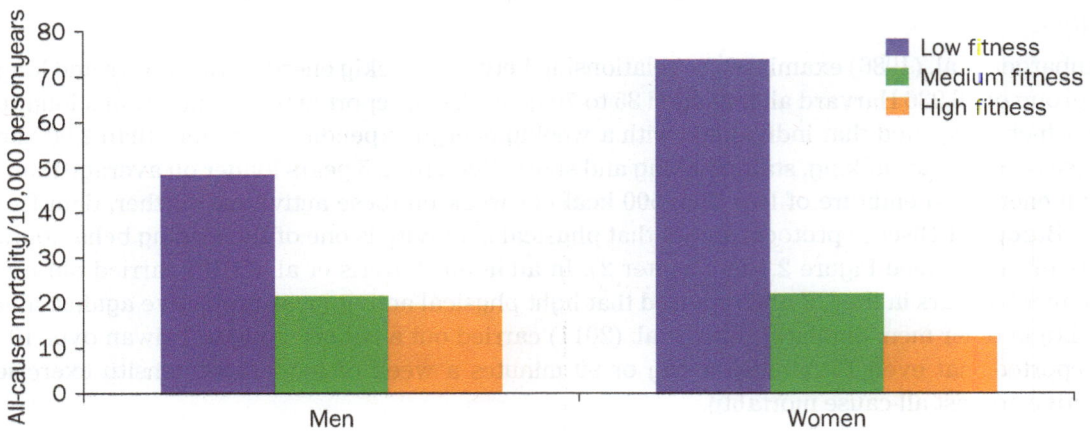

Figure 5.10 Mortality and fitness levels in individuals with a BMI > 25.4
SOURCE: Adapted from Blair (1993)

Table 5.1 and indicate that increased physical activity would seem to prevent many physical illnesses. The report also explored physical activity as a treatment for physical illness and the conclusions were less clear. It would seem that there is medium evidence for a moderate effect of physical activity for treating CHD, peripheral vascular disease, obesity/overweight and osteoarthritis and strong evidence for a strong effect for lower back pain. However, there was insufficient data or only weak evidence for the remaining conditions.

Exercise may also be of benefit for those with HIV. For example, Jaggers and Hand (2016) conducted a review of the literature and concluded that physical activity is both safe and effective in improving cardiorespiratory fitness, metabolic profile and quality of life among people living with HIV and AIDS.

TABLE 5.1 Physical activity as a cause or prevention of physical health problems

Physical illness	Level of evidence	Impact of physical activity
CHD	High	Strong
Stroke: occlusive	High	Moderate
Stroke: haemorrhagic	Medium	Weak
Obesity/overweight	Medium	Moderate
Type 2 diabetes	High	Strong
Osteoporosis	High	Strong
Lower back pain	Medium	Weak
Colon cancer	High	Strong
Rectal cancer	Medium	No effect
Breast cancer	High	Moderate
Lung cancer	Low	Moderate
Prostate cancer	Medium	Equivocal
Endometrial cancer	Low	Weak

SOURCE: Department of Health (2004)

Exercise may influence physical health in the following ways:

1 Increased muscular activity protects the cardiovascular system by stimulating the muscles that support the heart.

2 Increased exercise may increase the electrical activity of the heart.

3 Increased exercise may increase an individual's resistance to ventricular fibrillation.

4 Exercise may be protective against other risk factors for CHD (e.g. obesity, hypertension).

5 Exercise helps the laying down of calcium in the bones to prevent bone thinning.

6 Exercise strengthens muscles, improving body posture and thereby reducing back pain.

7 Exercise may improve immune functioning.

8 Exercise may help smoking cessation thereby reducing the risks of smoking-related diseases.

Subjective Health Status

Research has also addressed the impact of activity on subjective health. For example, Parkes (2006) carried out a large-scale longitudinal study of 314 industry employees to explore the role of both job activity and leisure activity on self-rated health (SRH) at five years follow-up. The results showed that an interaction between both job activity and leisure activity at baseline predicted follow-up SRH, indicating that the more active people were at the start of the study, the higher they rated their health at the end. Individually, however, leisure activity at baseline was only predictive of higher SRH in younger participants. In addition, active and strenuous jobs were predictive of lower SRH although the author argued that this could be due to the confounding effect of adverse work conditions.

Treatment for Chronic Fatigue Syndrome (CFS)

Exercise is used to manage obesity and in rehabilitation programmes for people with CHD (see Chapter 13). It is also used in varying degrees of intensity to help treat a number of other health problems such as back pain, injury, constipation, headaches and diabetes. One area that has received much interest over recent years is the use of exercise in the treatment of CFS. CFS is characterized by chronic disabling fatigue in the absence of any alternative diagnosis and prognosis is poor if it is not treated. The preferred treatment approach by patient groups is called adaptive pacing therapy (APT) which sees CFS patients as having a finite and reduced amount of energy (an envelope) which must be carefully used. Therefore APT encourages patients to limit their activity so as not to exhaust their energy supplies, to detect early warning signs as to when they might be becoming fatigued and to plan regular rest and relaxation and limit demands placed upon them. Up until recently, NICE guidelines recommended cognitive behavioural therapy (CBT) (see Chapter 8) and graded exercise therapy (GET), despite the fact that patient groups report that these approaches can be harmful. GET is based on the idea that people with CFS have become 'deconditioned' and intolerant to exercise and they therefore need to build up their strength and improve their energy levels through exercise. The treatment involves an identification of baseline levels and negotiated, incremental increases in activity levels, usually through walking. A large-scale randomized trial explored the impact of interventions based on either CBT, APT and GET compared to specialist medical care, alone or with the other treatments (White et al. 2011). The main outcome variables were fatigue and physical function and the results showed that after one year, compared to APT, both CBT and GET were associated with less fatigue and better physical function. Of the 641 patients, only 9 showed adverse reactions which were equally spread across the different groups. The authors concluded that both CBT and GET can be added to standard medical care to improve fatigue and that these treatments are both effective and safe. This illustrates the contrast between a deconditioning model of CFS which recommends exercise versus an envelope model of CFS which recommends energy preservation.

Exercise therefore influences longevity, mortality, subjective health status and chronic illnesses. It is also used as a treatment for many chronic and acute conditions.

THE PSYCHOLOGICAL BENEFITS

Research indicates that exercise may improve psychological well-being in terms of depression, positive and negative mood, responses to stress, body image and smoking withdrawal.

Depression

In line with recent research on the impact of inactivity on physical health, Zhai et al. (2015) conducted a meta-analysis on 24 studies and reported that sedentary behaviour was associated with an increased risk of depression. Over the past few decades research has also explored the impact of exercise on reducing depression. In 2012, Rimer et al. carried out a systematic review and meta-analysis, which is published as part of the Cochrane Reviews database. Their search criteria identified 32 randomized control trials (n = 1,858) which compared exercise to standard treatment, no treatment or a placebo treatment in adults (aged 18 and over) with depression, excluding postnatal depression. Thirty studies were included in the meta-analyses. When compared to no treatment or a control intervention the results showed a moderate clinical effect of exercise. However, when compared to CBT the results showed no added benefit of exercise. Further, when the analysis was redone on the four most robust trials the moderate effect was reduced to a small effect size. The authors concluded that exercise improves depression in adults diagnosed with depression but that these results should be treated with an element of caution given the methodological problems with some of the studies. In a similar vein, Larun et al. (2006) carried out a narrative review of the effectiveness of exercise for treating depression in children and adolescents. Their search identified 16 studies (n = 1,191) with participants aged 11 to 19 years of age. The sample of studies was very mixed in terms of type of exercise used in the interventions, definition and measurement of depression and the control group used, which limited their conclusion. They report, however, that there is some evidence that exercise has a small effect on depression in this population.

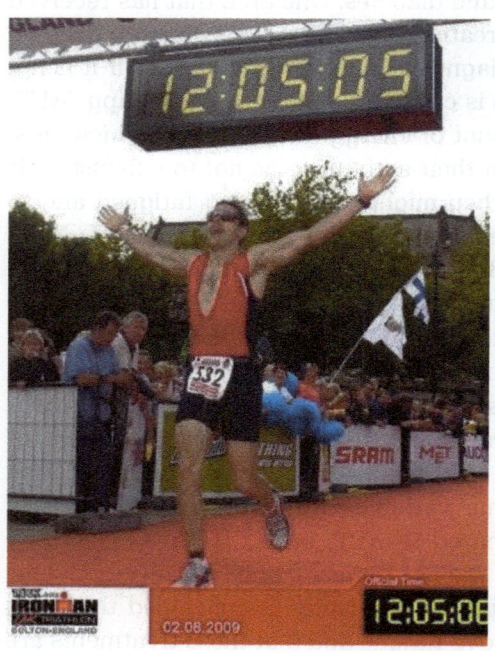

Exercise can enhance mood and create feelings of pleasure

Positive and Negative Mood

Research has also explored the impact of exercise on mood in general in terms of positive and negative mood and feelings of pleasure.

Crush et al. (2018) used a randomized controlled trial design to investigate the impact of exercise on mood in 352 healthy adults. The results showed that moderate-intensity exercise had a beneficial effect on feelings of depression, hostility and fatigue regardless of exercise duration and recovery period. Likewise, Hall et al. (2002) used an experimental design to explore the relationship between exercise and affect with 30 volunteers rating their affective state every minute as they ran on a treadmill. The results showed improvements in affect from baseline to follow-up. The results, however, also showed a brief deterioration in mood mid-exercise. The authors suggest that although prolonged exercise may improve mood, this dip in mood may explain why people fail to adhere to exercise programmes. Lind et al. (2008) also explored the impact of exercise on mood but differentiated between exercise at a desired level of intensity and that which exceeded this level. In their experimental study 25 middle-aged sedentary women took part in two treadmill sessions. For one they selected the desired speed and for one the speed was raised 10 per cent above the level selected. They then rated their pleasure. The results showed that pleasure ratings were stable for the selected speed but decreased in the raised speed condition. The researchers argued that new exercisers may experience displeasure if they are pushed too far and that this might explain non-adherence to exercise regimens. Parfitt et al. (2006) also explored the impact of exercise intensity on affect but focused on levels that were either self-selected or above or below the anaerobic threshold. Twelve participants took part in the three conditions in randomized order and the results showed that affective ratings during exercise were lowest in the above anaerobic threshold compared to the self-selected or below anaerobic threshold. This again suggests that pushing people too far may be a deterrent to exercise and that self-selected levels may be the most effective way to promote continued physical activity.

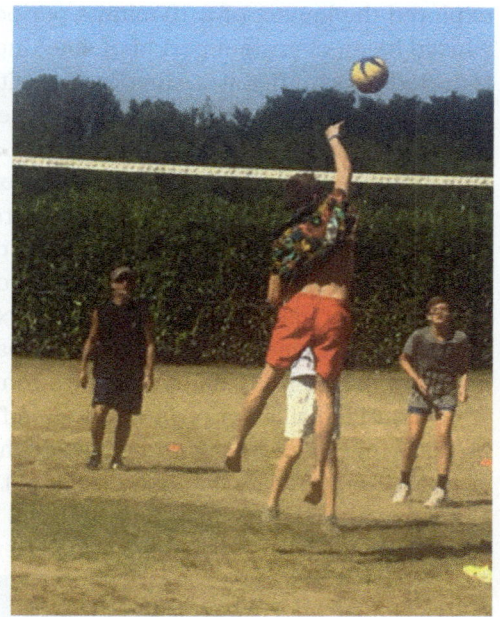

Exercise is an effective way to manage stress and let off steam

Response to Stress

Exercise has been presented as a mediating factor for the stress response (see Chapter 10). Exercise may influence stress either by changing an individual's appraisal of a potentially stressful event by distraction or diversion (e.g. 'This situation could be stressful but if I exercise I will not have to think about it') or may act as a potential coping strategy to be activated once an event has been appraised as stressful (e.g. 'Although the situation is stressful, I shall now exercise to take my mind off things'). Burg et al. (2017) examined the bi-directional relationship between stress and exercise and concluded that not only does increased exercise lead to stress reduction but also that increased stress leads to reduced exercise.

Body Image and Self-Esteem

It has also been suggested that exercise may enhance an individual's psychological well-being by improving body image and self-esteem. Many studies have been carried out on the links between body image and exercise and in 2006 Hausenblas and Fallon carried out a meta-analysis of the results. They identified 121 studies using either cross-sectional designs (i.e. exercisers versus non-exercisers), experimental designs (i.e. before and after an exercise intervention compared to a control group) or cohort studies (i.e. before and after exercise). Overall, the results indicated small effect sizes indicating a moderate impact of exercise. However, exercisers had a more positive body image than non-exercisers, exercise resulted in improved body image compared to a control group and body image improved from before to after exercise. There are many possible explanations for this effect, including the impact of exercise on mood (which in turn influences body image), changes in actual body shape and size and changes in energy levels.

Smoking Withdrawal

Many people experience withdrawal symptoms such as agitation, irritability and restlessness when they have stopped smoking, even for just a few hours. Some research has explored the effectiveness of exercise at reducing withdrawal symptoms following smoking cessation. For example, Ussher et al. (2001)

explored the impact of a 10-minute period of exercise of moderate intensity on withdrawal symptoms caused by an overnight period of smoking cessation. The results showed that those who had exercised reported a significant reduction in withdrawal symptoms while exercising, which lasted up to 15 minutes post-exercise. In a similar vein, Daniel et al. (2006) examined the impact of either light intensity or moderate intensity exercise and reported that only moderate intensity exercise reduced withdrawal symptoms. As a means to explore why exercise might have this effect, the researchers compared exercise with a cognitive distraction task to see whether the benefits of exercise were due to exercise per se or just the process of doing something to take one's mind off smoking. The results showed that exercise was still more effective when compared to the distraction task. In addition, this effect was not just due to the impact of exercise on mood. In 2013, Haasova et al. carried out a systematic review and meta-analysis of the impact of acute physical activity on cigarette cravings measured as either the desire to smoke or the strength of the desire to smoke. Their search identified 19 studies which fulfilled their criteria and had sufficient information for analysis. They concluded from their analysis that there was strong evidence that physical activity reduces cigarette craving. Likewise, there is also some evidence that exercise might be a useful for those undergoing treatment for substance use (Fagan et al. 2021).

4 | WHAT FACTORS PREDICT EXERCISE?

Because of the potential benefits of exercise, research has evaluated which factors are related to exercise behaviour. The determinants of exercise can be categorized as demographic, social, cognitive and emotional (see Figure 5.11).

DEMOGRAPHIC DETERMINANTS

Dishman (1982) reported that non-modifiable factors such as age, education, smoking, ease of access to facilities, body fat/weight and self-motivation were good predictors of exercise. King et al. (1992) evaluated the factors predicting being active in leisure time. They described the profile of an active individual as younger, better educated, more affluent and more likely to be male. Aggio et al. (2018) conducted a large scale cohort study to investigate the predictors of physical activity during the transition

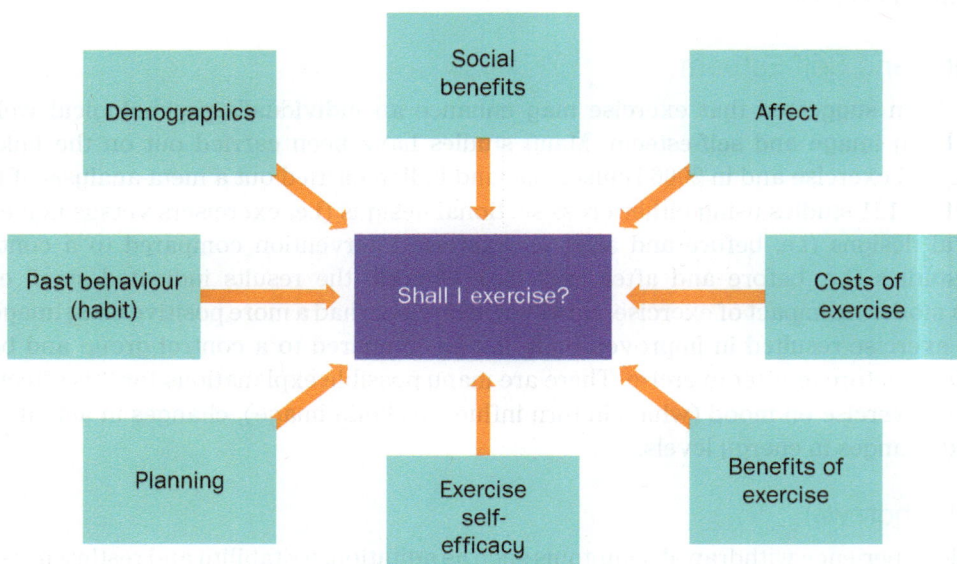

Figure 5.11 Predictors of exercise

into old age in men. Men (n = 7,735) aged 40–59 were recruited in 1978–80 and were followed up after 12, 16 and 20 years. The results showed that becoming less active as they got older was predicted by having a manual occupation, having never married or had children, residing in the Midlands or North of England, suffering from a range of health conditions, being a smoker/ex-smoker and never consuming breakfast cereal. Recently, Zaman et al. (2021) carried out a mixed-methods study to explore the determinants of exercise behaviour in individuals with Parkinson' disease (n = 30). The results showed that the best predictors of exercise were being male, married and enjoyment of exercise whereas fear of falling, negative perceptions of health, perception of Parkinson's disease symptoms, bad weather and lack of exercise partner were negative predictors of exercise.

SOCIAL DETERMINANTS

Research examining the predictors of exercise behaviour consistently suggests that the main factors motivating exercise are the beliefs that it is enjoyable and provides social contact. For example, Hardy and Grogan (2009) carried out a qualitative study to explore the reasons for exercising in older adults (aged 52–87) and concluded that although they exercised to prevent a decline in their health status, other key factors included the role of other people who helped keep them motivated. Beck et al. (2010) likewise reported a key role for social factors in their study of activity in retirement, alongside a need for a sense of purpose and a source of personal challenge. Further, Molloy et al. (2010)

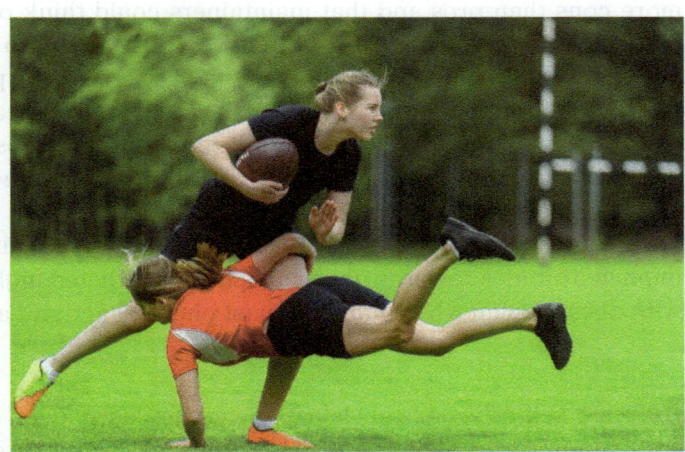

Social contact and fun encourage exercise

© Shutterstock/sportoakimirka

reported an important role for social support for physical activity in their study of 903 university students, particularly for women. Exercise therefore seems more likely to happen if it is a social activity which brings with it social benefits. Similarly, Lawman and Wilson (2014) reported that parental and neighbourhood support was associated with light physical activity in a sample of 181 overweight and obese adolescents but not with either moderate or vigorous physical activity.

COGNITIVE AND EMOTIONAL DETERMINANTS

Much research has explored the cognitive and emotional predictors of exercise using models such as the theory of planned behaviour (TPB), protection motivation theory (PMT), the COM-B and the stages of change model (SOC) (see Chapter 2 for details). Research has also explored differences in attitudes between those who exercise and those who do not, and the role of baseline variables in predicting exercise at follow-up. From these studies some key variables emerge as consistently predictive of exercise.

Costs and Benefits of Exercise

Exercisers have also been shown to differ from non-exercisers in their beliefs about the benefits of exercise. For example, a study of older women (aged 60–89) indicated that exercisers reported a higher rating for the health value of exercise, reported greater enjoyment of exercise, rated their discomfort from exercise as lower and perceived exercise programmes to be more easily available than non-exercisers (Paxton et al. 1997). Hausenblas et al. (2001) argued that it is not only the benefits of exercise that promote the activity but also the barriers to exercise that prevent uptake. They developed a questionnaire entitled the Temptation to Not Exercise Scale which measured two forms of barrier: 'affect' and 'competing demands'. Subjects are asked to rate a series of answers following the statement 'Please indicate how tempted you are not to exercise in the following situations . . .'. The answers include 'when I am angry' and 'when I am satisfied' to reflect 'affect', and 'when I feel lazy' and 'when I am busy' to reflect competing interests. The authors argue that such temptations are central to understanding exercise uptake and should be used alongside the SOC. Using a stages of change framework, Cropley et al. (2003) used a reasoning task to assess beliefs about the pros and cons of exercise and asked people to list 'as many advantages/disadvantages of taking part in exercise' as they could. They then explored how accessible these beliefs were by timing how long it took for people to think of their first pro or con and then assessed how many pros and cons could be generated in 60 seconds. Participants were then divided according to whether they were pre-contemplators or maintainers. The results showed that pre-contemplators could think of more cons than pros and that maintainers could think of more pros than cons. In addition, the pre-contemplators were quicker to think of their first pro reason. The authors concluded that while maintainers can think of lots of benefits of exercise, the pre-contemplators may not exercise because they can't think of any reason to do so. Some research has also used the COM-B to predict exercise. For example, Howlett et al. (2019) used a prospective design and concluded that capability and motivation were the key predictors of moderate-to-vigorous physical activity in 186 healthy adults. Some research also shows a role for implicit rather than explicit attitudes to exercise. For example, Chevance et al. (2018) concluded from their prospective study that baseline favourable implicit attitudes towards physical activity predicted higher levels of physical activity in participants with obesity even when age, BMI, past physical activity and intentions were controlled for.

Self-Efficacy

Exercise self-efficacy consistently emerges as a good predictor of exercise. For example, in an early study, Sallis et al. (1986) indicated that exercise self-efficacy, attitudes to exercise and health knowledge were the best predictors of initiation and maintenance of vigorous/moderate exercise for one year. Jonas et al. (1993) followed up 100 men and women and reported the best predictors of intentions to participate in exercise programmes and actual participation were attitudes to continued participation, perceived social norms and perceived behavioural control (similar to self-efficacy). Similarly, Sniehotta et al. (2005) used a longitudinal design to explore physical activity in 307 cardiac rehabilitation patients and concluded that self-efficacy was an important mediator between intentions to exercise and actual exercise at four months follow-up. Further, Lippke and Plotnikoff (2009) and Plotnikoff et al. (2009) concluded that self-efficacy was a key predictor in their longitudinal study of Canadian adults. However, following a workplace intervention, Keller et al. (2016) concluded that self-efficacy was not a predictor of physical activity.

Past Behaviour and Habit

Much exercise is habitual and Norman and Smith (1995) found that, although most of the TPB variables were related to exercise, the best predictor of future behaviour was past behaviour. Similarly, Kaushal et al. (2017) conducted a prospective study to investigate the role of habit in different phases of exercise and found that behavioural intentions and habit were both correlated with observed exercise 6 weeks later. Similarly, Brickell et al. (2006) used a TPB framework to explore past behaviour and spontaneous implementation intentions to predict physical activity over a three-week period. The results showed that past behaviour predicted future behaviour. However, this was reduced if participants generated implementation intentions in the interim. Further, implementation intentions only predicted future behaviour in those who showed low levels of activity in the past. Likewise, in a recent RCT exploring exercise in patients with breast cancer, An et al. (2020) concluded that aerobic fitness was the most consistent predictor of longer-term exercise behaviour.

Therefore, past behaviour predicts future behaviour (i.e. we are creatures of habit), but implementation intentions can help break this pattern in those who haven't done much exercise before. This links in with research on planning.

Planning

In line with much research on bridging the intention–behaviour gap (see Chapter 2), research has addressed the role of planning and implementation intentions in predicting and promoting exercise and consistently shows that both spontaneous (i.e. made by the participant unprompted) and researcher-prompted plans to do exercise (e.g. 'I will walk up the stairs at work tomorrow') are good predictors of physical activity (Scholz et al. 2008; Molloy et al. 2010; Keller et al. 2016).

Affect

Many theories of health behaviours, including physical activity, have been criticized for focusing on cognitions and ignoring emotion. One version of emotion that has been studied is the construct 'affective judgement' which relates to feelings such as pleasure, enjoyment or feeling happy. Rhodes et al. (2009) carried out a review and meta-analysis and concluded that 83 out of the 85 correlational studies reviewed showed a significant relationship between affective judgements and physical activity that was consistent regardless of sample, measures used or the quality of the study.

Exercise is therefore predicted by a combination of demographic, cognitive and emotional factors. The relationship between cognitions and physical activity is not always consistent, however. For example, Hardeman et al. (2011) carried out a study in primary care of 252 sedentary adults at risk of Type 2 diabetes and reported that TPB variables failed to predict either absolute brisk walking or an increase in brisk walking by 12 months follow-up. Similarly, Scott et al. (2007) explored the role of TPB variables in predicting walking while wearing a pedometer and concluded that although the variables predicted intentions to walk, they did not predict actual walking as measured by the pedometer.

5 | IMPROVING EXERCISE BEHAVIOUR

Given the physical and psychological benefits of exercise and based upon our understanding of the predictors of exercise uptake and maintenance, research has also addressed ways in which people can be encouraged to exercise more. This has involved social and political changes and the use of behavioural strategies to encourage exercise.

SOCIAL AND POLITICAL FACTORS

An increased reliance on technology and reduced daily activity in paid and domestic work has resulted in an increase in the number of people having relatively sedentary lifestyles (see Figures 5.1 to 5.9). In addition, a shift towards a belief that exercise is good for an individual's well-being and is relevant for everyone has set the scene for social and political changes in terms of emphasizing exercise. Since the late 1960s many government initiatives have aimed to promote sport and exercise including:

- Initiatives such as 'Sport for All', 'fun runs' and targets for council facilities, such as swimming pools and sports centres.
- Rethinking town planning to make walking easier and the introduction of street lighting and cycle paths
- Increasing the number of pedestrianized areas in cities.
- Charging more for car use in residential areas and encouraging the use of public transport, cycling or walking.

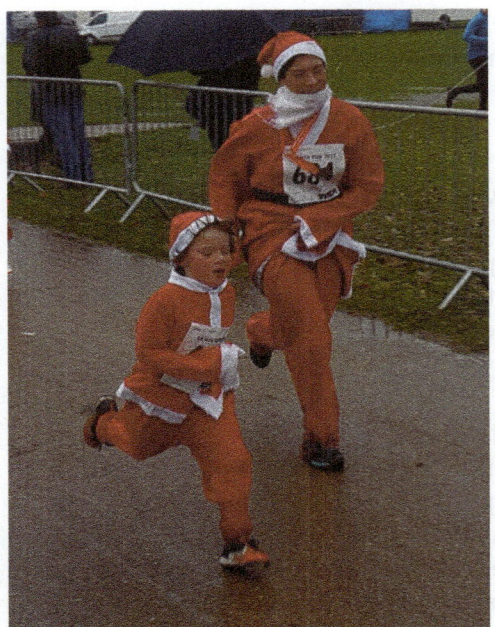

Local organised events can promote exercise

- Limiting the use of lifts or escalators to those who cannot use the stairs.
- Some cities now have bikes available that can be hired and used as and when they are needed.
- There is currently talk about changing traffic lights in cities to make them green for pedestrians until a car approaches as a means to discourage driving and encourage walking.

Some of these approaches encourage exercise through the use of sports facilities. Many, however, attempt to make small changes to people's daily lives that can be sustainable, such as walking or changing a person's usual mode of transport. Evidence for the effectiveness of these approaches is still forthcoming but any effort to make people less sedentary and more active in their daily lives would predictably be of benefit.

Exercise Prescription Schemes

One recent approach to increasing exercise uptake is the exercise prescription scheme whereby GPs refer targeted patients for exercise. This could take the form of vouchers for free access to the local leisure centre, an exercise routine with a health and fitness adviser or recommendations from a health and fitness adviser to follow a home-based exercise programme, such as walking.

Stair Climbing

An alternative and simpler approach involves the promotion of stair rather than escalator or lift use. Interventions to promote stair use are cheap and can target a large population. In addition, they can target the most sedentary members of the population who are least likely to adopt more structured forms of exercise. This is in line with calls to promote changes in exercise behaviour that can be incorporated into everyday life (Dunn et al. 1998). Research also indicates that stair climbing can lead to weight loss, improved fitness and energy expenditure and reduced risk of osteoporosis in women (e.g. Boreham et al. 2000). Some research has therefore attempted to increase stair use. For example, motivational posters between stairs and escalators or lifts have been shown to increase stair walking (e.g. Andersen et al. 1998; Kerr et al. 2001). In a more detailed study, Kerr et al. (2001) explored what characteristics of poster prompts were most effective and whether this varied according to message, gender and setting. The results showed that larger posters were more effective at promoting stair use, that effectiveness was not related overall to whether the message emphasized time and health (i.e. 'stay healthy, save time, use the stairs') or just health (i.e. 'stay healthy, use the stairs'), but that whereas the message including time was more effective for women in a train station, it was more effective for men when presented at a shopping centre.

BEHAVIOURAL STRATEGIES

Many behavioural strategies are available for the promotion of exercise in both healthy and unhealthy populations (see Chapter 7). These include those derived from learning theory (e.g. modelling, reinforcement, incentives) and social cognition theory (e.g. planning, implementation, intentions) and have taken place in the community, via the mass media (e.g. advertising campaigns, TV, billboards) or using new technologies (e.g. texts, email). Most interventions utilize a number of different approaches and over the past few years there have been a series of key systematic reviews of the evidence for promoting exercise (Dishman et al. 1998; Marcus et al. 1998; Tudor-Locke et al. 2001; Rubak et al. 2005; Vandelanotte et al. 2007). These highlight several factors as effective in promoting exercise as follows.

Social Support

Research indicates that local support groups, 'buddy' systems, walking groups and exercise contracts can promote exercise (Kahn et al. 2002).

Learning and Social Cognition Strategies

Planning, goal-setting, self-reward schemes, relapse prevention and tailoring interventions to the needs of the individual can be effective approaches (Sniehotta et al. 2006; Conner et al. 2010).

Self-Monitoring

The use of pedometers is a simple and easy to use form of self-monitoring and may promote exercise. As noted earlier, Australia encourages a 10,000 steps a day target, but although evidence shows that wearing a pedometer can increase walking (Rooney et al. 2003), it has been argued that this is too low for children and too high for sedentary adults (Tudor-Locke et al. 2001). Freak-Poli et al. (2020) carried out a systematic review of 14 studies to evaluate the effectiveness of pedometer interventions in the workplace. The authors concluded that some immediate positive effects were observed at the end of the intervention but these effects were not consistent and not always sustained over time.

School-based Interventions

Evidence shows that simply increasing time spent on physical exercise at school can increase activity without damaging academic achievement. For example, Dauenhuer et al. (2016) evaluated a school-based intervention and found that 30 minutes each week of group sessions based around goal setting and social support significantly increased daily step counts in the children by 2,349 steps and also increased their cardiovascular fitness. This resulted in an overall decline in the prevalence of overweight and obesity from 59.6 per cent to 53.5 per cent. However, whether or not this influences activity outside school remains unclear (Kahn et al. 2002). In addition, changing the structure of school playgrounds and the introduction of extra equipment can also increase activity (Stratton et al. 2008).

Work-based Interventions

Work-based interventions are a useful way to target large numbers of the population, improve the well-being of a workforce and promote social support. For example, Keller et al. (2016) conducted a workplace intervention to improve health and well-being among 1,063 of their employees by improving their physical activity. Findings indicated an increase in self-efficacy, planning and physical activity following the intervention. Some interventions, however, show improvements in absenteeism and productivity but no significant improvements in fitness or physical activity (Dishman et al. 1998; Engbers et al. 2005).

Mass Media Campaigns

Social marketing approaches have been used to change exercise behaviour via TV, billboards and magazines. Reviews show that although people can recall the messages, they have little impact on actual behaviour (Finlay and Faulkner 2005; Marcus et al. 2009).

Technologies

Mobile phones, laptops, smartphones and the internet all provide new opportunities to prompt healthier behaviour. Although evidence in this area is still in its infancy, there is some promising evidence that this approach might be effective for encouraging activity both through texts, websites and telephoning (Sirriyeh Lawton and Ward 2010; Fanning et al. 2012; Cadmus-Bertram et al. 2015). In

2019, Webb et al. carried out a randomized controlled trial which showed that a print-based 'Move More' pack supported by internet tools (costed at £8.19 per person) improved physical activity in adult cancer survivors by 36.9 per cent over 12 weeks compared to 9.1 per cent in the control group and that this change was maintained by 24 weeks. In 2018, Muellmann et al. carried out a systematic review of 20 studies to compare the effectiveness of eHealth interventions promoting physical activity in adults aged 55 years and above, with either no intervention or a non-eHealth intervention. The authors concluded that while eHealth interventions are effective in the short term, more evidence is needed regarding sustained changes. Likewise, Laranjo et al. (2021) also carried out a systematic review and meta-analysis and concluded that mobile apps or trackers with automated and continuous self-monitoring and feedback are an effective means to promote physical activity but, again, longer term studies were lacking.

6   EXERCISE ADHERENCE

Given the impact of exercise on physical and mental well-being, it is key not only to try exercise but to continue with exercise and adhere to recommendations of physical activity for the longer term. Research has therefore examined which variables predict exercise adherence. For example, Jefferis et al. (2014) conducted a large-scale study of 1,593 men and 857 women between the ages of 70 and 93 to investigate adherence to physical activity. They found that those who adhered to exercise guidelines were generally younger, healthier with fewer chronic health conditions, less depressed, had less severe mobility limitations, had higher exercise self-efficacy and exercise outcome expectations. They also rated their local environment to be high for social activities and leisure facilities and they left the house more times a week, were more likely to use active transport (e.g. walk rather than take the car) and were more likely to regularly walk a dog. Further, using a stages of change approach, Ingledew et al. (1998) explored which factors were important for the transition between the earlier stages of adoption and the later stages of continued behaviour and concluded that continued exercise was predicted by intrinsic motives, specifically enjoyment. Similarly, Kwasnicka et al. (2016) conducted a systematic review of behaviour change maintenance in general, including physical activity, and concluded that enjoyment of an activity leads to a greater likelihood of that becoming maintained over time. Some research has also explored predictors of relapse and drop-out rates from exercise programmes. For example, Dishman et al. (1985) concluded that relapse was highest among blue-collar workers, smokers and those who believe that exercise is an effort, and lowest in those who report a history of past participation, have high self-motivation, the support of a spouse, those who report having the available time, those who have access to exercise facilities and those who report a belief in the value of good health.

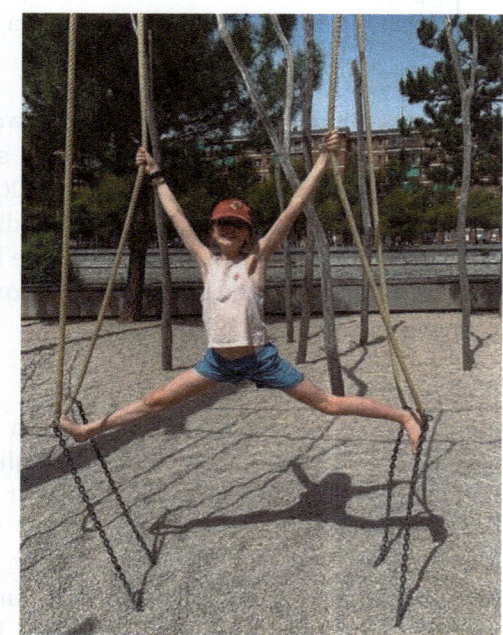

Recently, Dunton et al. (2022) argued that we need to reconceptualize the way we think about exercise uptake and maintenance and developed a new conceptual model of physical activity maintenance with 'inflection points' at different stages. These 'inflection points' highlight points of change at which changes in physical activity are underpinned by changes in the accompanying psychological processes. They also argue that researchers need to redefine and clarify these 'inflection points' in order to maximize the benefit of research to the development of policy and intervention development.

Exercise adherence is increased if it is enjoyable

BOX 5.1
Critical Approaches to Health Psychology

Research exploring exercise highlights some of the bigger issues with research in health psychology:

The individual vs the social vs the political: Exercise takes place within and because of our social and political worlds. We can only cycle because we have bikes, go to the gym because we have gyms and run round parks because they are there and are safe. And we only can do exercise for pleasure if we are not totally physically exhausted from our daily lives. Health psychology tries to capture this complexity through simple constructs such as 'opportunity' or 'social context' but we cannot measure this without simply asking individuals what they think about the world they live in which is very different. Much of our research therefore takes places in a social and political vacuum.

A snapshot in time: Exercise is a complex behaviour varying from fidgeting, to standing, to walking, to running (my speed) to running fast. When we measure it we capture a person's beliefs about what they do (self report) or we take an objective measurement from a movement monitor. None of these can capture the complexity of all the different types of exercise and how they may well vary from the second the measurement is taken to the next second when it is not. Our measurement tools are always going to be problematic.

Individual differences: Research often explores differences between people according to demographics (gender, sexuality, body weight, social class, etc.). This imposes a false dichotomy upon variables which are often more fluid that this. It also assumes that these demographics tell us something useful about the individual concerned.

.7 THINKING CRITICALLY ABOUT EXERCISE

There are many problems with exercise research which are similar to other health-related behaviours such as eating, smoking and alcohol use.

SOME CRITICAL QUESTIONS

When reading or thinking about research in the area of exercise, ask yourself the following questions.

- Why is measuring exercise so difficult?
- Psychological research focuses on the individual when explaining exercise behaviour. What other factors might be important?
- Many studies in this area only have short-term follow-ups. Why might this be a problem for understanding the impact of exercise?
- Some studies have much longer follow-ups. Why might this also be a problem for understanding the impact of exercise?

SOME PROBLEMS WITH. . .

Below are some specific problems with research in this area that you may wish to consider.

Measurement: Measuring exercise behaviour is difficult as some exercise takes the form of structured, organized activity such as sport, whereas some takes the form of behaviour which is integrated in a person's daily life such as walking and stair climbing. Self-report measures may be inaccurate and more objective measures (e.g. monitors) may actually change behaviour.

Research synthesis: Exercise can promote both psychological (e.g. well-being) and physiological (e.g. heart rate) changes. Working out how these changes interact is complicated. Further, combining research is made difficult as some studies focus on psychological outcomes while others rely upon physiological outcomes.

Are we in control?: Exercise is mostly studied as a behaviour that is under the control of the individual, that is, we explore whether a person's beliefs, emotions or motivations determine whether or not they exercise. However, it is also a behaviour that is very much determined by the environment, which may not be controllable. For example, structural factors such as safe paths, street lighting, free access to sports centres and town planning may have an enormous impact upon activity levels. Research needs to incorporate such factors into the models used.

TO CONCLUDE

As we become an increasingly sedentary society, there has been an increased emphasis on understanding and promoting exercise. This chapter has covered who exercises and described the physical and psychological benefits of exercise and the harms of prolonged sitting and a sedentary lifestyle. It has then explored the predictors of exercise with a focus on demographics, social determinants and cognitive and emotional factors. The chapter then described possible ways to increase exercise uptake and adherence with a focus on social and political factors and behavioural strategies. Finally, this chapter has described some of the problems with research in this area.

QUESTIONS

1 Evaluate the evidence for the physical benefits of exercise.
2 What are the psychological benefits of exercise?
3 To what extent can we predict exercise behaviour?
4 How can psychological theories be used to promote exercise behaviour?
5 To what extent is our sedentary lifestyle a social and political problem rather than a psychological problem?
6 Making people more active is easier than getting them to exercise. Discuss.
7 Exercise behaviour has to be an integrated part of people's lives. Discuss.
8 Describe a possible research project designed to predict attendance at an exercise class.
9 Why is exercise difficult to define and measure?
10 What are some of the problems with research in this area?

FOR DISCUSSION

Consider your own exercise behaviour and discuss the extent to which this relates to your social and political world versus your health beliefs.

FURTHER READING

Biddle, S.J.H., Gorely, T. and Mutrie, N. (2015) *Psychology of Physical Activity: Determinants, Wellbeing and Interventions, 3rd* edn. London: Routledge.
An excellent book that provides a thorough and expert guide to the literature of physical activity.
Faulkner, G.E.J. and Taylor, A.H. (eds) (2005) *Exercise, Health and Mental Health.* London: Routledge.
A comprehensive edited collection of chapters that cover the impact of exercise on a range of physical health problems including cancer, heart failure, HIV and schizophrenia. It provides a good summary of the existing research and a useful summary chapter at the end.

Hallal, P.C., Andersen, L.B., Bull, F.C., et al. (2012) Global physical activity levels: surveillance progress, pitfalls, and prospects. *The Lancet,* **380:** 247–57.
This was part of a special issue published in the *The Lancet* prior to the 2012 Olympics and is worth a read as it covers the risks of inactivity and benefits of exercise and gives a global perspective.

O'Donovan, G., Lee, I., Hamer, M. and Stamatakis, E. (2017) Association of 'Weekend Warrior' and other leisure time physical activity patterns with risks for all-cause, cardiovascular disease, and cancer mortality, *JAMA Internal Medicine,* **177**(3): 335–42. Doi:10.1001/jamainternmed.2016.8014
This is an interesting study which evaluates the impact of a modern phenomenon – the weekend warrior – which describes those who sit all week and exercise all weekend. Very relevant to modern life.

Perry, J. (2020) *The Psychology of Exercise.* London: Routledge.
This is a great little book that covers the research and theories of exercise in an accessible way.

Rhodes, R.E., Boudreau, P., Josefsson, K.W. and Ivarsson, A. (2021) Mediators of physical activity behaviour change interventions among adults: a systematic review and meta-analysis, *Health Psychology Review,* **15**(2): 272–86. Doi: 10.1080/17437199.2019.1706614
This is a great review of the recent literature on activity.

6
Sex

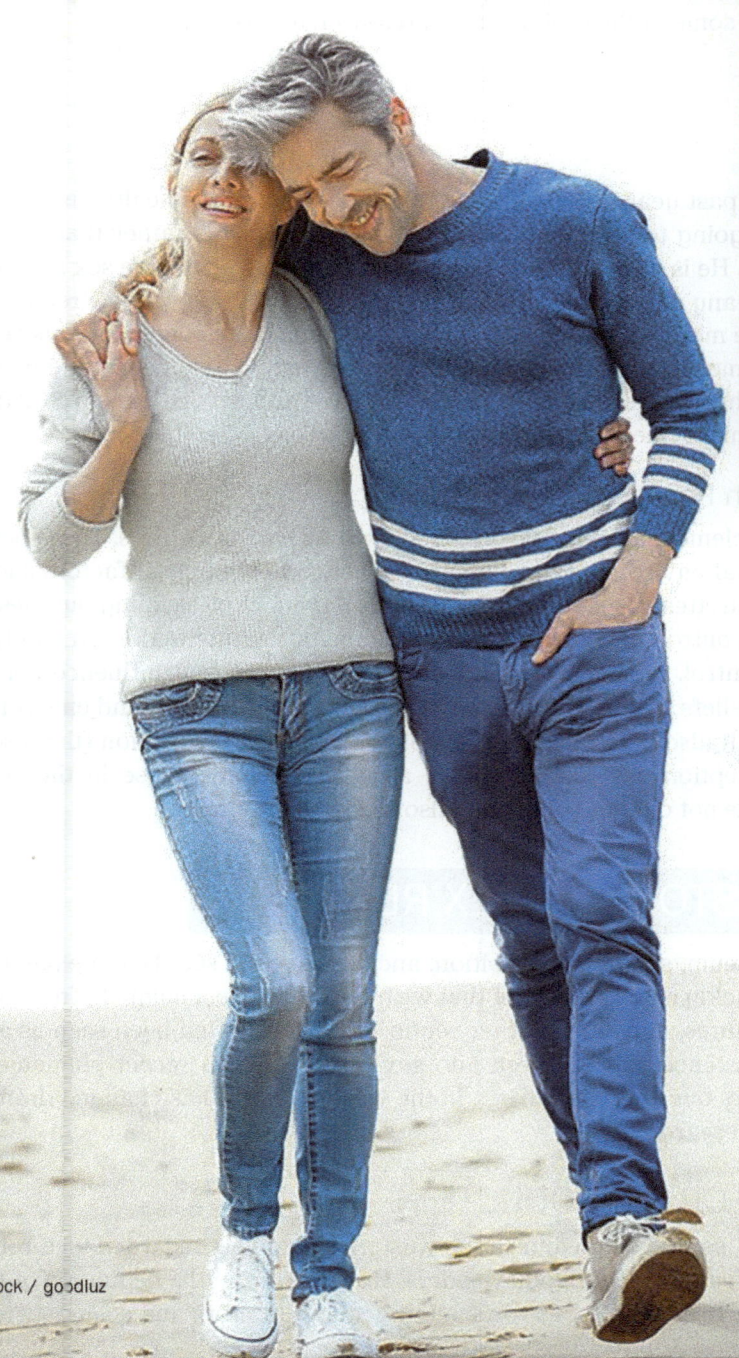

Learning Objectives

To understand:
1. A Brief History of Sex Research
2. Contraception Use for Pregnancy Avoidance
3. Sex in the Context of HIV/AIDS
4. Sex and Risk Perception
5. Sex as an Interaction
6. Sex Education
7. Thinking Critically about Sex Research

CHAPTER OVERVIEW

This chapter first provides a brief history of the literature on sex, illustrating the shift from early discussions of biology and sex for reproduction, to debates about sexual pleasure, to an emphasis on sex as a risk behaviour in the context of pregnancy avoidance, STDs, HIV and AIDS towards the recent focus on sexual health as being a state of physical, emotional and social well-being and the increasing focus on the breadth of sexualities and a recognition of the needs of both heterosexual and LGBTQ+ communities. The chapter then explores psychological research within these different perspectives including predicting contraception use, a focus on condoms in the context of HIV, sex and risk perception, sex as an interaction and the role of negotiation, power and social norms and the role of sex education from both the government and at school. Finally, the chapter explores some of the problems with research in this area.

CASE STUDY

Adrian is 22 and gay. Over the past year he has decided to take control of his health and has stopped smoking, started running and going to the gym and cooking his own meals rather than eating take-aways or going out all the time. He is also aware of the risks associated with unsafe sex and so always insists on using a condom with any new partner. He has just met a man, Chris, who he really likes and this seems as if it could become more serious than his usual partners. They laugh a lot, talk really well and seem to have a lot in common. They also really fancy each other. Chris doesn't like condoms as he says they ruin the feeling. Chris also says that he has been tested and isn't HIV positive. After much discussion Adrian agrees that this is fine and they have unprotected sex.

Through the Eyes of Health Psychology. . .

Most behaviours have a social element as we often drink, smoke and eat with others. These behaviours also take place within our social environment and so are influenced by external factors such as the availability of food, cost of cigarettes or alcohol. But at the very moment of carrying out these behaviours we have some degree of control. In contrast, sex is all about social interaction. And at times this can interfere with personal control. Adrian's story illustrates the factors that influence condom use in the context of HIV such as beliefs (wanting to be healthy), risk (of unsafe sex) and emotions (wanting to please his new partner). It also illustrates the key role of sex as an interaction (the discussion). This chapter explores contraception use for pregnancy avoidance, condom use in the context of HIV/AIDS and highlights the role not only of beliefs but also sex as an interaction.

1 | A BRIEF HISTORY OF SEX RESEARCH

Any visit to an art gallery, museum, sculpture exhibition, ancient caves to see the cave paintings or a read of the *Kama Sutra* will quickly expel any belief that we have a become a uniquely free and adventurous generation. In other cultures, and across other centuries, sex has often been seen as a fun and pleasurable part of human existence. Yet research into sex seems to be a recent phenomenon and over the past few hundred years our approach to sex in the western world has changed dramatically. Below is a brief history of sex research.

SEX AS BIOLOGICAL, FOR REPRODUCTION

Prior to the nineteenth century, sexual behaviour in the western world was regarded as a religious or spiritual concern and guidance came from religious leaders. However, from the beginning of the 1800s sexuality and sexual behaviour became a focus for scientific study. Doctors and scientists took over the responsibility for teaching about sex and it was subsequently studied within medicine and biological sciences. Sex was viewed as a biological function alongside eating and drinking.

During the nineteenth century, much was written about sexual behaviour and attempts were made to develop criteria to describe sexual normality and abnormality. Generally, behaviours linked to reproduction were seen as normal and those such as masturbation and homosexuality as abnormal. This is illustrated by the Victorian concern with sexual morality, movements proclaiming sexual puritanism and attempts to control prostitution. Sex was seen as a biological drive that needed to be expressed but which should be expressed within the limitations of its function: reproduction.

SEX AS BIOLOGICAL, FOR PLEASURE

From the beginning of the twentieth century, there was a shift in perspective. Although sex was still seen as biological, the emphasis was now on sexual behaviour rather than on outcome (reproduction). This involved a study of sexual desire, sexual pleasure and orgasms. It resulted in a burgeoning literature on sex therapy and manuals on how to develop a good sex life. This emphasis is illustrated by the classic survey carried out by Kinsey in the 1940s and 1950s, the research programmes developed by Masters and Johnson in the 1960s and the Hite Reports on sexuality in the 1970s and 1980s.

The Kinsey Report

Kinsey interviewed and analysed data from 12,000 white Americans and his attempts to challenge some of the contemporary concerns with deviance were credited with causing 'a wave of sexual hysteria' (e.g. Kinsey et al. 1948). He developed his analysis of sexual behaviour within models of biological reductionism and argued that sex was natural and therefore healthy. Kinsey argued that the sexual drive was a biological force and the expression of this drive to attain pleasure was not only acceptable but desirable. He challenged some of the contemporary concerns with premarital sex and argued that, as animals do not get married, there could be no difference between marital and premarital sex. He emphasized similarities between the sexual behaviour of men and women and argued that if scientific study could promote healthy sex lives, then this could improve the quality of marriages and reduce divorce rates. His research suggested that a variety of sexual outlets were acceptable and emphasized the role of sexual pleasure involving both sexual intercourse and masturbation for men and women.

Masters and Johnson

This emphasis on the activity of sex is also illustrated by the work of Masters and Johnson in the 1960s. They used a variety of experimental laboratory techniques to examine over 10,000 male and female orgasms in 694 white middle-class heterosexuals (e.g. Masters and Johnson 1966). They recorded bodily contractions, secretions, pulse rates and tissue colour changes and described the sexual response cycle in terms of the following phases: (1) excitement; (2) plateau; (3) orgasm; and (4) resolution. They emphasized similarities between men and women and argued that stable marriages depended on satisfactory sex. According to Masters and Johnson, sexual pleasure could be improved by education and sex therapy and again their research suggested that masturbation was an essential component of sexuality – sex was for pleasure, not for reproduction.

The Hite Reports

Shere Hite (1976, 1981, 1987) published the results from her 20 years of research in her reports on female and male sexuality. Her research also illustrates the shift from the outcome of sex to sex as an activity. Hite's main claim is that 'most women (70 per cent) do not orgasm as a result of intercourse', but she suggests that they can learn to increase clitoral stimulation during intercourse to improve their sexual enjoyment. She describes her data in terms of women's dislike of penetrative sex ('Perhaps it could be said that many women might be rather indifferent to intercourse if it were not for feelings towards a particular man') and discusses sex within the context of pleasure, not reproduction.

Segal (1994) has criticized Hite's interpretation of the data and argues that the women in Hite's studies appear to enjoy penetration (with or without orgasm). Although this is in contradiction to Hite's own conclusion, the emphasis is still on sex as an activity.

SEX AS A RISK TO HEALTH

In the late twentieth century there was an additional shift in the literature on sex. Although research still emphasized sex as an activity, this activity was viewed as increasingly risky and dangerous. As a consequence, sex was discussed in terms of health promotion, health education and self-protection. This shift has resulted in a psychological literature on sex as a risk both in terms of pregnancy avoidance and in the context of STDs/HIV preventive behaviour.

SEX AND WELL-BEING

Since the turn of the twenty-first century there has been an additional shift in the ways in which sex is conceptualized. Although much work still continues to explore how to prevent unwanted pregnancy or STDs, sexual research has begun to incorporate a notion of the benefits of sex, not just the costs. There has therefore been an increasing interest in sex as pleasure, masturbation, fantasy and the role of a sexual life within a more holistic view of the individual. This is reflected in the World Health Organization (WHO) definition in 2006 which stated that sexual health is: 'a state of physical, emotional, mental and social well-being in relation to sexuality; it is not merely the absence of disease, dysfunction or infirmity. Sexual health requires a positive and respectful approach to sexuality and sexual relationships, as well as the possibility of having pleasurable and safe sexual experiences, free of coercion, discrimination and violence. For sexual health to be attained and maintained, the sexual rights of all persons must be respected, protected and fulfilled' (WHO 2006).

This approach is also reflected in Robinson et al.'s (2002) all-inclusive sexual health model which locates sex within the context of physical and mental health, relationships and culture. Although this was developed within the context of HIV prevention it has implications for thinking about sexual behaviour across all domains of any individual's life. The model is illustrated in Figure 6.1.

How sex sits within our lives has therefore changed from a narrow focus on biology, health or risk to a much broader focus on mental and physical well-being. In addition, over the past decade or so, research has also broadened the notion of who is having sex and with whom from a narrow dichotomous classification of either heterosexual or homosexual sex to a much more flexible notion of sexuality. This reflects not only the recognition of many different versions of sexuality, to include heterosexual and gay people and all members of the LGBTQ+ community, but also recognizes how these classifications can themselves be restrictive with people increasingly moving between these limited definitions. Therefore, in line with gender classifications (see Chapter 15), definitions of sexuality are also becoming more fluid.

IN SUMMARY

Early literature emphasized sex as a biological process and the focus was on reproduction. From the start of the twentieth century, however, sex was no longer described as a biological means to an end but as an activity in itself. Discussions of 'good sex', orgasms and sexual pleasure emphasized sex as action; however, even as an activity sex remained predominantly biological. Kinsey regarded sex as a drive that was natural and healthy, Masters and Johnson developed means to measure and improve the sexual experience by examining physiological changes and Hite explained pleasure with descriptions of physical stimulation. By the end of the twentieth century, however, discussions had shifted towards a more negative model of sex with the emphasis being on risk and danger and a focus on pregnancy avoidance and STDs, particularly in the light of HIV/AIDS. Nowadays a new shift is occurring towards a more integrated model of sex in terms of well-being, which includes not only a sense of physical health but also one of pleasure and a sense that sexuality and sexual behaviour are central to how people feel

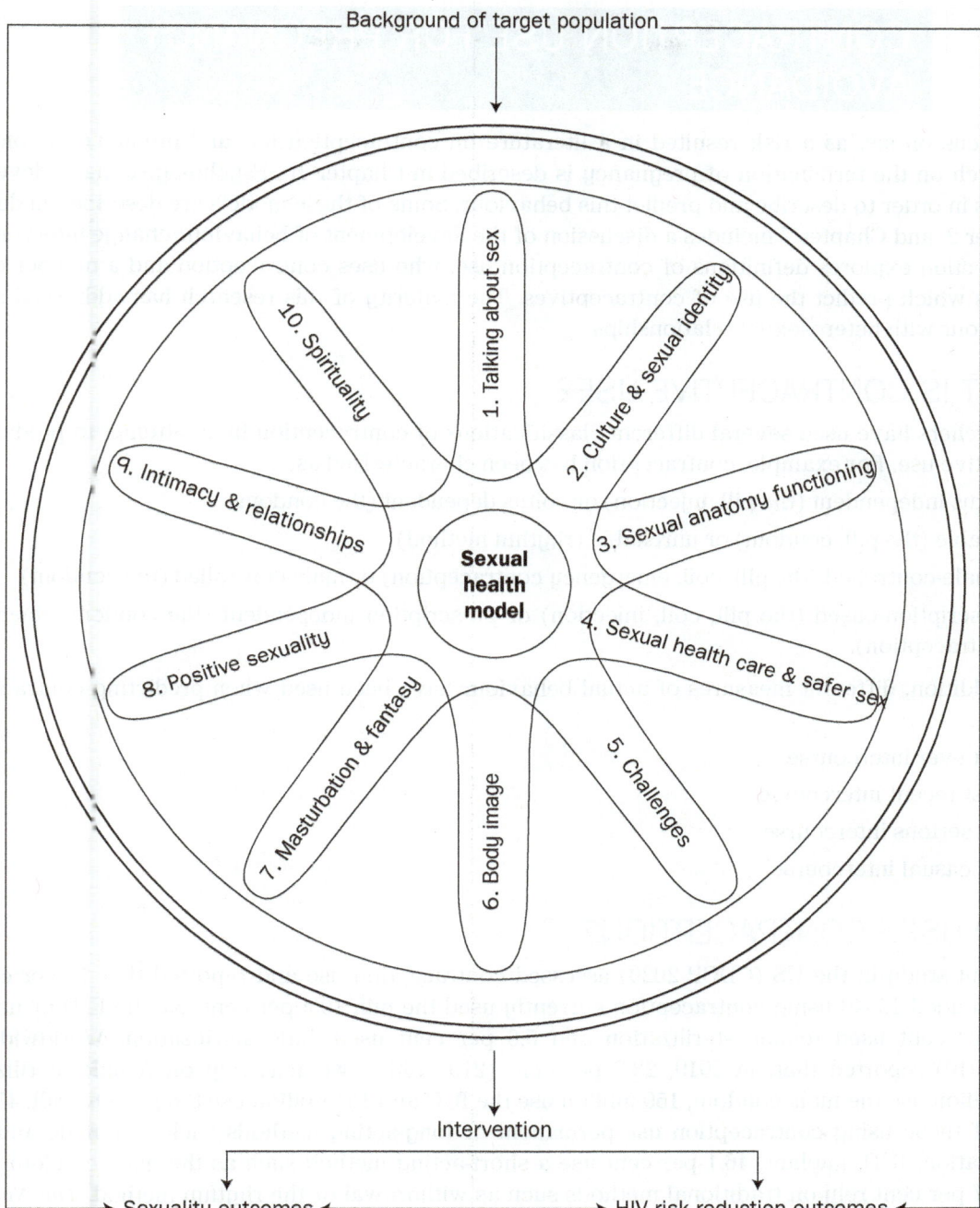

Figure 6.1 The sexual health model

SOURCE: Robinson et al. (2002), reproduced by permission of Oxford University Press

about themselves. Furthermore, this broader model of sex has also expanded both the definitions of what sex is and the classifications of the people involved in having it!

Over the past few decades these different perspectives have generated a number of different strands of research. These include an analysis of contraception use for pregnancy avoidance, condom use in the context of HIV and STDs, sex and risk perception, sex as an interaction and the role of negotiation, power and social norms, and sex education from the government and schools. These will now be described.

2   CONTRACEPTION USE FOR PREGNANCY AVOIDANCE

The focus on sex as a risk resulted in a literature on contraception use and pregnancy avoidance. Research on the termination of pregnancy is described in Chapter 15. Psychologists have developed models in order to describe and predict this behaviour. Some of these models are described in detail in Chapter 2, and Chapter 7 includes a discussion of the development of behaviour change interventions. This section explores definitions of contraception use, who uses contraception and a number of key factors which predict the use of contraceptives. The majority of this research has addressed sexual behaviour with heterosexual relationships.

WHAT IS CONTRACEPTIVE USE?

Researchers have used several different classifications of contraception in an attempt to predict contraceptive use. For example, contraception has been characterized as:

- coitus independent (the pill, injection) or coitus dependent (the condom)
- reliable (the pill, condom) or unreliable (rhythm method)
- female-controlled (the pill, coil, emergency contraception) or male-controlled (the condom)
- prescription-based (the pill, coil, injection) or prescription independent (the condom, emergency contraception).

In addition, different measures of actual behaviour have been used when predicting contraceptive use at:

- first ever intercourse
- most recent intercourse
- last serious intercourse
- last casual intercourse.

WHO USES CONTRACEPTION?

A recent study in the US (CDCP 2020) assessed contraception use and reported that 14 per cent of women aged 15–49 using contraception currently used the pill, 10.4 per cent use the IUD or implant, 18.1 per cent used female sterilization and 5.6 per cent used male sterilization. Worldwide, the UN (2019) reported that, in 2019, 23.7 per cent (219 million women) rely on female sterilization, 189 million use the male condom, 159 million use the IUD and 151 million use the pill. Overall, 45.2 per cent of those using contraception use permanent or long-acting methods such as female and male sterilization, IUD, implant, 46.1 per cent use a short-acting method such as the male condom or the pill, 8.7 per cent rely on traditional methods such as withdrawal or the rhythm method. *The National Survey of Sexual Attitudes and Lifestyles* (Wellings et al. 1994) examined the sexual behaviour of nearly 20,000 men and women across Britain. This produced a wealth of data about factors such as age at first intercourse, homosexuality, attitudes to sexual behaviours and contraception use. For example, Figure 6.2 shows the proportion of respondents who used no contraception at first intercourse. These results indicate that the younger someone is when they first have sex (either male or female), the less likely they are to use contraception.

The results from this survey also show what kinds of contraception people use at first intercourse. The data for men and women aged 16–24 years are shown in Figure 6.3 and suggest that the condom is the most popular form of contraception; however, many respondents in this age group reported using no contraception, or unreliable methods, such as withdrawal or the safe period.

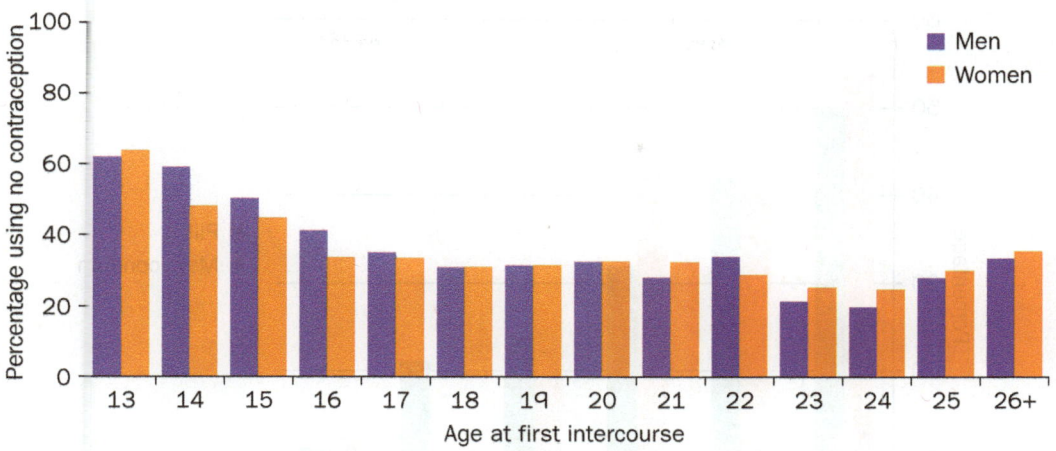

Figure 6.2 Percentage using no contraception at first intercourse, by age at first intercourse

SOURCE: Adapted from Wellings et al. (1994)

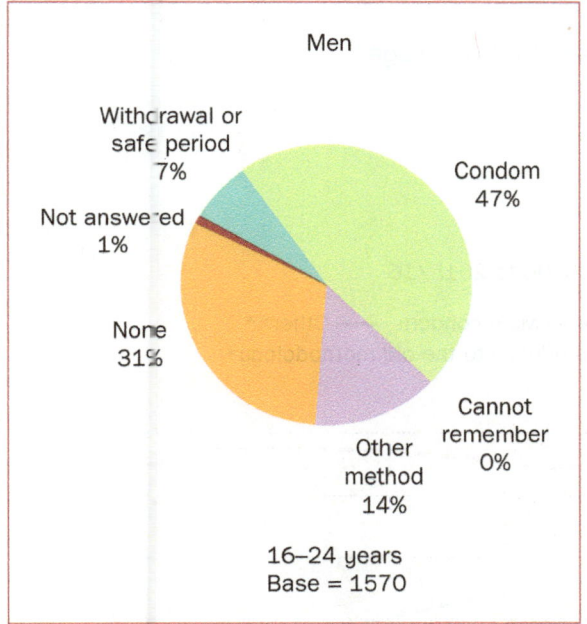

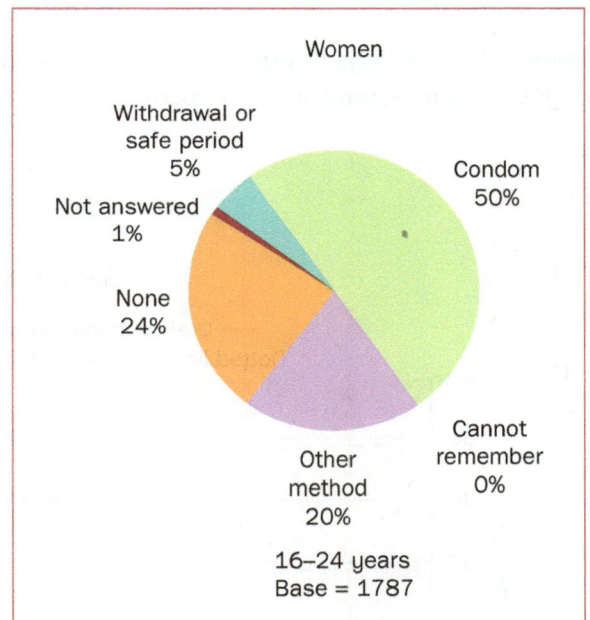

Figure 6.3 Contraception use at first intercourse in those aged 16–24

SOURCE: Adapted from Wellings et al. (1994)

In 2008/9 the Office for National Statistics published data on condom and pill use in women under 50 and these are shown in Figure 6.4. The results show that whereas the pill is the preferred mode of contraception for women in their early twenties and thirties, women in their early forties are more likely to use the male condom. However, Mosher et al. (2004) calculated that 1.43 million women could be at risk of unplanned pregnancy in the USA, with the highest risk groups being sexually active Hispanic and black women.

Research also shows changes in contraceptive choice over time and indicates a decline in condom use and an increase in the contraceptive pill (see Figure 6.5).

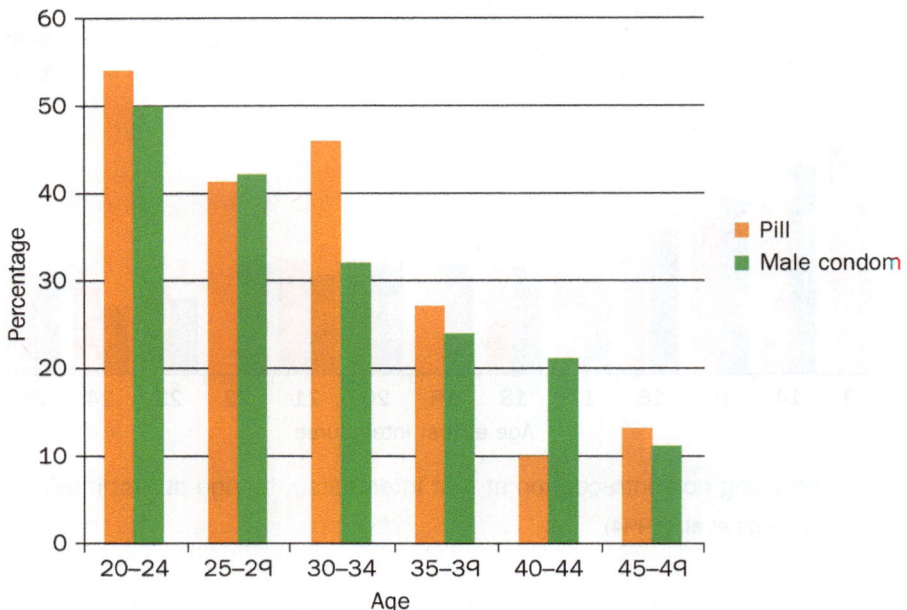

Figure 6.4 Percentage of women using the pill or male condom by age

SOURCE: Office for National Statistics (2009)

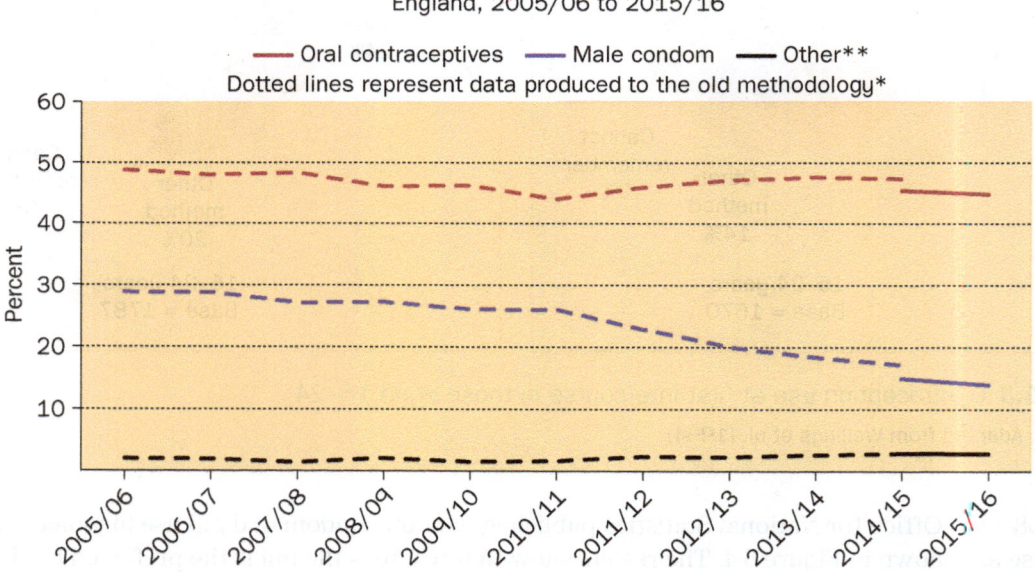

*This chart uses data produced using an old methodology for determining a woman's main method, which is still deemed suitable for illustrating relative change in main method uptake. See appendix C for details of the methodological change that occurred in 2014/15.
**Includes female condom, contraceptive patch, natural family planning, cap, diaphragm, spermicides and vaginal ring.

Figure 6.5 Changes in contraception choice over time

SOURCE: NHS Digital (2016)

PREDICTING CONTRACEPTION USE

Research exploring contraceptive use for pregnancy avoidance has drawn upon a number of different models (see Chapter 2 for details of some of these models). These include Lindemann's (1977) three-stage theory which describes the transition from the 'natural' to 'expert' stage of contraception use; Rains' (1971) model which places contraception use within the context of sexuality and self-concept; Subjective Expected Utility Model (Edwards 1954), which when applied to contraception use predicts that individuals weigh up the possible costs and benefits of contraception and pregnancy before making a decision (Luker 1975); social cognition models such as the HBM and TPB (Lowe and Radius 1982); the Sexual Behaviour Sequence Model developed by Byrne et al. (1977) which adds sexual arousal and emotional responses to sex to the TRA; and Herold and McNamee's (1982) model which emphasizes the general context of social norms and the context of the relationship.

Sheeran et al. (1991) argued that these models can be combined and that the best way to understand contraceptive use is as a product of: (1) background; (2) intrapersonal; (3) interpersonal; and (4) situational factors, as follows.

Background Factors

Research indicates that contraception use varies according to a number of background variables such as age, sex, ethnicity, social class and education (see Figures 6.2 to 6.4; Wellings et al. 1994; Bentley et al. 2009; NHS Digital 2016). Whether this effect is direct or through the effect of other factors such as knowledge and attitudes is unclear. In a recent study, involving 41,508 men and women living in the USA, Anderson (2017) found that an adverse childhood environment which included growing up with someone who was mentally ill, or an alcoholic, or had served time in prison, or had divorced parents or having experienced sexual trauma predicted an increased likelihood of engaging in risky sexual behaviours, suggesting a role for background factors in the broadest sense. Kara et al. (2019) explored the contraception use among female undergraduates (n = 347) in Tanzania and reported that while 96 per cent were aware of contraception this was predicted by age, marital status and religion, with 32.3 per cent giving religion as a reason for not using contraception. Similarly, Sait et al. (2021) assessed contraception use in men in Saudi Arabia (n = 243). About 79 per cent of the men were aware of contraception and 55 per cent reported using at least one type of contraception. Actual usage was predicted by being a government employee, having a smaller number of children, higher educational degree and higher monthly income, but was not associated with age, duration of marriage, marital status or having multiple marriages.

Intrapersonal Factors

Contraception use is also predictive by intrapersonal factors such as knowledge, cognitions, attitudes and personality.

1 *Knowledge:* Whitley and Schofield (1986) analysed the results of 25 studies of contraceptive use and reported a correlation of 0.17 between objective knowledge and contraceptive use in both men and women, suggesting that knowledge is poorly linked to behaviour. However, ignorance about contraception has also been shown by several studies. For example, Cvetkovich and Grote (1981) reported that, of their sample, 10 per cent did not believe that they could become pregnant the first time they had sex, and 52 per cent of men and 37 per cent of women could not identify the periods of highest risk in the menstrual cycle. In addition, Lowe and Radius (1982) reported that 40 per cent of their sample did not know how long sperm remained viable. Further, in their study of men in Saudi Arabia, Sait et al. (2021) reported that while 83 per cent thought that condoms were safe to use, 62 per cent believed that vasectomy was associated with complications and 14 per cent believed that contraception could lead to irreversible sterility. Further, a leaflet-based intervention showed that a leaflet and questions could improve knowledge about the contraceptive pill (Little et al. 1998).

2 *Attitudes:* Fisher (1984) reported that positive attitudes towards contraception parallel actual use. Negative attitudes included beliefs that 'it kills spontaneity', 'it's too much trouble to use' and that there

are possible side-effects. In addition, carrying contraceptives around is often believed to be associated with being promiscuous (e.g. Lowe and Radius 1982). Free and Ogden (2005) also reported a role for attitudes with users of emergency contraception reporting more positive attitudes than non-users. Further, Bryant (2009) concluded from her survey of diverse female college students that more positive attitudes to contraception were associated not only with contraception use but also consistent and effective use. This is particularly important as research indicates that many people show only partial adherence to contraception recommendations (see Chapter 10 for discussion of adherence).

3   *Cognitions:* research has identified a role for cognitions using the TRA (e.g. Albarracin et al. 2001; Muoz-Silva et al. 2007), HBM (Winfield and Whaley 2002) and TPB (Espada et al. 2015; Chowdhuri et al. 2019). Espada et al. (2015) conducted a cross-sectional study on 410 sexually experienced adolescents aged 13–18 and reported that the TPB, specifically condom use intention, was the most suitable model for predicting the frequency of condom use in young people compared to other models. Likewise, DeMaria et al. (2019) used the TPB to explore women's intention to change from the contraceptive pill to long-acting reversible contraceptive and reported a prediction role for attitudes, perceived behavioural control and self-identity.

4.   *Personality:* many different personality types have been related to contraceptive use. This research assumes that certain aspects of individuals are consistent over time and research has reported associations between the following types of personality:

- *Conservatism and sex role* have been shown to be negatively related to contraceptive use (e.g. McCormick et al. 1985).

- *An internal locus of control* appears to correlate with contraceptive use but not with choice of type of contraception (Morrison 1985). Further, Silva and Lopes (2020) reported that students who used contraceptive methods at first sexual encounter had higher 'externality powerful others' and those who used coitus interruptus who scored higher on 'externality chance'.

- *Sex guilt and sex anxiety* positively relate to use and consistency of use of contraception (Herold and McNamee 1982).

- *Personality* is often measured using the big-five factors (Goldberg 1999). These are *agreeableness, conscientiousness, emotional stability, extraversion* and *intellect*. Ingledew and Ferguson (2007) explored the role of personality in predicting riskier sexual behaviour. The results showed that agreeableness and conscientiousness reduced riskier behaviour. The results also showed that this effect was related to different forms of motivation. Beltz et al. (2019) however, found no differences in personality between women who relied on the oral contraceptive and those who defined their method as naturally cycling (NC).

Interpersonal Factors

Research also highlights a role for interpersonal factors reflecting the interactive nature of sex:

1   *Partner:* aspects of the relationship may influence contraception use including duration of relationship, intimacy, type of relationship (e.g. casual versus steady), exclusivity and ability to have overt discussions about contraception. For example, increased partner support was related to the use of emergency contraception (Free and Ogden 2005) and contraception in general (Coleman and Ingham 1998; Lalas et al. 2020). In a large nationally representative longitudinal data of Ugandan women aged 15–49, Sarnak et al. (2021) reported that not discussing pregnancy avoidance doubled the relative risk of stopping contraception by follow up and that partner support for future contraceptive use at baseline was associated with a nearly three-fold increased odds of contraceptive adoption. Interestingly, however, it may be that women's perceptions of their partner's approval may be the better predictor of contraception use than their partner's actual approval (Hernandez et al. 2022).

2   *Parents:* there is some evidence to suggest that increased parental communication about contraception is related to contraception use. For example, Widman et al. (2016) conducted a meta-analysis of 52 studies (n = 25,314) investigating the effect of parent-adolescent sexual communication on safer

sex behaviour among adolescents. They found that sexual communication with parents, particularly mothers, plays a small protective role for safer sexual behaviour among adolescents. The effect was stronger for girls than boys. Research also indicates, however, that parents tend to underestimate their child's sexual activity which may place that child at risk of pregnancy (or STDs) if parents don't encourage them to use contraception (Jones et al. 2005; O'Donnell et al. 2008).

3 *Peers:* increased contraceptive use relates to peer permissiveness and peers' own contraceptive behaviour (e.g. Herold 1981). For example, Calhoun et al. (2022) carried out a large scale cross-sectional study of contraceptive use among young men (n = 1279) and women (n = 1191) in Kenya. The results showed that both young men and women are more likely to report using condoms if they believe that their peers are using contraceptives. Similarly, data from the National Longitudinal Study of Adolescent to Adult Health showed that having friends who were accepting of adolescent sex increased contraceptive use in later life and that having friends who held negative attitudes toward contraceptive use during adolescence were more likely to be non-users in later life (Dehingia et al. 2022). Peer norms have also been assessed within the framework of using social cognition models to predict contraception use (e.g. Albarracin et al. 2001).

In 2015, Amialchuk and Gerhardinger conducted a study to explore contraceptive use for pregnancy avoidance in a sample of 3,717 adolescents. Their results provide evidence for a variety of interpersonal factors; 'going out' with their sexual partner increased contraception consistency among males; discussing the use of contraception before sexual intercourse increased contraception use for both genders; discussing contraception with parents increased contraception use for females. Likewise a qualitative study of adolescent girls in Nigeria (Sanchez et al. 2022) found that discussions with both parents and peers were considered the most import factors in determining contraception use rather than discussions with their partner.

Situational Factors

Situational factors also contribute to contraceptive use, including the following:

1 *The spontaneity of sex:* spontaneity is often given as a reason for not using contraception (e.g. Holland et al. 1990b).

2 *Substance use prior to sex:* taking substances such as drugs or alcohol prior to sex may relate to risky sex (Cooper 2002; NCASA 2011). For example, Best et al. (2021) reported that of 210 women attending an antenatal clinic for substance use disorder, 64 per cent reported unintended pregnancies and only a minority had attended antenatal (11 per cent) and postpartum (35 per cent) contraception counselling.

3 *The accessibility of contraception:* research has examined whether easy access to contraception both in general (i.e. the provision of condom machines in pubs) and at the time of contemplating sex predicts contraception use (e.g. Sable et al. 2000).

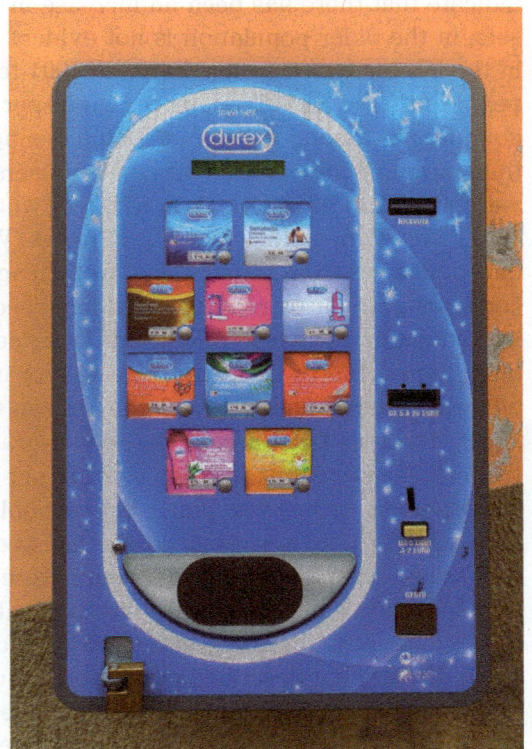

Easy access to condoms can improve condom use

SOURCE: © Shutterstock / Christian Mueller

IN SUMMARY

Contraception use can therefore be seen as a result of demographics (background) (e.g. age, experience), intrapersonal variables (e.g. knowledge and attitudes), interpersonal variables (e.g. partner support) and the situation (e.g. accessibility, substance use). These different variables interact in order to predict contraception use. This approach reflects a combination of individual and social variables and highlights how sexual behaviour is an interaction between two people and how any explanation needs to include a role for the individual's social context. The impact of sex as an interaction in terms of negotiation, power dynamics and cultural norms is addressed later in this chapter.

3 | SEX IN THE CONTEXT OF HIV/AIDS

The HIV virus was identified in 1983 (see Chapter 12 for a discussion of HIV and AIDS). Since the beginning of the HIV/AIDS epidemic, sex as a risk has taken on a new dimension – the dimension of chronic illness and death. Research has therefore focused on the role of condoms in preventing STDs, HIV and AIDS. Early campaigns emphasized monogamy or at least cutting down on the number of sexual partners. Campaigns also promoted non-penetrative sex and suggested alternative ways to enjoy a sexual relationship. However, since the late 1980s campaigns have emphasized safe sex and using a condom. As a result, research has examined the prerequisites to safer sex and condom use in an attempt to develop successful health promotion campaigns. This is particularly pertinent given that rates of other STDs have increased over the past 20 years. This section will explore condom use in different populations and the predictors of condom use.

DO PEOPLE USE CONDOMS?

Young People

Since the late 1980s governments have funded several mass media campaigns to promote condom use in young people, yet during this time there has been an increase in STDs. For example, in the UK, data indicate that there has been an increase in chlamydia and that the dramatic reduction in gonorrhoea seen in the older population is not evident among younger people. Furthermore, new cases of STDs in the UK increased from 669,291 in 1991 to 1,332,910 in 2001 and by 2001 1,025 out of every 100,000 people suffered an STD compared to 350 per 100,000 in 1991. Richard and van der Pligt (1991) examined condom use among a group of Dutch teenagers and reported that only 50 per cent of those with multiple partners were consistent condom users. In an American study, 30 per cent of adolescent women were judged to be at risk from STDs, of whom 16 per cent used condoms consistently (Weisman et al. 1991). The Women, Risk and AIDS Project (WRAP) (e.g. Holland et al. 1990b) interviewed and collected questionnaires from heterosexual women aged 16–19 years and reported that 16 per cent of these used condoms on their own, 13 per cent had used condoms while on the pill, 2 per cent had used condoms in combination with spermicide and 3 per cent had used condoms together with a diaphragm. Overall, only 30 per cent of their sample had ever used condoms, while 70 per cent had not. Sui et al. (2021) analysed a large data set from the Taiwan Global School-Based Student Health Survey, consisting of 27,525 students from across the school grades. The results showed that condom use rate decreased from 57.07 per cent at first sex to 25.72 per cent at last sex and that the condom use rate for first sex (in ascending order) was junior high school (37.67 per cent), night school (55.83 per cent), vocational high school (61.13 per cent), comprehensive school (62.83 per cent) and senior high school (68.38 per cent) suggesting that younger students were much less likely to use condoms the first time they had sex than older students. Hatherall et al. (2006) also explored condom use in young people and reported that 62 per cent said that they had used a condom in their most recent sexual experience. However, of these, 31 per cent described putting on the condom after penetration at least once in the previous six months and 9 per cent reported having penetration after the condom had been removed. This suggests that even when condoms are used, they are not always used in the most effective way. Furthermore, Stone et al. (2006) explored the use of condoms during oral sex (which is recommended for the prevention of STD transmission) and the results showed that of those who had had oral sex only 17 per cent reported ever using a condom and only 2 per cent reported consistent condom use. Reasons for non-use included reduced pleasure and lack of motivation and reasons for use included hygiene and avoidance of the 'spit/swallow dilemma'. Figure 6.5 shows that condom use had gradually declined compared to the contraceptive pill over the past decade. Condom use in the previous year by age and sex is shown in Figure 6.6 (ONS 2013). This indicates that men use condoms more often than women and that they are most commonly used by the younger age groups.

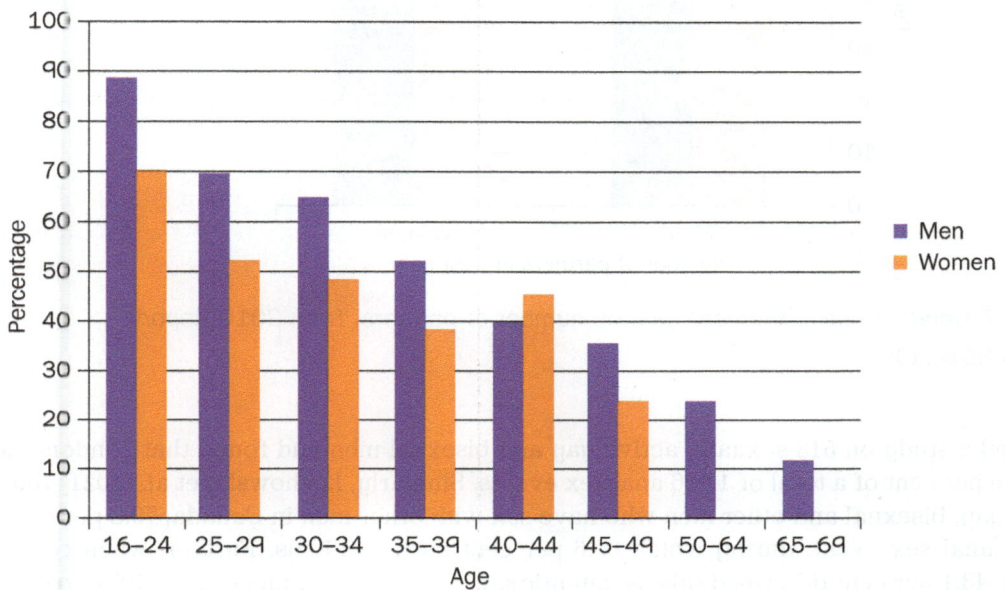

Figure 6.6 Condom use in the previous year by age and sex, from 2010 Report
SOURCE: ONS (2013)

The ONS (2013) survey also asked about condom use and number of partners. These data are shown in Figure 6.7 The results from this analysis indicate that condom use is more common in both men and women who have had more than one partner in the past year.

Gay Men

Research has examined condom use among men who have sex with men (MSM). Weatherburn et al. (1991) interviewed 930 homosexually active men in England and Wales and reported that 270 of them had had insertive anal intercourse in the preceding month, with 38.9 per cent reporting always using a condom, 49.6 per cent never using a condom and 11.5 per cent sometimes using a condom. Of the 254 who reported having receptive anal sex in the preceding month, 42.5 per cent had always used a condom, 45.7 per cent had never used a condom and 11.8 per cent had sometimes used a condom. Weatherburn et al. reported that condom use was associated with casual, not regular, sexual partners and was more common in open and non-monogamous relationships. Research also shows that there was a consistent increase in condom use among gay men from the mid 1980s to the late 1990s following the identification of HIV and the subsequent recognition that condom use was the most effective form of prevention. Recent data, however, suggest that this trend is reversing with an increasing number of gay men practising unprotected anal sex (known as 'bare backing', see Ridge 2004) in both the USA and the UK (Chen et al. 2002; Dodds and Mercey 2002). For example, Lachowski et al. (2016)

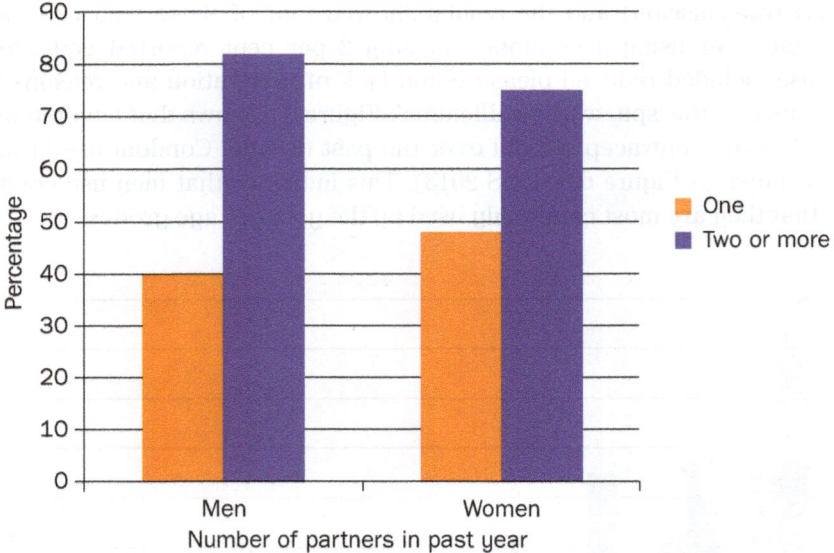

Figure 6.7 Condom use in the past year by number of partners, from 2010 Report

SOURCE: ONS (2013)

conducted a study on 513 sexually active gay and bisexual men and found that condoms were used in only 56 per cent of a total of 1,196 anal sex events. Similarly, Lachowsky et al. (2021) reported that of 1,830 gay, bisexual and other men who have sex with other men in Canada, 79.8 per cent reported a recent anal sex event, during which 60.6 per cent used condoms. Further, when condoms were not used, 43.1 per cent described this as 'intentional'. Likewise, Swann et al. (2019) carried out a longitudinal study with data collected in 2007, 2010 and 2015 to assess changes from late adolescence to adulthood. Overall, the results showed that younger MSM were engaging in less anal sex, but also less likely to use a condom whereas as they got older they were more likely to use a condom but also engaged in more anal sex. For example, at age 17, 57 per cent of an average of 10.17 anal sex acts were condomless, whereas by age 26, 30 per cent of an average of 19.53 anal sex acts were condomless, or an average of 5.86 CAS acts. Therefore, within this high-risk group, condom use is low. In addition, research indicates that gay men who have unsafe sex talk about their behaviour in terms of a number of factors which justify or perpetuate the non-use of condoms. These include condom fatigue, unsafe sex as a sign of intimacy and optimistic beliefs about the effectiveness of treatments for HIV (Adam et al. 2005; Martin 2006).

Over the last decade, the risk of contracting HIV has been greatly reduced by the introduction of medication called PrEP (pre-exposure prophylaxis). When taken as prescribed PrEP can reduce the risk of acquiring HIV up to 99 per cent. In 2021 Ayerdi Aguirrebengoa et al. assessed the impact of PrEP on condom use for anal intercourse, number of sexual partners, sexualized drug use and STI incidence. The results showed that 78.2 per cent of PrEP users reported a reduction in condom use for anal intercourse and that while before PrEP, 85.4 per cent used condoms usually in anal intercourse; 10.0 per cent occasionally and 4.5 per cent never; after PrEP, only 30.0 per cent used condoms usually, 50.0 per cent occasionally and 20.0 per cent never.

Bisexuals

Boulton et al. (1991) asked 60 bisexual men about their sexual behaviour and their condom use. Over the previous 12 months, 80 per cent had had male partners, 73 per cent had had female partners and 60 per cent had had at least one male and one female partner. In terms of their condom use with their current partner, 25 per cent reported always using a condom with their current male partner, 12 per cent reported always using a condom with their current female partner, 27 per cent reported sometimes/never using a condom with their male partner and 38 per cent reported sometimes/never using a condom with their female partner. In terms of their non-current partner, 30 per cent had had unprotected sex with a man and 34 per cent had had unprotected sex with a woman. Schnarrs et al. (2021) examined HIV prevention practices according to sexual subcultural community using a social and sexual networking smartphone app and reported that of 2533 who identified as bisexual, 57.7 per cent reported condom use whereas 42.3 per cent reported not using condoms. Fernandes et al. (2015) conducted a cross-sectional study with 430 men who have sex with men and transgender women to investigate syphilis infection, sexual practices and bisexual behaviour. Results found that bisexual men having sexual intercourse with a woman was a protective factor for developing syphilis due to increased condom use, compared with bisexual men having sexual intercourse with a man.

Transsexuals

Some research has also started to explore condom use in transsexuals. For example, Yi et al. (2019) explored consistent condom use among sexually-active transgender women (n = 1202) in Cambodia, specifically who reported having anal sex with at least one non-commercial male partner in the past three months. The results showed that 41.5 per cent reported always using condoms with male non-commercial partners and that consistent condom use was predicted by living in an urban community and having at least 10 years of formal education. Likewise, Wang et al. (2020) reported that the rate of consistent condom use in transgender women in China (n = 198) was 47.0 per cent. More research is needed in this group.

PREDICTING CONDOM USE

Simple models using 'knowledge only' have been used to examine condom use yet show that knowledge is not enough to predict using condoms (eg. Wang et al. 2020) as a focus on knowledge only ignores the individual's beliefs and assume that simply increasing knowledge about HIV will promote safe sex. In order to incorporate an individual's cognitive state, models such as HBM, TPB and the COM-B have been applied to condom use in the context of HIV and AIDS (see Chapter 2 for a discussion of these models). These models are similar to those used to predict other health-related behaviours, including contraceptive use for pregnancy avoidance, and illustrate varying attempts to understand cognitions in the context of the relationship and the broader social context.

Using Models of Health Beliefs and Behaviour

A number of models have been used to predict condom use in heterosexual and homosexual populations. For example, research has used the COM-B to develop an intervention for the prevention of HIV and STIs (Bru-Garcia et al. 2022), the HBM has been used for gay men (McCusker et al. 1989) and for heterosexual men and women (Winfield and Whaley 2002), and studies have used the TRA and TPB to predict condom use (e.g. Fisher 1984; Boldero et al. 1992; Albarracin et al. 2001). Research has also explored the relative usefulness of different models for predicting condom use (Espada et al. 2015) and in framing interventions to promote condom use (Montanaro and Bryan 2014; Bru-Garcia et al. 2022). In general, results from these studies indicate the following:

- *The role of habit:* the most reliable predictor of future condom use behaviour is past condom use.
- *The role of norms:* peer, partner and social norms are good predictors of condom use. It remains more normal for men than women to carry condoms.
- *Support is important:* partner support is a good predictor of condom use.
- *Self-efficacy:* self-efficacy predicts condom use highlighting the need for skills training as a means to promote self-efficacy.

- *Perception of risk:* risk perception can predict condom use but this comes with the problems of a ceiling effect and a floor effect.
- *A ceiling effect:* there is a consensus of perceptions of severity for HIV which presents the problem of a ceiling effect with only small differences in ratings of this variable.
- *A floor effect:* although people appear to know about HIV, its causes and how it is transmitted, feelings of immunity and low susceptibility ('it won't happen to me') are extremely common. This presents the problem of a floor effect with little individual variability (see later for discussions of risk perceptions).
- *Safer sex requires long-term maintenance of behaviour:* the HBM, TRA, TPB and COM-B may be good predictors of short-term changes in behaviour (e.g. taking up an exercise class, stopping smoking in the short term), but safer sex is an ongoing behaviour which requires an ongoing determination to adopt condom use as a habit.

Problems with using health belief and behaviour models

Using models such as the HBM, TPB and COM-B provides some insights into the predictors of condom use but has its problems in common with the use of these models in general (see Chapter 2). In addition, this approach neglects a number of key factors that might explain why people do or do not use condoms:

1 *Inconsistent findings:* the research examining condom use has not produced consistent results. Different studies have used very different populations (gay, heterosexual, adolescents, adults). Perhaps models of condom use should be constructed to fit the cognitive sets of different populations. Attempts to develop one model for everyone may ignore the multitude of different cognitions held by different individuals within different groups.

2 *Sex as a result of individual cognitions:* models that emphasize cognitions and information processing intrinsically regard behaviour as the result of information processing – an individualistic approach to behaviour. In particular, early models tended to focus on representations of an individual's risks without taking into account their interactions with the outside world. Furthermore, models such as the HBM emphasize this process as rational. However, recent models have attempted to remedy this situation by emphasizing cognitions about the individual's social world (the normative beliefs) and by including elements of emotion (the behaviour becomes less rational).

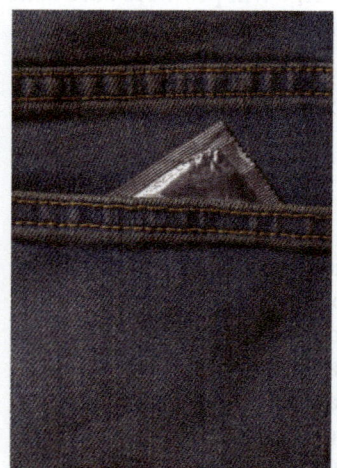

Social norms predict condom use. But it's still more normal for men to carry condoms than women (is this a man or a woman?)

SOURCE: © Shutterstock / Bobkov Evgeniy

3 *Perception of susceptibility:* in addition, these models predict that, because people appear to know that HIV is an extremely serious disease, and they know how it is transmitted, they will feel vulnerable (e.g. 'HIV is transmitted by unprotected sex, I have unprotected sex, therefore I am at risk from HIV'). This does not appear to be the case and many people underestimate their risk of HIV. Furthermore, the models predict that high levels of susceptibility will relate to less risk-taking behaviour (e.g. 'I am at risk, therefore I will use condoms'). Again this association is problematic.

4 *Sex as an interaction between individuals – the relationship context:* models of condom use focus on cognitions. In attempts to include an analysis of the place of this behaviour (the relationship), variables such as peer norms, partner norms and partner support have been added. However, these variables are still accessed by asking one individual about their beliefs about the relationship. Perhaps this is still only accessing a cognition, not the interaction.

But sex is an interaction between people and condom use requires some degree of communication and negotiation.

5 *Sex in a social context:* sex also takes place within a broader social context, involving norms about sexual practices, gender roles and stereotypes, the role of illness and theories of sexual behaviour. Cognitive models cannot address this broader context.

6 *Sex is emotional and involves a level of high arousal:* these factors are omitted in these models.

The remainder of this chapter will address some of these issues.

4 SEX AND RISK PERCEPTION

Having sex today involves a relationship to risk that is different from that seen previously. However, one of the most consistent findings to emerge from the research is the perception of personal invulnerability to HIV across all different sexualities. These feelings of invulnerability are shown by quantitative studies that have examined ratings of perceived susceptibility and unrealistic optimism (see Chapters 2 and 12). For example, Abrams et al. (1990) concluded from their survey in 1988 that young people 'have a strong sense of AIDS invulnerability which seems to involve a perception that they have control over the risk at which they place themselves'. More recently, Mwaba et al. (2020) explored gender differences in the perceived risk of contracting HIV and AIDS among sexually active unmarried young people in Zambia. The results showed that 61 per cent of females and 64.4 per cent of males reported a low perceived risk of contracting HIV and that low risk perception was predicted by wealth index, exposure to media, consistent use of condoms with all partners and drinking alcohol. Further, a study of young people in Ghana (n = 706) found that only 20.5 per cent perceived themselves to be at risk of HIV infection (Afriyie and Essilfie 2019). Clifton et al. (2016) conducted a study on 13,751 sexually active men and women in Britain which investigated the relationship between HIV risk behaviour, risk perception and HIV testing. They found that a higher perception of the risk of HIV was associated with greater sexual risk behaviours and with HIV testing. However, they also found that the majority of those who perceived themselves to be at a high risk of HIV had not been tested in the past year. Furthermore, of those who were gay men and black Africans (the groups most affected by HIV), while the majority reported sexual risk behaviours, they did not perceive themselves to be at risk of HIV and had not been tested for HIV. In a similar vein, a cross-sectional study described perception of risk of HIV among transgender women in Colombia (n = 620). The results showed that higher risk perception was associated with being single, working in prostitution, had sexually transmitted infections in the last year, avoiding health services and using cocaine (Ramos-Jaraba et al. 2021). Further, Biello et al. (2019) reported that among men who have sex with men, at a STI clinic those who perceived themselves to be at higher risk of HIV were more likely to express interest in PrEP although higher perception of risk to HIV was not related to lower risk of other rectal STIs.

Qualitative methods have also been used to further examine whether individuals feel that they are at risk from HIV. In an early study, carried out during the AIDS epidemic, Woodcock et al. (1992) interviewed 125 young people aged 16–25 about their sexual behaviour and examined how these individuals evaluated their own risk factors. The authors reported that many of the interviewees endorsed risky behaviour and gave reasons both acknowledging their own risk or denying that they had put themselves at risk. Their ways of coping with risk were as follows:

1 *Acknowledging risk:* one subject acknowledged that their behaviour had been risky, saying, 'I'm a chancer and I know I'm a chancer . . . with this AIDS thing, I know that I should use a condom.' However, most subjects, even though they acknowledged some degree of risk, managed to dismiss it in terms of 'it would show by now', 'it was in the past' or 'AIDS wasn't around in those days' (from a 21-year-old interviewee).

2 *Denying risk:* most commonly, people denied that they had ever put themselves at risk and the complex ways in which their sexual behaviour was rationalized illustrates how complicated the concept of susceptibility and 'being at risk' is. Woodcock et al. (1992) presented many ways of rationalizing risky behaviour. These included believing 'it's been blown out of proportion', that 'AIDS is a risk you take in living' and the authors reported that 'the theme of being run over, particularly by buses' was common and believing that 'it doesn't affect me' was also apparent. In addition, the interviewees evaluated their own risk in the context of the kinds of people with whom they had sex. For example, 'I don't go with people who go around a lot', 'He said, I've only slept with you in the last six months', and 'I do not have sex in risky geographical areas' – one interviewee said, 'London is the capital: has to be more AIDS.'

Some research has also used qualitative methods to explore risk perception in men who have sex with men. For example, Flowers et al. (1998) explored how gay men feel about sex in the context of HIV and argued that although they are aware of their risk in the abstract, this 'somewhat distant threat of HIV' can lose its meaning in the immediate context of sex and other more pertinent desires or concerns. Similarly, it has been argued that gay men have 'actual' rather than 'hypothetical' sexual encounters and that the rational decision to minimize the threat of HIV can get lost in the moment of having sex (Westhaver 2005; Martin 2006). In 2020, Tan et al. used a qualitative approach to explore which factors influence perceptions of risk of HIV or other STIs in gay, bisexual, and other men who have sex with men. The results showed that participants drew upon a range of factors including past experiences of risk, perceived trust and familiarity with their sexual partners, and situational factors such as their familiarity with the venues where sexual activity took place.

Most health belief models emphasizing rational information processing suggest that condom use is related to feelings of susceptibility and being at risk from HIV. However, many people do not appear to believe that they themselves are at risk, which is perhaps why they do not engage in self-protective behaviour, and even when some acknowledgement of risk is made, this is often dismissed and does not always relate to behaviour change.

5 | SEX AS AN INTERACTION

Studying sexual behaviour is not straightforward from a psychological perspective as it presents a problem – of interaction. Social psychologists have spent decades emphasizing the context within which behaviour occurs. This is reflected in the extensive literature on areas such as conformity to majority and minority influence, group behaviour and decision-making, and obedience to authority. Such a perspective emphasizes that an individual's behaviour occurs as an interaction both with other individuals and with the broader social context. Sex highlights this interaction as it is inherently an interactive behaviour. Health psychology, however, draws on many other areas of psychology (e.g. physiological, cognitive, behavioural), which have tended to examine individuals *on their own*. In addition, psychological methodologies such as questionnaires and interviews involve an individual's experience (e.g. I felt, I believe, I think, I did). Even if individuals discuss their interactions with other individuals (e.g. we felt, we believe, we think, we did), or place their experiences in the context of others (e.g. I felt happy because she made me feel relaxed), only their own individual experiences are accessed using the psychological tools available. This problem of interaction is exacerbated by the psychological methodologies available (unless the researcher simply observes two people having sex!). The problem of the interaction has been addressed in terms of the process of negotiation, the power relations between men and women and the social norms of the LGBTQ+ community.

THE PROCESS OF NEGOTIATION

In 1990, a large scale project called the WRAP study interviewed 150 women from London and Manchester about their sexual histories and sexual behaviour and described the factors that related to the negotiation of condom use. Holland et al. (1990b) stated that during sex *'words are likely to be the most difficult things to exchange'* and suggested that the negotiation of condom use is far more complex than *'a simple, practical question about dealing rationally with risk, it is the outcome of negotiation between potentially unequal partners'*. They suggested that although the process of negotiation may be hindered by embarrassment as suggested by some of the health promotion campaigns, this *'embarrassment over using condoms is not simply a question of bad timing but indicates a very complex process of negotiation'*. Therefore they place condom use within the context of the relationship and, rather than see the interaction between individuals as only one component of the process of condom use, they place this interaction centrally.

The results from the WRAP study provide some insights into the process of negotiation and the interaction between individuals. Some of the interviewees reported no difficulties in demanding safe sex, with one woman saying, 'If they don't want to wear a condom, then tough, you know, go and find someone else'. Another woman said, 'He really hates using them, so I used to say to him, "look, right, look, I have no intention of getting pregnant again and you have no intention to become a father so you put one of these on".' However, other women described how difficult it was to suggest safe sex to their partner with reasons for this relating to not wanting to hurt their boyfriend's feelings, not wanting to 'ruin the whole thing', and not being able to approach the subject. One woman said, 'When I got pregnant I thought to myself, "I'm not using a condom here, I'm not using anything" but I just couldn't say, just couldn't force myself to say, "look you know"'. Holland et al. (1990b) argued that safe sex campaigns present condoms as neutral objects, which can be easily negotiated prior to sex and that this did not appear to be the case with the women they interviewed. The qualitative data from the WRAP study provide some insights into the process of negotiation; they also emphasize sex as an interaction. In addition, these data provide a relationship context for individual beliefs and cognitions.

In line with the WRAP study, Debro et al. (1994) examined the strategies used by 393 heterosexual college students to negotiate condom use and concluded that they used reward, emotional coercion, risk information, deception, seduction and withholding sex. Noar et al. (2002) built upon Debro et al.'s work and developed and validated a measure to quantify negotiation strategies called the Condom Influence Strategy Questionnaire (CISQ). They conceptualized negotiation in terms of six strategies: withholding sex, direct request, education, relationship conceptualizing, risk information, and deception, and indicated that these factors account for variance in a range of safer sex variables such as behavioural intentions and actual condom use. Stone and Ingham (2002) also explored partner communication in the context of predicting the use of contraception at first intercourse. The study involved a survey of 963 students aged between 16 and 18 and explored the role of a range of individual, contextual and background factors. The results showed that communication with a partner was a significant predictor of contraception use for both men and women. In particular, young men's contraception use was predicted by discussing contraception beforehand, giving an intimate reason for having sex the first time (e.g. they loved their partner as opposed to losing their virginity) and having parents who portrayed sexuality positively. For young women, contraception use was predicted by discussing contraception beforehand, being older, expecting to have sex, comfort and ease of interacting with boys and not having visited a sexual health service provider prior to having sex (this last result was in contrast to much previous work). Wilkinson et al. (2002) also highlighted a role for partner cooperation. They asked 398 unmarried students to rate both their sexual behaviour and their perception of how cooperative their partner had been to practise safer sex. The results showed that partner cooperation was linked to safer sexual behaviour. Likewise, Amialchuk and Gerhardinger (2015) reported that adolescents who were 'going out' with their partner were more likely to use contraception as were those who discussed contraception before sex suggesting a role for relationships and negotiation. Similarly, Ajayi et al. (2019) reported that condom use by students in Nigeria was predicted by the ability to discuss HIV and STIs with their sexual partner and Catelan et al. (2021) explored condom-protected sex among transgender men (n = 68) and transgender women (n = 192) and reported a key role for condom negotiation self-efficacy in predicting condom use.

Qualitative and quantitative research has emphasized the importance of negotiation which seems to have been taken on board by health education campaigns with advertisements highlighting the problem of raising the issue of safer sex (e.g. when would you mention condoms?). However, do interviews really access the interaction? Can the interaction be accessed using the available (and ethical) methodologies? (It would obviously be problematic to observe the interaction!) Are qualitative methods actually accessing something different from quantitative methods? Are interviews simply another method of finding out about people's cognitions and beliefs? Debates about methodology (quantitative versus qualitative) and the problem of behaviour as an interaction are relevant to all forms of behaviour but are particularly apparent when discussing sex.

POWER RELATIONS BETWEEN SEXUAL PARTNERS

Sex is an interaction between people and using contraception, particularly condoms, emerges out of this interaction, with or without explicit negotiation. But relationships between people are often unequal and research has explored the impact of power relations between sexual partners, both between men and women and between men and men.

Men and Women

Holland et al. (1990b) argued that condom use 'must be understood in the context of the contradictions and tensions of heterosexual relationships' and the 'gendered power relations which construct and constrain choices and decisions'. They presented examples of power inequalities between men and women and the range of ways in which inequality can express itself, from coercion to rape. For example, one woman in their study said, 'I wasn't forced to do it but I didn't want to do it' and another explained her ambivalence to sex as 'like, do you want a coffee? Okay, fine, you drink the coffee, because you don't really like drinking coffee but you drink it anyway.' In fact, empirical research suggests that men's intentions to use condoms may be more likely to correlate with actual behaviour than women's, perhaps because women's intentions may be inhibited by the sexual context (Abraham et al. 1996). Likewise, a large-scale analysis of data from the African Cohort Study (n = 2482), (Analogbei et al. 2020) reported that partner disapproval of condom use or actual refusal to use a condom was a consistent driver of condom non-use among participants who were HIV-infected, female and aged 18 to 24 years. Sex should therefore also be understood within the context of gender and power.

Men and Men

Studies indicate that between one-fifth to one-third of men report having experienced some form of sexual coercion in their relationships with men (see Flowers et al. 1998; Ratner et al. 2003; Ridge 2004). Gavey et al. (2009) carried out focus groups with 40 gay and bisexual men in New Zealand to explore how coercion was experienced and its impact on safer sex practices and highlighted issues relating to drugs and alcohol, power and experience. Gavey et al. (2009) concluded that safe sex practices require choice and control and a process of negotiation, but that power relations between men can result in coercion which undermines these behaviours. Likewise, Kubicek et al. (2015) conducted a qualitative study with young gay and bisexual men to understand their relationship challenges and experiences of intimate partner violence. The participants described power as stemming from a variety of sources within the relationship such as sexual positioning, gender roles, income, education, internalized homophobia and prior relationship experiences. All believed that power and sexual behaviour are interwoven.

Transsexuals' experiences

Sexual coercion has also been reported by transsexual men and women. For example, Bungener et al. (2020) described sexual and romantic development during and after gender-affirmative treatment (n = 113). The results showed that 13.6 per cent of transgender young adults reported negative sexual experiences, which was equivalent for transwomen and transmen. Likewise, a large-scale study by Heino et al. (2020) compared sexual experiences of trans youth with their cisgender peers. The results showed that after adjusting for sex, age and honesty, transgender youth had increased odds for both sexual coercion and dating violence perpetration. Power relations can also exist between patients and health care professionals and interestingly, Yan et al. (2019) also reported that transgender women in China are less likely to go for HIV and STI testing due to fear of discrimination and stigma at testing sites.

Sex is therefore an interaction between people which should be understood within the context of power. This is perfectly illustrated by a sex education video created by Thames Valley Police (2015) which compares having sex with having a cup of tea and describes how if someone doesn't want a cup of tea you don't force them to have one. Please do watch this video!

SOCIAL NORMS OF THE LGBTQ+ COMMUNITY

Sex also occurs within the context of the LGBTQ+ communities, which have their own sets of norms and values. Studies by Flowers et al. (1997, 1998) explored 'the transformation of men who come to find themselves within a specific gay culture, one in which there are clear values which structure their new social world, shaping their relationships and their sexual behaviour'. Flowers et al. asked the question 'How do the social norms and values of the gay community influence gay men's sexual practices?' They interviewed 20 gay men from a small town in northern England about their experiences of becoming gay within a gay community. The results provided some interesting insights into the norms of gay culture and the impact of this social context on an individual's behaviour. First, the study describes how men gain access to the gay community: 'through sex and socialising they come to recognise the presence of other gay men where once . . . they only felt isolation'; second, the study illustrates how simply having a gay identity is not enough to prepare them for their new community and that they have 'to learn a gay specific knowledge and a gay language'; and third, the study describes how this new culture influences their sexual behaviour. For example, the interviewees described how feelings of romance, trust, love, commitment, inequality within the relationship, lack of experience and desperation resulted in having anal sex without a condom even though they had the knowledge that their behaviour was risky.

There are also norms relating to the use of drugs for sex. For example, Ahmed et al. (2016) interviewed 30 gay men who had used illicit substances either immediately before or during intercourse to investigate the social norms surrounding 'chemsex' – the combining of drugs and sex. The results showed that those who engaged in chemsex described exaggerated beliefs about the popularity and normality of chemsex, suggesting that they overestimated the norm for this behaviour. Similarly, Hibbert et al. (2019) explored sexualized drug use among women who have sex with women (WSW). The results showed that 39 per cent reported any drug use and 17 per cent reported sexualized drug use and that those who reported sexualized drug use were more likely to identify as bisexual, have had more than five female sexual partners and have left education at 16 years or less. In 2020, Pienaar et al. carried out 32 qualitative interviews in Australia to explore the use of drugs in the LBBTQ+ community. The results indicated that not only can drug use enhance sexual pleasure but it can also facilitate gender expression and at times help to ameliorate bodily discomfort. Sexual behaviour therefore also occurs within the context of specific communities with their own sets of norms and values.

IN SUMMARY

Sex is therefore an interaction between two people which provides a problem for research, particularly psychology, with its focus on the individual and the use of models which emphasize cognitions. This interaction is illustrated by research which has focused on the process of negotiation, the role of power and the impact of the norms of any given community.

6 | SEX EDUCATION

The decision to use contraception or condoms is informed by sex education that comes from a variety of different sources, including sexual health services, government health education campaigns, school sex education programmes and an individual's social world. These four sources of information will now be examined further.

SEXUAL HEALTH SERVICES

Specialist family planning clinics, genito-urinary clinics, general practitioners (GPs), the chemist and nurse practitioners all provide sexual health services offering access to contraception and sexual health information and advice. Even condom machines in public toilets and free condoms in youth clubs act as a form of sexual health service. Research shows that, to be effective, sexual health services must be user friendly, non-judgemental, accessible, approachable and confidential (Allen 1991; Stone and Ingham 2000). For example, Allen (1991) evaluated three new family planning and pregnancy counselling projects for young people set up in 1987 and subsequently monitored their use over an 18-month period. This evaluation identified a range of factors that made contraception services more or less acceptable to young people, including inconvenient opening times, embarrassment at being seen by other people while seeking sexual health advice, not feeling comfortable with the staff, judgemental or unhelpful staff, fear of the services not being confidential and having to give personal details. In a similar vein, Harden and Ogden (1999b) asked 967 16–19-year-olds about their beliefs and use of contraception services and reported that the chemist and the condom machine had been used by the largest number of respondents, with men favouring the condom machine and women favouring the GP or family planning clinic. In terms of beliefs, the condom machine was regarded as the easiest and most comfortable to use but the least confidential, with men reporting higher ratings for ease of use than women. Much research shows that young people in particular do not use sexual health services and often report finding contraceptives difficult (Stone and Ingham 2000). Stone and Ingham (2003) gave a questionnaire to 747 attendees at a youth-targeted sexual health service to investigate why they used the service. The results showed that 29 per cent had used a service before having ever had sex, 'to be prepared', but that the remainder had only used a service after having sex. The most common reasons for non-use of services were being embarrassed or scared, concern about confidentiality or not knowing how to access services.

Research also shows similar concerns from members of the LGBTQ+ community. For example, a qualitative study in Tasmania by Lea et al. (2019) reported that whilst most gay and bisexual men interviewed were satisfied with their care at public sexual health services, barriers to use included concerns about anonymity and privacy in small communities and perceived stigma and discrimination. Yan et al. (2019) also reported that transgender women are reluctant to go for HIV and STI testing for fear of discrimination and stigma at testing sites. Similarly, Tan et al. (2020) concluded from their qualitative study of gay, bisexual or queer men that sexual health clinics can be stigmatizing and can impose 'deviant' identities on individuals who access them. Knight et al. (2019) explored men who have sex with men's experiences of *GetCheckedOnline.com* (GCO) compared to clinic-based testing. The results showed that many men preferred the online approach due to convenience, privacy and control over specimen collection (doing your own throat or anal swab) and preferred receiving their results online rather than by phone or email follow-up by clinic staff. However, attending a clinic was seen as better than GCO for addressing other co-occurring health issues such as mental health problems or substance use disorders. Almost all of the participants anticipated using both GCO and clinic-based services in the future.

Sexual health services are therefore key to promoting sexual health, yet many people anticipate or actually experience them in ways that prevent them from using them when necessary.

GOVERNMENT HEALTH EDUCATION CAMPAIGNS

In light of the AIDS epidemic in the 1980s and the increased awareness of the need for safer sex to prevent HIV transmission, a number of government health campaigns were introduced. Ingham et al. (1991) examined UK campaigns that promoted safe sex and suggested that slogans such as 'Unless you're completely sure about your partner, always use a condom', 'Nowadays is it really wise to have sex with a stranger?' and 'Sex with a lot of partners, especially with people you don't know, can be dangerous' emphasize knowing your partner. They interviewed a group of young people in the south of England to examine how they interpreted 'knowing their partners'. The results suggest that 27 per cent of the interviewees had had sex within 24 hours of becoming a couple, that 10 per cent of the sample reported having sex on the first ever occasion on which they met their partner, and that over 50 per cent reported having sex within two weeks of beginning a relationship. In terms of 'knowing their partner', 31 per cent of males and 35 per cent of females reported knowing nothing of their partner's sexual history, and knowing was often explained in terms of 'she came from a nice family and stuff', and having 'seen them around'. The results from this study indicate that promoting 'knowing your partner' may not be the best way to promote safe sex as knowledge can be interpreted in a multitude of different ways. In addition, safer sex campaigns emphasize personal responsibility and choice in the use of condoms, and condoms are presented as a simple way to prevent contraction of the HIV virus. This presentation is epitomized by government health advertisement slogans such as, 'You know the risks: the decision is yours'. This view of sex and condom use is in contradiction with the research suggesting that people believe that they are not at risk from HIV and that condom use involves a complex process of negotiation. In December 2017, Public Health England launched 'Protect against STIs', which was the first government sexual health campaign in 8 years and was aimed at reducing STI rates in 16–24 year olds through condom use. It was a nationwide digital advertising campaign which involves various real people talking about their own experiences of having an STI. In 2022, Fearce et al. reviewed 19 studies assessing the effectiveness of campaigns to promote uptake of chlamydia screening in young people aged 15 to 24 years. The quantitative evaluation indicated that while the campaigns increased the overall number of tests, the trend was not as clear for tests that were positive, indicating that the campaign may not be addressing the right audience. The qualitative evaluation indicated that for the campaigns to be effective they needed to have clear, relevant messaging that displayed the full range of testing options and must reassure the public of their anonymity. Government campaigns however, are not always relevant to everyone and Binse (2021) explored how sexual health promotion in England represents women who have sex with women (WSW) and their STI risk. They analysed five policy documents and 42 campaign materials and concluded that the androcentric and heteronormative framing of sexual health promotion results in the erasure of WSW which perpetuates false narratives of low STI risk which acts as a form of symbolic annihilation of this group and can be considered a form of symbolic violence. This also reflects evidence that lesbian women are less likely to receive contraceptive counselling at pregnancy tests, but more likely to be offered a STD test, and that lesbian women without male partners were less likely to have a counselling session about condom use at STD-related visits compared with heterosexual women (Everett et al. 2019).

SCHOOL SEX EDUCATION PROGRAMMES

Information about sex also comes from sex education programmes at school. Holland et al. (1990a) interviewed young women about their experiences of sex education and concluded that such education in schools is impersonal, mechanistic and concerned with biology. The women in their study made comments such as 'it was all from the book, it wasn't really personal' and 'nobody ever talks to you about the problems and the entanglements, and what it means to a relationship when you start having sex'. It has been argued that this impersonal and objective approach to sex education is counterproductive (Aggleton 1989) and several alternatives have been suggested. Aggleton and Homans (1988) argued for a 'socially transformatory model' for AIDS education, which would involve discussions of: (1) ideas about sex; (2) social relations; (3) political processes involved; and (4) the problem of resource allocation. This approach would attempt to shift the emphasis from didactic teachings of facts and knowledge to a discussion of sex within a context of relationships and the broader social context. An additional solution to the problem of sex education is a skills training approach recommended by Abraham and Sheeran (1993). They argued that individuals could be taught a variety of skills, including buying condoms, negotiation of condom use and using condoms. These skills could be transmitted using tuition, role-play, feedback, modelling and practice. They are aimed at changing cognitions, preparing individuals for action and encouraging people to practise different aspects of the sequences involved in translating beliefs into behaviour. Sell et al. (2021) carried out a systematic review of process evaluation studies of school-based sex education and highlighted a number of factors to maximise their effectiveness, with a focus on transforming gender norms and empowerment. These included a key role of the skill and training of the facilitator, the need to be flexible and adapt to students' needs, having a supportive school environment, student participation, student-facilitator relationship-building, and open discussions concerning gender and power. Such approaches are all far away from a more traditional focus on biology. Likewise, Ingham (2005) provides a detailed analysis of sex and relationship education and argues for the importance of teaching young people about desire and pleasure and how these are important both to physical and mental health. In particular, Ingham suggests that by learning about their bodies and how to achieve sexual pleasure, young people may feel more empowered to have healthier and happier sexual relationships. He argues that 'if young people are enabled to feel more relaxed about their own bodies, and about bodily pleasures then they may be less affected by the pressures to engage in sexual activity against their wishes or in ways that they do not feel comfortable about' (p. 385). Ingham then suggests that the use of small group teaching, organized around friendship groups with people at similar stages of sexual development and experience, could enable a deeper and more focused discussion of both the 'factual' and pleasure aspects of sex. Recently, Gillespie et al. (2022) carried out in-depth interviews with 17 lesbian, gay, bisexual, and other sexual minority (LGB−) individuals, aged 18–23 years, about their experiences of first same sex/gender sex. The results indicated that participants, particularly women, reported difficulty defining sex between same-sex/gender partners, that men mostly met their partners online and that many were motivated by factors such as affirmation of personal sexual identity, sexual exploration, social expectation and spontaneity. Further, many participants felt that they had not been prepared for their first same-sex/gender sex and felt that their sex and relationship education had not included any relevant information. They therefore had turned to more experienced partners, pornography and social media. The authors concluded that sex education needs to better recognize sexual diversity to prepare LGB+ young people for their early sexual encounters.

In contrast to this more liberal perspective, over the past decade or so some countries have been promoting an abstinence only approach which has been particularly apparent across the US. Hall et al. (2019) analysed the content of school-based sex education policies of all 50 states of the US and concluded that most state policies emphasized abstinence from sexual behaviour and did not require education about contraception to prevent either pregnancy or STIs. Only half of the states addressed relationship issues such as healthy relationships, sexual decision-making and sexual violence; only a few states required content on communication about sexual consent and eight states explicitly stigmatized homosexuality. In contrast, 12 states were found to be inclusive of diverse sexual orientations and 7 states were inclusive of diverse gender identities. In line with this approach, Rabbitte and Enrique (2019) reviewed the evidence for the impact of policy on sexual health education and concluded that while abstinence was the best way to avoid both unwanted pregnancies and STIs, promoting abstinence only in schools was ineffective in delaying sexual initiation or decreasing teenage pregnancy or STI rates whereas comprehensive sex education programmes were effective at both delaying sex initiation and decreasing unwanted pregnancies.

An Individual's Social World

Information about sex also comes from an individual's broader social world and Holland et al. (1990a) argued that sex education and the process of learning about sex occur in the context of five key sources: school, peers, parents, magazines, and partners and relationships. Holland et al. argued that through these different sources, individuals learn about sex and their sexuality and suggested that 'the constructions which are presented are of women as passive, as potential victims of male sexuality or at best reproductive' (p. 43). However, they also argued that women do not simply passively accept this version of sexuality but are in a 'constant process of negotiating and re-negotiating the meaning which others give to their behaviour' (p. 43). . They therefore redefined the 'problem of sex education' as something that is broader than acquiring facts and that the resulting knowledge not only influences an individual's own knowledge and beliefs but also creates their sexuality.

In line with this, much research highlights the key role of learning from peers. For example, from their scoping review Dias et al. (2019) concluded that adolescents are influenced by their peers in decision-making around romantic and/or sexual relationships and that peers are the main source of information about sexual health. Likewise, Muraleetharan and Brault (2021) carried out a qualitative study of students living on campus and concluded that students turn to their friends for trusted information about sexual health services to share both logistical and emotional experiences.

In summary

Sex education therefore impacts upon sexual behaviour and can influence the decision to start having sex, choices about who to have sex with and the use of contraception for either pregnancy avoidance or the prevention of STIs. Sex education comes from a variety of different sources, including sexual health services government health education campaigns, school sex education programmes and an individual's social world. Any understanding of sexual behaviour should therefore take place within an understanding of the social context of sex education in the broadest sense.

BOX 6.1
Critical Approaches to Health Psychology

Research exploring sexual behaviour highlights some of the bigger issues with research in health psychology:

Gender differences: Much research exploring sexual behaviour focuses on gender differences particularly between men and women. This ignores the complexity of gender and assumes that this dichotomous approach tells us something about the people we are studying.

Sexuality: Research also classifies people as gay, heterosexual, bisexual, transsexual and assumes that these are fixed categories. It also assumes that these boxes are important and tell us something about how people think, feel and behave.

Making sense of data: When we collect data we collect it from individuals. But to describe it to others and make sense of it we need to analyse it and this mostly means looking for differences of similarities between groups. By doing this we impose false dichotomies upon the population being studied and risk creating or reinforcing stereotypes. But if we don't do this we just have hundreds of data points which would be meaningless. This is a dilemma for researchers!

The problem of power: This chapter has explored the role of power in sex and highlighted how power dynamics can exist between individuals. In the main, research exploring power has focused on power inequalities due to gender, age or economic factors. But power is a complex issue and may result from a vast array of other factors such as attractiveness, sexual experience, sexual confidence, past history, height, hair colour, education, status, having hair, size of breasts, penis size etc. Therefore, understanding power dynamics should involve exploring not only the traditional causes of power but all the possible factors that may influence a sexual dynamic.

7   THINKING CRITICALLY ABOUT SEX RESEARCH

Although sex is a behaviour like any other, researching sex and associated behaviours such as contraception and condom use has its own specific problems.

SOME CRITICAL QUESTIONS

When thinking about research in this area ask yourself the following questions.

* Why is sexual behaviour so difficult to measure?
* How does the interactive nature of sex pose a problem for researchers?
* Why does sex research mostly focus on the problems?
* Can sex research ever be unbiased and separate to the researcher's own values?

SOME PROBLEMS WITH. . .

Thinking critically about sex research involves recognizing the following problems:

Interaction: Sexual behaviour involves two people and therefore results out of an interaction between two sets of beliefs, emotions and behaviours. Although ultimately all behaviour is located in its social context, sexual behaviour explicitly illustrates this and therefore results in specific problems in terms of understanding and measuring what factors relate to whether someone has sex or not and whether they engage in risky behaviours.

A very personal area: Sexual behaviour can generate embarrassment and is considered a sensitive and personal area of research. This can lead to problems gaining ethical approval and in encouraging people to speak openly and honestly.

A problem: Most sexual behaviour research focuses on the problems associated with sex such as STDs and HIV. To date, little research in health psychology has highlighted sex as a healthy and pleasurable activity. In part, this is due to issues of embarrassment and in part due to funders' emphasis on health problems.

Research bias: Sexual behaviour research can be loaded with ideological perspectives in terms of whether people believe abstinence is the way forward, whether they are judgemental of homosexual behaviour, whether they believe in monogamy and whether they are critical of 'promiscuity'. Research may therefore be biased in terms of the areas of research selected, the data collected and funded and ways in which the research is interpreted and presented.

Stereotyping: Research exploring sexual behaviour tends to group people according to their sexuality (i.e. gay or heterosexual or bisexual or transsexual). While this reflects the breadth of sexualities it can also result in stereotyping and creating false dichotomies between different groups which may well not be as discrete or as different as we often treat them.

TO CONCLUDE

This chapter provided a brief history of sex research and documented the shift from sex as a biological function whose outcome was reproduction, to sex for pleasure, to sex as a risk towards a broader model which locates sexual behaviour within an individual's physical, mental and social well-being. This chapter explored contraception use for pregnancy avoidance with a focus on intrapersonal, interpersonal and situational factors. It then described research relating to condom use in the context of HIV/AIDS and STIs which has tended to emphasize individual cognitions. Sex, however, is intrinsically an interactive behaviour which presents a problem for psychologists. It also exists within a broader social context. This chapter has therefore explored this context in terms of perceptions of risk, the process of negotiation, power relations, the social norms of the LGBTQ+ community and sex education. Finally, this chapter has described some of the issues with carrying out research in this area.

QUESTIONS

1 Outline changes in the ways in which sex has been described over the past 200 years.
2 Why do people not use contraception?
3 To what extent can models such as the TPB and COM-B predict condom use?
4 How can qualitative research contribute to an understanding of condom use?
5 In what ways does the social context impact upon contraception and condom use?
6 Why can talking about contraception be difficult?
7 How might power influence sexual behaviour?
8 What are sexual norms of different communities and how might they influence sexual behaviour?
9 To what extent do the problems highlighted by the sex literature relate to other health behaviours?
10 Why is researching sex more difficult than other health behaviours?

FOR DISCUSSION

Watch the sex education campaign called 'Tea and sex', produced by Thames Valley Police (2015) and discuss what it is trying to achieve and whether you think it works.

FURTHER READING

Barker, M.J. (2018) *The Psychology of Sex*. London: Routledge.

This is a great little book that covers the theories and research around sex and sexuality in a accessible way.

Holland, J., Ramazanoglu, C. and Scott, S. (1990) Managing risk and experiencing danger: tensions between government AIDS health education policy and young women's sexuality, *Gender and Education*, **2**: 125–46.

The WRAP study was an impressive piece of qualitative work that changed the ways in which people thought about sexual behaviour. This paper presents some of the results from the WRAP and examines how young women feel about their sexuality in the context of HIV.

Ingham, R. and Aggleton, P. (eds)(2005) *Promoting Young People's Sexual Health*. London: Routledge.

This book provides an excellent analysis of the practical and ideological barriers to enhancing sexual health in young people and offers a detailed account of cross-cultural differences and the problems faced in developing countries.

Lee, E., Clements, S., Ingham, R. and Stone, N. (2004) *A Matter of Choice? Explaining National Variations in Teenage Abortion and Motherhood*. York: Joseph Rowntree Foundation.

This book provides a detailed analysis of young people's sexual behaviour and their decisions about becoming a parent.

Robinson, B.B., Bockting, W.O., Rossner, BR. et al. (2002) The sexual health model: application of a sexological approach to HIV prevention, *Health Education Research*, 17: 43–57.

This paper presents the sexual health model described at the start of this chapter and illustrates a broader way of thinking about sex, condom use and sex as a core part of people's lives.

7

Changing Health Behaviours

CHAPTER OVERVIEW

Chapter 2 explored factors that help us to understand and predict health-related behaviours. Chapters 3–6 then focused on individual health behaviours. This chapter explores a number of different approaches that have been developed to change health-related behaviours. Although there are a multitude of strategies that can be used to change individual behaviour, this chapter describes those that have been informed by four main theoretical perspectives: (1) learning and cognitive theory leading to behavioural strategies, cognitive behavioural therapy and relapse prevention; (2) social cognition theory and the use of social cognition models to frame interventions, planning, implementation intentions and information; (3) stages of change theory (SOC) and the development of stage matched interventions and motivational interviewing; (4) theories of affect and the use of fear appeals, visualization and self-affirmation. The chapter finally explores how these different approaches have been integrated through the creation of a science of behaviour change interventions, the use of modern technologies, the mass media and a focus on sustained behaviour change.

CASE STUDY

Sapphira is a dietician and works with patients with diabetes. Many of her patients are overweight and some take medication. Her role is to encourage them to eat a healthy diet, do more exercise, stop smoking and take their medication. This is not an easy task as many of their unhealthy habits have been entrenched for many years. In addition, she only sees them for 50 minutes every month. She does, however, always see the same patients and over time manages to build a relationship with them. During these consultations she finds that trying to understand their behaviour from their own perspective, listening rather than just giving advice, setting doable short-term goals which involve small changes that fit into their lives, rewarding them whenever they try to make a difference and keeping positive, work the best. She has also learned from experience that being disappointed or irritated when patients don't follow her advice just means that they don't come back. After many years in her job, Sapphira believes that the most important part of her role is to build a good relationship with her clients so that they keep coming back.

Through the Eyes of Health Psychology. . .

Changing behaviour is difficult as many behaviours are habitual and have become embedded over many years. Sapphira's story illustrates the difficult task faced by those trying to help others change their behaviour, which is far more complex than simply telling patients what to do. This chapter will describe the key theoretical approaches to behaviour change that highlight some of the behaviour change strategies illustrated above, such as reinforcement (rewarding patients and keeping positive); planning (setting doable goals); and tailored approaches (small changes that fit into their lives). It will then describe how these approaches have been integrated for use by different professionals and across the different health behaviours.

1   THE NEED TO CHANGE BEHAVIOUR

Before the twentieth century, the most common causes of death were childbirth or acute illnesses, such as tuberculosis or flu, caused by bacteria or viruses. Over the past 100 years this has changed and now most people in the developed world die as a result of chronic conditions such as heart disease, cancer, diabetes or obesity. Furthermore, the majority of those seeking medical help may not only have these more common chronic conditions but others including chronic back and joint pain, asthma, multiple sclerosis (MS), fibromyalgia, inflammatory bowel disorder (IBD), HIV/AIDS, high blood pressure, fatigue and headaches. These chronic conditions illustrate a key role for behaviour and why changing health behaviour is central to health care management:

- **To prevent illness:** Behaviour change is key to preventing chronic conditions. For example, stopping smoking can prevent lung cancer, eating a healthier diet can prevent bowel cancer and doing more exercise can prevent heart disease. This is sometimes called primary prevention.

- **To manage illness:** Once diagnosed with a chronic condition, behaviour change is also key to illness management. For example, dietary change plays a core role in the management of obesity and diabetes, increased exercise is central to the management of patients post heart attack and encouraging medication adherence is important for many illnesses such as asthma and those with high blood pressure. This is sometimes known as secondary prevention.

- **To reduce physical symptoms:** Chronic conditions can result in a multitude of physical symptoms such as fatigue, pain, nausea and bowel problems. Behaviour change can help to reduce these symptoms. For example, dietary change may reduce nausea or bowel problems and exercise may reduce fatigue and pain.

- **To improve well-being:** Having cancer, being diagnosed with heart disease or living with MS, fibromyalgia, asthma or IBD can be miserable and reduce a person's sense of well-being and quality of life. Behaviour change can also help to improve well-being. In particular, being more active has positive effects on mood (see Chapter 5) and can lead to more social support if people join group activities. Further, eating a healthier diet may or may not improve physical health outcomes for cancer but it can help people feel more in control of their lives and that they can make a difference in a small way.

Behaviour change is therefore central to many aspects of health. Research has explored ways to help people change their behaviour.

Behaviour change can be seen as being either conscious and effortful, whereby the individual makes choices about how and whether to change their behaviour (e.g. joining a gym) *or* effortless, whereby behaviour change occurs with no conscious processing (e.g. buying wholewheat bread as that is all that is on offer). Most psychological approaches encourage effortful changes in behaviour through interventions targeted at the individual. In contrast, public health interventions focus more on structural and environmental changes that bring about shifts in behaviour without the individual necessarily knowing they are involved in an intervention or even that they have changed their behaviour. Community events can encourage behaviour change by providing the right environment for a behaviour and then encouraging an individual the make the choice to take part. A good example of this is parkrun which takes place every Saturday morning at 9 o'clock. It happens in many different countries across the world and people of all abilities run a timed 5 km together. Similarly, local fun runs can get people running who have never run before.

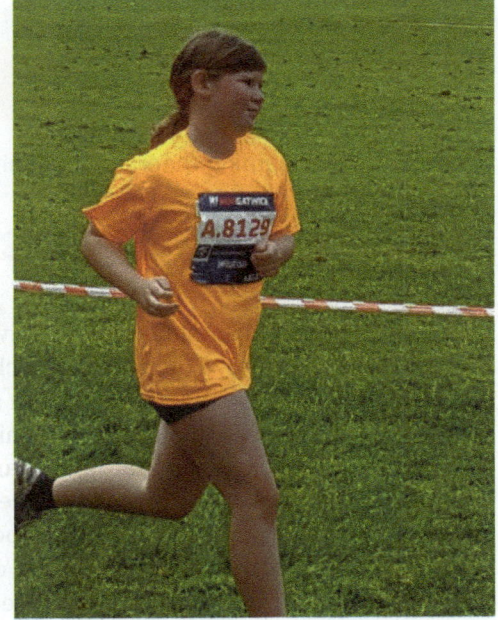

This chapter will explore both effortful and effortless behaviour change strategies in the context of both individual and public health approaches to behaviour change. It will also explore how a range of strategies have evolved from a number of key psychological theories (see Chapter 3 for details on smoking- and alcohol-specific interventions).

Community events can help to change behaviour

Most psychology-based interventions fall within the framework of four main theoretical perspectives: learning and cognitive theory; social cognition theory; stage models; the role of affect. These will now be explored together with attempts to integrate these approaches and generate integrated models of behaviour change.

2   LEARNING AND COGNITIVE THEORY

Learning theory forms the basis of much psychological work with its emphasis on associative learning, reinforcement and modelling. From this perspective we eat chocolate when we are feeling fed up because we associate chocolate with feeling special from when we were children (associative learning), because our parents commented how lucky we were when they gave it to us (reinforcement) and because we saw them eat it (modelling). Cognitive theory then adds to this approach by exploring how people think as well as how they behave. These theoretical perspectives have informed a number of therapeutic approaches which have been used to promote behaviour change. This chapter first describes those approaches informed by learning theory (reinforcement, incentives, modelling, associative learning, exposure). It then describes those informed by both learning and cognitive theories (cognitive behavioural therapy (CBT) and relapse prevention). These different approaches are shown in Figure 7.1.

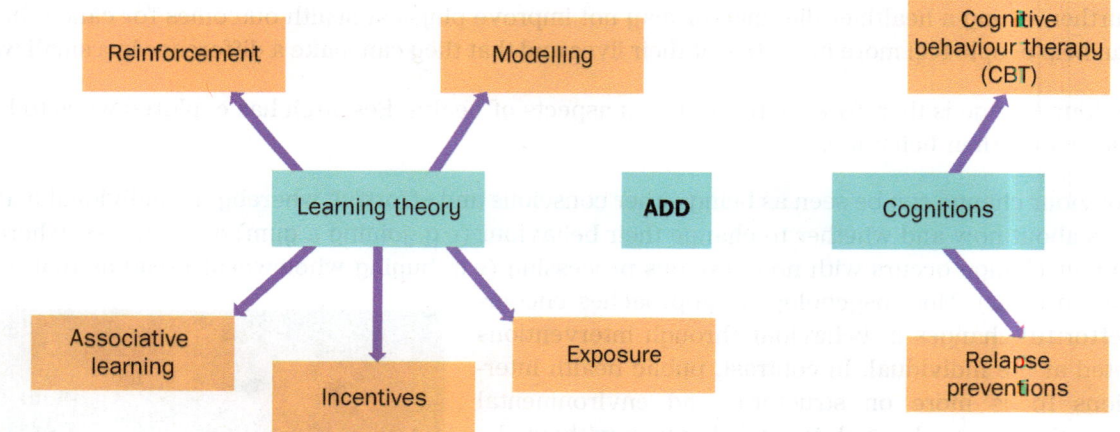

Figure 7.1 How learning theory and cognitive theory inform behaviour change

LEARNING THEORY APPROACHES

Reinforcement

One way to change behaviour is to positively reinforce the desired behaviour and ignore or punish the less desired behaviour. For example, a child is more likely to eat fruit and vegetables if their parent smiles while they are eating them and an adult is less likely to return for a screening test if they found the last one embarrassing and painful. This process has been assessed by a number of different experimental studies and interventions. For example, Barthomeuf et al. (2007) explored whether the emotion expressed on people's faces could influence food preferences. Men and women were exposed to a series of pictures of liked and disliked foods that were either on their own or accompanied by people eating them and expressing one of three emotions: disgust, pleasure or neutrality. The results showed that the expression of the eater influenced ratings of preference. Therefore, pairing a food with emotion changes the preference for that food. Similarly, Gwozdz et al. (2020) conducted a field experiment in ten primary schools in five European countries and concluded that smiley stamps promoted fruit and vegetable eating among children in some but not all countries. Likewise, Harne-Britner et al. (2011) conducted a trial to improve healthcare workers' hand hygiene using positive reinforcement with a sticker reward system. The results showed a 15.5 per cent increase in hand hygiene compliance during the first month. They also found, however, that this effect was not sustained in the longer term. Further, in 2019, Fazzino et al.'s systematic review of 10 studies concluded that reinforcement-based interventions were effective in promoting positive outcomes in substance use. The role of reinforcement is also implicit with several medical approaches to managing behaviour. For example, the drug Antabuse induces sickness if the individual also consumes alcohol and the drug orlistat causes anal leakage if taken with fatty foods. Both these consequences act as a deterrent for future behaviours (Ogden and Sidhu 2006; Hollywood and Ogden 2016). Furthermore, research indicates that people often change their behaviour in the longer term when the old unhealthy behaviour is no longer functional. For example, people stop smoking when it no longer offers them a way to spend time with friends or change their diet when they find different foods more enjoyable (Ogden and Hills 2008).

Incentives

Research has also explored the impact of financial incentives as a means to change behaviour. Incentivizing behaviour is rooted in a notion of reinforcement and has long been the standard tool of the retail industry which aims to encourage consumers to purchase a particular brand rather than a competitor's brand. It is also linked to the notion of a token economy, In the context of health-related behaviours, incentivizing can take the form of centralized changes to the cost of products such as cigarettes, fatty foods and fizzy drinks or directly paying people to lose weight, stop smoking or be more physically active. Over the past few years research has addressed the effectiveness of these simple (and fairly crude) approaches and indicates that, in general, changes in cost and direct financial rewards can effectively change behaviour. For example, increased taxes on both alcohol and cigarettes over the past few decades have been linked with a reduction in drinking and alcohol (Sutherland et al. 2008) and current ongoing direct payment schemes include giving pregnant women in the UK £20 food vouchers for one-week smoking cessation, £40 after four weeks and £40 after one year (North East Essex NHS Trust 2009); paying men and women $45 in Tanzania to have regular tests for sexually transmitted diseases (World Bank 2008) and giving points to children in Scotland for eating healthy school meals which can be exchanged for donations to a Save the Children project abroad (East Ayrshire Council 2011). Marteau et al. (2009) reviewed the evidence for incentivizing behaviour change and concluded the following:

- The greater the incentive, the greater the likelihood of behaviour change.
- Incentives are better at producing short-term rather than longer-term changes.
- The impact of the incentive depends upon the financial state of the individual.
- Incentives are more effective if the money is paid as close as possible to that target behaviour.
- Incentives work better for discrete and infrequent behaviours such as having vaccinations rather than repeated habitual behaviours such as diet or smoking.

Marteau et al. (2009) also concluded that there may be three unintended consequences of incentivizing behaviour. These are:

- Incentives may undermine an individual's intrinsic motivation for carrying out a behaviour (e.g. 'I ate healthily but now I don't really like healthy foods').
- Incentives are a form of bribery which undermine an individual's informed consent and autonomy.
- Incentives may change the doctor–patient relationship if the patient is paid by the doctor to behave in certain ways.

Incentives therefore seem to change behaviour through a crude version of reinforcement. However, they may also have unintended consequences which may undermine changes in behaviour in the longer term.

Modelling

Modelling healthy behaviour can also change behaviour: a child is more likely to smoke if their parents smoke and less likely to take up exercise if they see their parents sitting on the sofa watching TV (see Chapters 3 and 4). Research shows that adolescents are more likely to eat breakfast if their parents do (Pearson et al. 2009) and that adolescents are more likely to eat for emotional reasons such as boredom or comfort if their parents do this as well (Snoek et al. 2007). An intervention study explicitly used modelling to change children's eating behaviour (Lowe et al. 1998). This series of studies used video material of 'food dudes' – older children enthusiastically consuming refused food – which was shown to children with a history of food refusal. The results showed that exposure to the 'food dudes' significantly changed the children's food preferences and specifically increased their consumption of fruit and vegetables as the participants modelled their behaviour on that of the 'food dudes' in the video. The Food Dudes healthy eating programme has now been adopted in parts of England and the Republic of Ireland and is based upon the three 'Rs': role modelling, repeated tasting, and rewards. Marcano-Olivier et al. (2021) evaluated the intervention and reported an increase in children's intake of fruit, vegetables, vitamin C and E and a decrease in their total energy consumption of fat, saturated fat and sodium intake in the intervention school but not in the control school. Similarly, Sanderson and Yopyk (2007) showed young people a video consisting of other young people with positive attitudes towards condoms who modelled strategies for using them appropriately. The results showed increased intentions to have safe sex, higher self-efficacy to refuse unsafe sex and higher condom use four months later. Further, using a qualitative method, Deliens et al. (2015) reported that university students identified the behaviour of their social networks as the key determinants of their own physical activity and sedentary behaviours.

Associative Learning

Associative learning involves pairing two variables together so that one variable acquires the value or meaning of the other. For example, in the classic early studies Pavlov's dogs heard a bell ring whenever they were given food and after a while they started to salivate when they heard the bell (even without the food). Similarly, Van den Akker et al. (2017) paired time and chocolate and showed that the repeated consumption of chocolate at a specific time of day over 15 days increased the desire to eat chocolate at this time. One form of associative learning is *evaluative conditioning* whereby an attitude object is paired repeatedly with an object which is either viewed positively or negatively as a means to make the attitude object either more positive or negative. This method is frequently used in marketing as a means to make relatively neutral objects (e.g. perfume, cigarettes, pet food, air freshener) seem more positive by pairing them with something that is inherently attractive (e.g. attractive people, green fields, romantic music, etc.). Gibson (2008) tested this process experimentally and reported that evaluative conditioning could make participants predictably choose between Coca-Cola or Pepsi depending on which one had been paired with positive meaning. In terms of health, Hollands et al. (2011) used an evaluative conditioning procedure to increase the negative value attached to unhealthy snacks such as crisps and chocolate. Participants were shown images of unhealthy snacks interspersed with aversive unhealthy images of the body for the experimental condition (e.g. artery disease, obesity, heart surgery), or a blank screen for the control condition. The results showed that the intervention resulted in more positive implicit attitudes compared to the control condition. In addition, those in the experimental condition also chose fruit rather than high calorie snacks in a behavioural task. But whether these changes are sustained in the longer term remains unknown.

Exposure

One of the best predictors of future behaviour is past behaviour (see Chapter 2), as having already performed a behaviour makes that behaviour seem familiar and can increase an individual's confidence that they can carry out the behaviour again. Therefore, one of the simplest ways to change behaviour is through exposure to the behaviour, practice or skills training. In terms of eating habits, research shows that we eat what we are familiar with and have been exposed to. For example, Wardle et al. (2003) carried out a study whereby children aged 2–6 identified a vegetable they least liked and then were exposed to this vegetable for 14 days (compared to children who were either given information or were in the control group). The results showed that daily exposure resulted in the children eating more of the vegetable in a taste test and reporting greater preference for the vegetable than those in the other two groups. Similarly, research indicates that children can identify and are willing to taste vegetables if their parents purchase them (Busick et al. 2008). Simple exposure can therefore change intake and preference. In a similar vein, actually performing a behaviour once can increase the chances that this behaviour will occur again in the future. For example, as part of sexual education interventions, research shows that basic skills training in negotiating how to ask for a condom, putting a condom on or buying a condom, which involves rehearsing these behaviours in a safe environment, improves the likelihood of these behaviours in the future (e.g. Weisse et al. 1995; see Chapter 6). Furthermore, not only does past behaviour predict future behaviour but

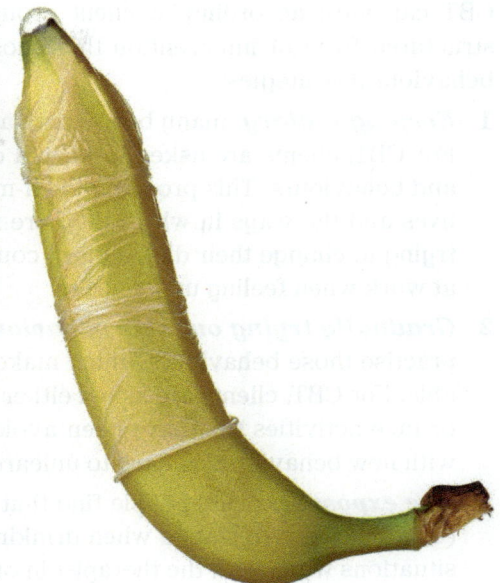

Skills training for condom use can promote health behaviours through exposure to those behaviours in a safe context (This is a banana!)

SOURCE: © Shutterstock / pics five

it also predicts and changes cognitions that then predict behaviour (Gerrard et al. 1996). For example, if I think 'condoms are difficult to put on' and my behaviour is 'I don't use condoms' and then I put one on a banana during a skills training session, my cognition will shift to 'actually I can use condoms' and my behaviour will change as well to 'I now use condoms'.

ADDING COGNITIVE THEORY

Reinforcement, incentives, modelling, associative learning and exposure are behaviour change approaches derived from learning theory. Adding cognitive theory leads to cognitive behaviour therapy (CBT) and relapse prevention.

Cognitive Behavioural Therapy (CBT)

Interventions to change behaviour tend to combine cognitive and behaviour strategies into cognitive behavioural therapy (CBT). Freeman (1995) describes how CBT emphasizes the following:

- The link between thoughts and feelings.
- Therapy as a collaboration between patient and therapist.
- The patient as scientist and the role of experimentation.
- The importance of self-monitoring.
- The importance of regular measurement.
- The idea of an agenda for each session set by both patient and therapist.
- The idea that treatment is about learning a set of skills.
- The idea that the therapist is not the expert who will teach the patient how to get better.
- The importance of regular feedback by both patient and therapist.

CBT can vary according to client group and the problem being addressed, but involves a more structured form of intervention than most therapies and often includes the following cognitive and behavioural strategies:

1 *Keeping a diary:* many behaviours and thoughts occur without people being fully aware of them. For CBT, clients are asked to keep a diary of significant events and associated feelings, thoughts and behaviours. This process of self-monitoring enables clients to understand the patterns in their lives and the ways in which they are responding to whatever is happening to them. For someone trying to change their diet, a diary could reveal that they eat while watching the TV or turn to food at work when feeling under stress.

2 *Gradually trying out new behaviours:* many behaviours are habitual and over time we learn to practise those behaviours which make us feel good and avoid those that make us feel uncomfortable. For CBT, clients are asked either on their own or with the therapist to try out new behaviours or face activities that have been avoided. This enables people to build confidence and familiarity with new behaviours and try to unlearn old behaviours.

3 *Cue exposure:* many people find that unhealthy behaviours can be triggered by certain situations (e.g. the desire to smoke when drinking alcohol). For CBT, clients are sometimes exposed to such situations when with the therapist in order to help them learn new coping responses and extinguish the old unhealthy reactions to these situations. For example, people addicted to drugs may be gradually exposed to the paraphernalia of drugs (e.g. silver foil, needles, cigarette papers, etc.) as a means to change their response to them.

4 *Relaxation techniques:* clients may use music, repeated clenching and relaxing of muscles, recordings of soothing voices or recordings of subliminal messages as a means to aid relaxation. This can help them to reduce their anxiety and negative thoughts about aspects of their lives.

5 *Distraction techniques:* distraction can be a powerful method for managing anxiety or preventing unhealthy responses to certain situations. In CBT, clients can be helped to find distraction strategies that work for them. For example, if a person feels the need to smoke when with certain friends, they can be taught how to focus on other aspects of their lives at these times or encouraged to use a telephone help line.

6 *Cognitive restructuring:* central to CBT is the notion that behaviour is maintained through a series of distorted cognitions and a vicious cycle between thoughts and behaviours which is perpetuated by irrational self-talk. Such distorted cognitions are:

- *Selective abstraction,* which involves focusing on selected evidence (e.g. 'drinking alcohol is the only way I can unwind after work').
- *Dichotomous reasoning,* which involves thinking in terms of extremes (e.g. 'If I am not in complete control, I will lose all control').
- *Overgeneralization,* which involves making conclusions from single events and then generalizing to all others (e.g. 'I failed last night so I will fail today as well').
- *Magnification,* which involves exaggeration (e.g. 'Stopping smoking will push me over the brink').
- *Superstitious thinking,* which involves making connections between unconnected things (e.g. 'If I do exercise, I will have another heart attack').
- *Personalization,* which involves making sense of events in a self-centred fashion (e.g. 'They were laughing, they must be laughing at me').

CBT then uses a number of cognitive strategies to challenge and change these distorted cognitions and replace them with more helpful ones. The main approach involves Socratic questions, with the therapist challenging the client's cognitions by asking for evidence and attempting to help the client to develop a different perspective. Questions could include: 'What evidence do you have to support your thoughts?'; 'How would someone else view this situation?'; 'When you say "everyone", who do you mean?';

'When you say "all the time", can you think of times when this is not the case?' To aid this process the therapist can use role play and role reversal so that the client can watch and hear someone else using their cognitions and learn to see how unhelpful and irrational they are.

There is much evidence to support the use of CBT for behaviour change. For example, Rüther et al. (2018) used CBT to promote smoking cessation using a RCT with 155 smokers aged 18–70. They found that those in the intervention group reduced smoking significantly more compared to controls, but this effect was not maintained over time. Likewise, Çelik and Sevi's (2020) systematic review of 20 studies concluded that CBT-based treatments promoted smoking cessation, especially when combined with medication and nicotine replacement therapy. Further, Vinci's (2020) review concluded that CBT was effective for smoking cessation for special populations (e.g., low SES; pregnant smokers) when delivered via mhealth/ehealth. Similarly, Riper et al. (2014) conducted a meta-analysis of 12 studies comprising 1,721 patients investigating the effectiveness of combined CBT and motivational interviewing (MI) for alcohol use disorder. They found that the combination of CBT and MI has a small but clinically significant impact on decreased alcohol use and depression symptoms compared with treatment as usual. This is also supported by Hadjistavropoulos et al.'s (2020) systematic review of 14 studies which compared internet-delivered CBT (ICBT) and therapist-guided therapy (TCBT) for alcohol misuse. The results indicated that while small effects were found for ICBT, small to large effects were found to TCBT.

CBT and Chronic Illness

Antoni and colleagues (Antoni et al. 2001, 2002) have developed structured guidelines for using CBT with patients with a range of chronic illnesses including those with HIV and cancer as a means to change cognitions and promote behaviour change. For example, beliefs that HIV or cancer are terminal illnesses and that nothing can be done will change a person's help seeking, and feelings of hopelessness and helplessness will change their mood and quality of life. They outline a detailed system for changing irrational thoughts using rational thought replacement, which they call the ABCDE system. This is as follows:

Awareness: because much of our self-talk is automatic, the first step is to become aware of the cognitions we hold and the ways in which these impact upon emotional and physical responses. This awareness process can involve diary-keeping, reflection and talking to a therapist.

Beliefs: clients are then asked to rate their beliefs about each of the self-talk processes they hold to identify how strong their cognitions are. They should ask themselves 'How much do I believe that each of these cognitions is true?'.

Challenge: clients challenge their thoughts through questions which ask for evidence or encourage the client to think through what other people would think or do in the same situation.

Delete: Antoni and colleagues then argue that clients need to delete these self-statements and replace them with constructive cognitions. This can involve thinking through alternative explanations and different ways of making sense of what happens to them.

Evaluate: the final stage is for the client to evaluate how they feel after the cognitions have been deleted and whether they feel the process has been successful.

CBT has been most commonly used within the mental health domain to treat problems such as panic disorders, obsessive compulsive disorder (OCD) and eating disorders. It is also used in health psychology, particularly for a number of chronic conditions, to change behaviours such as physical activity, diet, safe sex practices, smoking and alcohol intake (Antoni et al. 2001, 2002, 2006). For example, Vanderlinden et al. (2012) evaluated the effectiveness of CBT delivered for 1 day a week for an average of 7 months to patients with obesity and binge eating disorder. The results showed improvement in eating behaviours, weight and psychological parameters that lasted up to 3 and a half years post treatment. Similarly, Bennebroek Evertsz et al. (2017) investigated the effectiveness of CBT for patients with inflammatory bowel disease and showed improvements in quality of life, anxiety and depression. Further, Aricó et al. (2016) conducted a review of 16 studies on the effectiveness of CBT for insomnia in breast cancer survivors and concluded that CBT was effective at improving insomnia, but also improved mood, general and physical fatigue, and global and cognitive dimensions of quality of life.

Relapse Prevention

CBT describes a number of cognitive and behavioural strategies to help people change their behaviour. Marlatt and Gordon (1985) developed a relapse prevention model to explore the processes that occur when a change in behaviour fails to last and people relapse. This model was developed in the context of addictions to substances such as nicotine, alcohol and drugs but has implications for understanding all other forms of behaviour change that may or may not be sustained. The relapse prevention model was based on the following concept of addictive behaviours:

- Addictive behaviours are learned and therefore can be unlearned; they are reversible.
- Addictions are not 'all or nothing' but exist on a continuum.
- Lapses from abstinence are likely and acceptable.
- Believing that 'one drink = a drunk' is a self-fulfilling prophecy.

   Marlatt and Gordon distinguished between a lapse, which entails a minor slip (e.g. a cigarette, a couple of drinks), and a relapse, which entails a return to former behaviour (e.g. smoking 20 cigarettes, getting drunk). They examined the processes involved in the progression from abstinence to relapse and in particular assessed the mechanisms that may explain the transition from lapse to relapse (see Figure 7.2). These processes are described below.

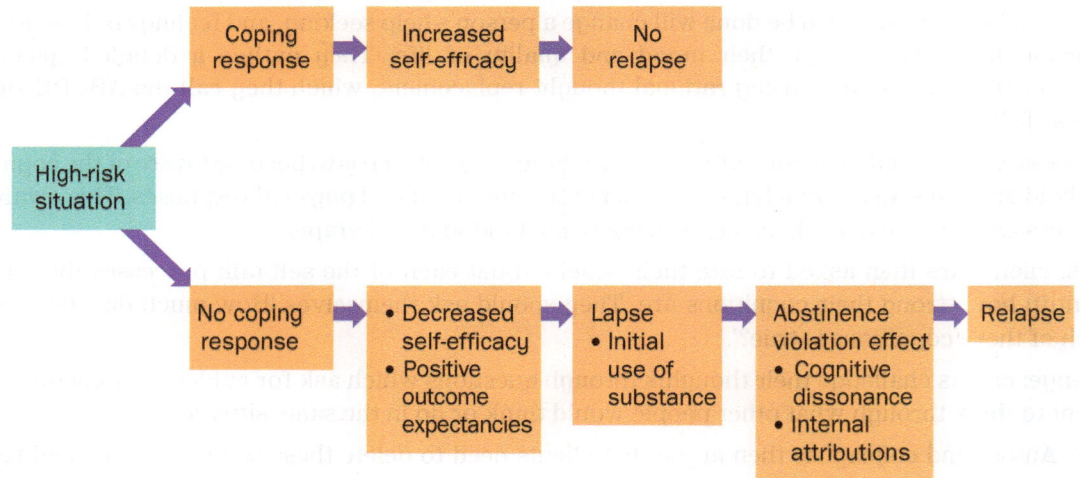

Figure 7.2 The relapse process

SOURCE: Adapted from Marlatt and Gordon (1985)

Baseline State

Abstinence. If an individual sets total abstinence as the goal, then this stage represents the target behaviour and indicates a state of behavioural control.

Pre-Lapse State

High-risk situation. A high-risk situation is any situation that may motivate the individual to carry out the behaviour. Such situations may be either external cues, such as someone else smoking or the availability of alcohol, or internal cues, such as anxiety. Research indicates that the most commonly reported high-risk situations are negative emotions, interpersonal conflict and social pressure

(Marlatt and Gordon 1985). This is in line with social learning theories, which predict that internal cues are more problematic than external cues.

Coping behaviour. Once exposed to a high-risk situation the individual engages the coping strategies. Such strategies may be behavioural, such as avoiding the situation or using a substitute behaviour (e.g. eating), or cognitive, such as remembering why they are attempting to abstain.

Positive outcome expectancies. According to previous experience the individual will either have positive outcome expectancies if the behaviour is carried out (e.g. 'smoking will make me feel less anxious') or negative outcome expectancies (e.g. 'getting drunk will make me feel sick').

No Lapse or Lapse?

Marlatt and Gordon (1985) argue that when exposed to a high-risk situation, if an individual can engage good coping mechanisms and also develop negative outcome expectancies, the chances of a lapse will be reduced and the individual's self-efficacy will be increased. However, if the individual engages poor coping strategies and has positive outcome expectancies, the chances of a lapse will be high and the individual's self-efficacy will be reduced.

- *No lapse:* good coping strategies and negative outcome expectancies will raise self-efficacy, causing the period of abstinence to be maintained.

- *Lapse:* poor or no coping strategies and positive outcome expectancies will lower self-efficacy, causing an initial use of the substance (the cigarette, a drink). This lapse will either remain an isolated event and the individual will return to abstinence, or will become a full-blown relapse. Marlatt and Gordon describe this transition as the abstinence violation effect (AVE).

The Abstinence Violation Effect (AVE)

The transition from initial lapse to full-blown relapse is determined by dissonance conflict and self-attribution. Dissonance is created by a conflict between a self-image as someone who no longer smokes or drinks and the current behaviour (e.g. smoking/drinking). This conflict is exacerbated by a disease model of addictions, which emphasizes 'all or nothing', and minimized by a social learning model, which acknowledges the likelihood of lapses.

Having lapsed, the individual is motivated to understand the cause of the lapse. If this lapse is attributed to the self (e.g. 'I am useless, it's my fault'), this may create guilt and self-blame. This internal attribution may lower self-efficacy, thereby increasing the chances of a full-blown relapse. However, if the lapse is attributed to the external world (e.g. the situation, the presence of others), guilt and self-blame will be reduced and the chances of the lapse remaining a lapse will be increased.

Marlatt and Gordon developed a relapse prevention programme based on cognitive behavioural techniques to help prevent lapses turning into full-blown relapses. This programme involved the following procedures:

- Self-monitoring (what do I do in high-risk situations?).
- Relapse fantasies (what would it be like to relapse?).
- Relaxation training/stress management.
- Skills training ('How will I say "No" to a drink?').
- Contingency contracts ('When offered a cigarette I will . . .').
- Cognitive restructuring (learning not to make internal attributions for lapses).

In the image below the transition from 'high risk situation' through to 'no coping response' and the ultimate 'AVE' can be seen running across the middle. A relapse prevention programme would use the techniques described above to help the individual deal with each of these stages. How these procedures relate to the different stages of relapse is illustrated in Figure 7.3.

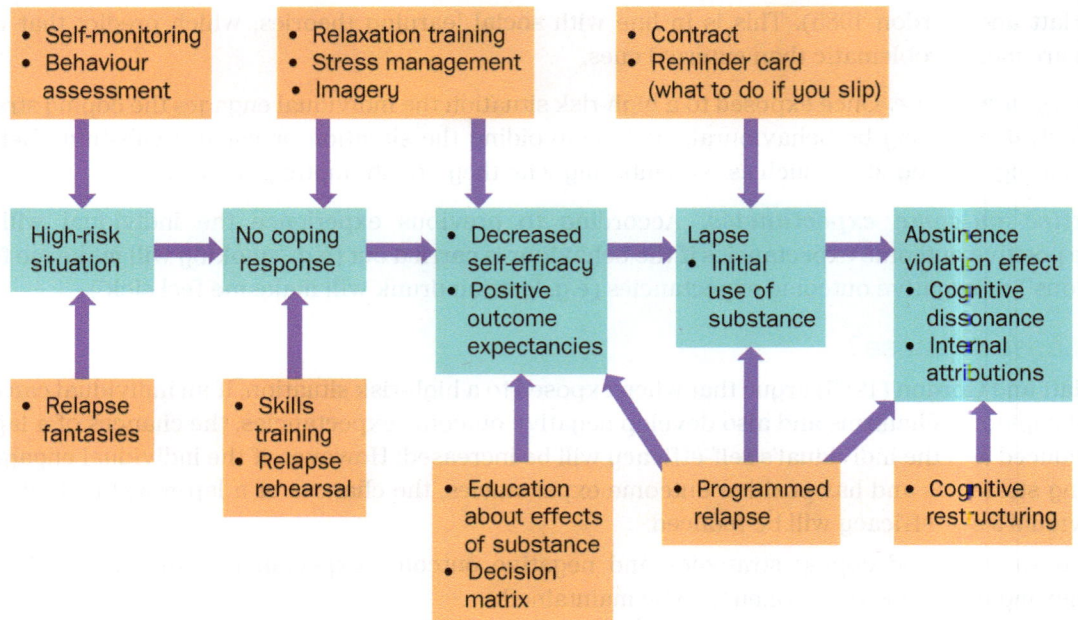

Figure 7.3 Relapse prevention intervention strategies

SOURCE: Adapted from Marlatt and Gordon (1985)

Relapse prevention has been used in a multitude of different contexts as a means to change behaviour either on its own or as part of a complex intervention. For example, Roske et al. (2008) explored the impact of a smoking cessation intervention using relapse prevention techniques in women post-pregnancy. The results showed that the intervention predicted both non-smoking and improved self-efficacy by six months. But by one year the intervention group showed smoking levels similar to the control group. Likewise, Bowen et al. (2014) conducted a randomized control trial with 286 participants and found that compared with psycho-education, mindfulness-based relapse prevention led to participants having a significantly lower risk of relapse for drug use and heavy drinking.

Learning theory (along with cognitive theory) therefore forms the basis of many interventions to change behaviour. Some of these take the form of behavioural strategies with their emphasis on reinforcement, modelling and associative learning. Many incorporate both cognitive and behavioural strategies such as CBT (with its emphasis on behaviour change) and relapse prevention (with its emphasis on sustaining change and preventing relapse).

3   SOCIAL COGNITION THEORY

Social cognition theory was described in Chapter 2 and emphasizes expectancies, incentives and social cognitions (e.g. Bandura 1986). Expectancies include beliefs such as 'a poor diet can cause heart disease', 'if I changed my diet I could improve my health' and 'I could change my diet if I wanted to'. Incentives relate to the impact of the consequences of any behaviour and are closely aligned to reinforcements. For example, a healthy diet would be continued if an individual lost weight or had more energy but stopped if they became bored. Finally, social cognitions reflect an individual's representations of their social world in terms of what other people around think about any given behaviour. These constructs form the basis of social cognition models such as the theory of planned behaviour (TPB) and were described in Chapter 2 in the context of predicting how people behave and the intention-behaviour gap. This approach has been used to develop interventions to change cognitions as a means to change subsequent behaviour and to close the intention-behaviour gap. These different types of intervention are shown in Figure 7.4 and will now be considered.

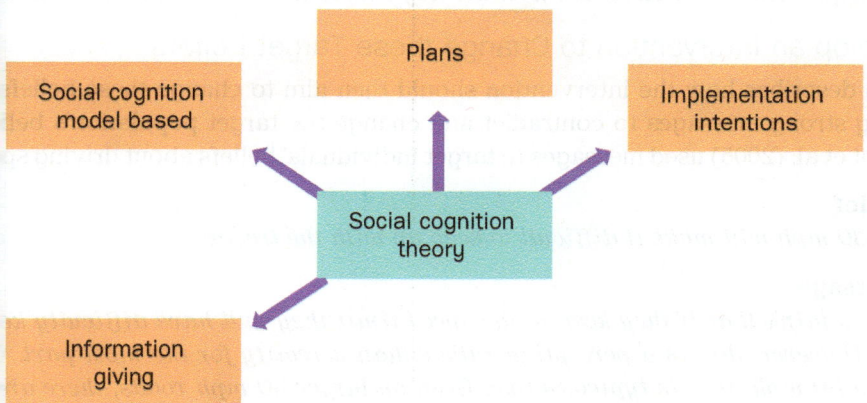

Figure 7.4 Behaviour change interventions derived from social cognition theory

SOCIAL COGNITION MODEL BASED INTERVENTIONS

Sutton (2002b, 2010) described a series of steps to develop an intervention based upon the TPB, although he argued that the steps could also be applied to other social cognition models.

Step 1: Identify Target Behaviour and Target Population

Sutton argued that it is crucial that the target population and behaviour are clearly defined so that all measures used can be specific to that behaviour and population. This is in line with Ajzen's (1988) notion of correspondence or compatibility. For example, the behaviour should not just be 'healthy eating' but 'eating lettuce with my sandwich at lunchtime in the work canteen'. Accordingly the target behaviour should be defined in terms of action (eat healthily), target (lettuce), time (lunchtime) and context (at work).

Step 2: Identify the Most Salient Beliefs about the Target Behaviour in the Target Population Using Open-Ended Questions

Sutton then suggests that those developing the intervention carry out an elicitation study to identify the most salient beliefs about the target behaviour in the target population being studied. Elliot et al. (2005) designed an intervention to encourage drivers' compliance with speed limits and asked questions such as 'What do you think are the advantages of keeping within the speed limit while driving in a built-up area?' The most common beliefs are known as *modal beliefs* and form the basis for the analysis. A modal belief in this situation might be 'to avoid accidents with pedestrians'.

Step 3: Conduct a Study Involving Closed Questions to Determine which Beliefs Are the Best Predictors of Behavioural Intention. Choose the Best Belief as the Target Belief

To further help to decide which beliefs to target in the intervention, Sutton (2002b, 2010) suggests carrying out a quantitative study including the salient beliefs identified in Step 2 involving the target population. These data can then be analysed to explore the best predictors of behavioural intentions as a means to decide whether all or only some of the TPB variables need to be included in the intervention.

Step 4: Analyse the Data to Determine the Beliefs that Best Discriminate between Intenders and Non-Intenders. These Are Further Target Beliefs

Next, Sutton suggests that the same data set be used to assess which beliefs (including those identified in Step 2) differentiate between either intenders versus non-intenders or those who either do or do not carry out the target behaviour. These are now the key beliefs to be addressed in the intervention.

Step 5: Develop an Intervention to Change these Target Beliefs

Finally, Sutton describes how the intervention should then aim to change these beliefs which mostly involves giving strong messages to contradict and change the target population's beliefs. Using this approach, Elliot et al. (2005) used messages to target individuals' beliefs about driving speed as follows:

Target belief
Keeping to 30 mph will make it difficult to keep up with the traffic.

Strong message
Many drivers think that if they keep to the speed limit they will have difficulty keeping up with the traffic. However, this is a perception rather than a reality for the most part. Consider what driving in a 30 mph area is typically like. Even on larger 30 mph roads, there are roundabouts, traffic lights, pedestrian crossings and other things that make it necessary for traffic to slow down or stop. If a vehicle in front starts to pull away from you, you will often find that by maintaining a speed of 30 mph you will catch up with that vehicle further up the road, because they have had to stop or slow down. They will have saved no significant amount of time and they will have gained little or no advantage.

From this perspective the TPB can be used as a framework for developing a behaviour change intervention. However, as Sutton (2002b, 2010) points out, although this process provides clear details about the preliminary work before the intervention, the intervention itself remains unclear. Hardeman et al. (2002) carried out a systematic review of 30 papers which used the TPB as part of an intervention and described a range of frameworks that had been used. These included persuasion, information, increasing skills, goal-setting and rehearsal of skills. These have recently been developed and integrated into a causal modelling approach for the development of behaviour change programmes (Hardeman et al. 2005). Sutton (2002b) indicates that two additional frameworks could also be useful. These are guided mastery experiences, which involve getting people to focus on specific beliefs, and the 'elaboration likelihood' model (Petty and Cacioppo 1986), which involves the presentation of 'strong arguments' and time for the recipient to think about and elaborate upon these arguments. Studies have also used a range of methods for their interventions including leaflets, videos, lectures and discussions.

Evidence for Social Cognition Model Based Interventions

There are some problems with using social cognition models for interventions, as follows.

- *How to change beliefs.* As Hardeman et al. (2002) found from their systematic review, although many interventions are based upon theory, this is often used for the design of process and outcome measures and to predict intention and behaviour rather than to design the intervention itself. Using the TPB for behaviour change interventions describes which beliefs should be changed but not how to change them.

- *Does behaviour change?* A TPB-based intervention assumes that changing salient beliefs will lead to changes in behaviour. However, studies indicate that there is an attenuation effect whereby any changes in beliefs are attenuated by the other variables in the model which reduce their impact upon behaviour (Armitage and Conner 2001; Sniehotta 2009). Further, although there is some evidence that theory-based interventions are successful, whether the use of theory relates to the success of the intervention remains unclear. For example, Hardeman et al. (2002) reported that the use of the TPB to develop the intervention was not predictive of the success of the intervention.

- ***Do they miss other important factors?*** Sniehotta (2009) described the 'bottleneck' whereby interventions using the TPB assume that all changes in behaviour will be mediated through intentions. This, he argues, misses the opportunity to change other relevant factors that may influence behaviour directly, such as changes in the environment, and which do not need to pass through behavioural intentions.

Social cognition models have therefore been used to develop behaviour change interventions. To date, however, although they provide a clear structure for evaluating an intervention, the actual intervention and the means to be used to change beliefs require further attention.

MAKING PLANS AND IMPLEMENTATION INTENTIONS

Much research indicates that although an individual may make an intention to carry out a behaviour this intention is not always translated into practice. This is known as the intention–behaviour gap (see Chapter 2) and appears to result from intenders who do not act rather than non-intenders who do act (Sheeran 2002). Research has highlighted a number of ways that this gap can be closed and in 1993 Gollwitzer defined the notion of implementation intentions which involve the development of simple but specific plans, after intentions, as to what an individual will do given a specific set of environmental factors. Therefore implementation intentions describe the 'what' and the 'when' of a particular behaviour. For example, the intention 'I intend to stop smoking' will be more likely to be translated into 'I have stopped smoking' if the individual makes the implementation intention 'I intend to stop smoking tomorrow at midday when I have finished my last packet'. Further, 'I intend to eat healthily' is more likely to be translated into 'I am eating healthily' if the implementation intention 'I will start to eat healthily by having a salad tomorrow at lunchtime' is made. Implementation intentions are quite similar to the notion of SMART goals that are used in other disciplines, and which stand for goals that are S – Specific, M – Measurable, A – Achievable, R – Reasonable and T – Timebound.

Evidence for Implementation Intention Interventions

Some experimental research has shown that encouraging individuals to make implementation intentions can actually increase the correlation between intentions and behaviour for a range of behaviours such as adolescent smoking (Conner and Higgins 2010), adult smoking (Armitage 2007b), fruit consumption (Armitage 2007a), fruit and vegetable consumption (Gratton et al. 2007), taking a vitamin C pill (Sheeran and Orbell 1998), reducing alcohol intake (Armitage 2009a) and reducing dietary fat (Armitage 2004). Gollwitzer and Sheeran (2006) carried out a meta-analysis of 94 independent tests of the impact of implementation intentions on a range of behavioural goals and concluded that implementation intentions had a medium to large effect on goal attainment. In 2013, Bélanger-Gravel et al. conducted a meta-analysis of 26 studies investigating the effects of implementation intentions on physical activity. The overall effect size was small to medium and they concluded that implementation intentions were particularly effective among student and clinical populations. Implementation intentions therefore provide a simple and easy way to promote and change health-related behaviours. There have, however, been some criticisms of this approach, as follows:

- ***Do people make plans when asked to?*** Research indicates that between 20 and 40 per cent of people do not make implementation intentions when they are asked to (Skar et al. 2008). This must influence the effectiveness of any intervention.

- ***The impact of existing plans.*** Implementation intention interventions ask people to make plans and then explore the impact of this on their behaviour. This assumes that people have not already made plans. Sniehotta et al. (2005) suggest that we need to differentiate between spontaneous plans and those made in response to the interventions.

- ***Do people own their plans?*** If people have made their own spontaneous plans they may well feel more ownership of these plans, making them more motivated to carry them out. This is not usually assessed in intervention studies.

- *Is all behaviour change volitional?* Central to a social cognition model approach to behaviour and the use of implementation intentions is the assumption that behaviour is volitional and under the control of the individual. Much behaviour, however, may be either habitual or in response to environmental changes. These aspects are not addressed within this framework.

- *Not all plans are the same.* Sniehotta (2009) argues that research often treats all types of plans as the same but that it is important to differentiate between *action plans* and *coping plans*. Action plans involve choosing the behaviour that will achieve the goal (the where, when and how of the behaviour) and are what have been called implementation intentions. In contrast, coping plans prepare an individual for successfully managing high-risk situations in which strong cues might encourage them to engage in unwanted habits (without intention) or new unhealthy behaviours (with intention). Sniehotta et al. (2006) explored the relative impact of action and coping plans in promoting physical activity post-heart attack and concluded that those in the combined planning group did more activity than those in either the action planning group or the usual care group.

INFORMATION-GIVING

If a person believes 'I smoke but I am not at risk of getting lung cancer' or 'I eat a high fat diet but my heart is healthy', then the obvious first starting point to change their behaviour would be to improve their knowledge about their health. This has been the perspective of health education and health promotion campaigns for decades and has resulted in information provision through leaflets, billboards, TV advertisements and group-based seminars and lectures. Some research has evaluated the impact of information-giving using a range of mediums. For example, O'Brien and Lee (1990) manipulated knowledge about pap tests for cervical cancer by showing subjects an informative video and reported that not only did the video improve knowledge but that the resulting increased knowledge was related to future healthy behaviour. Further, Hammond et al. (2003) examined the effectiveness of the warning labels on cigarette packets and showed that the intention to stop smoking in the next six months and the number of quit attempts was higher in those who reported reading, thinking about and discussing the labels with other people. Similar results were also found in adolescents who were either established or occasional smokers (White et al. 2008; Germain et al. 2010). The provision of information is often incorporated into more complex interventions such as CBT, relapse prevention and psychoeducational interventions with people in rehabilitation (e.g. Dusseldorp et al. 1999; Sebregts et al. 2000; Rees et al. 2004). In 2017, Collins et al. carried out a systematic review of six systematic reviews investigating the impact of providing risk information regarding cardiovascular disease. They concluded that while increasing the accuracy of risk perception in adults, there was no evidence that information giving reduced the incidence of cardiovascular disease. Generally it is accepted that giving information is not sufficient to change behaviour but that it is a useful and necessary adjunct to any other form of behaviour change strategy.

Social cognition theory has therefore informed much research on predicting and explaining health-related behaviours (see Chapter 2). It has also been the basis for behaviour change interventions, particularly through the use of the TPB and planning in the form of implementation intentions. In addition, interventions often use information and education as a means to improve knowledge and change cognitions. Such approaches are not without their problems, however, particularly in terms of their narrow focus on intentions and behaviour and the focus on behaviour as a response to intentions and other related cognitions.

4   STAGE MODELS

Strategies to change behaviour based upon both learning theory and social cognition theory conceptualize behaviour as a continuum and change behaviour by encouraging people to move along the continuum from unhealthy to healthy ways of acting. In contrast, stage models of behaviour such as the Stages of Change (SOC) and the health action process approach (HAPA) emphasize differences between people who are at different stages (see Chapter 2). Stage models have influenced behaviour change interventions in two ways: the use of stage-matched interventions and the development of motivational interviewing.

STAGE-MATCHED INTERVENTIONS

A stage model approach to behaviour highlights how people show different levels of motivation to change their behaviour at different stages. Therefore, someone at the pre-contemplation stage is less likely to attend a smoking cessation clinic or wear a nicotine replacement patch than someone at the contemplation or action stages. A stage approach has often been combined with the many strategies derived from learning and cognitive theory or social cognition theory described above so that interventions can be targeted to people according to where they are in the process of change. This has taken the form of either tailored or stage-matched interventions. Participants are initially asked to rate their motivation as a means to assess their stage and then the intervention is delivered accordingly. At times this results in people being refused entry into the study as they are at the pre-contemplation stage and deemed not ready to change. Overall, it means that interventions tend to be more effective as the intervention makes more sense to the individual and those who would not have responded to the intervention are removed from the study. Stage-matched interventions have been used across a number of behaviours such as smoking cessation (Di Clemente et al. 1991; Aveyard et al. 2006) and cervical cancer screening (Luszczynska et al. 2010). For example, Lu et al. (2019) carried out a nurse-led smoking cessation stage-matched intervention in patients with coronary heart disease or diabetes and concluded that it resulted in successful smoking reduction and abstinence at 3 and 6 months. Stage-matched interventions are often used in conjunction with a range of intervention approaches such as CBT, counselling, implementation intentions and planning.

MOTIVATIONAL INTERVIEWING (MI)

If people are at a stage when they are unmotivated to change their behaviour, then there seems little point in offering them an intervention or including them in a study, particularly as motivation is a consistently good predictor of behavioural intentions and behaviour (e.g. Jacobs et al. 2011). Motivational interviewing (MI) was developed by Miller and Rollnick (2002) as a way to help people consider changing their behaviour and to increase their motivation to change. From a stages of change perspective it takes people from a pre-contemplation to a contemplation stage in the behaviour change process. MI therefore doesn't show people *how* to change but encourages them to think about their behaviour in ways that may make them realize that they *should* change. MI was originally used with people with addictions but is now used across all health care settings and has become a core part of the toolkit of any health professional. The process of MI is based upon the idea that cognitive dissonance is uncomfortable and that people are motivated to get out of a state of dissonance by changing their cognitions (Festinger 1957). For health-related behaviours, conflicting beliefs such as 'My drug addiction lost me my job' and 'I like taking drugs' or 'My weight makes it difficult for me to move' and 'I like eating a lot' cause cognitive dissonance and are uncomfortable. The aim of MI is to encourage people to focus on these conflicting beliefs and therefore feel the discomfort more strongly. Questions asked would include:

'What are some of the good things about smoking/eating a lot/taking drugs?'
'What are the not so good things about smoking/eating a lot/taking drugs?'

The client is then encouraged to elaborate on the costs and benefits of their behaviour which are then fed back to them by the health professional to highlight the conflict between these two sets of cognitions:

'So your smoking makes you feel relaxed but you are finding it hard to climb stairs?'
'So taking drugs helps you cope but you have lost your job because of them?'

Next, the client is asked to describe how this conflict makes them feel and to consider how things could be different if they changed their behaviour. It is hoped that by focusing on their cognitive dissonance they will be motivated to change both their cognitions and behaviour as a means to resolve this dissonance. Obviously it is hoped that they will change towards being healthier, although this may not always be the case as the process could encourage people to see the benefits of their behaviour and decide to continue as they are.

Miller and Rollnick (2002) are very clear that their approach should be non-confrontational and should encourage people to think about the possibility of change rather than persuading them to change. This is particularly important for clients who may have already met much frustration and anger at their behaviour from other professionals or family members and may be very reluctant to speak openly. Miller and Rollnick also emphasize that professionals using MI should be empathic and non-judgemental and should assume that the client is responsible for the decision to change when and if they want to make that decision. A systematic review shows that MI is an effective tool for use by non-specialists for drug abuse treatment (Dunn et al. 2001). Research also shows that MI is effective across a number of areas including promoting attendance at a drug treatment programme (Heslop et al. 2001), enhancing medication compliance in people with schizophrenia (Bellack and DiClemente 1999), treating eating disorders (Killick and Allen 1997), reducing problem drinking in inpatients with psychiatric problems (Hulse and Tait 2002), promoting healthy eating (Resnicow et al. 2001), promoting a short-term increase in physical activity in a primary care setting (Harland et al. 1999) and training pharmacists to deliver smoking cessation (Caponnetto et al. 2017). Recently, however, several systematic reviews have found mixed results for the effectiveness of MI. For example, Morton et al. (2015) conducted a systematic review to investigate the impact of MI on health behaviour change in primary care settings. They included 33 papers focusing on physical activity, dietary behaviours and/ or alcohol intake and found that around 50 per cent of studies reported a positive effect of MI on the health behaviours. However, they also concluded that the efficacy of MI remains unclear due to the inconsistency of MI descriptions and intervention components. Likewise, Lindson et al.'s (2019) systematic review of 37 studies evaluated the efficacy of MI for smoking cessation and found mixed results and Michalopoulou et al. (2022) concluded from their systematic review and meta-analysis of 46 studies suggested that there is no evidence that MI increases effectiveness of behavioural weight management programmes in controlling weight.

Stage models have therefore influenced behaviour change interventions through the use of tailored or stage-matched interventions and the development of motivational interviewing as a means to move people to a stage where they might consider entering an intervention to change their behaviour.

5 | THE ROLE OF AFFECT

One of the main criticisms of many psychological theories of behaviour and the strategies used to change behaviour is that they do not address an individual's emotions and consider people to be rational processors of information (van der Pligt et al. 1998; van den Berg et al. 2005). Some studies, however, have included a role for affect and this has taken various forms including fear appeals, visualization and self-affirmation interventions. These are illustrated in Figure 7.5.

USING FEAR APPEALS

In recognition of the role that emotion plays in behaviour, many health promotion campaigns include fear appeals which are designed to raise fear as a means to change how people behave. For example, in the 1980s tombstone images were used to promote awareness about the dangers of AIDS, pictures of emaciated and wasted people were used in the 2000s to discourage drug use and cigarette warnings on packets show images of cancer or describe the problems of impotency or harm to unborn children.

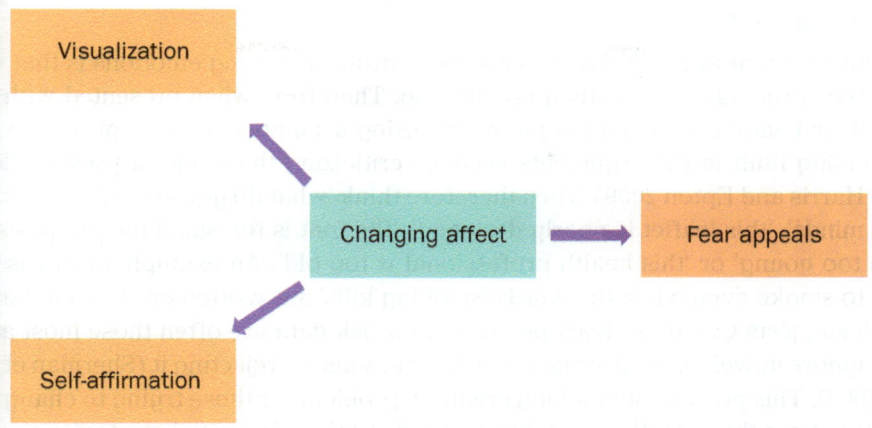

Figure 7.5 Behaviour change interventions based on a changing affect

Fear appeals typically provide two types of message relating to fear arousal and safety conditions as follows:

1 Fear arousal which involves:

- There is a threat: *'HIV infection', 'lung cancer'*.
- You are at risk: *'Unsafe sex or sharing needles puts you at risk of HIV'*.
- The threat is serious: *'HIV kills', 'Lung cancer kills'*.

2 Safety conditions which involve:

- A recommended protective action: *'Use condoms', 'Don't share needles', 'Stop smoking'*.
- The action is effective: *'Condoms prevent HIV', 'Stopping smoking prevents lung cancer'*.
- The action is easy: *'Condoms are easy to buy and easy to use'*.

Together, fear arousals and safety conditions are designed to generate an emotional response (i.e. fear) and offer a simple way to manage the threat (i.e. behaviour change). However, research indicates that it is not clear whether, when or how fear appeals work. For example, originally it was believed that fear had a U-shaped impact on behaviour with maximum change resulting from moderate fear, while low fear caused no effect and high levels of fear resulted in denial, defensiveness and inaction (Janis 1967). Subsequent research, however, indicates that a more linear relationship may exist with greater levels of fear being the most effective at changing behaviour, although this might be due to the kinds of fear that can be generated in the laboratory setting (Ruiter et al. 2001). For example, Tannenbaum et al. (2015) conducted a meta-analysis on 127 papers investigating the impact of fear appeals on attitudes, intentions and behaviour change. They concluded that fear appeals positively influence attitudes, intentions and behaviours and are more effective when they depict high levels of fear, include an efficacy message and stress severity and risk. Fear appeals also seemed to be more effective for women and when they recommended one-time only behaviours.

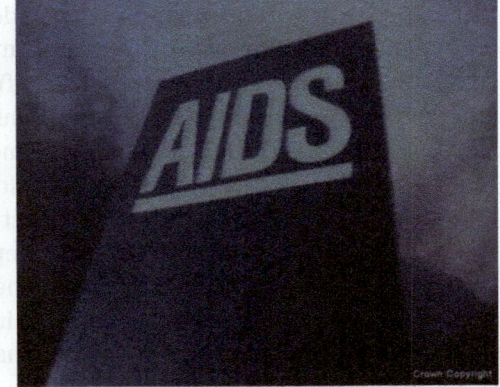

Fear appeals: this gravestone advertisement was one of the first health promotion attempts after the identification of the HIV virus

SOURCE: © Department of Health, Reproduced under the Open Government Licence v3.0. https://www.nationalarchives.gov.uk/doc/ open-government-licence/version/3/

The Problem of Blocking

The key problem with fear appeals and the process of arousing strong emotions is that when aroused, people tend to block the information they are hearing. Therefore, when presented with messages trying to change their behaviour, many people resist, using a number of strategies such as avoidance, ignoring and finding fault in the arguments used, or criticizing the mode of presentation (Jacks and Cameron 2003; Harris and Epton 2009). They therefore think 'what do you know?', 'scientists are always changing their minds', 'this leaflet is poorly designed', 'the font is too small on that poster', 'this health professional is too young' or 'this health professional is too old'. An example of this is smokers' ability to continue to smoke even when the words 'smoking kills' are written on their packet of cigarettes. In fact research suggests that those least persuaded by risk data are often those most at risk and that they can either ignore unwelcome information or find reasons for rejecting it (Sherman et al. 2000; Jacks and Cameron 2003). This process of blocking creates a problem for those trying to change behaviour as the message cannot get through. Research has highlighted three potential strategies to counteract this tendency to block: the use of visual images, self-affirmation and focusing on benefits to someone else.

Using Visual Images

The saying 'a picture paints a thousand words' reflects the belief that visual images may be more effective at conveying information or changing beliefs compared to language-based messages. This forms the basis of most advertising, marketing and health education campaigns and is central to the use of diagrams and illustrations throughout education. Some research has explored the impact of visual images in health research (see Chapter 9 for a discussion of imagery and changes in illness cognitions). For example, Hammond et al. (2003) examined the effectiveness of the cigarette warning labels and reported an association between reading and discussing the labels with a higher intention to stop smoking, more quit attempts and a reduction in smoking. Shahab et al. (2007) also reported that showing smokers images of their carotid arteries with a plaque compared to an artery without a plaque increased intentions to stop smoking in those with higher self-efficacy and Kang and Lin (2015) showed that visual fear appeals reduced optimistic bias in smokers. Further, Karamanidou et al. (2008) reported that showing patients with renal disease a plastic container in which they could see how their phosphate binding medication would work in their stomachs changed their beliefs about treatment. In a similar vein, Lee et al. (2011) used a web-based intervention to show participants images of heart disease (with or without text) and concluded that imagery caused more changes than text alone but that a combination of the two forms of information was the most effective. To further unpack the impact of images, Byrne et al. (2019) compared full-colour graphic warning images (GWI) about the harms of smoking vs black and white GWIs vs prominent text-only warnings vs brand images. The results showed that both youth and adult smokers paid more attention to full-colour GWIs than black-and-white GWIs; that for adults, images (regardless of colour) generated more negative affect than text only, and that text only generated more negative affect than brand imagery; and that in young smokers the colour of the image made no difference, but they reported greater negative affect after the warning images compared to the brand images. Images therefore seem to change cognitions and behaviour but to date little is known about the mechanisms behind this process. However, researchers have begun to theorize about this process and have suggested that images may be processed more rapidly than text and may be more memorable over time. In addition, images may also have a greater impact upon affect than text which in turn influences behaviour (Cameron 2008, 2009; Cameron and Chan 2008). Accordingly, visual images may be a means to prevent blocking when people are presented with emotional information.

Using Self-affirmation

Self-affirmation theory is grounded in the idea of 'self-integrity' and argues that people are inherently motivated to maintain their self-integrity and their sense of self as being 'adaptively and morally adequate' (Steele 1988). If a person's integrity is challenged by information indicating that their behaviour is damaging, then they resist this information as a means to preserve their sense of self. This perspective provides a framework for understanding the process of blocking. It also highlights a way to encourage people to stop blocking and respond to the message in the desired way. In particular, self affirmation theory indicates that resistance can be reduced if the individual is encouraged to enhance their self-integrity by affirming their self-worth by focusing on other factors that are core to how they see themselves but unrelated to the threat (Harris and Epton 2009).

A self-affirmation intervention can take many forms and studies have used methods such as providing positive feedback on a test, asking participants to rate themselves on a series of key values, writing an essay on their most important value or asking a series of questions about a universally valued construct such as kindness (e.g. 'Have you ever forgiven another person when they have hurt you?'). Therefore, if presented with information that threatens their sense of self, they behave defensively and either ignore or reject it. However, if given the opportunity to self-affirm in another domain of their lives, then their need to become defensive is reduced. For example, if a smoker thinks that they are a sensible person, when confronted with a message that says that smoking is not sensible, their integrity is threatened and they behave defensively by blocking the information. If given the chance, however, to think about another area in which they are sensible, then they are less likely to become defensive about the anti-smoking message.

Epton et al. (2015) conducted a meta-analysis of 144 experimental tests of self-affirmation on health message acceptance, intentions to change, and subsequent behaviour. They found that, in general, deploying self-affirmation had a positive effect on all outcomes although effect sizes were small but comparable to others found in meta-analyses of other health behaviour interventions. In particular, they showed that self-affirmation can increase message acceptance for information relating to caffeine consumption, smoking, sun safety, alcohol intake and safe sex (e.g. Sherman et al. 2000; Harris and Napper 2005; Harris et al. 2007). It can change affect (Harris and Napper 2005; Harris et al. 2007) and attitudes (Jessop et al. 2009) and in general cause increases in behavioural intentions (Harris et al. 2007). The review also indicates that self-affirmation interventions can change behaviour in the short term (e.g. immediately taking a leaflet or buying condoms) but to date there is little evidence on longer-term changes in behaviour. Further, those most at risk (e.g. heavy drinkers, heavy smokers) seem to be more responsive to self-affirmation interventions than those less at risk.

Focusing on benefit to someone else

When someone is asked (or told) to change their behaviour they can feel affronted as it challenges their sense of self and personal integrity. They can therefore block this information and may denigrate the messenger by thinking 'what do you know?', 'scientists are always changing their minds', 'the leaflet is poorly designed'. Some people also resort to their sense of freedom and might think 'it's my body I can do what I like', 'it's my choice' and may even decide to 'live fast die young'. One possible way to combat this 'inner libertarian' is by encouraging people to think about someone else rather than themselves. Interestingly, the smoking ban could be implemented once we started to understand the risks of passive smoking; the inner libertarian voice saying 'it's my body' no longer worked. Likewise, the law enforcing seatbelt wearing in the back of a car could be brought in once advertising showed us that people in the back not wearing seatbelts could kill people in the front (Ogden 2014). To date, there is not much research within health psychology focusing on the benefits of focusing on others but within environmental psychology some research points to the benefits of moral motives, biospheric and altruistic (self-transcendent) values and moral norms (i.e. being good) as more effective at changing behaviour than selfishly motivated benefits, such as saving money (i.e. being greedy) (eg. Bolderdijk et al. 2013). This would be a useful avenue for research to address.

USING AFFECT EFFECTIVELY

Health psychology (and even psychology in general) is often criticized for ignoring emotion. Fear appeals use emotion to change behaviour yet can be met with resistance with people blocking the information as it challenges their sense of integrity. Visual images, self-affirmation and focusing on others are useful approaches to limit this process of blocking. How fear appeals, visual images, self affirmation and focusing on others can work together is shown below, with the example of someone who is living with obesity:

- *Fear appeal:* 'Being overweight can cause heart disease'.
- *Emotional response:* 'Anxiety'.
- *Resistance:* Ignoring the message/thinking 'research is always wrong', 'that leaflet isn't very well designed' or 'it's my life and I can live it however I want to'.
- *Self-affirmation intervention:* 'Think of times when you have been kind to others'.
- *Visual image:* Here is an image of fatty deposits on an artery.
- *Focusing on others*: 'Being healthier would also help your children to be healthier'.
- *Emotional response:* 'I am reassured', 'I am a good person', 'I am a good parent'.
- *Reaction to fear appeal:* 'Maybe I should lose some weight'.

Affect can therefore be used to change behaviour. This can involve fear appeals which generate strong emotions, the use of visual images, the use of self-affirmation and taking the focus away from the self to counter the voice of the 'inner libertarian'.

6   INTEGRATED APPROACHES

So far this chapter has outlined the wide range of different behaviour change strategies based upon four theoretical frameworks: learning and cognitive theory; social cognition theory; stage models and the use of affect. Over recent years there has been a call to integrate these different perspectives to deliver more successful interventions. This has taken four different approaches: creating a science of behaviour change interventions; the use of modern technologies; the use of mass media and understanding sustained behaviour change.

CREATING A SCIENCE OF BEHAVIOUR CHANGE INTERVENTIONS

Over the past decade there has been a call to improve intervention research in the following ways: to improve the reporting of interventions to make the process more transparent and easier to synthesize and replicate; to identify which aspects of behaviour change interventions are effective; to improve the design and therefore effectiveness of behaviour change interventions (e.g. Abraham and Michie 2008; Michie et al. 2009; Michie and Wood, 2015; West et al. 2010). This call for a science of behaviour change interventions has involved two key approaches: (i) the integration of theories of behaviour change; and (ii) the development of a taxonomy of behaviour change techniques (BCTs). This drive for a science of behaviour change will now be described.

1. The Integration of Theories of Behaviour Change

Due to the proliferation of theories of health behaviour (see Chapter 2) and the number of theoretical approaches to behaviour change described in this chapter, Michie and colleagues proposed an integrated approach to behaviour change (e.g. Abraham and Michie 2008; Michie et al. 2011b; Michie et al. 2014b; Atkins et al. 2015; Michie and Wood 2015). This has resulted in the following:

The COM-B

Following a cross disciplinary review of theories of behaviour and behaviour change including 83 theories and 1,659 constructs, the COM-B was created to reflect a comprehensive and parsimonious approach to behaviour and the factors necessary for behaviour change to occur. The COM-B highlights the key role of **C**apability (derived from the individual's psychological or physical ability to enact the behaviour), **O**pportunity (reflecting the physical and social environment that enables the behaviour) and **M**otivation (describing the reflective and automatic mechanisms that activate or inhibit the behaviour). In turn, these factors predict **B**ehaviour. This is discussed further in Chapter 2 and illustrated in Figure 7.6.

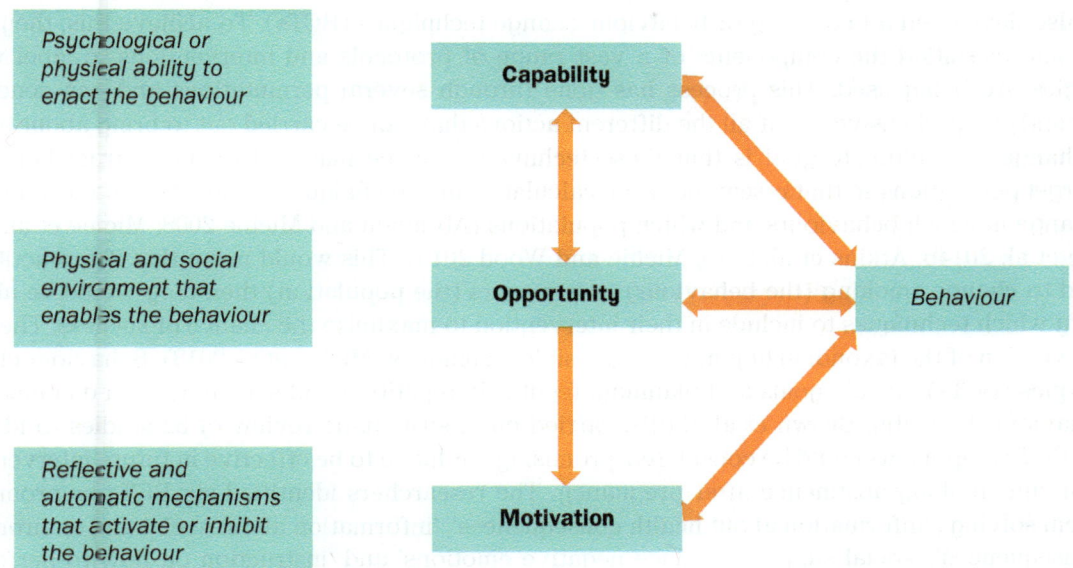

Figure 7.6 The COM-B

SOURCE: Michie et al. (2011b)

The COM-B finds reflection in the models used in a number of domains such as criminology (the opportunity, motive, capability triad) and workplace and environmental interventions (Motivations, opportunities ability model, MOA) and has been used to predict and explain a multitude of behaviours including physical activity, weight loss, hand hygiene, dental hygiene, diet, smoking, medication adherence, prescribing behaviours, condom use, female genital mutilation and hygiene practices during the COVID pandemic (e.g. Jackson et al. 2014; Brown et al. 2015; Bailey et al. 2016; Chadwick and Benelam 2013; Asimakopoulou and Newton 2015; Gibson Miller et al. 2020; Heneghan et al. 2020; Willmott et al. 2021; see Michie and Wood 2015; Atkins et al. 2015 and Michie et al. 2014b for reviews).

The Theoretical Domains Framework (TDF)

In addition to the COM-B, Michie and colleagues have developed the Theoretical Domains Framework (TDF) as a means to synthesize across the different theories that psychologists use to predict behaviour and design and evaluate behaviour change interventions (see Atkins et al. 2017 for a review). The TDF was initially developed in the context of health professional behaviour and involved the synthesis of 33 theories of behaviour and behaviour change which were clustered into 14 domains (Michie et al. 2005; Cane et al. 2012). It was then extended to patient behaviours in general (e.g. Kolehmainen et al. 2011; Taylor et al. 2013). More recently the researchers have identified 33 theories and 128 theoretical constructs which have also been grouped into a similar structure of 14 domains and a guide has been developed for the use of the TDF in the development of interventions (Davis et al. 2015; Atkins et al. 2017). These domains include social influences, environmental context and resources, physical skills, emotion, memory, attention and decision processes, knowledge, beliefs about consequences and beliefs about capabilities.

The COM-B and the TDF have therefore been developed as a means to integrate existing theories of behaviour and behaviour change and provide a framework for developing and evaluating interventions.

Together they have been used to frame a wide range of interventions focusing on issues such as nutritional adherence in performance sport and cervical screening (e.g. Bentley et al. 2019; O'Donovan et al. 2021).

2. The Development of a Taxonomy of Behaviour Change Techniques (BCTs)

As part of the drive to improve the reporting and effectiveness of interventions, Michie and colleagues have also developed a taxonomy of behaviour change techniques (BCTs). To achieve this, they have coded and classified the components of a vast range of protocols and interventions to label which strategies are being used. This process has gone through several permutations and has generated a long and comprehensive list of all the different actions that can be carried out to bring about behaviour change. The ultimate goal is that these techniques can be matched to their target behaviour and target populations so that researchers can calculate which techniques are most effective at producing change in which behaviours and which populations (Abraham and Michie 2008; Michie et al. 2011; Michie et al. 2014b; Atkins et al. 2015; Michie and Wood 2015). This would mean that if a practitioner wanted to change smoking (the behaviour) in teenagers (the population) then they would be able to identify which techniques to include in their intervention to maximize the chance of success. The most recent version of the taxonomy highlights 93 possible techniques (Michie et al. 2013). Behaviour change techniques (BCTs) include goals and planning, feedback, repetition and substitution, and comparison of behaviour. Recently, Brown et al. (2019) carried out a systematic review of 32 studies to identify which BCT components could be considered 'promising', or likely to be effective in future interventions to maintain smoking abstinence after pregnancy. The researchers identified six BCTs as promising: 'problem solving', 'information about health consequences', 'information about social and environmental consequences', 'social support', 'reduce negative emotions' and 'instruction on how to perform a behaviour'. They also concluded that tailored self-help approaches, with or without counselling, may be the most effective modes of delivery of these BCTs.

The Behaviour Change Wheel (BCW)

Michie and colleagues have therefore integrated existing theories of behaviour change to produce the COM-B and the TDF. They have also identified and coded a wide range of BCTs as a means to improve both the reporting and effectiveness of interventions and also to target specific techniques at specific behaviours and populations. In 2011, Michie et al. carried out a synthesis of all the different types of taxonomy as a means to identify essential conditions for behaviour change and how these could be turned into actual behaviour change. From this process, the researchers created a behaviour change wheel with three levels illustrating the translational process from essential conditions, through intervention functions, to policy (see Figure 7.7).

- *Essential conditions:* the researchers identified three conditions which are deemed essential for behaviour and behaviour change: capability, motivation and opportunity. These constructs reflect the COM-B.
- *Intervention functions:* it is argued that changing behaviour requires a change in these essential conditions and that a series of intervention functions can bring this change about. The nine functions identified in the behaviour change wheel reflect a synthesized version of the many strategies that are used to change behaviour and were derived from a detailed coding process. These reflect the BCTs.
- *Categories of policy:* finally, the researchers argue that policy changes are needed to enable the interventions to occur.

The end result of the behaviour change wheel would be that the policy enables interventions to occur, which in turn change the essential *conditions* of behaviour which bring about *changes* in behaviour. The model can be used to describe and understand why interventions do or do not work. It could also be used to design more effective interventions which could be linked to policy or even used to promote new policy.

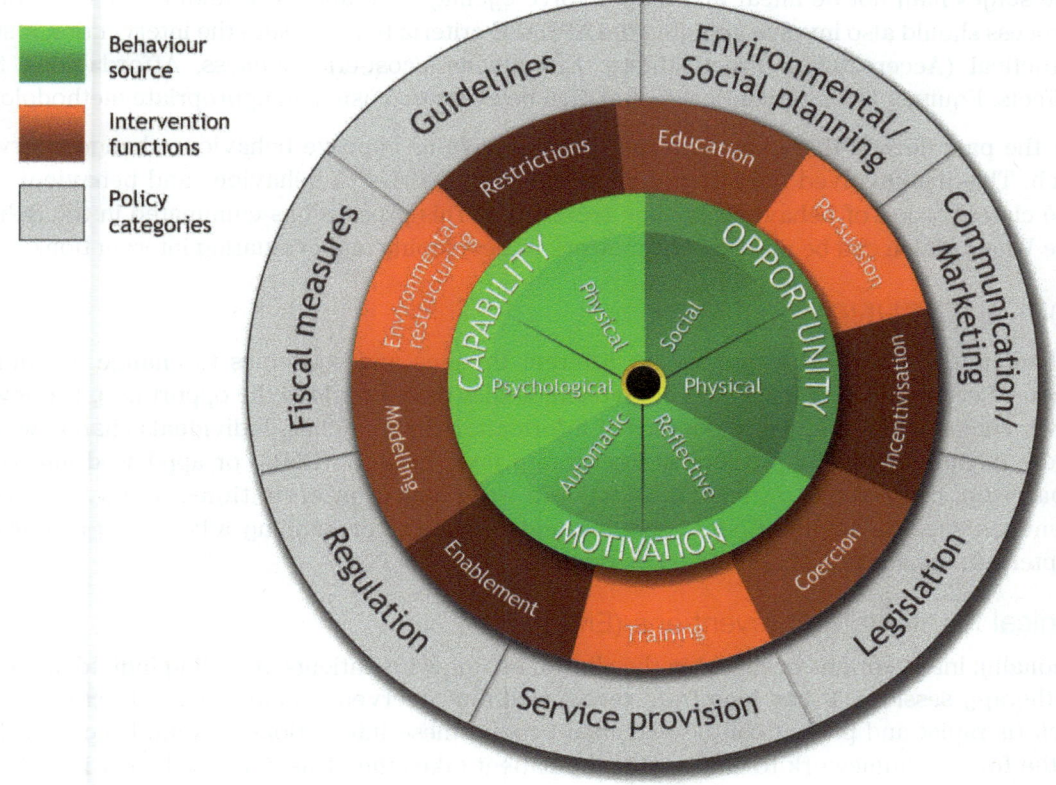

Figure 7.7 The behaviour change wheel

SOURCE: Michie et al. (2011b)

Case Study Using the Science of Behaviour Change to Develop and Test an Intervention

West and Michie (2015) provide the following simple step-by-step guide to using the science of behaviour change for developing and evaluating an intervention based upon their longer book (Michie et al. 2014a). This could be to bring about a change in any behaviour (diet, exercise, help seeking, screening, shopping) or for any population (well, ill, old, young, British, African, European). Recently, West et al. (2020) and Lunn et al. (2020) also suggested that the principles of behaviour change could be used to reduce the transmission of COVID-19. The steps are as follows, and reflect moving from the inner ring of the Behaviour Change Wheel outwards:

1 **Behavioural target specification:** Specify what behaviour needs to change, in what way and for whom.

2 **Behavioural diagnosis:** Use the COM-B to determine what factors would change the specified behaviour (i.e. Capability, Opportunity, Motivation).

3 **Intervention strategy selection:** From the COM-B decide what 'intervention functions' to use (e.g. Education, Persuasion, Incentivisation, Coercion).

4 **Implementation strategy selection:** Choose from the possible policy options (e.g. Fiscal policy, Legislation, Regulation).

5 **Selection of specific behaviour change techniques:** Select the appropriate behaviour change techniques from the taxonomy to design the intervention.

6 **Drafting the full intervention specification:** Write a detailed intervention.

These stages may not be linear and may involve cycling back and forth until the task is complete. This process should also involve applying the APEASE criteria to make sure the intervention is suitable and practical (Acceptability, Practicability, Effectiveness/cost-effectiveness, Affordability, Safety/side-effects, Equity). The intervention should then be evaluated using an appropriate methodology.

Over the past decade there has therefore been a drive to improve behaviour change intervention research. This has involved the integration of existing theories of behaviour and behaviour change and the classification of behaviour change techniques. This process has culminated in the Behaviour Change Wheel which can be used as a framework to developing and evaluating interventions.

MODERN TECHNOLOGIES

This chapter has described a number of different theories and strategies to change health-related behaviour. Recent developments in modern technologies have provided the opportunity for new ways to deliver such strategies and new sources of information that may help individuals change what they do. These include the use of 'ecological momentary interventions' (EMIs) or app-based interventions (via palmtop computers or smarthones) and web-based interventions. Behaviour change interventions such as smoking bans, taxation and restricting or banning advertising are described in Chapter 3 in the context of addictive behaviours.

Ecological Momentary Interventions (EMIs)

Traditionally, interventions occurred in the clinical setting with patients attending individual or group-based therapy sessions. It has long been recognized that interventions are more effective if contact between therapist and patient can be extended beyond these interactions and until recently this has taken the form of homework to ensure that the patient takes the ideas discussed back into their day-to-day lives, or telephone helplines so that people can ring up whenever they need extra support when their resilience is weakened and additional motivation is needed. The development of new technologies, such as smartphones and palmtop computers, provides a simple and cost-effective way to extend therapy beyond the consultation and patients become accessible at all times. The term EMI refers to treatments provided to people during their everyday lives (i.e. in real time) and in natural settings (i.e. in the real world). Such treatments/interventions include text messaging and apps and have been used for a wide range of behaviours such as smoking cessation, weight loss, anxiety, alcohol use, dietary change and exercise promotion. They have also been used across a number of different chronic illnesses including obesity (Ogden et al. 2019) diabetes, coronary heart disease (CHD) and eating disorders (see Heron and Smyth 2010 for a comprehensive review). They are particularly useful for hard-to-reach groups, such as adolescents who would usually avoid contact with health professionals. For example, Sirriyeh et al. (2010) explored the impact of affective text messages and instrumental texts for promoting physical activity in adolescents, with those in the intervention groups receiving one text per day over a two-week period. The results showed that all participants increased their activity levels over the course of the study. In addition, affective texts such as 'exercise is enjoyable' were particularly effective at changing behaviour in those who were most inactive at baseline. For their review of the evidence, Heron and Smyth (2010) identified 27 interventions using EMIs to change behaviour and drew three conclusions. First, at the most practical level EMIs can be easily and successfully delivered to the target group. Second, this new approach is acceptable to patients, even those who are hard to reach such as adolescents, and third, EMIs are effective at changing a wide range of behaviours. Recent systematic reviews indicate that text messaging can be effective for smoking (Whittaker et al. 2019), physical activity (King et al. 2008), a reduction in calorie intake (Joo and Kim 2007), weight management (Alamnia et al. 2022), pain management (Fritsch et al. 2020) and diabetes self-management (Sahin et al. 2019), although most changes seem to be in the shorter rather than longer term and reviews often conclude that effect sizes can be small. Recently, research has also used virtual representations (i.e. digital twins) to promote behaviour change as these encourage participants to further engage with the image on the app or who they are and who they could become (see Taylor et al. 2022 for a review). They represent a combination of a wide range of behaviour change techniques as well as visual imagery and information tailored to the individual. EMIs are a relatively new approach but offer a simple and cost-effective means to change behaviour for a wide section of the population.

Web-based Interventions

New developments in technologies have also led to the use of web-based interventions so that patients who may be unable or unwilling to attend face-to-face consultations can now engage in a range of therapeutic strategies from their own home to fit in with their own time frame. For example, packages of web-based interventions have been developed for patients with a range of chronic illnesses such as diabetes, asthma, coronary heart disease, AIDS/HIV to deliver treatments such as cognitive behaviour therapy (CBT), relapse prevention, education and goal-setting. Many also address psychological problems such as depression and anxiety, obsessive compulsive disorder (OCD) and body image disturbance. Rosser et al. (2009) carried out a systematic review of novel technologies for the management of chronic illnesses (both psychological and physical) and identified that most utilized web-based interventions (53 per cent), with other technologies being interactive CD-ROM programmes, online message boards, video presentations, email contact or virtual reality delivery. From this review they highlighted a number of packaged interventions such as 'MoodGYM', 'Diabetes Priority Programme', 'Beating the Blues' and 'CHESS'. Rosser et al. (2009) made three key observations about the studies they included in their review. First, they noted that sample sizes for the studies were extremely high (mean size at start of study n = 780), reflecting the ease with which patients can be targeted with this approach. Second, they highlighted the extremely high level of dropouts over the course of the studies as patients stopped engaging with the interventions (range, 0–84 per cent, mean sample size after dropouts n = 258). Finally, they noted that although the interventions were delivered remotely (i.e. by computer or email), 73 per cent still included some involvement with a therapist and that greater involvement with a therapist was associated with lower dropout rates. Overall, therefore, web-based interventions can reach large numbers of people who may not want to, or be able to, come into a consultation. They may be effective but they have high attrition rates and still seem to require therapist involvement to be more successful.

THE MASS MEDIA

The mass media also illustrate the ways in which different theories and strategies are integrated to change behaviour. Television, the internet, magazines and outdoor advertising all constantly bombard us with information about what to buy, what to see and what to do. This has a major impact upon our health behaviours in both negative and positive ways. For example, after Eyton's *The F Plan Diet* (1982), which recommended a high fibre diet, was featured in a number of magazine articles and on numerous television programmes, sales of bran-based cereals rose by 30 per cent, wholewheat bread sales rose by 10 per cent, wholewheat pasta by 70 per cent and baked beans by 8 per cent. Similarly, when Edwina Curry, then junior health minister in the UK, said on television in December 1988 that 'most of the egg production in this country, sadly, is now infected with salmonella', egg sales fell by 50 per cent and by 1989 were still only at 75 per cent of their previous levels (Mintel 1990). Similarly, massive publicity about the health risks of beef in the UK between May and August 1990 resulted in a 20 per cent reduction in beef sales. The mass media can be used either as a means to make us more unhealthy or as a resource to help improve the health of the population.

The Media as a Negative Influence

Although cigarette and alcohol adverts have now been banned across the USA and most of Europe, food adverts are still considered acceptable. For example, Radnitz et al. (2009) analysed the nutritional content of food on TV aimed at children under 5 years and showed that unhealthy foods were given almost twice as much air time and were shown to be valued significantly more compared to healthy foods. Some research has explored the potential impact of TV adverts on eating behaviour. For example, Halford et al. (2004) used an experimental design to evaluate the impact of exposure to food-related adverts. Lean, overweight and obese children were shown a series of food and non-food-related adverts and their snack food intake was then measured in a controlled environment. The results showed that, overall, the obese children recognized more of the food adverts than the other children and that the degree of recognition correlated with the amount of food consumed. Furthermore, all children ate more after exposure to the food adverts than the non-food adverts. Similarly, King and Hill (2008) showed children adverts for healthy or less healthy foods and measured their hunger, food choice and product recall. No effects were found for hunger or food choice but children could remember more of the less healthy than the healthy foods.

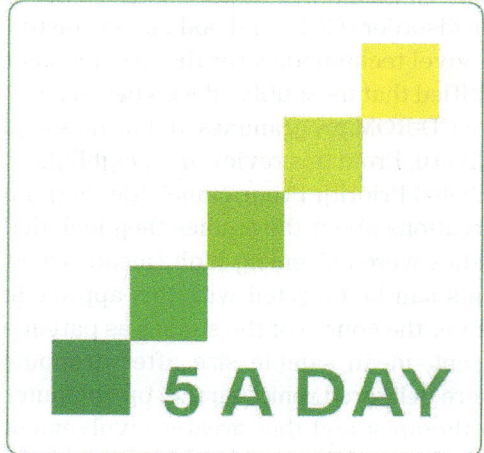

Just Eat More
(fruit & veg)

Five a day: just eat more. A simple and memorable message

SOURCE: © Department of Health

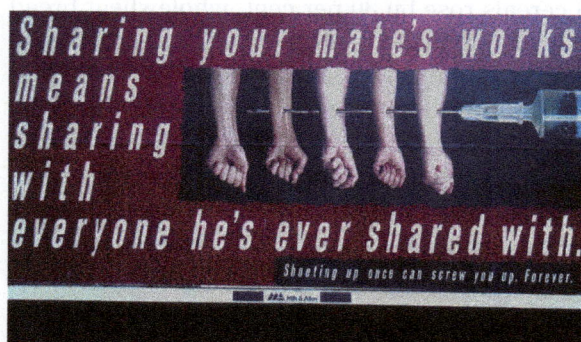

A powerful image to discourage needle sharing

SOURCE: © Christine Osborne/Photographers Direct

The Media as a Resource for Positive Change

The media has also been used by government and health promotion campaigns as a means to reach a wide audience and promote health behaviour. To date there is very little evidence as to whether these campaigns have been effective and it has been argued that perhaps such initiatives should be about raising awareness rather than changing behaviour (Stead et al. 2002). It is also possible that whereas individual campaigns may only raise awareness, repeated ongoing campaigns over many years may cause change through a 'drip drip effect' as successive generations gradually become accustomed to a new way of thinking or behaving. This is particularly apparent in the reduction in drink driving over the past decade. No one particular campaign may have made this happen but negative attitudes towards drink driving in the new generation of drivers may be a response to always having been aware that this was not an acceptable thing to do (Shinar et al. 1999).

One way to understand the impact of mass media campaigns is to identify those which are memorable and explore why this might be. Memorable campaigns over recent years include:

- *'Five a day: just eat more':* this is a simple message using simple words and imagery and aims to promote healthy eating. Interestingly, it encourages doing more rather than less of something which minimizes the chance of a rebound effect which is a common response to many other forms of dietary advice (see Chapter 5). It also offers clear rules of what to eat which are set slightly higher than the average intake but are also realistic.

- *'Most people are killed by someone they know':* this was the basis of an advert to promote seat-belt wearing in the front and back of cars to prevent those in the back seat from being thrown into the front during an accident.

One advert involved a group of young men buying pizzas and setting off in the car without doing up their seat belts. They crashed and the ones in the back were flung forward and killed the ones in the front. The message was very simple. The imagery was powerful and the solution it offered required very little effort. Also the target audience was clearly represented in the advert.

- **'Sharing your mate's works means sharing with everyone he's ever shared with':** this campaign showed a picture of a needle going through a series of arms and was designed to discourage needle-sharing in drug users for HIV prevention. It was effective as it illustrated rather than described the notion of needle-sharing. However, it also had implications for safe sex as it illustrated the idea that even though you might have sex with one person, this one person could connect you with a long line of other 'one persons'.

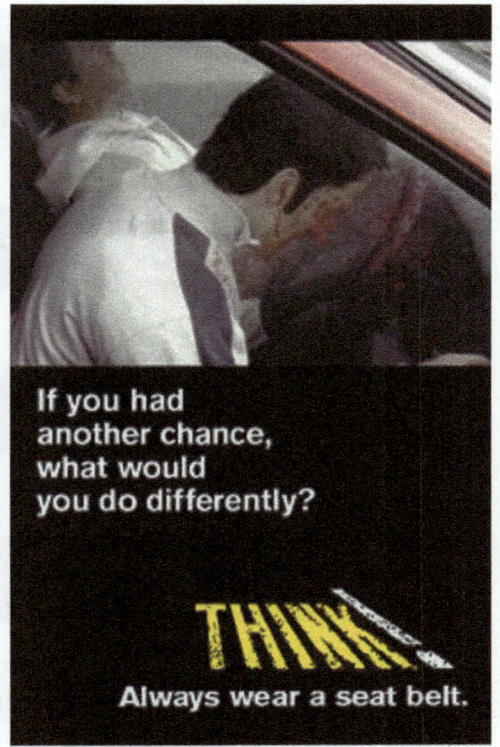

If you had another chance, what would you do differently?

THINK

Always wear a seat belt.

Promoting wearing seat belts in the back and front seats of a car

SOURCE: © Department of Transport

Understanding Media Campaigns

Media campaigns use a number of the psychological strategies described above to encourage us to change our behaviour. These include modelling (i.e. using people who are like us), fear appeals (i.e. being shocking), visual imagery (i.e. to change affect and maybe reduce denial or resistance), targeting a specific audience (i.e. those at the right stage of change and with a good level of motivation) and encouraging people to focus on the negative aspects of what they do (i.e. in line with motivational interviewing to create cognitive dissonance). The elaboration likelihood model (ELM, Petty and Cacioppo 1986) was developed as a model of persuasion and provides a framework for understanding why some media campaigns might be more successful than others and how they could be improved. The ELM is shown in Figure 7.8.

The ELM is a popular model in the area of persuasion across a range of fields including political persuasion, media influence and health behaviour change. It argues that in order for people to change their beliefs and behaviour, they need to do the following:

- Be motivated to receive the argument.
- Centrally process the argument.

This will occur if:

- The message is congruent with their existing beliefs.
- The message is personally relevant to them.
- The individual can understand the argument.

This central processing involves an assessment of arguments being presented which are then incorporated into the person's existing belief systems. This can result in a strong change in beliefs and longer-term changes in behaviour if this central processing determines that the case being made is strong and relevant. Only weak changes will occur that will not persist, however, if the case is deemed to be weak and not personally relevant. For example, if an overweight person has started to find it hard to climb the stairs and has realized that her clothes no longer fit, then she will be motivated to change

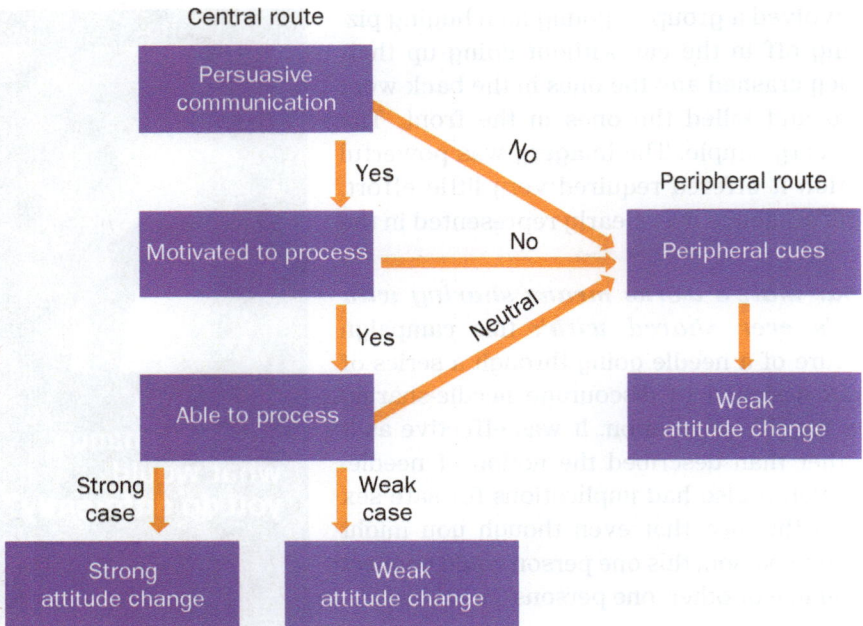

FIGURE 7.8 The elaboration likelihood model (ELM)

SOURCE: Adapted from Petty & Cacioppa, (1997)

and a message could be centrally processed. Such a message could be 'Eating less fat and more fruit and vegetables can help you lose weight, fit into your clothes and have more energy'.

But what if a person is not motivated in the first place? Given that most media campaigns are aimed at changing behaviour in those who are not already performing this behaviour, then many of these people will not fulfil the criteria for central processing as they will not be motivated. If this is the case, the ELM offers another route called 'peripheral processing'. This involves the following:

- Using direct cues and information.
- Maximizing the credibility of the source of the message.
- Maximizing the attractiveness of the source of the message.

For an overweight person who suffers no symptoms of breathlessness and has a wardrobe of larger clothes, the message above will not work. The campaign will therefore need to work harder to make a difference. For example, it could use indirect cues and information such as 'Weight loss clubs can be fun and are a good way to meet people'. It could increase the credibility of the message by using a more scientific approach (e.g. people in white coats, charts, data) and could make the message more attractive (e.g. a good-looking person in a white coat, images of friendly-looking people at a club, a smiling person selling fruit and vegetables). According to the ELM, messages using this peripheral processing route can change beliefs and behaviour but are likely to be less effective or long-lasting.

UNDERSTANDING SUSTAINED BEHAVIOUR CHANGE

Even though there has been much research and a multitude of interventions, many people continue to behave in unhealthy ways. For example, although smoking in the UK has declined, a substantial minority of the population still continue to smoke (see Chapter 3). Similarly, the prevalence of diet- and exercise-related problems, particularly obesity and overweight, is rising (see Chapters 4, 5 and 13).

Further, even though many people show initial changes in their health-related behaviours, rates of sustained behaviour change are poor, with many people reverting to their old habits. For example, although obesity treatments in the last 20 years have improved rates of initial weight loss, there has been very little success in weight loss maintenance in the longer term with up to 95 per cent of people returning to baseline weights by 5 years (see Chapter 13). Similarly, nearly half of those smokers who make a quit attempt return to smoking within the year (see Chapter 3). If real changes are to be made to people's health status, then research needs to address the issue of behaviour change in the longer term. To date, however, most research has focused on the onset of new behaviours or changes in behaviour in the short term due to the use of quantitative methods, with prospective designs that have follow-ups varying from a few weeks only to a year, as longer-term follow-ups require greater investment of time and cost. Some research, however, has addressed the issue of longer-term behaviour change maintenance, particularly for weight loss, smoking cessation and exercise.

- *Weight loss maintenance:* research indicates that although the majority of people with obesity regain the weight they lose, a small minority show weight loss maintenance. The factors that predict this are described in detail in Chapter 13 and illustrate a role for profile characteristics such as baseline body mass index (BMI), gender and employment status, historical factors such as previous attempts at weight loss, the type and amount of help received and psychological factors including motivations and individuals' beliefs about the causes of their weight problem. In addition, research also shows a role for behaviour change and a recent systematic review by Paixão et al. (2020) of 52 studies concluded that weight loss maintenance was related to increased physical activity, decreased total energy and fat intake. Further, research also suggests that longer-term weight loss maintenance is often initiated after a life event, a 'teachable moment' or 'epiphany', which can disrupt normal life, creates a shift in the costs and benefits of the behaviour and is associated with a behavioural model of obesity whereby behaviour is seen as central to both its cause and solution (Ogden and Sidhu, 2006; Ogden and Hills 2008; Ogden 2000, 2018).

- *Smoking cessation:* in terms of smoking cessation, much research has drawn upon a stage model approach and suggests that smoking cessation relates to factors such as action plans, goal-setting and the transition through stages (e.g. Prochaska and Velicer 1997, see Chapter 3). In contrast, however, West and Sohal (2006) asked almost 2,000 smokers and ex-smokers about their quit attempts and reported that nearly half had made quit attempts that were unplanned and that unplanned attempts were more likely to succeed than planned ones. They argue that longer-term smoking cessation may not always be the result of plans and the transition through stages and is often the result of 'catastrophes' which suddenly motivate change.

- *Exercise:* as with changes in diet and smoking, much research exploring exercise uptake has focused on short-term changes. From this perspective most research shows that exercise is related to social factors and enjoyment rather than any longer-term consideration of health goals (see Chapter 5). Armitage (2005) aimed to explore the problem of exercise maintenance and examined the predictors of stable exercise habits over a 12-week period. This study used the standard TPB measures and indicated that perceived behavioural control predicted behaviour in terms of both initiation and maintenance. Some research also indicates a link between smoking cessation and exercise, indicating that improvements in behaviour in one domain may create improvements in other domains that last in the longer term (Sohlberg and Bergmark 2020).

In general, it would seem that there is a role for a range of demographic, psychological and structural factors in understanding longer-term changes in behaviour and that, while some changes in behaviour may result from the 'drip drip effect' illustrated by stages and plans, other forms of change are the result of more sudden shifts in an individual's motivation. To date, however, there remains very little research on longer-term changes in behaviour. Further, the existing research tends to focus on behaviour-specific changes rather than factors that may generalize across behaviours.

BOX 7.1
Critical Approaches to Health Psychology

Research exploring behaviour change highlights some of the bigger issues with research in health psychology:

A snapshot of behaviour: For behaviour change to be effective and useful it needs to be sustained into the longer term. Most research, however, doesn't have the funding, time or staffing to carry out research over many years. Therefore it is difficult to know whether any of our interventions really last.

The individual vs social vs political: Behaviour change research in health psychology mostly focuses on the role of individual level variables such as cognitions and emotions. But all behaviours exist within a broader social and political context. Exercise can be increased through the availability of community events or open spaces, smoking cessation can be facilitated through government-backed smoking bans and alcohol drinking can be reduced through reducing work stress or increasing the price of alcohol. Many of these wider level variables are ignored or minimized in our research or reduced to simple boxes such as 'social context', 'social norms' or 'opportunity'.

Stereotyping: Behaviour change interventions should be tailored to the individual in order to work effectively. To do this the individual is assessed according to who they are and offered the most appropriate approach. This often means describing them according to their demographics: they are a young, black man or a middle-aged white woman, etc. Much as this is done with good intentions, it can end up stereotyping people according to group variables which don't actually tell us that much about the individual.

7 | THINKING CRITICALLY ABOUT CHANGING HEALTH BEHAVIOURS

This chapter has described the many theories and models used to inform research and develop interventions to change health behaviours. There are several problems with the literature in this area that need to be considered (see Ogden 2003, 2015, 2016a, 2016b, 2019 for further analysis).

SOME CRITICAL QUESTIONS

When thinking about research in the area of behaviour change, ask yourself the following questions:

- Are our beliefs really as separate and discrete as described by our models?
- Why is measuring health behaviour so difficult?
- What factors might influence behaviour change other than our beliefs?
- What is the problem with models that are too simple?
- What is the problem with models that are too complex?

SOME PROBLEMS WITH. . .

Here are problems with research in the area of behaviour change.

Problems with the Theories and Models

Research exploring behaviour change is subject to the same conceptual problems found in the research on health beliefs which are described in Chapter 2. In particular:

Stage models: these assume stages are qualitatively different to each other rather than seeing behaviour as being on a continuum.

Social cognition models: these suffer from issues of whether they measure or change beliefs, whether the constructs they describe are separate from each other or tautological and whether the theories can ever be rejected.

Integrated models: models such as the COM-B and TDF reflect an integration of other theories and models. They illustrate the tensions between being either too specific or too inclusive, being designed for the expert (and therefore complex) or for the lay reader (and therefore too simple) and being designed now (when evidence is still weak but when we need a new approach) or in the future (when evidence is stronger but causing a delay to the development of new interventions). They also illustrate the problem with trying to systematize research and practice and the implications of this for creativity and tailored interventions which are professional and patient specific.

Problems with Research Methodology

Research in this field is also subject to some common methodological problems:

Research design: the gold standard design for evaluating the effectiveness of an intervention is the randomized controlled trial (RCT) which enables conclusions about causality to be drawn and can control for confounding variables whether or not they have been measured. Due to funding issues, time and the involvement of researchers (who have limited time and energy) much research in this area is limited by poor research designs which use only short-term follow-ups, cross-sectional or longitudinal designs. Even the RCT, however, has its problems, as it can only tell us what works for some of the people some of the time. Further, it cannot highlight which component of any intervention is particularly effective and which adds nothing to improving health outcomes.

Sampling: research aims to involve representative samples so that the results can be generalized beyond the study. Unfortunately this is very rarely the case with studies including only those who are approached to take part *and* who consent to take part *and* who complete the study for all follow up time points. These people are often very different from the wider population.

Measures: constructs need to be clearly conceptualized and then operationalized in ways that researchers can be confident that they are measuring what they are supposed to be measuring. Sometimes in behaviour change research the different constructs are very similar. When these constructs are then analysed it is not clear whether we are associating like with like or what is really predicting what when the different things being measured overlap.

Problems with the Assumptions behind this Research Area

Research exploring behaviour change also makes some assumptions which are problematic:

The science of behaviour is the same as that of behaviour change: often research assumes that if we know what predicts and causes behaviour then we can use these variables to change behaviour. This may not always be the case.

Behaviour is rational: much research focuses on the cognitive predictors of behaviour and behaviour change. Humans beings, however, can be irrational, random, emotional and unpredictable and are often governed by unconscious factors. These rarely feature in research in this area.

People change their behaviour because of what is done to them: evaluations of the active ingredients of interventions assess what the intervention involves and then assess change in behaviour. However, there are many other less tangible and less obvious components to any intervention that may also be important, such as the relationship between the client and professional, smiling, warmth or even raising an eyebrow that might make a difference. These are never, and cannot ever, all be measured.

Professionals do what they are told to do by the protocol: evaluations of the effectiveness of interventions often code the protocol to see what the intervention entailed and then assess whether behaviour changed. This assumes that what is in the protocol is what was delivered in the intervention. But those delivering the intervention are human beings, delivering the intervention to another human being. It is unlikely that the protocol was perfectly adhered to given that the interaction between human beings generates a whole other level of intervention (relationship, smiling, warmth, eyebrow raising, etc.) not in the protocol and dependent upon what happens moment by moment in the intervention.

TO CONCLUDE

Chapters 2–6 have described different health behaviours and the factors that predict them. This chapter has examined how health behaviours can be changed drawing upon a number of different theoretical perspectives. First, it described learning theory and how together with cognitive theory this illustrates a role for reinforcement, modelling, associative learning, CBT and relapse prevention. Second, it described interventions derived from social cognition theory such as the use of the TPB to develop interventions, the role of planning and implementation intentions. Next it explored interventions influenced by stage models including the use of stage-matched interventions and motivational interviewing. The chapter then explored the role of emotions in behaviour change which are used in fear appeals, visual images and self-affirmation. The chapter then explored the ways in which these theoretical approaches have been integrated. In particular, the chapter addressed the drive to create a science of behaviour change interventions with the use of the COM-B, TDF, BCTs and BCW. It then explored how different approaches are integrated in interventions using modern technology and the media. Finally, the chapter described ways to think critically about this area of research in terms of theories and models, the methods used and the key assumptions underlying behaviour change research.

QUESTIONS

1 What is the evidence for behavioural strategies for changing health behaviour?
2 How can cognitive theories add to learning theory approaches to promote behaviour change?
3 In what ways can social cognitive theory inform behaviour change interventions?
4 Are implementation intentions effective for changing behaviour?
5 Can affect be changed and would this aid behaviour change?
6 What is the evidence for self-affirmation-based interventions?
7 Can behaviour change be made into a proper science and what would this mean?
8 What factors might predict behaviour change that aren't captured by any of our models?
9 What problems are there with our models of behaviour change?
10 How does knowing how people have already changed their behaviour add to the development of behaviour change interventions?

FOR DISCUSSION

People make small changes in their behaviour often without realizing it. Think of the last time you changed your behaviour (e.g. tried out a new clothes shop, had something different for breakfast, started to do more exercise) and think of all the reasons for this and explore how much these reasons related to the psychological theories and strategies described in this chapter.

FURTHER READING

Conner, N. and Norman, P. (eds) (2015) *Predicting and Changing Health Behaviour: Research and Practice with Social Cognition Models,* 3rd edn. New York: McGraw Hill.
This is an excellent book that describes the different theoretical approaches to behaviour and behaviour change. It is up to date and provides a balanced view of the field

Gardner, B. (2015) A review and analysis of the use of 'habit' in understanding, predicting and influencing health-related behaviour. *Health Psychology Review, 9,* 277–295. https://doi.org/10.1080/17437199.2013.876238
This is a great review of the theories and research focusing on habit and habit change and is relevant to any attempt to change any behaviour.

Hagger, M.S. , Cameron, L.D., Hamilton, K., Hankonen, N., and Lintunen, T. (eds) (2020) *The Handbook of Behaviour Change.* New York, NY: Cambridge University Press (pp 599–616).
This is an extremely comprehensive book which covers pretty much all the theories and all the research on behaviour change.

Michie, S., Atkins, L. and West, R. (2014) *The Behaviour Change Wheel: A Guide to Designing Interventions.* London: Silverback Publishing.
This book describes the vast volume of research over recent years attempting to develop a science of behaviour change.

Ogden, J. and Hills, L. (2008) Understanding sustained changes in behaviour: the role of life events and the process of reinvention, *Health: An International Journal,* 12: 419–37.
This is one of my papers. I have included it here because it uses qualitative methods to explore how people make sense of their own successful changes in behaviour in terms of weight loss and smoking cessation. Work on success stories provides a different angle on what works for individuals. This paper focuses on the notion of identity shifts and reinventions which can be triggered by life events which make people see their futures differently.

Thaler, R.H. and Sunstein, C.A. (2008) *Nudge: Improving Decisions about Health, Wealth, and Happiness.* New Haven, CT: Yale University Press.
This is a fairly accessible book which has generated much interest over the past couple of years. It describes the notion of 'nudge' and the ways in which small changes can 'nudge' people into changing aspects of their lives including their behaviour. The UK government has set up a 'nudge unit' to consider ways to nudge people to improve their behaviour. Roger Ingham suggested in the *The Guardian* that if they turn their attention to sexual health, this should be called 'the nudge nudge unit' (see www.guardian.co.uk/theguardian/2010/nov/15/say-no-more-nudge-wink).

PART THREE
Becoming Ill

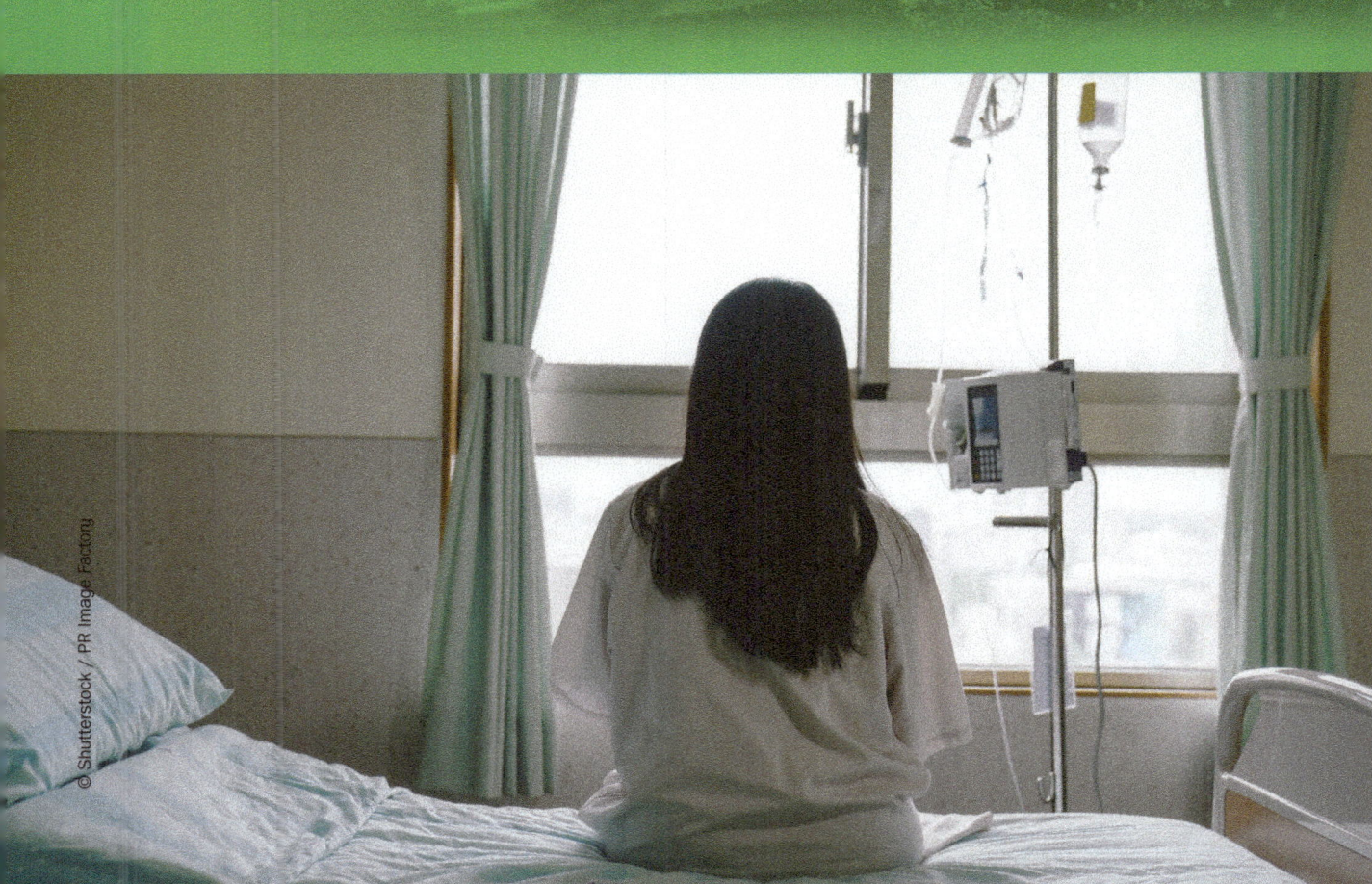

8

Illness Cognitions

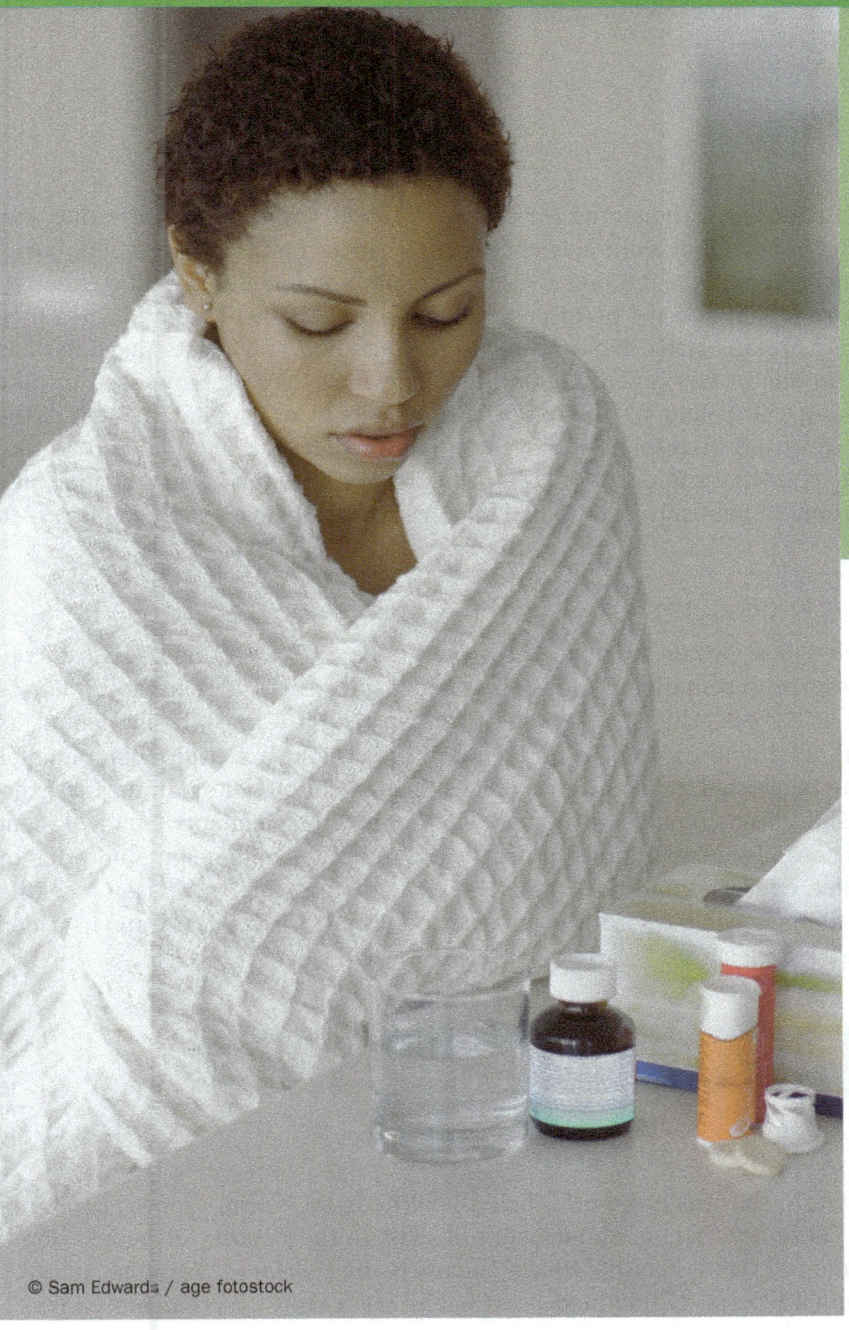

© Sam Edwards / age fotostock

Learning Objectives

To understand:

1. Making Sense of Health and Illness
2. What are Illness Cognitions?
3. The Self Regulatory Model
4. Stage 1: Interpretation
5. Stage 2: Coping
6. Predicting and Changing Health Outcomes
7. Thinking Critically about Illness Cognitions

> ## CHAPTER OVERVIEW
>
> Chapter 2 described health beliefs and their relationship to health behaviours. Individuals, however, also have beliefs about illness. This chapter examines what it means to be 'healthy' and what it means to be 'sick', and reviews these meanings in the context of how individuals cognitively represent illness (their illness cognitions). The chapter then assesses how illness cognitions can be measured and places these beliefs within Leventhal's self-regulatory model, with its focus on symptom perception, illness cognitions and coping. The relationship between these factors is then discussed and the association between illness cognitions and health outcomes explored with a focus on the central role of coherence. The chapter then describes interventions to change illness cognitions and their impact on patient health.

CASE STUDY

Meg-John is 25 and has been diagnosed with asthma for 5 years. Most of the time they are fine, can carry on their life as normal and believe that asthma is not a very serious condition that will go away in time. They also think that they can manage it themselves by not smoking and doing gentle exercise. Sometimes, however, they can suddenly become breathless and have had about 10 attacks when they have been unable to catch their breath. These have been very frightening and twice Meg-John has been admitted into hospital. The doctor has given them an inhaler which they are supposed to take every day, regardless of how they are feeling, to prevent further attacks from happening. Most of the time, however, Meg-John feels fine and therefore will not take their medication. They have read that medicines can do harm if taken over time and the patient information leaflet listed some worrying side effects. They also don't like to think of themselves as an ill person who needs help and feel embarrassed to use their inhaler in public.

Through the Eyes of Health Psychology. . .

People have beliefs about their illness which influence how they behave. We call these illness cognitions, illness beliefs or illness representations. Meg-John's story illustrates a number of illness cognitions about factors such as the severity of a condition (thinks they are fine), beliefs about its consequences (it will go away), its emotional impact on the sufferer (attacks are frightening, inhaler is embarrassing), whether it can be treated by medication (self-management by not smoking and exercise), whether medication has side effects (can do harm) and whether it can be managed by the patient themselves (doing exercise). These illness cognitions in turn relate to how people behave in terms of their health behaviours (e.g. diet, exercise) and how they decide to manage their condition (seeking help, taking medication). This chapter will explore what illness cognitions are and the ways in which they can impact upon someone's health status.

1	MAKING SENSE OF HEALTH AND ILLNESS

WHAT DOES IT MEAN TO BE HEALTHY?

For the majority of people living in the western world, being healthy is the norm – most people are healthy for most of the time. Therefore, beliefs about being ill exist in the context of beliefs about being healthy (e.g. illness means not being healthy, illness means feeling different from usual, etc.). The World Health Organization (WHO) (1947) defined good health as 'a state of complete physical, mental and social well being'. This definition presents a broad multidimensional view of health that departs from the traditional medical emphasis on physical health only.

Over the past few decades this multidimensional model has emerged throughout the results of several qualitative studies from medical sociology that have asked lay people the question, 'What does it mean to be healthy?' For example, Blaxter (1990) asked 9,000 individuals to describe someone whom they thought was healthy and to consider, 'What makes you call them healthy?' and 'What is it like when you are healthy?' A qualitative analysis was then carried out on a sub-sample of these individuals. For some, health simply meant not being ill. However, for many, health was seen in terms of a reserve, a healthy life filled with health behaviours, physical fitness, having energy and vitality, social relationships with others, being able to function effectively and an expression of psychosocial well-being. Blaxter also examined how a concept of health varied over the life course and investigated any sex differences. Calnan (1987) also explored the health beliefs of women in England and argued that their models of health could be conceptualized in two sets of definitions: positive definitions including feeling energetic, plenty of exercise, feeling fit, eating the right things, being the correct weight, having a positive outlook and having a good life/marriage; and negative definitions including not getting coughs and colds, only in bed once, rarely go to the doctor and have check-ups – nothing wrong.

The issue of 'What is health?' has also been explored from a psychological perspective with a particular focus on health and illness cognitions. For example, Lau (1995) found that when young healthy adults were asked to describe in their own words 'what being healthy means to you', their beliefs about health could be understood within the following dimensions:

- *physiological/physical,* for example, good condition, have energy
- *psychological,* for example, happy, energetic, feel good psychologically
- *behavioural,* for example, eat, sleep properly
- *future consequences,* for example, live longer
- *the absence of illness,* for example, not sick, no disease, no symptoms.

Lau argued that most people show a positive definition of health (not just the absence of illness), which also includes more than just physical and psychological factors. He suggested that healthiness is most people's normal state and represents the backdrop to their beliefs about being ill. Psychological studies of the beliefs of the elderly (Hall et al. 1989), those suffering from a chronic illness (Hays and Stewart 1990) and children (Schmidt and Frohling 2000) have reported that these individuals also conceptualize health as being multidimensional. This indicates some overlap between professional (WHO) and lay views of health (i.e. a multidimensional perspective involving physical and psychological factors).

WHAT DOES IT MEAN TO BE ILL?

In his study of the beliefs of young healthy adults, Lau (1995) also asked participants 'What does it mean to be sick?' Their answers indicated the dimensions they use to conceptualize illness:

- *not feeling normal,* for example, 'I don't feel right'
- *specific symptoms,* for example, physiological/psychological
- *specific illnesses,* for example, cancer, cold, depression
- *consequences of illness,* for example, 'I can't do what I usually do'
- *time line,* for example, how long the symptoms last
- *the absence of health,* for example, not being healthy.

These dimensions of 'what it means to be ill' have been described within the context of illness cognitions (also called illness beliefs or illness representations).

2 | WHAT ARE ILLNESS COGNITIONS?

Leventhal and his colleagues (Leventhal et al. 1980, 2007a, 2007b; Leventhal and Nerenz 1985) defined illness cognitions as 'a patient's own implicit common sense beliefs about their illness'. They proposed that these cognitions provide patients with a framework or a schema for *coping with* and *understanding their illness,* and *telling them what to look out for if they are becoming ill.* Using interviews with patients suffering from a variety of different illnesses, Leventhal and his colleagues identified five cognitive dimensions of these beliefs (see Figure 8.1).

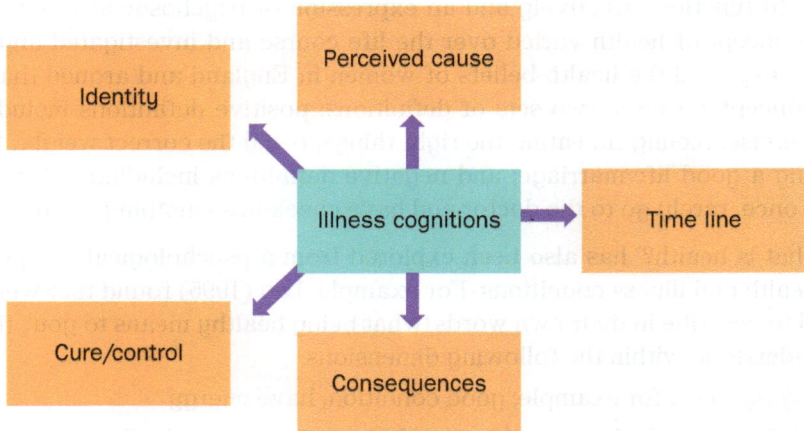

Figure 8.1 Illness cognitions: the five core dimensions
SOURCE: Adapted from Leventhal et al. (1980)

Some of these dimensions are similar to those described by attribution theory in Chapter 2:

1 *Identity:* this refers to the label given to the illness (the medical diagnosis) and the symptoms experienced (e.g. I have a cold – 'the diagnosis', with a runny nose – 'the symptoms').

2 *The perceived cause of the illness:* these causes may be biological, such as a virus or a lesion, or psychosocial, such as stress- or health-related behaviour. In addition, patients may hold representations of illness that reflect a variety of different causal models (e.g. 'My cold was caused by a virus', 'My cold was caused by feeling run down').

3 *Time line:* this refers to the patient's beliefs about how long the illness will last, whether it is acute (short term) or chronic (long term) (e.g. 'My cold will be over in a few days').

4 *Consequences:* this refers to the patient's perceptions of the possible effects of the illness on their life. Such consequences may be physical (e.g. pain, lack of mobility), emotional (e.g. loss of social contact, loneliness) or a combination of factors (e.g. 'My cold will prevent me from playing football, which will prevent me from seeing my friends').

5 *Curability and controllability:* patients also represent illnesses in terms of whether they believe that the illness can be treated and cured and the extent to which the outcome of their illness is controllable either by themselves or by powerful others (e.g. 'If I rest, my cold will go away', 'If I get medicine from my doctor, my cold will go away').

EVIDENCE FOR THE DIMENSIONS OF ILLNESS COGNITIONS

The extent to which beliefs about illness are constituted by these different dimensions has been studied using both qualitative and quantitative methodologies.

Qualitative Research

Leventhal and his colleagues carried out interviews with individuals who were chronically ill, those who had been recently diagnosed as having cancer and with healthy adults. The resulting descriptions of illness suggest underlying beliefs that are made up of the aforementioned dimensions. Leventhal argued that interviews are the best way to access illness cognitions as this methodology avoids the possibility of priming the subjects. For example, asking a subject 'To what extent do you think about your illness in terms of its possible consequences?' will obviously encourage them to regard consequences as an important dimension. However, according to Leventhal, interviews encourage subjects to express their own beliefs, not those expected by the interviewer. Since then, a multitude of qualitative studies have been carried out to explore how people make sense of common and less common chronic conditions including Spinal Cord injury, Inflammatory Bowel Disease (IBD), Mild Traumatic Brian Injury (MtBI), varicose veins, incurable cancer, fibromyalgia and leg ulcers (Dibb et al. 2014; Tollow and Ogden 2016; Tollow et al. 2020; Matini and Ogden 2016; Hudson et al. 2015; Brunger and Ogden 2013; Theadom and Cropley 2010). Fairly consistently, research illustrates that illness cognitions for a wide range of conditions tend to reflect the original five dimensions of identity, timeline, cause, consequences and control.

Quantitative Research

Other studies have used more artificial and controlled methodologies, and these too have provided support for the dimensions of illness cognitions. Lau et al. (1989) used a card-sorting technique to evaluate how subjects conceptualized illness. They asked 20 subjects to sort 65 statements into piles that 'made sense to them'. These statements had been made previously in response to descriptions of 'your most recent illness'. They reported that the subjects' piles of categories reflected the dimensions of identity (diagnosis/symptoms), consequences (the possible effects), time line (how long it will last), cause (what caused the illness) and cure/control (how and whether it can be treated).

A series of experimental studies by Bishop and colleagues also provided support for these dimensions. For example, Bishop and Converse (1986) presented subjects with brief descriptions of patients who were experiencing six different symptoms. Subjects were randomly allocated to one of two sets of descriptions: high prototype in which all six symptoms had been previously rated as associated with the same disease, or low prototype in which only two of the six symptoms had been previously rated as associated with the same disease. The results showed that subjects in the high prototype condition labelled the disease more easily and accurately than subjects in the low prototype condition. The authors argued that this provides support for the role of the identity dimension (diagnosis and symptoms) of illness representations and also suggested that there is some consistency in people's concept of the identity of illnesses. In addition, subjects were asked to describe in their own words 'What else do you think may be associated with this person's situation?' They reported that 91 per cent of the given associations fell into the dimensions of illness representations as described by Leventhal. However, they also reported that the dimensions of consequences (the possible effects) and time line (how long it will last) were the least frequently mentioned.

There is also some evidence for a similar structure of illness representations in other cultures. Weller (1984) examined models of illness in English-speaking Americans and Spanish-speaking Guatemalans. The results indicated that illness was predominantly conceptualized in terms of contagion and severity. Lau (1995) argued that contagion is a version of the cause dimension (i.e. the illness is caused by a virus) and severity is a combination of the magnitude of the perceived consequences and beliefs about time line (i.e. how will the illness affect my life and how long will it last?) – dimensions that support those described by Leventhal. Hagger and Orbell (2003) carried out a meta-analysis of 45 empirical studies which used Leventhal's model of illness cognitions. They concluded from their analysis that there was consistent support for the different illness cognition dimensions and that the different cognitions showed a logical pattern across different illness types.

MEASURING ILLNESS COGNITIONS

Leventhal and colleagues originally used qualitative methods to assess people's illness cognitions. Since this time other forms of measurement have been used. These will be described in terms of questionnaires that have been developed and methodological issues surrounding measurement.

The Use of Questionnaires

Measuring Illness Beliefs

Although it has been argued that the preferred method to access illness cognitions is through interview, interviews are time-consuming and can only involve a limited number of subjects. In order to research further into individuals' beliefs about illness, researchers in New Zealand and the UK have developed the Illness Perception Questionnaire (IPQ) (Weinman et al. 1996). This questionnaire asks subjects to rate a series of statements about their illness. These statements reflect the dimensions of identity (e.g. a set of symptoms such as pain, tiredness), consequences (e.g. 'My illness has had major consequences on my life'), time line (e.g. 'My illness will last a short time'), cause (e.g. 'Stress was a major factor in causing my illness') and cure/control (e.g. 'There is a lot I can do to control my symptoms'). This questionnaire has been used to examine beliefs about illnesses such as chronic fatigue syndrome, diabetes and arthritis and has been translated in a number of different languages. A revised version of the IPQ has now been published (the IPQR; Moss-Morris et al. 2002) which has better psychometric properties than the original IPQ and includes three additional subscales: cyclical time line perceptions, illness coherence and emotional representations. A brief IPQ has also been developed which uses single items and is useful when participants don't have much time or when they are completing a large battery of different measures (the B-IPQ; Broadbent et al. 2006). In 2015, Broadbent et al. conducted a systematic review and meta-analysis of 188 papers using the B-IPQ. They concluded that the scale has good concurrent and predictive validity and that the subscales were predictive of a wide range of health outcomes. In addition, researchers have created a version of the IPQ-R for use with healthy people (Figueiras and Alves 2007). The IPQ even has its own website now.

Measuring Treatment Beliefs

People also have beliefs about their treatment, whether it is medication, surgery or behaviour change. In line with this, Horne (1997; Horne et al. 1999) developed a Beliefs about Medicine Questionnaire (BMQ) which conceptualized such beliefs along four dimensions. Two of these are specific to the medication being taken: 'specific necessity' (to reflect whether their medicine is seen as important) and 'specific concerns' (to reflect whether the individual is concerned about side-effects); and two of these are general beliefs about all medicines: 'general overuse' (to reflect doctors' overuse of medicines) and 'general harm' (to reflect the damage that medicines can do). These two core dimensions of necessity and concerns have been shown to describe people's beliefs about anti-retroviral therapy for HIV/AIDS (V. Cooper et al. 2002; Horne et al. 2004) and to be relevant to a range of beliefs about medicines for illnesses such as asthma, renal disease, cancer, HIV and cardiac failure (e.g. Horne and Weinman 1999). Research also shows that although individuals may report a consistent pattern of beliefs, this pattern varies according to cultural background (Horne et al. 2004). Nie et al. (2019) carried out a systematic review and meta-analysis of 58 studies using the BMQ in China and concluded that it was a reliable tool for assessing medication beliefs in the Chinese population and that the Necessity-Concerns Framework was a useful conceptual model to explain Chinese patients' medication adherence.

Measurement Issues

Although quantitative measures of illness and treatment beliefs are now commonly used, they are not without their limitations. Beliefs about illness can be assessed using a range of measures. Some research has used interviews (e.g. Leventhal et al. 1980, 2007a; Schmidt and Frohling 2000), some has used formal questionnaires (e.g. Horne and Weinman 2002; Llewellyn et al. 2003), some has used vignette studies (e.g. French et al. 2002a) and other research has used a repertory grid method (e.g. Walton and Eves 2001).

French and colleagues asked whether the form of method used to elicit beliefs about illness influenced the types of beliefs reported. In one study French et al. (2002a) compared the impact of eliciting beliefs using either a questionnaire or a vignette. Participants were asked either simply to rate a series of causes for heart attack (the questionnaire) or to read a vignette about a man and to estimate his chances of having a heart attack. The results showed that the two different methods resulted in different beliefs about the causes of heart attack and different importance placed upon these causes. Specifically, when using the questionnaire, smoking and stress came out as more important causes than family history, whereas when using the vignette, smoking and family history came out as more important causes than stress. In a similar vein French et al. (2001) carried out a systematic review of studies involving attributions for causes of heart attack and compared these causes according to method used. The results showed that stressors, fate or luck were more common beliefs about causes when using interval rating scales (i.e. 1–5) than when studies used dichotomous answers (i.e. yes/no). French et al. (2005b) also asked whether causal beliefs should be subjected to a factor analysis as a means to combine different sets of beliefs into individual constructs (e.g. external causes, lifestyle causes, etc.) and concluded that although many researchers use this approach to combine their data, it is unlikely to result in very valid groups of causal beliefs. In addition, the IPQ measures have been criticized for having ambiguous subscales, for being too general and not specific to the beliefs of each individual, and for not being sufficiently relevant for the characteristics of each individual condition (French and Weinman 2008).

In summary it appears that individuals may show consistent beliefs about illness that can be used to make sense of their illness and help their understanding of any developing symptoms. These illness cognitions have been incorporated into a model of illness behaviour to examine the relationship between an individual's cognitive representation of their illness and their subsequent coping behaviour. This model is known as the 'self-regulatory model of illness behaviour'.

3 THE SELF-REGULATORY MODEL

Leventhal incorporated his description of illness cognitions into his self-regulatory model (SRM) of illness behaviour (e.g. Leventhal et al. 1980; 2007a). This model is based on approaches to problem-solving and suggests that illness/symptoms are dealt with by individuals in the same way as other problems (see Chapter 9 for details of other models of problem solving). It is assumed that, given a problem or a change in the status quo, the individual will be motivated to solve the problem and re-establish their state of normality. Traditional models describe problem-solving in three stages: (1) interpretation (making sense of the problem); (2) coping (dealing with the problem in order to regain a state of equilibrium); and (3) appraisal (assessing how successful the coping stage has been). According to models of problem solving, these three stages will continue until the coping strategies are deemed to be successful and a state of equilibrium has been attained. In terms of health and illness, if healthiness is an individual's normal state, then any onset of illness will be interpreted as a problem and the individual will be motivated to re-establish their state of health (i.e. illness is not the normal state).

These stages have been applied to health using the SRM (see Figure 8.2) and are described briefly here and in more detail later on.

STAGE 1: INTERPRETATION

An individual may be confronted with the problem of a potential illness through two channels: *symptom perception* ('I have a pain in my chest') or *social messages* ('the doctor has diagnosed this pain as angina').

Once the individual has received information about the possibility of illness through these channels, according to theories of problem-solving, the individual is then motivated to return to a state of 'problem-free' normality. This involves assigning meaning to the problem. According to Leventhal, the problem can be given meaning by accessing the individual's illness cognitions. Therefore the symptoms

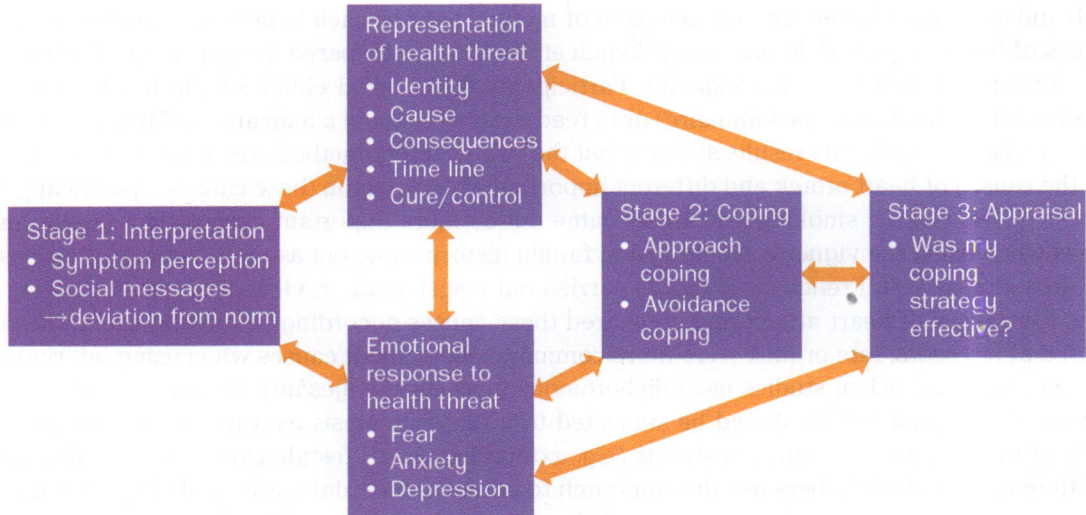

Figure 8.2 Leventhal's Self-Regulatory Model (SRM)

and social messages will contribute towards the development of illness cognitions, which will be constructed according to the following dimensions: identity, cause, consequences, time line, cure/control. These cognitive representations of the 'problem' will give the problem meaning and will enable the individual to develop and consider suitable coping strategies.

However, a cognitive representation is not the only consequence of symptom perception and social messages. The identification of the problem of illness will also result in changes in emotional state.

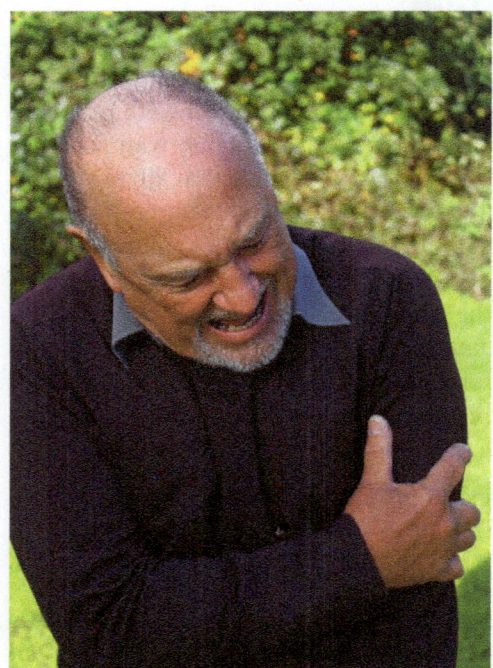

Experiencing symptoms can generate an emotional response and an illness representation

SOURCE: © Shutterstock / Giideon

For example, perceiving the symptom of pain and receiving the social message that this pain may be related to coronary heart disease (CHD) may result in anxiety. Therefore, any coping strategies have to relate to both the illness cognitions and the emotional state of the individual.

STAGE 2: COPING

The next stage in the SRM is the development and identification of suitable coping strategies. Coping can take many forms, which will be discussed in detail later in this chapter and in Chapter 10. However, two broad categories of coping have been defined that incorporate the multitude of other coping strategies: approach coping (e.g. taking pills, going to the doctor, resting, talking to friends about emotions) and avoidance coping (e.g. denial, wishful thinking). When faced with the problem of illness, the individual will therefore develop coping strategies in an attempt to return to a state of healthy normality.

STAGE 3: APPRAISAL

The third stage of the SRM is appraisal. This involves individuals evaluating the effectiveness of the coping strategy and determining whether to continue with this strategy or whether to opt for an alternative one.

WHY IS THE MODEL CALLED SELF-REGULATORY?

This process is regarded as self-regulatory because the three components of the model (interpretation, coping, appraisal) interrelate in order to maintain the status quo (i.e. they regulate the self). Therefore, if the individual's normal state (health) is disrupted (by illness), the model proposes that the individual is motivated to return the balance back to normality. This self-regulation involves the three processes interrelating in an ongoing and dynamic fashion. Therefore, interactions occur between the different stages. For example:

- Symptom perception may result in an emotional shift, which may exacerbate the perception of symptoms (e.g. 'I can feel a pain in my chest. Now I feel anxious. Now I can feel more pain as all my attention is focused on it.').

- If the individual opts to use denial as their coping strategy, this may result in a reduction in symptom perception, a decrease in any negative emotions and a shift in their illness cognition (e.g. 'This pain is not very bad' (denial); 'Now I feel less anxious' (emotions); 'This pain will not last for long' (time line); 'This illness will not have any serious consequences for my lifestyle' (consequences)).

- A positive appraisal of the effectiveness of the coping strategy may itself be a coping strategy (e.g. 'My symptoms appear to have been reduced by doing relaxation exercises' may be a form of denial).

PROBLEMS WITH ASSESSMENT

This dynamic, self-regulatory process suggests a model of cognitions that is complex and intuitively sensible, but poses problems for attempts at assessment and intervention. For example:

1   If the different components of the SRM interact, should they be measured separately? For example, is the belief that an illness has no serious consequences an illness cognition or a coping strategy?

2   If the different components of the SRM interact, can individual components be used to predict outcome or should the individual components be seen as co-occurring? For example, is the appraisal that symptoms have been reduced a successful outcome or is it a form of denial (a coping strategy)?

The individual processes involved in the SRM will now be examined in greater detail.

4 | STAGE 1: INTERPRETATION

The interpretation stage involves symptom perception and social messages. These result in the creation of illness cognitions and an emotional representation of the problem.

SYMPTOM PERCEPTION

It is often assumed that we experience symptoms in response to some underlying physical problem. For example, we think that our headache reflects something going on in our head and that the worse it feels, the worse the damage in our head must be. Research exploring symptom perception indicates that this simple stimulus – response model of symptoms ignores the wealth of psychological factors that can make symptoms either better or worse. Research has addressed individual differences in symptom perception and the role of mood, cognition and the social context. These are illustrated in Figure 8.3.

Individual Differences in Symptom Perception

Symptoms such as a temperature, pain, a runny nose or the detection of a lump may indicate to the individual the possibility of illness. However, symptom perception is not a straightforward process and research indicates much variability between people (see Chapter 11 for details of pain perception and see Chapter 9 for how symptom perception can influence help seeking and the role of thresholds). For example, what might be a sore throat to one person could be another's tonsillitis, and whereas a retired person might consider a cough a serious problem, a working person might be too busy to think

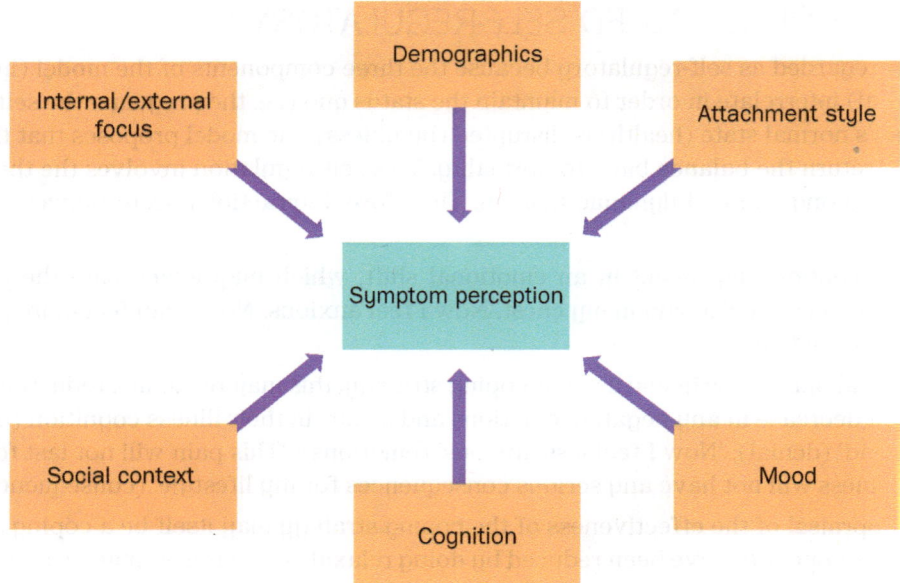

Figure 8.3 Symptom perception

about it. Research has addressed this variability in terms of an internal/external focus, demographics and attachment styles.

Internal/External Focus

Pennebaker (1983) has argued that there are individual differences in the amount of attention people pay to their internal states and that whereas some individuals may sometimes be internally focused and more sensitive to symptoms, others may be more externally focused and less sensitive to any internal changes. However, this difference is not always consistent with differences in how accurate people are at detecting their symptoms. For example, Pennebaker reported that individuals who were more focused on their internal states tended to overestimate changes in their heart rate compared with subjects who were externally focused. In contrast, Kohlmann et al. (2001) examined the relationship between cardiac vigilance and heart-beat detection in the laboratory and reported a negative correlation; those who stated they were more aware of their heart underestimated their heart rate. Being internally focused has also been shown to relate to a perception of slower recovery from illness (Miller et al. 1987) and to more health-protective behaviour (Kohlmann et al. 2001). Being internally focused may result in a different perception of symptom change, not a more accurate one.

Some research also indicates individual variability in the extent to which symptoms are considered discrete or whether they overlap. For example, Carter and Ogden (2021) explored the degree of interoceptive crossover between emotional symptoms, such as happy, calm or sad, and physical symptoms such as stomach pain, headache and abnormal heartbeat. The results showed that while there were some more predictable crossovers such as Afraid and Abnormal Heartbeat (74.5 per cent); Sad and Fatigue (29.4 per cent) and Afraid and Shortness of Breath (58.5 per cent), other crossovers were more surprising, such as Satisfied with Headache (1.2 per cent); Bored with Back Pain (5.95 per cent) and Happy and Back Pain (0.4 per cent). This might relate to trait variables such as alexithymia and indicates that people differ not only in whether they are internally or externally focused but also in whether they can differentiate between different types of symptoms.

Demographics

Research has also explored variability in symptom reporting by gender, time of day, day of week and family group (Michel 2006; 2007). For example, in one study parents and adolescents from 173 families completed measures of their somatic symptoms six times a day for seven consecutive days. The results showed that symptoms were more likely to be reported in the mornings and evenings than in the middle of the day and less likely to be reported on weekend evenings than week evenings. In addition, women reported more symptoms than men (during the day) and adolescents showed an increase in symptoms in the evenings compared to their parents (Michel 2007). In a parallel study, variation in symptom reporting was found at the individual level but not at the family level (Michel 2006).

Attachment Style

The notion of attachment style is derived from Bowlby's early work on how children internalize their interactions with their primary caregiver to form the basis for their beliefs and expectations of present and future interpersonal interactions (Bowlby 1973). Ainsworth et al. (1978) used this perspective to develop their three-factor model of attachment behaviour and classified attachment as secure ('my mother will respond to me'), anxious ambivalent ('my mother inconsistently responds to me') and avoidant ('my mother doesn't respond to me'). Attachment style has been used to inform much recent research across all areas of psychology including depression, stress, coping and anxiety. Within health psychology, research has identified a link between attachment style and symptom reporting and, in general, research indicates that those with secure attachment styles report fewer somatic symptoms than those with either anxious/ambivalent or avoidant styles (Taylor et al. 2000; Wearden et al. 2003). Research has also explored factors that may mediate this relationship and indicates that higher levels of symptoms may only relate to a less secure attachment style in those with either negative affect, lower social support or higher levels of suppressed anger (i.e. 'anger in', not 'anger out'), (Kidd and Sheffield 2005; Armitage and Harris 2006).

Mood, Cognition and Social Context

Skelton and Pennebaker (1982) suggested that symptom perception is also influenced by mood, cognition and the social context.

Mood

The role of mood in symptom perception is particularly apparent in pain perception with anxiety increasing self-reports of the pain experience. In addition, anxiety has been proposed as an explanation for placebo pain reduction, as taking any form of medication (even a sugar pill) may reduce the individual's anxiety, increase their sense of control and result in pain reduction (see Chapter 11 for a discussion of anxiety, pain and placebos. LeRoy et al. (2017) found that baseline loneliness predicted self-reported cold symptoms over time, more so than demographic variables, the season of participation (e.g. winter), and depressive affect. Likewise, Charles and Almeida (2006) explored the relationship between state negative affect and a wide range of somatic symptoms and using a lagged design focused on the direction of the relationships between these factors in an attempt to determine what comes first – symptom or low mood. The results were complex, with no simple story emerging, but showed that whereas pain (e.g. headaches, backaches and muscle soreness) seemed to lead to lowered mood, lowered mood seemed to lead to gastrointestinal symptoms such as poor appetite nausea/upset stomach or constipation.

The relationship between mood and physical symptoms, however, is not always clear cut. Zeiser et al. (2021) carried out a scoping review to explore the direction of the relationship between depression and eczema. Their analysis showed that while depression was correlated with atopic eczema symptoms, the effect of eczema symptoms on depression seemed stronger than the effect of depression on eczema symptoms. Contradictory results were observed for anxiety. Mora et al. (2007) also explored the role of negative affect on symptom perception and the processes underlying this relationship. Their study involved both a cross-sectional and longitudinal design and assessed trait and state negative affect in adults with moderate and severe asthma. The results showed that higher trait negative affect was related to higher reports of all symptoms whether or not they were related to asthma. In addition, the results showed that only those who were worried about their asthma attributed their asthma symptoms to asthma. This suggests that negative affect increases symptom perception and further that worrying about asthma enables the individual to associate their symptoms with their illness. Similarly, Hollier et al. (2019) found that while anxiety and depression were correlated with IBS symptom severity in children, this relationship was greater in those also showing somatization and pain catastrophizing.

In line with this relationship between mood and symptoms, one study explored the impact of manipulating psychological stress on symptom perception (Wright et al. 2005). Using an experimental design, 42 patients with heartburn and reflux were exposed either to a psychological stressor or a no-stress control condition. They then rated their state anxiety and symptom perception. In addition, objective ratings of reflux symptoms were taken. The results showed that the stressor resulted in increased subjective ratings of symptoms. The stressor, however, did not result in any increase in actual reflux. Therefore the stressor resulted in a greater dissociation between subjective and objective symptoms. This study is important as it not only illustrates the impact of stress on symptom perception but also illustrates that gap between objective and subjective accounts of symptoms. Further, a meta-analytic review of 244 observational studies of irritable bowel syndrome, non-ulcer dyspepsia, fibromyalgia and chronic fatigue syndrome reported a consistent impact of depression and anxiety on symptom perception (Henningsen et al. 2003) with parallel results also being reported for children and adolescents for stomach pain, headache and leg pain (Eminson 2007). Research therefore indicates a link between mood and symptom perception. Brosschot and Van der Doef (2006) explored whether a simple intervention could reduce this association. In their study, 171 teenagers were asked to record their 'worry' and any symptoms. In addition, half were asked to postpone their worry to a special 30-minute 'worry period' each day (the postponers) for six days and the results showed a reduction in their symptoms.

Cognition

An individual's cognitive state may also influence their symptom perception. This is illustrated by the placebo effect with the individual's expectations of recovery, resulting in reduced symptom perception (see Chapter 11). It is also illustrated by Stegen et al.'s (2000) study of breathing symptoms with expectations changing symptom perception. Ruble (1977) carried out a study in which she manipulated women's expectations about when they were due to start menstruating. She gave subjects an 'accurate physiological test' and told women either that their period was due very shortly or that it was at least a week away. The women were then asked to report any premenstrual symptoms. The results showed that believing that they were about to start menstruating (even though they were not) increased the number of reported premenstrual symptoms. This indicates an association between cognitive state and symptom perception. Pennebaker also reported that symptom perception is related to an individual's attentional state and that boredom and the absence of environmental stimuli may result in over-reporting, whereas distraction and attention diversion may lead to under-reporting (Pennebaker 1983). Some research provides support for Pennebaker's theory. For example, in one study, 61 women who had been hospitalized during pre-term labour were randomized to receive either information, distraction or nothing (van Zuuren 1998). The results showed that distraction had the most beneficial effect on measures of both physical and psychological symptoms, suggesting that symptom perception is sensitive to attention.

Some research has also explored which types of distraction are more effective for pain reduction. For example, Hudson et al. (2015) carried out a randomized controlled trial to explore the impact of different forms of distraction on pain during conscious varicose vein surgery. The results showed that talking to the nurse and playing with a stress ball were most effective and more effective than music. In a similar vein, Bascour-Sandoval et al. (2019) explored the impact of sensory modality on effectiveness. They found that while auditory distractors were effective for the reduction of acute pain in adults, they were not effective for healthy children and for adults with chronic pain. Further, visual distractors showed promising results for acute pain in adults and children and tactile and mixed distractors decreased acute pain in adults. Likewise, Gates et al. (2020) concluded from their systematic review and meta-analysis that digital distraction provides modest pain reduction for children undergoing painful procedures.

Social Context

Symptom perception is therefore influenced by mood and cognitions. It is also influenced by an individual's social context. Cross-cultural research consistently shows variation in the presentation of psychiatric symptoms such as anxiety, psychosis and depression. For example, Minsky et al. (2003) explored diagnostic patterns in Latino, African American and European American psychiatric patients and reported that not only did the diagnoses of major depression and schizophrenic disorders vary by ethnic group, but so did symptom presentation, with Latinos reporting a higher frequency of psychotic symptoms than the other groups. Similarly, a consensus statement by the International Consensus Group of Depression and Anxiety (Ballenger et al. 2001) concluded that there was wide cultural variation not only in the diagnosis and responsiveness to treatment for depression and anxiety but also significant variation in symptom presentation. A similar pattern of variation can also be found for somatic symptoms such as headaches, fatigue, constipation and back pain although research in this area is less extensive. For example, epidemiological studies indicate that while headache is a common symptom in the USA and Western Europe, its prevalence remains much lower in China and in African and Asian populations (e.g. Ziegler 1990; Stewart et al. 1996; Wang et al. 1997). Similarly, large surveys of primary care attenders report that those from countries in the Global South and from Latin America tend to report more somatic symptoms in general (Gureje et al. 1997; Piccinelli and Simon 1997). One study explored cataract patients' reports of visual function and the extent to which they were bothered by their cataract, and also explored differences by culture (Alonso et al. 1998). The results showed that, after controlling for clinical and sociodemographic characteristics, patients from Canada and Barcelona reported less trouble with their vision than patients from Denmark or the USA, suggesting cultural variation in the perception of visual symptoms. Symptom perception and diagnosis are therefore highly influenced by the individual's context and cultural background.

Mood, cognition and social context therefore influence symptom perception. These different factors may independently influence how symptoms are perceived, but often they interact together to make symptoms either worse or better. This is illustrated by three conditions: 'medical student disease', medically unexplained symptoms and post-traumatic stress symptoms.

A large component of the medical curriculum involves learning about the symptoms associated with a multitude of different illnesses. More than two-thirds of medical students incorrectly report that at some time they have had the symptoms they are being taught about. This was described by Mechanic (1962) as 'medical student disease'. Perhaps this phenomenon can be understood in terms of the following:

- *Mood:* medical students become quite anxious due to their workload. This anxiety may heighten their awareness of any physiological changes, making them more internally focused.

- *Cognition:* medical students are thinking about symptoms as part of their course, which may result in a focus on their own internal states.

- *Social context:* once one student starts to perceive symptoms, others may model themselves on this behaviour.

Research exploring symptom perception highlights how the severity and impact of symptoms can be changed by a number of factors such as demographics, internal or external focus, mood, cognitions and the individual's social context. This assumes that there is the 'nugget' of a symptom there which is then made worse or better by the way we think about it. It is possible, however, that some symptoms might actually be created without this 'nugget'. From this perspective, not only can the way we think change the severity of any symptom, it might also generate the symptom in the first place. Pennebaker (1982) explored this question and using an experimental design reported that people were more likely to start scratching if they sat next to a confederate who was also scratching. In a similar vein, research indicates that both smiling and yawning can be contagious (Wild et al. 2001; Platek et al. 2005; Schurman et al. 2005). This suggests that seeing a symptom may help to generate that symptom elsewhere. In 2009, Ogden and Zoukas carried out a similar experimental study to explore whether feeling itchy, cold or pain could be created by watching a film. Participants viewed a film showing either headlice in a head of hair (itchy), people swimming in icy water and running in snow (cold) or people sustaining broken limbs as part of football or boxing matches (pain). Participants then rated their symptoms and were observed for symptom-related behaviour (e.g. scratching, shivering, flinching). The results showed that the films did indeed generate their matched symptom (itchiness, cold, pain) on both subjective and objective measures but that cold symptoms were more easily generated than either itchiness or pain.

Symptom perception is therefore not a simple process and is influenced by a number of factors including mood, cognitions and social context. These factors can make symptoms worse or better. They may also be able to create symptoms in the first place.

SOCIAL MESSAGES

Information about illness also comes from other people in the form of a formal diagnosis from a health professional or a positive test result from a routine health check. Such messages may or may not be a consequence of symptom perception. For example, a formal diagnosis may occur after symptoms have been perceived, when the individual has subsequently been motivated to go to the doctor and has been given a diagnosis. However, screening and health checks may detect illness at an asymptomatic stage of development and therefore attendance for such a test may not have been motivated by symptom perception. Information about illness may also come from other lay individuals who are not health professionals. Before (and after) consulting a health professional, people often access their social network, which has been called their 'lay referral system' by Freidson (1970). This can take the form of colleagues, friends or family and involves seeking information and advice from multiple sources. For example, coughing in front of one friend may result in the advice to speak to another friend who had a similar cough, or a suggestion to take a favoured home remedy. Alternatively, it may result in a lay diagnosis or a suggestion to seek professional help from the doctor. In fact, Scambler et al. (1981) reported that three-quarters of those taking part in their study of primary care attenders had sought advice from family or friends before seeking professional help. In contrast, a study of men with symptoms of prostate disease such as dribbling, needing to urinate in the night and urgency showed that their delay in seeking help with their symptoms was related to the absence of any social messages from their friends or family as they were able to hide their symptoms due to a need to live up to traditional images of masculinity (Hale et al. 2007). Therefore, people may get or not get social messages which will influence how they interpret the 'problem' of illness and whether they decide to seek help.

The language used by the doctor is also an important source of information. Some research has explored how such language can influence how a patient feels about their problem. Ogden et al. (2003) explored the relative effect of calling a problem by its lay term (i.e. sore throat/stomach upset) or by its medical term (i.e. tonsillitis/gastroenteritis) and showed that whereas the medical terms made the patient feel that their symptoms were being taken seriously and reported greater confidence in the doctor, the lay terms made the patient feel more ownership of the problem which could be associated with unwanted responsibility and blame. Similarly, Tayler and Ogden (2005) explored the relative effect of describing a problem as either 'heart failure' or the doctors' preferred euphemism for the symptoms that are considered as heart failure – 'fluid on your lungs as your heart is not pumping hard enough'. The results showed that manipulating the name of the problem in this way resulted in significant shifts in people's beliefs about the problem. In particular, the term 'heart failure' resulted in people believing that the problem would have more serious consequences, would be more variable over time, would last for longer and made them feel more anxious and depressed about their problem compared to the euphemism. A recent study also explored the impact of words on patients with Poly Cystic Ovary Syndrome (PCOS). In this retrospective study, Ogden and Bridge (2022) asked patients with PCOS to recall the words used in their original diagnostic consultation and to then rate their current well-being. The results showed that lower communication comfort during the diagnostic consultation and greater use of the word 'raised' predicted poorer current body esteem and poorer quality of life, greater use of the word 'irregular' predicted greater current concerns about fertility and greater focus on appearance predicted greater current concerns about hirsutism. People therefore receive social messages about the nature of their problem which influence how they represent this problem and subsequently how they then behave.

People receive information about their health problem through symptom perception and social messages. This then leads to the formation of a cognitive representation of the problem in the form of illness cognitions and their different dimensions (identity, causes, control, consequences, time line) which have been described in detail above. It also leads to an emotional representation which might take the form of fear, denial, depression or anxiety. Compared to illness cognitions, the emotional response to symptom perception and social messages remains a much-neglected part of the SRM.

5 | STAGE 2: COPING

There is a vast literature on how people cope with a range of problems including stress, pain and illness. Coping with stress and pain is covered in Chapters 10 and 11. This section will examine three approaches to coping with illness: (1) coping with the crisis of illness; (2) adjustment to physical illness and the theory of cognitive adaptation; (3) benefit-finding and post-traumatic growth. These different theoretical approaches have implications for understanding the differences between adaptive and maladaptive coping, and the role of reality and illusions in the coping process. They therefore have different implications for understanding the outcome of the coping process (see Figure 8.4).

1. COPING WITH THE CRISIS OF ILLNESS

Being diagnosed with a physical illness has been understood within the framework of crisis theory and the need to return to a state of equilibrium (Moos and Schaefer 1984).

What Is Crisis Theory?

Crisis theory has been generally used to examine how people cope with major life crises and transitions and has traditionally provided a framework for understanding the impact of illness or injury. The theory was developed from work done on grief and mourning and a model of developmental crises at transition points in the life cycle. In general, crisis theory examines the impact of any form of disruption on an individual's established personal and social identity. It suggests that psychological systems

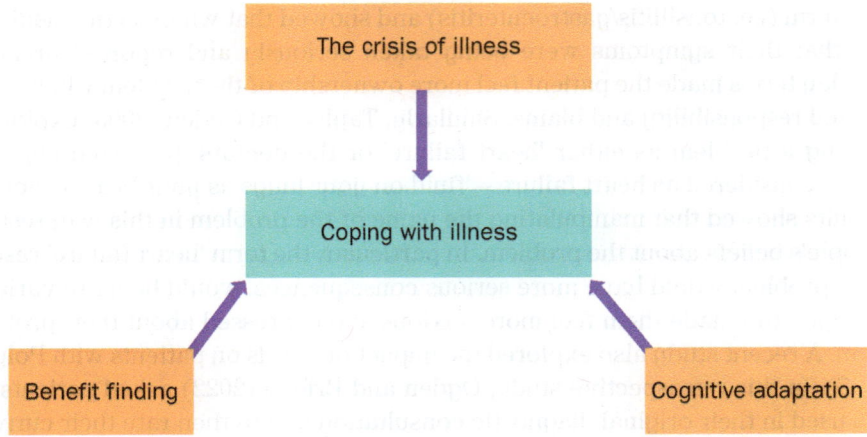

Figure 8.4 Coping with illness

are driven towards maintaining homeostasis and equilibrium in the same way as physical systems. Within this framework, any crisis is self-limiting as the individual will find a way of returning to a stable state; individuals are therefore regarded as self-regulators.

Physical Illness as a Crisis

Moos and Schaefer (1984) argued that physical illness can be considered a crisis as it represents a turning point in an individual's life. They suggest that physical illness causes the following changes, which can be conceptualized as a crisis:

- *Changes in identity:* illness can create a shift in identity, such as from carer to patient, or from breadwinner to person with an illness.
- *Changes in location:* illness may result in a move to a new environment such as becoming bed-ridden or hospitalized.
- *Changes in role:* a change from independent adult to passive dependent may occur following illness, resulting in a changed role.
- *Changes in social support:* illness may produce isolation from friends and family, effecting changes in social support.
- *Changes in the future:* a future involving children, career or travel can become uncertain.

In addition, the crisis nature of illness may be exacerbated by factors that are often specific to illness such as:

- *Illness is often unpredicted:* if an illness is not expected then the individual will not have had the opportunity to consider possible coping strategies.
- *Information about the illness is unclear:* much of the information about illness is ambiguous and unclear, particularly in terms of causality and outcome.
- *A decision is needed quickly:* illness frequently requires decisions about action to be made quickly (e.g. should we operate? Should we take medicines? Should we take time off from work? Should we tell our friends?).
- *Ambiguous meaning:* because of uncertainties about causality and outcome, the meaning of the illness for an individual will often be ambiguous (e.g. is it serious? How long will it affect me?).
- *Limited prior experience:* most individuals are healthy most of the time. Therefore illness is infrequent and may occur to individuals with limited prior experience. This lack of experience has implications for the development of coping strategies and efficacy based on other similar situations (e.g. I've never had cancer before, what should I do next?).

Many other crises may be easier to predict, have clearer meanings and occur to individuals with a greater degree of relevant previous experience. Within this framework, Moos and Schaefer considered illness a particular kind of crisis, and applied crisis theory to illness in an attempt to examine how individuals cope with this crisis.

The Coping Process

Once confronted with the crisis of physical illness, Moos and Schaefer (1984) described three processes that constitute the coping process: (1) cognitive appraisal; (2) adaptive tasks; and (3) coping skills. These processes are illustrated in Figure 8.5.

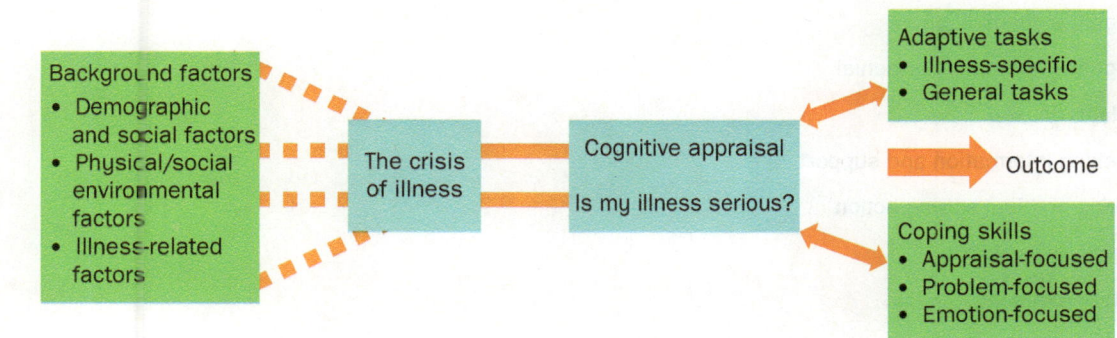

Figure 8.5 Coping with the crisis of illness

Process 1: Cognitive Appraisal

At the stage of disequilibrium triggered by the illness, an individual initially appraises the seriousness and significance of the illness (e.g. Is my cancer serious? How will my cancer influence my life in the long run?). Factors such as knowledge, previous experience and social support may influence this appraisal process. In addition, it is possible to integrate Leventhal's illness cognitions at this stage in the coping process because such illness beliefs are related to how an illness will be appraised.

Process 2: Adaptive Tasks

Following cognitive appraisal, Moos and Schaefer describe seven adaptive tasks that are used as part of the coping process. These can be divided into three illness-specific tasks and four general tasks and are illustrated in Table 8.1.

TABLE 8.1 Adaptive tasks

Illness-related tasks
• Dealing with pain and other symptoms
• Dealing with the hospital environment and treatment procedures
• Developing and maintaining relationships with health professionals
General tasks
• Preserving an emotional balance
• Preserving self-image, competence and mastery
• Sustaining relationships with family and friends
• Preparing for an uncertain future

Process 3: Coping Skills

Following both appraisal and the use of adaptive tasks, Moos and Schaefer described a series of coping skills that are accessed to deal with the crisis of physical illness. These coping skills can be categorized into three forms: (1) appraisal-focused coping; (2) problem-focused coping; and (3) emotion-focused coping (see Table 8.2).

TABLE 8.2 Coping tasks

Appraisal-focused
• Logical analysis and mental preparation
• Cognitive redefinition
• Cognitive avoidance or denial
Problem-focused
• Seeking information and support
• Taking problem-solving action
• Identifying rewards
Emotion-focused
• Affective regulation
• Emotional discharge
• Resigned acceptance

Therefore, according to this theory of coping with the crisis of a physical illness, individuals appraise the illness and then use a variety of adaptive tasks and coping skills which in turn determine the outcome.

Evidence for Coping with the Crisis of Illness

Much research has used the notion of crisis theory and coping with the crisis of illness to explore, predict and change how people respond to illness. In particular, research has explored the relative impact of different types of coping on a range of psychological outcomes following illness. For example, research exploring coping with rheumatoid arthritis suggests that active and problem-solving coping are associated with better outcomes whereas passive avoidant coping is associated with poorer outcomes (Manne and Zautra 1992; Newman et al. 1996). For patients with chronic obstructive pulmonary disease (COPD), wishful thinking and emotion-focused coping were least effective (Buchi et al. 1997). Similarly, research exploring stress and psoriasis shows that avoidant coping is least useful (e.g. Leary et al. 1998). Further, for women at risk of ovarian cancer, problem-focused coping predicted higher distress over time (in those with high levels of perceived control) and poorer attendance at screening appointments (Fang et al. 2006). Pollard and Kennedy (2007) explored changes in coping strategies, depression and anxiety following traumatic spinal cord injury and reported that all three variables were fairly stable over a 10-year period. In addition, the results indicated that although two-thirds of patients showed no signs or symptoms of depression, the level of depression at year 10 was predicted by more adaptive coping strategies at week 12 post-injury. A parallel link between adaptive coping and psychological morbidity was also found in a similar study but with a much larger sample across six European countries (n = 237) with a one-year follow up (Kennedy et al. 2010). Further, from a systematic review of coping in IBS, David et al. (2021) concluded that emotion-focused coping was associated with worse psychological outcomes, that problem-focused coping was not always associated with better psychological outcomes and that catastrophizing was negatively associated with health-related quality of life. Overall, reviews of the impact of coping indicate that poorer health outcomes tend to be predicted by avoidant coping strategies and ones which involve inhibiting emotional expression (de Ridder et al. 2008), although venting emotions per se does not always seem to be most effective either. Further a review by Finkelstein-Fox and Park (2019) concluded that while problem-focused coping may lead to better outcomes in patients with chronic illness compared to emotion-focused coping, this is only the case in situations that are appraised as controllable. Therefore trying to problem solve in an uncontrollable situation may lead to worse outcomes, suggesting that patients should use a range of coping strategies across the different components of their illness (e.g., medication management, pain symptoms, worries about the future) rather than consistently using the same approach.

In line with this, some research has also attempted to change the way people cope through coping skills training which aims to help them adjust to their illness, particularly through improving self-efficacy and encouraging individuals to prioritize coping resources towards those aspects of the illness which are most controllable and amenable to change. This approach has been used for a range of illnesses including HIV (Antoni et al. 2000, 2006), arthritis (Carson et al. 2006), diabetes (Grey et al. 2000) and sickle cell disease in children (Gil et al. 2001).

Implications for the Outcome of the Coping Process

Within this model, individuals attempt to deal with the crisis of physical illness via the stages of appraisal, the use of adaptive tasks and the employment of coping skills. The types of tasks and skills used may determine the outcome and such an outcome may be psychological adjustment or may be related to longevity or quality of life (see Chapter 10 for a discussion of coping and stress outcomes). According to crisis theory, individuals are motivated to re-establish a state of equilibrium and normality. This desire can be satisfied by either short-term or long-term solutions. Crisis theory differentiates between two types of new equilibrium: *healthy adaptation,* which can result in maturation, and a *maladaptive response* resulting in deterioration. In this perspective, healthy adaptation involves reality orientation, adaptive tasks and constructive coping skills. Therefore, according to this model of coping, the desired outcome of the coping process is reality orientation.

2. ADJUSTMENT TO PHYSICAL ILLNESS AND THE THEORY OF COGNITIVE ADAPTATION

In an alternative model of coping, Taylor and colleagues (e.g. Taylor 1983; Taylor et al. 1984) examined ways in which individuals adjust to threatening events. Based on a series of interviews with rape victims and cardiac and cancer patients, they suggested that coping with threatening events (including illness) consists of three processes: (1) a search for meaning; (2) a search for mastery; and (3) a process of self-enhancement. They argued that these three processes are central to developing and maintaining illusions and that these illusions constitute a process of cognitive adaptation. Again, this model describes the individual as self-regulatory and as motivated to maintain the status quo. In addition, many of the model's components parallel those described earlier in terms of illness cognitions (e.g. the dimensions of cause and consequence). This theoretical perspective will be described in the context of their results from women who had recently had breast cancer (Taylor et al. 1984) and is shown in Figure 8.6.

A Search for Meaning

A search for meaning is reflected in questions such as 'Why did it happen?', 'What impact has it had?' and 'What does my life mean now?' A search for meaning can be understood in terms of a search for causality and a search to understand the implications. Attribution theory suggests that individuals need to understand, predict and control their environment (e.g. Weiner 1986). Taylor et al. (1984) reported

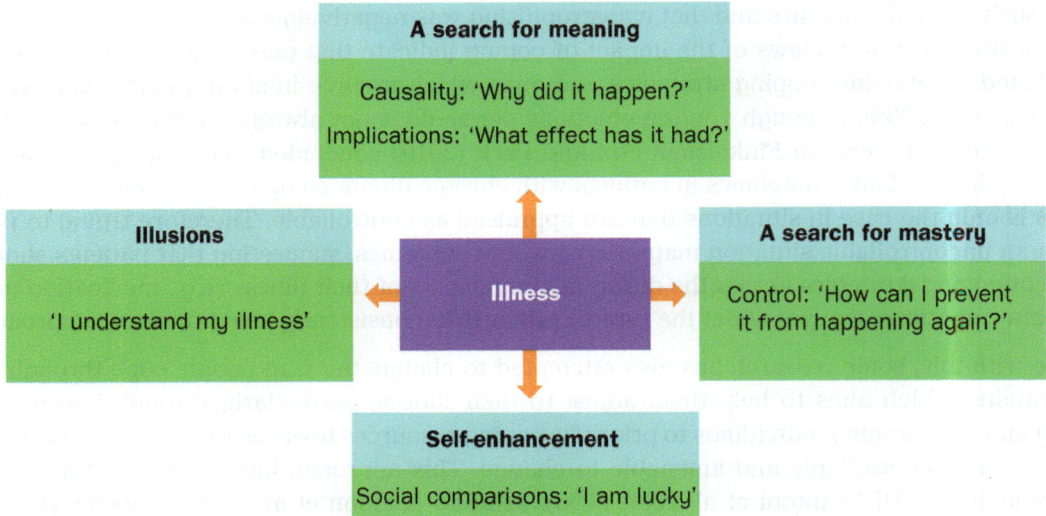

Figure 8.6 Cognitive adaptation theory
SOURCE: Adapted from Taylor et al. (1984)

that 95 per cent of the women they interviewed offered an explanation of the cause of their breast cancer. For example, 41 per cent explained their cancer in terms of stress, 32 per cent held carcinogens such as the birth control pill, chemical dumps or nuclear waste as responsible, 26 per cent saw hereditary factors as the cause, 17 per cent blamed diet and 10 per cent considered a blow to the breast to blame. Several women reported multiple causes. Taylor (1983) suggested that no one perception of cause is better than any other, but that what is important for the process of cognitive adaptation is the search for any cause. People need to ask, 'Why did it happen?' Taylor (1983) also argued that it is important for the women to understand the implications of the cancer for their life now. Accordingly, over 50 per cent of the women stated that the cancer had resulted in them reappraising their life, and others mentioned improved self-knowledge, self-change and a process of reprioritization.

A Search for Mastery

A search for mastery is reflected in questions such as 'How can I prevent a similar event reoccurring?' and 'What can I do to manage the event now?' Taylor et al. (1984) reported that a sense of mastery can be achieved by believing that the illness is controllable. In accordance with this, 66 per cent of the women in the study believed that they could influence the course or reoccurrence of the cancer. The remainder of the women believed that the cancer could be controlled by health professionals. Taylor reported that a sense of mastery is achieved either through psychological techniques such as developing a positive attitude, meditation, self-hypnosis or a type of causal attribution, or by behavioural techniques such as changing diet, changing medications, accessing information or controlling any side-effects. These processes contribute towards a state of mastery, which is central to the progression towards a state of cognitive adaptation.

The Process of Self-Enhancement

Following illness, some individuals may suffer a decrease in their self-esteem. The theory of cognitive adaptation suggests that individuals attempt to build their self-esteem through a process of self-enhancement. Taylor et al. (1984) reported that only 17 per cent of the women in their study reported only negative changes following their illness, whereas 53 per cent reported only positive changes.

To explain this result, Taylor developed social comparison theory (Festinger 1957). This theory suggests that individuals make sense of their world by comparing themselves with others. Such comparisons may either be downward comparisons (e.g. a comparison with others who are worse off: 'At least I've only had cancer once'), or upward comparisons (e.g. a comparison with others who are better off: 'Why was my lump malignant when hers was only a cyst?'). In terms of their study of women with breast cancer, Taylor et al. (1984) reported that, although many of the women had undergone disfiguring surgery and had been diagnosed as having a life-threatening illness, most of them showed downward comparisons in order to improve their self-esteem. For example, women who had had a lumpectomy compared themselves with women who had had a mastectomy. Those who had had a mastectomy compared themselves with those who had a possibility of having generalized cancer. Older women compared themselves favourably with younger women, and younger women compared themselves favourably with older women. Taylor suggested that the women selected criteria for comparison that would enable them to improve their self-esteem as part of the process of self-enhancement. The role of social comparisons in coping is further discussed in terms of the response shift in Chapter 14.

The Role of Illusions

The search for meaning and mastery and the improvement of self-esteem involves developing illusions. Such illusions are not necessarily in contradiction to reality but are positive interpretations of that reality. For example, although there may be little evidence for the real causes of cancer, or for the ability of individuals to control the course of their illness, those who have suffered cancer wish to hold their own illusions about these factors (e.g. 'I understand what caused my cancer and believe that I can control whether it comes back'). Taylor and her colleagues argued that these illusions are a necessary and essential component of cognitive adaptation and that reality orientation (as suggested by other coping models) may actually be detrimental to adjustment.

The need for illusions raises the problem of disconfirmation of the illusions (what happens when the reoccurrence of cancer cannot be controlled?). Taylor argued that the need for illusions is sufficient to enable individuals to shift the goals and foci of their illusions so that those illusions can be maintained and adjustment can persist. The notion of illusions is similar to benefit-finding which is discussed later in this chapter.

Evidence for Cognitive Adaptation Theory

Research has used a cognitive adaptation theory approach to explore, predict and change the ways in which people cope with illness. For example, research indicates that forms of cognitive adjustment are linked to illness progression in people with HIV/AIDS (Reed et al. 1994, 1999; Bower et al. 1998), that cognitive adaptation influences how people manage cancer (Taylor 1983) and that it reflects the ways in which women respond to having a termination (Goodwin and Ogden 2007). In 2013, Christianson et al. explored the role of sense making in adjustment in 80 late stage cancer patients and concluded that greater meaning predicted greater quality of life. Likewise, Czajkowska et al. (2013) used the cognitive adaptation index scale with 57 patients with non-melanoma skin cancer and reported that adaptation predicted 60 per cent of the variance in patient distress.

Implications for the Outcome of the Coping Process

According to this model of coping, the individual copes with illness by achieving cognitive adaptation. This involves searching for meaning ('I know what caused my illness'), mastery ('I can control my illness') and developing self-esteem ('I am better off than a lot of people'). These beliefs may not be accurate but they are essential to maintaining illusions that promote adjustment to the illness. Therefore, in this perspective the desired outcome of the coping process is the development of illusions, not reality orientation.

3. POST-TRAUMATIC GROWTH AND BENEFIT-FINDING

Most theories of coping emphasize a desire to re-establish equilibrium and a return to the status quo. Effective coping is therefore seen as that which enables adjustment to the illness and a return to normality. Some research, however, indicates that some people perceive benefits from being ill and see themselves as being better off because they have been ill. For example, Laerum et al. (1988) interviewed 84 men who had had a heart attack and found that although the men reported some negative consequences for their lifestyle and quality of life, 33 per cent of them considered their life to be somewhat or considerably improved. Similarly, Collins et al. (1990) interviewed 55 cancer patients and also reported some positive shifts following illness. Sodergren and colleagues have explored positivity following illness and have developed a structured questionnaire called the Silver Lining Questionnaire (SLQ) (Sodergren et al. 2002). They concluded from their studies that the positive consequences of illness are varied and more common than often realized. They also suggest that positivity can be improved by rehabilitation. Such research has been framed within a number of different theoretical perspectives and has been given a range of names resulting from extensive debates about the nature of the construct. For example, research has focused on stress-related growth (Park 2004), benefit-finding (Tennen and Affleck 1999), meaning-making (Park and Folkman 1997), growth-orientated functioning and crisis growth (Holahan et al. 1996), and existential growth (Janoff-Bulham 2004). Tedeschi and Calhoun (2004) developed a self-regulatory model of post-traumatic growth in an attempt to draw together the existing literature on trauma and coping and described the role of factors including personality, optimism, social support and meaning-making.

Evidence for Post-Traumatic Growth and Benefit-Finding

The positive consequences of traumatic events have been explored in terms of the experience of positive growth, the correlates of positive growth, the predictors of positive growth and the role of positive growth in predicting patient outcomes. This will now be described.

The Experience of Positive Growth

Research has explored the ways in which individuals make sense of trauma and their experiences of growth or thriving. In particular, Tedeschi and Calhoun have carried out much work in this area and their synthesis of the literature concluded that post-traumatic growth was a more progressed form of positive adjustment than either just resilience or optimism, and involved a process of transformation. Further, they highlighted five main areas of growth which were: perceived changes in self; closer family relationships; changed philosophy in life; a better perspective in life; and a strengthened belief system (Tedeschi and Calhoun 2004, 2006). Recently, Hefferon et al. (2009) carried out a systematic review of the qualitative research and argued that traumas could be conceptualized as either external (e.g. natural disasters, bereavement, war) or internal (e.g. physical illness or injury), and that different types of trauma may result in different experiences. For their review they identified 57 qualitative papers which assessed the experience of physical illness and highlighted four key themes across the different studies. These were: reappraisal of life and priorities; trauma equals development of self; existential re-evaluation; and new awareness of the body. In addition, they concluded that the latter theme, in particular, was unique to internal rather than external trauma and that although there existed common elements to positive growth across traumas, there were also differences.

The Correlates of Positive Growth

Some research indicates a strong overlap between post-traumatic growth and other aspects of sense making and coping. For example, a systematic review and meta-analysis by Shand et al. (2015) on 48 studies found that PTG was associated with decreases in distress and depression and increases in social support, optimism, positive reappraisal, spirituality and religious coping. Some research has also explored the association between post-traumatic growth and illness cognitions. For example,

Lau et al. (2017) conducted a study on a sample of 225 newly diagnosed HIV-positive men who have sex with men (MSM) and found illness cognitions relating to coherence, treatment control, personal control, and attribution to carelessness were positively associated with PTG while illness cognitions relating to timeline, consequence, identity, attribution to God's punishment/will and attribution to chance/luck were negatively associated with PTG.

Predicting Post-Traumatic Growth

Research has also explored the role of different factors in predicting positive growth after trauma. For example, Tedeschi and Calhoun (2004) argued that the degree of post-traumatic growth relates to symptom severity, time elapsed since the event, age, gender, social support and a clear cause to the event. Similarly, McMillen (2004) emphasized the role of available support for recovery and Harvey et al. (2004) highlighted the positive and negative responses of others. Furthermore, when evaluating post-traumatic growth following cancer diagnosis, Cole et al. (2008) emphasized the role of spirituality and Cordova et al. (2001) reported that growth after breast cancer was related to talking about and assigning meaning to the experience as well as financial stability. Further, Dunn et al. (2011) reported that benefit-finding after cancer was associated with being a woman, greater optimism, high intrusive thinking and high social support. Likewise, Zsigmond et al. (2019) concluded that over 97 per cent of the patients with breast cancer in their study experienced post-traumatic growth 3 years post diagnosis and that PTG was predicted by psychological immune competence after treatment, emotional severity of post-traumatic stress symptoms and social support. From a review of 281 studies, Henson et al. (2021) concluded that PTG was predicted by a wide range of factors including sharing negative emotions, cognitive processing or rumination, positive reappraisal, agreeableness and resilience. Research has also addressed growth following non-illness-related trauma. For example, McMillen et al. (1997) explored growth following a mass killing, surviving a tornado and a plane crash and reported that growth was predicted by being able to find benefit in the event and a stronger fear of death during the event.

The Role of Post-Traumatic Growth and Health Outcomes

Other studies have explored the role of post-traumatic growth in predicting patient outcomes. For example, Milam (2006) concluded that post-traumatic growth following a diagnosis of HIV was protective against certain physical illnesses and Reed et al. (1994) reported how 'realistic acceptance' of their HIV diagnosis illustrated by statements such as 'I tried to accept what has happened' and 'I prepare for the worst' was related to a higher chance of death at follow-up.

Implications for the Outcome of the Coping Process

Most models of coping emphasize a return to the status quo and the re-establishment of an equilibrium to back to where the individual was at the start of the process. In contrast, a post-traumatic growth or benefit-finding perspective illustrates how at times the individual ends up in a better place than they were before whatever traumatic event happened. The event, whether it might be an illness or a life event such as a divorce or a serious accident, is coped with in such a way that the individual is able to find the positives in the event and incorporate these into a more fruitful future.

IN SUMMARY

Coping research therefore explores the ways in which individuals manage and respond to any change in their lives. Health psychology draws upon coping with the crisis of illness and cognitive adaptation theories which emphasize how people are motivated to return to a state of normality. In contrast, research on post-traumatic growth and benefit-finding highlights how an illness may have positive consequences for the individual, and this is in line with recent developments within the positive psychology movement. This final approach is also similar to some work on sustained changes in behaviour following life events or 'epiphanies', which is described in Chapter 7.

6   PREDICTING AND CHANGING HEALTH OUTCOMES

The self-regulatory model describes a transition from interpretation, through illness cognitions, emotional response and coping to appraisal. Early research used the model to ask the question: 'How do illness cognitions relate to coping?' More recent research, however, has also explored the impact of illness cognitions on psychological and physical health outcomes with a focus on adherence to treatment and recovery from illnesses including stroke, rheumatoid arthritis and myocardial infarction (MI – heart attack).

HOW DO ILLNESS COGNITIONS RELATE TO COPING?

Much correlational research has explored the links between the different components of the SRM with a focus on the associations between illness cognitions and coping across a number of different health problems. For example, Kemp et al. (1999) reported a link between perception of control over illness and problem-focused coping in patients with neuroepilepsy and Lawson et al. (2007) concluded that more positive personal models (i.e. greater control, shorter time line, less consequences) were associated with more effective coping strategies in people with Type 1 diabetes. Likewise, Hill and Frost (2020) reported a correlation between illness cognitions and coping with Lyme's disease and Rocholl et al. (2021) reported a link between illness cognitions and coping in patients with Eczema. Searle et al. (2007) argued that rather than just focusing on coping cognitions, research should also address coping behaviours in terms of what people actually *do* (e.g. taking medication, diet, physical activity). They then explored associations between illness cognitions, coping cognitions and coping behaviours in patients with Type 2 diabetes. The results showed that illness cognitions predicted both aspects of coping. In addition the results showed that the link between illness cognitions and coping behaviours was direct and not mediated through coping cognitions. They argue that if we want to change people's behaviour (i.e. taking medication, diet, physical activity), it might be better to try and change their illness cognitions rather than their coping cognitions. Recent meta-analyses of the links between illness cognitions and coping indicate that in general a strong illness identity is associated with the use of avoidant coping strategies and those involving emotional expression, that perceived controllability of an illness is related to cognitive reappraisal, expressing emotions and problem-focused coping strategies and that avoidant and expressing emotion coping strategies are also correlated with perceptions of a chronic time line, serious consequences and ratings of a multitude of symptoms (Hagger and Orbell 2003; French et al. 2006a).

PREDICTING ADHERENCE TO TREATMENT

Beliefs about illness in terms of the dimensions described by Leventhal et al. (1980, 1997) have been shown to relate to coping. They have also been associated with whether or not a person takes their medication and/or adheres to suggested treatments. Some research shows that symptom perception is directly linked to adherence to medication. For example, Halm et al. (2006) explored asthmatics' beliefs about their problem, their perception of symptoms and their adherence to medication. The study involved 198 adults who had been hospitalized for their asthma over a 12-month period and identified a 'no symptoms, no asthma' belief, whereby people only believed they had asthma when they had symptoms, rather than seeing it as a chronic illness that is ongoing regardless of the level of symptomatology. Further, the results showed that those who held the 'acute asthma belief' were also less likely to take their medication. In a similar vein, Brewer et al. (2002) examined the relationship between illness cognitions and both adherence to medication and cholesterol control in patients with hypercholesterolaemia (involving very high cholesterol). The results showed that a belief that the illness has serious consequences was related to medication adherence. In addition, actual cholesterol control was related to the belief that the illness was stable, asymptomatic with serious consequences.

Some research has also included a role for treatment beliefs. For example, Horne and Weinman (2002) explored the links between beliefs about both illness and treatment and adherence to taking medication for asthma in 100 community-based patients. The results showed that non-adherers reported more doubts about the necessity of their medication, greater concerns about the consequences of the medication and more negative beliefs about the consequences of their illness. Overall, the analysis indicated that illness and treatment beliefs were better predictors of adherence than both clinical and demographic factors. In a similar study, Llewellyn et al. (2003) explored the interrelationships between illness beliefs, treatment beliefs and adherence to home treatment in patients with severe haemophilia. The results showed that poor adherence was related to beliefs about the necessity of the treatment, concerns about the consequences of treatment and beliefs about illness identity. Some research has also explored adherence in a broader sense. In 2016, Aujla et al. carried a systematic review and meta-analysis of 52 studies investigating the role of illness cognitions in predicting adherence to self-management behaviours. The results showed that cognitions relating to identity, timeline acute – chronic, consequences, personal control, treatment control, cure control and illness coherence all significantly prospectively predicted adherence, however the effect sizes were all very small. Likewise, Jones et al. (2016) conducted a systematic review of nine studies using the SRM to design interventions to improve adherence. The results showed that six studies reported improvements in adherence behaviours and that cure/control cognitions were particularly found to improve adherence.

PREDICTING ILLNESS OUTCOMES

Research has also used the SRM to understand and predict illness outcomes for a range of conditions including rheumatoid arthritis (Carlisle et al. 2005), diabetes (Lawson et al. 2007; Knowles et al. 2021), asthma (Achstetter et al. 2019), chronic fatigue syndrome (Deary 2008) and renal disease (Karamanidou et al. 2008). In 2015, Dempster et al. conducted a meta-analysis of illness cognitions and physical health conditions and found that across a range of illnesses, beliefs about the consequences of illness and emotional representations were consistently most associated with outcomes such as depression, anxiety and quality of life. Research has particularly explored the role of illness cognitions in predicting recovery from stroke and myocardial infarction (MI), which will now be described.

Recovery from Stroke

Partridge and Johnston (1989) used a prospective study and reported that individuals' beliefs about their perceived control over their problem predicted recovery from residual disability in stroke patients at follow-up. The results showed that this relationship persisted even when baseline levels of disability were taken into account. Van Mierlo et al. (2015) focused on life satisfaction post stroke and found that acceptance, helplessness and perceiving benefits were significantly associated with life satisfaction at both two months and two years post stroke. Further, they found that illness cognitions two months post stroke and changes in illness cognitions predicted life satisfaction two years post stroke. In line with this, Johnston et al. (2006) specifically explored the relationship between perceived control and recovery from stroke and followed up 71 stroke patients one and six months after discharge from hospital. In addition, they examined the possible mediating effects of coping, exercise and mood. They asked the questions, 'Does recovery from stroke relate to illness cognitions?' and 'If so, is this relationship dependent upon other factors?' The results showed no support for the mediating effects of coping, exercise and mood but supported earlier work to indicate a predictive relationship between control beliefs and recovery. This was also supported by a further study which explored the role of a range of clinical, demographic and psychological factors to predict functional recovery three years following a stroke. The results showed that perceptions of control at baseline added to the variance accounted for by both clinical and demographic variables (Johnston et al. 2004). To further assess the factors that may relate to recovery from stroke, Johnston et al. (2006) developed a workbook-based intervention which was designed to change cognitions about control in patients who had just had a stroke. In particular, the intervention focused on coping skills, encouraged self-management and offered encouragement. The results showed that at six months' follow-up, those receiving the intervention showed better disability recovery than those in the control group. However, it was unclear how the intervention had worked as the intervention group showed no significant changes in any psychological process variables apart from confidence in recovery, which did not itself relate to actual disability recovery. Research therefore indicates that control cognitions may relate to recovery from stroke. Further, an intervention to change such cognitions seems to improve recovery. It is not clear, however, which processes are involved in this change as the intervention did not actually change stroke patients' beliefs about control.

Recovery from MI

Research suggests that an individual's beliefs about their work capacity (Maeland and Havik 1987), helplessness towards future MIs (called 'cardiac invalidism') (Riegel 1993) and general psychological factors (Diederiks et al. 1991) relate to recovery from MI as measured by return to work and general social and occupational functioning. Using a self-regulatory approach, research has indicated that illness cognitions relate to recovery from MI. For example, the Heart Attack Recovery Project, which was carried out in New Zealand, followed 143 first-time heart attack patients aged 65 or under at 3, 6 and 12 months following admission to hospital. The results showed that those patients who believed that their illness had less serious consequences and would last a shorter time at baseline were more likely to have returned to work by six weeks. Furthermore, those with beliefs that the illness could be controlled or cured at baseline predicted attendance at rehabilitation classes (Petrie et al. 1996). Furthermore, those patients aged 73–98 who attribute their MI or stroke to old age are less likely to show lifestyle behaviour change and more likely to be hospitalized and show increased visits to the doctor up to three years later (Stewart et al. 2016).

One study not only explored the patients' beliefs about MI but also the beliefs of their spouse to discover whether congruence between spouse and patient beliefs was related to recovery from MI (Figueiras and Weinman 2003). Seventy couples in which the man had had an MI completed a baseline measure of the illness cognitions which were correlated with follow-up measures of recovery at 3, 6 and 12 months. The results showed that in couples who had similar positive beliefs about the identity and consequences of the illness, the patients showed improved recovery in terms of better psychological and physical functioning, better sexual functioning and lower impact of the MI on social and recreational activities. In addition, similar beliefs about time line were related to lower levels of disability and similar cure/control beliefs were associated with greater dietary changes. In a novel approach to assessing patients' beliefs about their MI, Broadbent et al. (2004) asked 69 patients who had just had an MI to draw their heart and how they felt it looked just after their heart attack. They also completed a series of questionnaires and repeated these drawings and measures at three and six months. The results showed that increases in the size of heart between baseline and three months were related to slower return to work, activity restriction and anxiety about having another MI as measured by a range of factors. The authors concluded that the increased size of the heart in the drawings may reflect the 'extent to which their heart condition plays on their mind'.

One study also explored the prevalence of PTSD in 44 patients who had either had an MI or a subarachnoid haemorrhage and examined the association with illness cognitions (Sheldrick et al. 2006). The results showed that the prevalence of PTSD was 16 per cent at two weeks, 35 per cent at six weeks and 16 per cent at three months after the medical event. The results also showed that beliefs relating to identity, time line, consequences and emotional representation were strongly correlated with PTSD symptoms at all time points. Further, the results indicated that baseline illness cognitions predicted PTSD at follow-up.

THE CENTRAL ROLE OF COHERENCE

Central to much research on illness beliefs and their relationship to outcome is the importance of a coherent model whereby beliefs about causes of the illness are consistent with beliefs about treatment (Leventhal et al. 1997). Leventhal and colleagues describe this association between causes and solutions in terms of the 'if. . . then rules'. For example, *if* I believe that breathlessness is caused by smoking, *then* I am more likely to decide to stop smoking. Similarly, *if* I believe that asthma symptoms are caused by bronchial constriction, *then* I am more likely to adhere to my medication that causes bronchial dilation. In contrast, an obese person who believes that their weight is caused by hormones rather than their diet is unlikely to eat less when advised to do so. Most research addressing the issue of coherence has focused on cross-sectional associations between the different sets of beliefs. For example, Horne and Weinman (2002) reported that adherence is more likely to occur when illness beliefs and treatment beliefs are coherent with each other. Similarly, Llewellyn et al. (2003) reported that adherence to medication for patients with haemophilia was also greater when beliefs about illness and treatment were matched. Some studies, however, have also explored whether or not beliefs can be changed to be more in line with each other. For example, although smoking increases the risk of cervical cancer, many women are not aware of this association. Therefore being told to stop smoking when having a cervical smear test makes no sense and women are therefore unlikely to take this advice on board – they do not have a coherent model of smoking as a cause of cervical cancer, and smoking cessation as a solution. In line with this, Hall et al. (2004) examined whether giving people a leaflet containing information about the link between smoking and cervical cancer, which provided them with a coherent model of this association, could change intentions to quit smoking. The results showed that the leaflet did increase women's coherent model of the association. Further, the results showed that perceptions of vulnerability to cervical cancer were associated with intentions to quit smoking but only in those with a coherent model.

Ogden and Sidhu (2006) also explored the notion of coherence in the context of taking medication for obesity. Many people with obesity deem their hormones or genetics to be responsible for their condition. They do not blame their diet and therefore do not change their diet. An obesity drug called orlistat can result in weight loss but also produces highly visual side-effects if taken with fatty foods, such as anal leakage and oily stools. Ogden and Sidhu explored the psychological mechanisms of the drug through interviews with patients and concluded that it can result in both adherence and behaviour change if the side-effects act as an education and bring people's beliefs about the causes of their obesity in line with a behavioural solution (see Chapter 13 for further details). People therefore see the side-effects after they have eaten fatty foods, realize the importance of their diet to their body weight and decide it is therefore worthwhile changing their diet.

Both these studies illustrate the importance of coherence and the benefits of changing beliefs. In contrast, Wright et al. (2003) explored the impact of informing smokers about their genetic pre-disposition towards nicotine dependence in terms of their choice of method for stopping smoking. In line with the studies described earlier, giving information did change beliefs. However, while those who believed that they were genetically prone to dependency were more likely to choose a medical form of cessation (a drug to reduce cravings), they were also likely to endorse relying upon their own willpower. Changing beliefs towards a more medical cause meant that smokers were less able to change their behaviour on their own and more in need of medical support. These results illustrate the importance of a coherent model, but they also illustrate that changing beliefs may not always be beneficial to subsequent changes in behaviour.

INTERVENTIONS TO CHANGE ILLNESS COGNITIONS

Research shows that people make sense of their illness and form illness cognitions which relate to their health outcomes. In line with this, interventions have been developed in an attempt to change illness cognitions and improve subsequent outcomes. Some interventions have used face-to-face consultations with a psychologist, while others, in line with the saying 'a picture paints a thousand words', have used visual information. (For a review of using the SRM for interventions see Wearden and Peters 2008 and related papers.)

Face-to-Face Consultations

Petrie et al. (2002) developed a three-session intervention for patients who had had an MI to change their beliefs about their condition and their health outcomes, which was evaluated using a randomized control trial. Session 1 focused on the nature of an MI in terms of its symptoms and explored patients' beliefs about the causes of the MI. Session 2 explored beliefs about causes, helped the patient to develop a plan to minimize the future risk of a further MI and tried to increase patient control beliefs about their condition. In the final session, concerns about medication were explored and symptoms that were part of the recovery process, such as breathlessness upon exercise, were distinguished from those that were indicative of further pathology such as severe chest pain. The results showed that patients who received the intervention reported more positive views about their MI at follow-up in terms of beliefs about consequences, time line, control/cure and symptom distress. In addition, they reported that they were better prepared to leave hospital, returned to work at a faster rate and reported a lower rate of angina symptoms. No differences were found in rehabilitation attendance. The intervention therefore seemed to change cognitions and improve patients' functional outcome after MI. Broadbent et al. (2009) repeated this intervention and expanded it to include partners of those who had had an MI. The results showed changes in the partners' beliefs and reflect research indicating the importance of social support and concordance between the patient and their partner in health outcomes (e.g. Figueiras and Weinman 2003).

Moss-Morris et al. (2007) also carried out an intervention to change the illness beliefs of patients with chronic pain as part of a cognitive behavioural pain management programme. The results showed that patients reduced both their perceptions of consequences and their emotional representations of their pain and increased their sense of coherence of their condition. In addition, improved physical functioning was predicted by reduced beliefs about consequences and improved mental functioning was predicted by greater coherence and reduced emotional representations.

A complex intervention has also been developed to change the illness cognitions and health outcomes of those with diabetes (Skinner et al. 2006; Davies et al. 2009). The trial was known as DESMOND (diabetes education and self-management for ongoing and newly-diagnosed) and used a group-based intervention to elicit patients' beliefs about their condition and help them to develop feasible self-management plans. The results showed that after a year patients who had received the intervention endorsed more serious consequences, a longer time line and greater personal control beliefs for their condition. They also showed improved levels of smoking cessation and weight loss than those who received standard care. Such face-to-face interventions generally aim to elicit patient beliefs, change these beliefs and bring them in line with the desired changes in behaviour and patient health outcomes. Central to this is the notion of coherence and the bringing together or beliefs about causes and solutions.

Research has also used mindfulness as a means to change illness cognitions and improve patient health outcomes. For example, Dalili and Bayazi (2019) used a randomized control trial to evaluate the impact of Mindfulness-Based Cognitive Therapy for people with rheumatoid arthritis and reported an improvement in illness perceptions in the intervention group compared to the control.

Imagery-Based Interventions

Research shows that people often form mental images as a way of making sense of any given problem. In terms of health problems, studies have explored the images of breast cancer survivors (Harrow et al. 2008), how people think about skin cancer (Cameron 2008) and how patients make sense of their heart attack (Broadbent et al. 2004). In addition, research indicates that visual images may be an effective means to raise awareness about the risks of behaviours such as smoking and sun-bathing. For example, Hammond et al. (2003) examined the effectiveness of the warning labels that became a standard feature on cigarette packets in 2000 in Canada. The results showed that the graphic images had effectively drawn participants' attention to the health warnings although this decayed over time as people habituated to the messages. In addition, those who reported reading, thinking about and discussing the labels with other people were more likely to report an intention to stop smoking in the next six months and showed more successful and unsuccessful quit attempts and a reduction in smoking over a three-month period. Similar results were also found in adolescents who were either established or occasional smokers (White et al. 2008; Germain et al. 2010). Further, Shahab et al. (2007) reported that showing smokers images of their carotid arteries with a plaque compared to an artery without a plaque increased their perceptions of risk for smoking-related illnesses. Further, in those with higher self-efficacy, the images also increased their intention to stop smoking. In terms of sun-bathing, Mahler et al. (2003, 2007) designed a series of studies to increase awareness about the impact of UV radiation in terms of skin damage and the risk of cancer. In the two experiments (Mahler et al. 2003), students and beachgoers were shown UV photos of their own skin or a photo-ageing video. The results showed that the personalized photo of their own skin was related to stronger intentions to use sun-screen in the future. (For reviews of the impact of visual images on perceptions of risk, see Hollands et al. 2010, 2011; Brown et al. 2021 (see Figure 8.7)).

In line with this, some research has also used images to change illness cognitions. For example, Karamanidou et al. (2008) used an imagery-based intervention to change beliefs about the importance

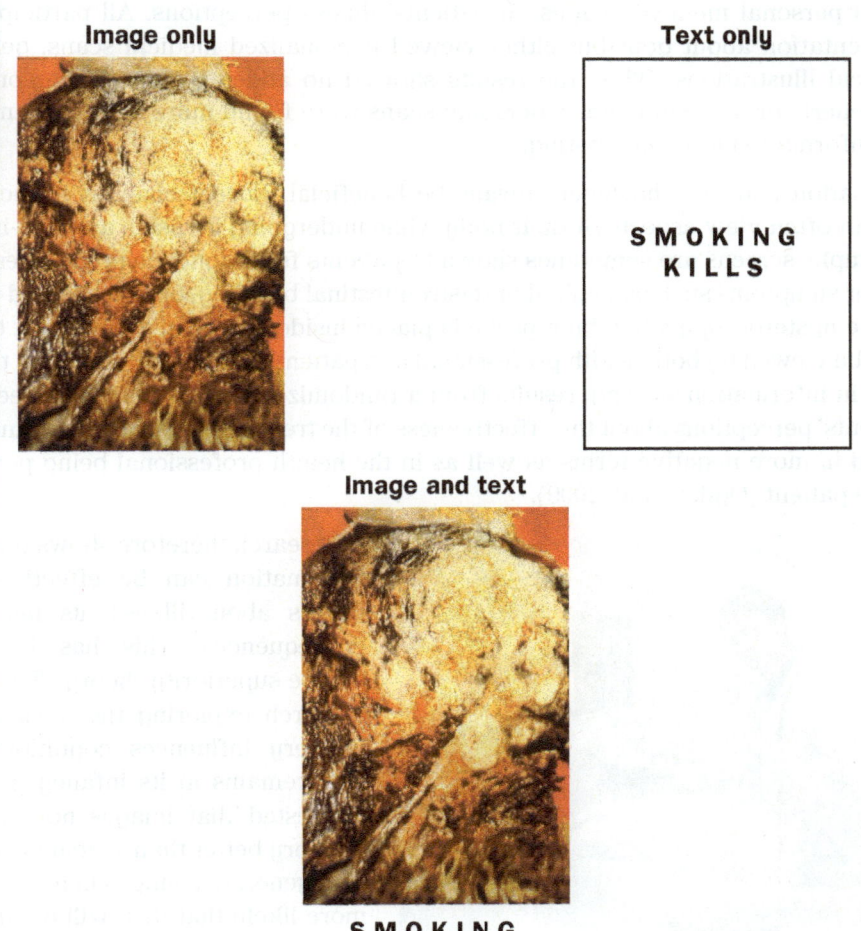

Figure 8.7 Using text and visual images to change beliefs and behaviour: Which is the most effective?

SOURCE: United States Government/Wikimedia Commons

of phosphate levels in patients with end-stage renal disease. Patients were shown a stomach-shaped container which illustrated the digestion process and showed how their phosphate binding medication could effectively bind with phosphates from the foods being eaten. The results showed that patients in the intervention group reported a more coherent understanding of their medication and greater beliefs in the ability of their medication to control their disease. In a similar vein, Lee et al. (2011) explored the relative impact of image-versus text-based information for changing beliefs about the risk of heart disease and subsequent health-related behaviours using a web-based intervention. The results showed that imagery had an immediate impact on illness cognitions, worry, behavioural intentions and mental imagery relating to heart disease and that an increased sense of coherence and worry were sustained by one month follow-up. Imagery also resulted in increased healthy diet efforts after two weeks. The results showed that text resulted in immediate changes in beliefs about causes, mental imagery relating to clogged arteries and worry and that by two weeks follow-up participants also showed increased physical activity, and a greater sense of coherence by one month. Overall, the results indicate that imagery resulted in more changes than text alone but that a combination of both approaches is probably the most effective means to change cognitions and behaviour. Similarly, research indicates that viewing images of internal body parts can influence beliefs about susceptibility to a health problem (Green et al. 2006) as well as illness coherence (Brotherstone et al. 2006). Krasnoryadtseva et al. (2020) carried out a randomized control trial to explore the effects of an educational intervention with embedded personal medical images on patients' illness perceptions. All participants viewed a 12-minute presentation about gout but either viewed personalized medical scans, generic scans or standard medical illustrations. While the results showed no added benefit of personalized images compared to generic or medical images, personal scans were found more helpful than generic scans and made the information more interesting.

Visual information may not, however, always be beneficial. Recent changes in technology mean that patients can often view aspects of their body while undergoing invasive and non-invasive procedures. For example, screens are sometimes shown to patients for diagnostic procedures searching for explanations for symptoms such as vaginal or gastrointestinal bleeding, or unexplained pain. One such procedure is the hysteroscopy whereby a probe is placed inside a woman's uterus via the vagina and the results can be viewed by both health professional and patient on a screen. Although this is regarded as an advance in information-sharing, results from a randomized trial indicate that seeing the screen can lower patients' perceptions about the effectiveness of the treatment, raise anxiety and result in pain being described in more negative terms as well as in the health professional being perceived as less receptive to the patient (Ogden et al. 2009).

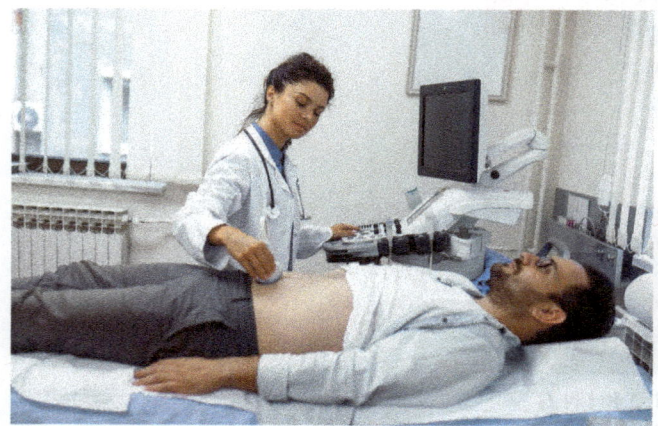

Seeing the screen during a procedure may change illness cognitions

SOURCE: © Shutterstock/Photoroyalty

Research therefore shows that image-based information can be effective at changing beliefs about illness, its management and consequences. This has been called the 'image superiority theory'. To date, however, research exploring the mechanisms of *how* imagery influences cognitions and behaviour remains in its infancy. But it has been suggested that images not only imprint on memory better than verbal messages but may also generate changes in mood which make it more likely that they will be turned into cues to action and subsequent changes in behaviour (Cameron 2009). It has also been argued that visual imagery may change implicit rather than explicit attitudes which in turn may change behaviour. Therefore, although the use of visual images is central to many existing health education interventions at both the individual and population level, how they work, and why they may work better than words is yet to be fully understood.

BOX 8.1
Critical Approaches to Health Psychology

Research and theories relating to illness cognition highlights some of the bigger issues in health psychology as follows:

The individual vs social vs political: Research exploring how people make sense of their health focus on their symptom perception, cognitions and feelings all of which are measured at the individual level. Yet these variables clearly exist within a social or political context. For example, a symptom will only feel worrying if we have enough capacity to think about it and are not struggling to stay alive due to poverty or war. Further, an illness will only make us feel we either do or do not have personal control over it if our culture, ethnicity and/or religion emphasizes personal agency rather than fate. And notions of health and illness will vary hugely between cultures dependent on factors such as life expectancy and rate of morbidity. It is hard to capture this level of complexity and variability in our research with our theories and our methods.

Individual differences: Research often explores differences in illness cognitions or symptoms or coping by individual factors such as gender, health status, age or ethnicity. This oversimplifies these constructs and puts people into boxes which helps analysis but is in danger of reinforcing stereotypes or imposing false dichotomies.

Mind–body relationships: Health psychology positions itself as conceptualizing the mind and body as interactive rather than discrete entities. But by measuring, labelling and analysing them separately to then assess their interaction they are also simultaneously being defined as discrete.

---

7   THINKING CRITICALLY ABOUT ILLNESS COGNITIONS

There are several problems with research exploring illness cognitions and their impact on health outcomes.

SOME CRITICAL QUESTIONS

When thinking about research in this area ask yourself the following questions:

- Do people have beliefs about their illness even before we have asked them?
- Could asking people about their symptoms change or even create their symptoms?
- Are beliefs about an illness different to how we cope with an illness?
- Some studies have short-term follow-ups to explore the impact of cognitions with health outcomes. What are the problems with this approach?
- Some studies have longer-term follow-ups. Are there also problems with this approach?

SOME PROBLEMS WITH. . .

Below are some problems with research in this area that you may wish to consider.

The mere measurement effect: Research often explores how people feel about their symptoms or illness by using existing questionnaires. It is possible that such measures change beliefs rather than simply access them (i.e. do I really have a belief about what has caused my headache until I am asked about it?). This is the same as the mere measurement effect described in Chapter 2.

Discrete constructs: Models of illness behaviour describe how the different constructs relate to each other (i.e. illness representations are associated with coping). It is not always clear, however, whether these two constructs are really discrete (e.g. 'I believe my illness is not going to last a long time' could either be an illness cognition or a coping mechanism).

The timing of measures: Many of the constructs measured as part of research on illness behaviour are then used to predict health outcomes such as illness beliefs and coping. It is not clear how stable these constructs are and whether they should be considered states or traits. As a self-regulatory model, the changing nature of these constructs is central. However, it presents a real methodological problem in terms of when to measure what and whether variables are causes or consequences of each other.

TO CONCLUDE

In the same way that people have beliefs about health, they also have beliefs about illness. Such beliefs are often called 'illness cognitions' or 'illness representations'. Beliefs about illness appear to follow a pattern and are made up of: (1) identity (e.g. a diagnosis and symptoms); (2) consequences (e.g. beliefs about seriousness); (3) time line (e.g. how long it will last); (4) cause (e.g. caused by smoking, caused by a virus); and (5) cure/control (e.g. requires medical intervention). This chapter examined these dimensions of illness cognitions and assessed how they relate to the way in which an individual responds to illness via their coping and their appraisal of the illness. Further, it described the SRM and its implications for understanding and predicting health outcomes and the central role for coherence. Finally, it described interventions to change illness cognitions involving face-to-face consultations or the use of visual images.

QUESTIONS

1 How do people make sense of health and illness?
2 Discuss the relationship between illness cognitions and coping.
3 Why is Leventhal's model 'self-regulatory'?
4 Symptoms are more than just a sensation. Discuss.
5 Discuss the role of symptom perception in adjusting to illness.
6 Discuss the role of coherence in illness representations.
7 Illness cognitions predict health outcomes. Discuss.
8 To what extent can illness cognitions be changed?
9 Design a research project to assess the extent to which illness severity predicts patient adjustment and highlight the role that illness cognitions may have in explaining this relationship.

FOR DISCUSSION

Think about the last time you were ill (e.g. headache, flu, broken limb, etc.). Consider the ways in which you made sense of your illness, how they related to your coping strategies and how you recovered.

FURTHER READING

Cameron, L. and Leventhal, H. (eds) (2003) *The Self-regulation of Health and Illness Behaviour.* London: Routledge.

This is a good book which presents a comprehensive coverage of a good selection of illness representations research and broader self-regulation approaches.

de Ridder, D.T.D., Adriaanse, M.A. and Fujita, Kentaro (2017) *Handbook of Self-Control in Health and Well-Being.* London: Routledge.
This is an excellent book that looks at different aspects of self control and their impact on health outcomes.

Eccleston, C. (2015) *Embodied: The psychology of physical sensation.* Oxford: Oxford University Press.
This is a novel book that covers how and why we experience symptoms such as pain, itch, breathing, fatigue and temperature. This is a great book based upon interviews with those suffering from extremes of these symptoms and concludes with a theoretical analysis of their experiences.

Petrie, K.J. and Weinman, J.A. (eds) (2006) *Perceptions of Health and Illness.* Amsterdam: Harwood.
This is an edited collection of projects using the SRM as their theoretical framework.

Taylor, S.E. (1983) Adjustment to threatening events: a theory of cognitive adaptation, *American Psychologist*, **38:** 1161–73.
This is an excellent example of an interview-based study. It describes and analyses the cognitive adaptation theory of coping with illness and emphasizes the central role of illusions in making sense of the imbalance created by the absence of health.

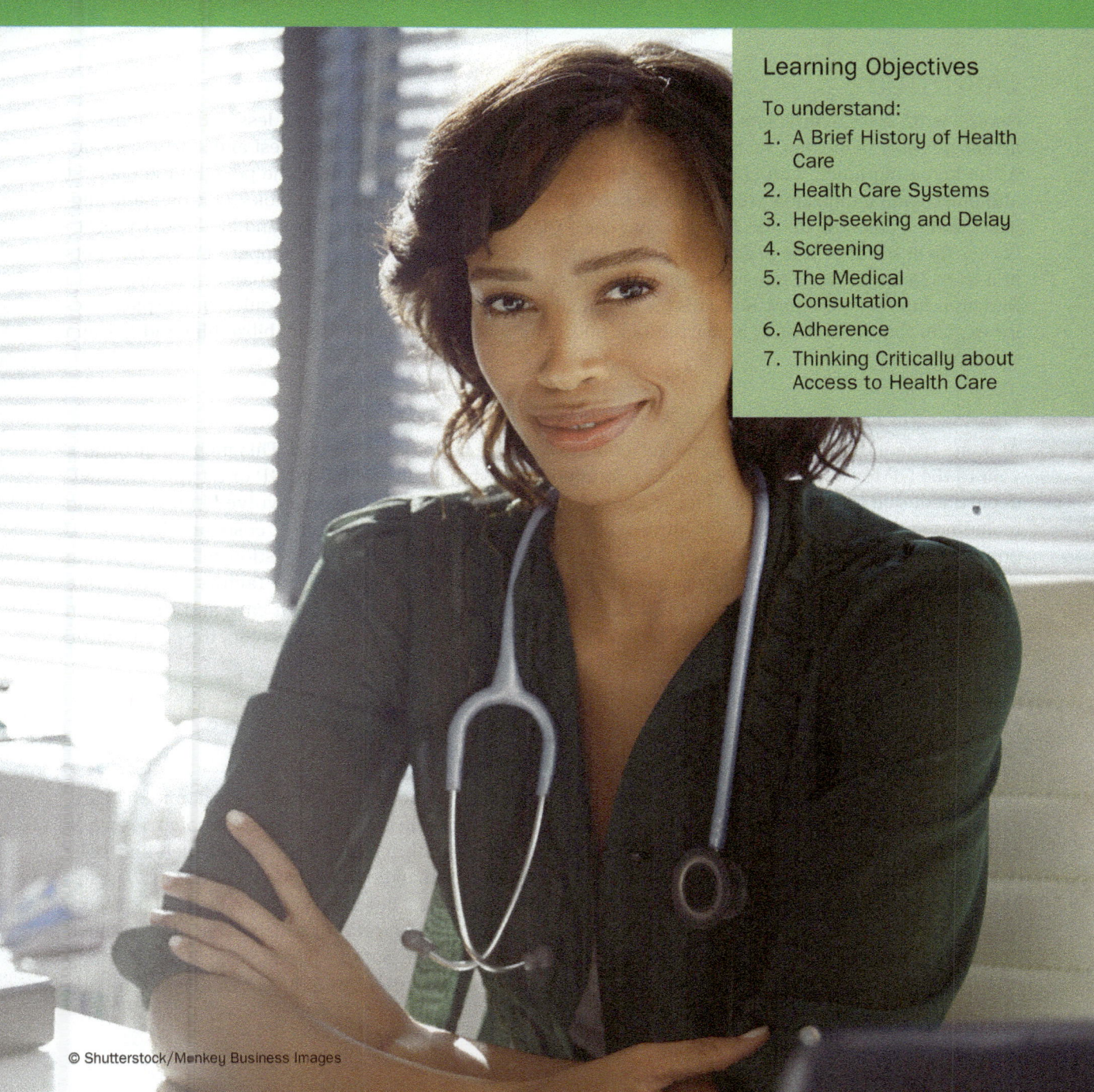

9
Accessing Health Care

Learning Objectives

To understand:
1. A Brief History of Health Care
2. Health Care Systems
3. Help-seeking and Delay
4. Screening
5. The Medical Consultation
6. Adherence
7. Thinking Critically about Access to Health Care

© Shutterstock/Monkey Business Images

CHAPTER OVERVIEW

This chapter describes a number of factors relating to accessing health care and the use of the health care system. First it describes help-seeking behaviour, the problem of delay and why people do or do not go to the doctor. It then describes research on screening and how people are brought into contact with health care through screening interventions. It next describes consultations between patients and health professionals and the role of diagnosis, referral and the impact of health professionals' own health beliefs. Finally it describes the problem of adherence and factors which influence whether patients do or do not follow medical advice.

CASE STUDY

George is 52, a bit overweight and although he used to be quite fit has become less and less active as he has got older. One day, on his way home from work, he feels a pain in his chest and starts to sweat. As he had a big lunch with colleagues he thinks it is probably indigestion, so he pops by the chemist and buys some indigestion pills. When he gets home his wife tells him that he looks a bit pale and suggests that he calls the doctor. He says that since COVID doctors are very busy and he doesn't want to bother them because it is probably just indigestion. She makes him a cup of peppermint tea and gets him to have a rest while she cooks dinner. Half an hour later she hears a scream and runs through to find him clutching his chest. She calls for an ambulance which is able to get there quickly. The paramedics explain that he is having a heart attack but fortunately they are able to stabilize him and get him to hospital.

Through the Eyes of Health Psychology. . .

At some time in their lives everyone has contact with the health care system. This may be through a visit to the GP for a cough, a hospital appointment following a referral by the GP or a trip to the A&E department due to an accident. George's case illustrates some of the factors involved in help-seeking including symptom perception ('it hurts'), illness cognitions ('it's not serious'), costs and benefits of going to the doctors (not wanting to be a nuisance), self-care (buying indigestion pills and having peppermint tea) and social support (have some tea and a rest) and how these factors can facilitate or delay help seeking. This chapter will describe the different types of health care and the ways in which people interact with the health care system in terms of help-seeking, screening, the consultation and adherence.

1 | A BRIEF HISTORY OF HEALTH CARE

Before the nineteenth century, the average life expectancy for most of the world was about 30 years. From the nineteenth century, life expectancy started to increase in early industrialized countries while it remained low in the rest of the world. This led to huge health inequalities between rich and poor countries. Since 1900, global average life expectancy has more than doubled and is now about 70 years. Much variability, however, still exists not only between countries, but also within countries by region, by gender and by social class. Some of this change is due to child mortality which accounted for such low life expectancy when many children did not reach 5 years old. But this change is also due to many other factors. This section will explore the role of medical interventions and the environment. The role of behaviour was described in Chapter 2.

THE ROLE OF MEDICAL INTERVENTIONS

From a medical perspective, variations in health and illness are explained with a focus on the success or failure of medical interventions and the availability of health care. Research indicates wide variations in health care provision and access in terms of the types and costs of medicines, the training and expertise of health care professionals, the distances needed to travel to access health care and the availability of free health care versus the need for health insurance.

New Medicines

A good example of the impact of medical interventions is that of HIV/AIDS. In the western world HIV/AIDS is now considered a chronic illness with many people living with the HIV virus having a normal Life expectancy. This change has been attributed to the antiretroviral medication HAART (see Chapter 12). In sub-Saharan Africa, however, where HAART is far less available, HIV/AIDS still shows the pattern of an acute terminal illness. Figures 9.1 and 9.2. show the differences in the number of deaths from AIDS between 1990-2019 where HAART was less available (Uganda) and more available (UK).

These figures illustrate that in non-African countries where medication is available, the life expectancy of a person with AIDS is similar to a person without AIDS. In stark contrast, however, in African countries where medication is not so easily accessible, a huge gap exists between the life expectancy of these two populations: medical intervention directly impacts upon the life expectancy of people with this condition, translating it from an acute to a chronic disorder.

Availability of Vaccinations

There is also worldwide variation in vaccinations for illnesses such as measles. Figure 9.3 shows vaccination for measles by WHO region and indicates changes over time since 1990. The highest rates are in Europe and America while the lowest are in Africa and the eastern Mediterranean region. Such variation will obviously impact upon the health of any given population.

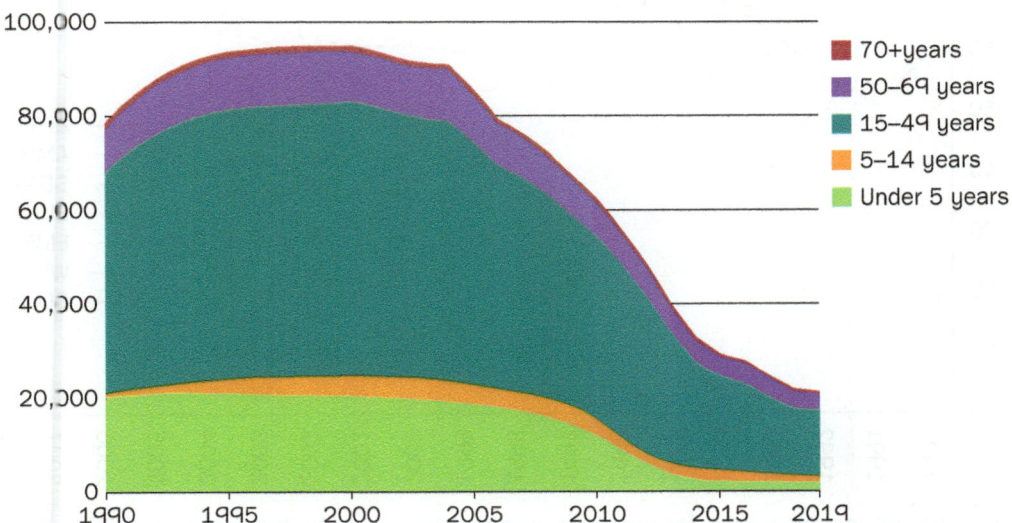

Figure 9.1 Deaths from AIDS 1990–2019 in Uganda where access to haart mediation was limited

SOURCE: Our World in Data (2022)

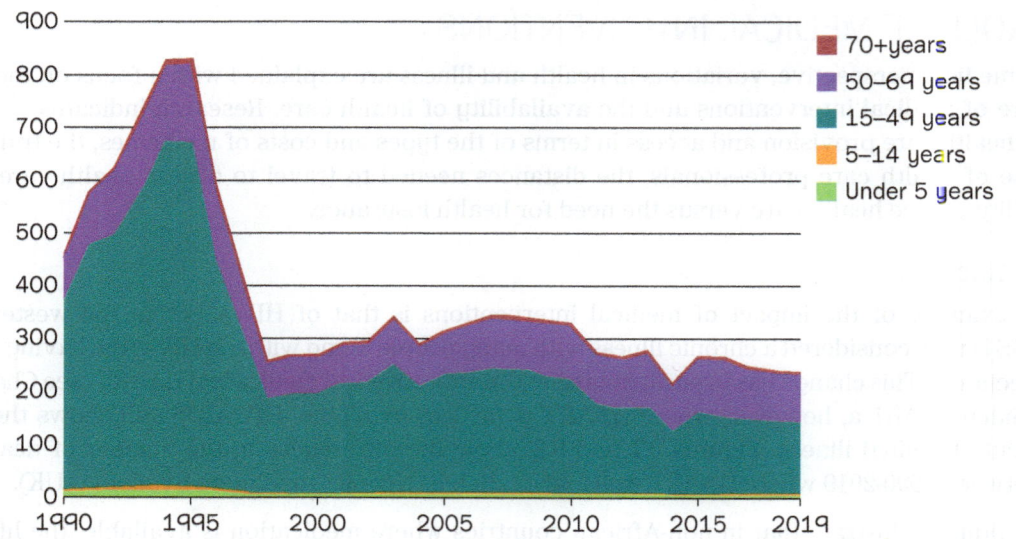

Figure 9.2 Deaths from aids in the UK 1990–2019 where HAART was more easily available

Reproduced under the creative commons attribution 4.0 International (CC by 4.0 License) https://creativecommons.Org/licenses/by/4.0/

SOURCE: Our World in Data 2022

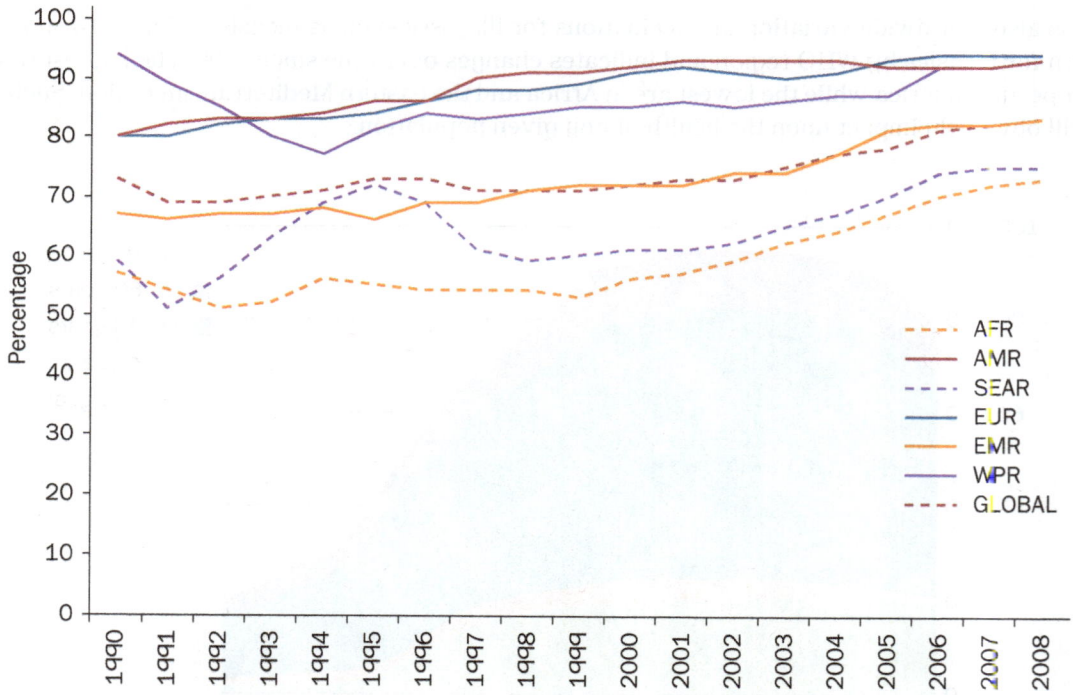

Figure 9.3 Variation in vaccination for measles among 1-year-olds by WHO region, 1990–2008

SOURCE: WHO (2010)

Availability of Skilled Health Professionals

Child mortality rates vary by geographical region. One possible reason is the presence of a skilled health professional at the birth. This does not happen universally, however, and in the WHO African

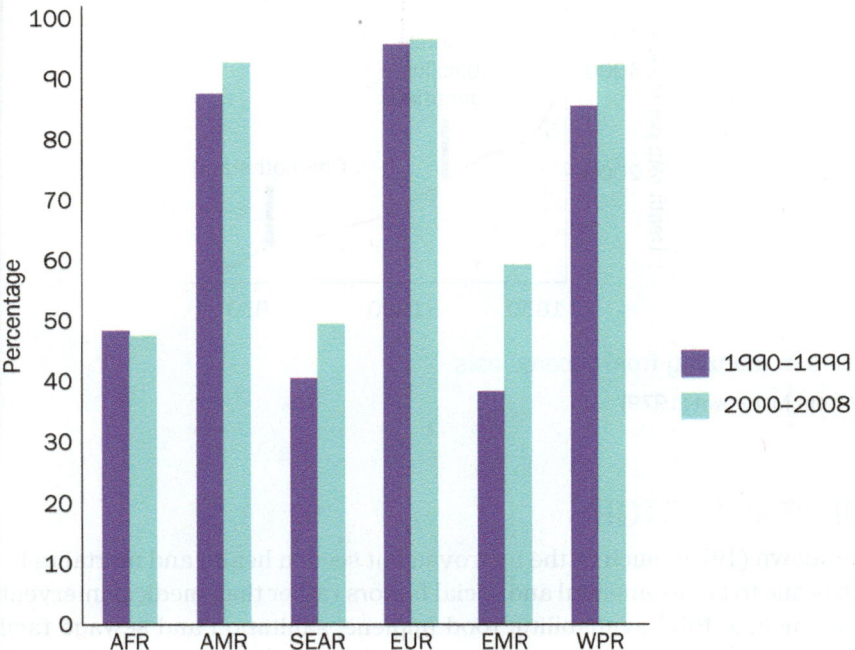

Figure 9.4 Births attended by a skilled health professional by WHO region, 1990–2008
SOURCE: WHO (2010)

and South-East Asian regions less than 50 per cent of women received skilled care during childbirth in 2008 (see Figure 9.4).

The availability and use of medicines and skilled health professionals may therefore explain some of the variation in health and illness.

Not Just Medical Interventions

The impact of medicine on health and illness is not, however, always this clear, particularly in the Global North. In his book *The Role of Medicine,* Thomas McKeown (1979) examined the impact of medicine on health since the seventeenth century. In particular, he evaluated the widely held assumptions about medicine's achievements and the role of medicine in reducing the prevalence and incidence of infectious illnesses, such as tuberculosis, pneumonia, measles, influenza, diphtheria, smallpox and whooping cough. McKeown argued that the commonly held view was that the decline in illnesses, such as tuberculosis, measles, smallpox and whooping cough, was related to medical interventions such as chemotherapy and vaccinations – for example, that antibiotics were responsible for the decline in illnesses such as pneumonia and influenza. He showed, however, that the reduction in such illnesses was already underway before the development of the relevant medical interventions. This is illustrated in Figure 9.5 (for tuberculosis). McKeown therefore claimed that the decline in infectious diseases seen throughout the past three centuries is best understood not in terms of medical intervention, but in terms of social and environmental factors 'predictably improved nutrition, better hygiene and contraception' (McKeown 1979: 117).

Health status therefore varies over time, by geographical location, gender and social class. Some of this variation can be explained by medical interventions in terms of the availability of medicines and vaccinations and free access to skilled health professionals. However, an alternative analysis focuses on the role of the environment.

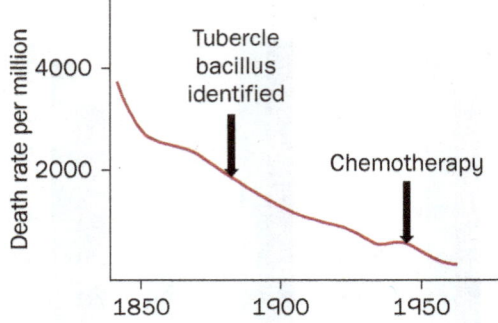

Figure 9.5 Decline in mortality from tuberculosis

SOURCE: Adapted from McKeown (1979)

ENVIRONMENTAL FACTORS

According to McKeown (1979) much of the improvement seen in health and mortality in the countires in the Global North is due to environmental and social factors rather than medical interventions. Such environmental factors include food availability, food hygiene, sanitation and sewage facilities, and clean water. These basic requirements vary by country and may contribute to health inequalities. In terms of sanitation facilities, in 2008 the WHO reported that 2,600 million worldwide were not using 'improved sanitation facilities' and that 1,100 million were still defecating in the open, which raises the risk of worm infestation, hepatitis, cholera, trachoma and environmental contamination. The use of improved sanitation facilities by WHO region is shown in Figure 9.6, which indicates that the lowest rates of use of improved sanitation facilities were in the African and South-East Asian regions.

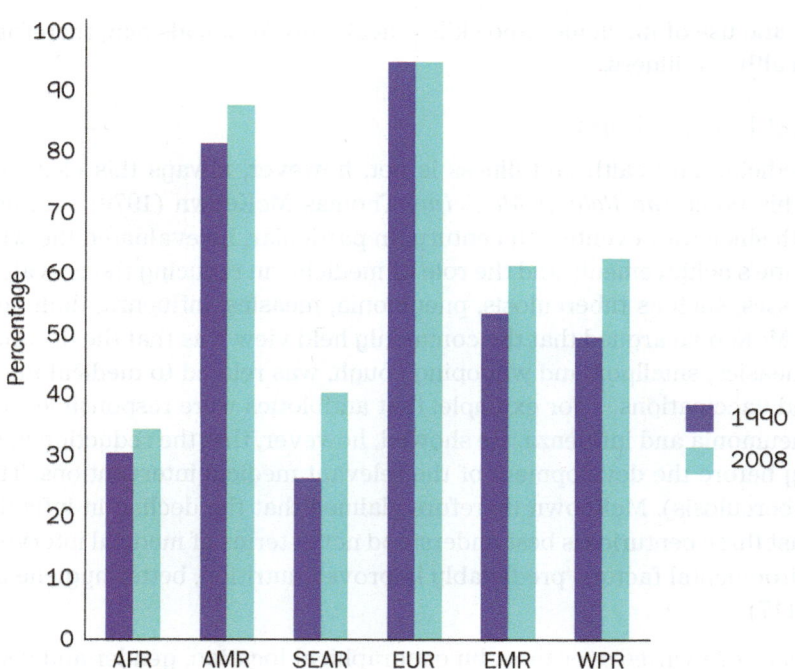

Figure 9.6 Use of improved sanitation facilities by WHO region, 1990, 2008

SOURCE: WHO (2010: 19)

The state of drinking water is also linked to health and poor water is associated with illnesses such as vomiting, sickness, diarrhoea and cholera. Data from the WHO show that the lowest levels of safe drinking water are in the African and South-East Asian regions (see Figure 9.7).

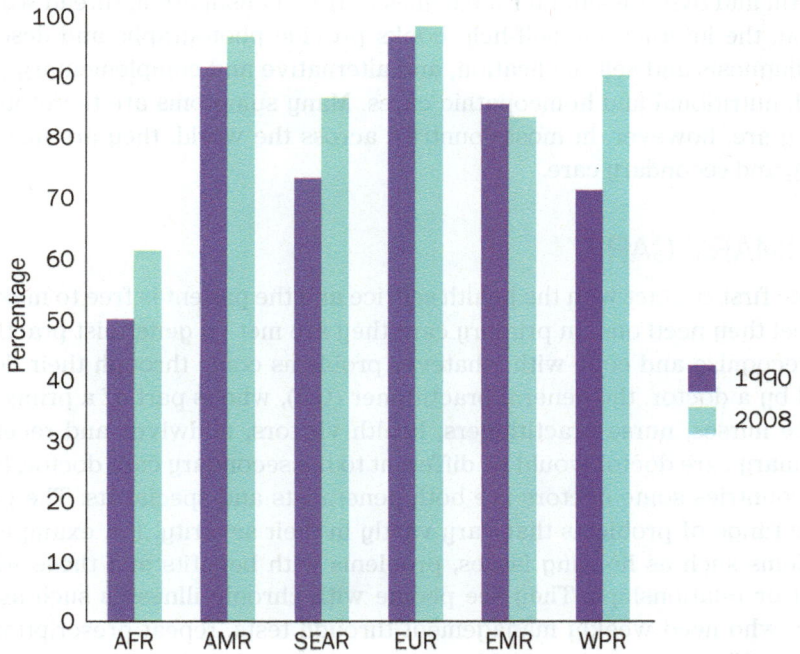

Figure 9.7 Use of improved drinking facilities by WHO world region, 1990, 2008

SOURCE: WHO (2010: 18)

All these data therefore show variation in key environmental factors which are linked to health and may help to explain health inequalities. In the Global North, where these basic requirements tend to be met, our health may still be influenced by our environment in terms of the quality of food available, easy access to unhealthy ultra high-processed and fast food, working environments that encourage a sedentary lifestyle, town planning which makes walking unsafe or difficult, and using the car the norm, with the absence of walkways or cycle paths and poor street lighting (see Chapter 13 for a discussion of the obesogenic environment).

IN SUMMARY

Health status varies over time, by geography and by gender and social class. From a medical perspective the main analysis of this variability focuses on the availability of medicines and access to skilled health professionals. The remainder of this chapter addresses the ways in which people access health care with a focus on help-seeking, screening, the consultation and adherence to medication. It is important to remember, however, that medical developments cannot explain all changes in health and that there is also a key role for the environment. Further, there is also a key role for health behaviour as described in Chapters 2–7. In addition, all medicines have side effects and some do more harm than good. This is discussed in detail in the 'Thinking critically about access to health care' section at the end of this chapter.

2   HEALTH CARE SYSTEMS

In essence there are three levels to any health care system although the details and structure of these systems vary between countries.

LEVEL 1: SELF-CARE

Many symptoms and illnesses are managed through self-care with no need for professional input. Most homes have cupboards with plasters and creams for cuts and bruises, pain relief pills for headaches, colds and flu and over-the-counter medicines to treat constipation, thread worms, allergies and thrush. In addition, the internet and self-help books provide photographs and descriptions of symptoms to aid self-diagnosis and self-medication, and alternative and complementary practitioners offer a range of herbal, nutritional and homeopathic cures. Many symptoms are therefore not taken to the doctor. When they are, however, in most countries across the world, they are met with a two-tiered system of primary and secondary care.

LEVEL 2: PRIMARY CARE

Primary care is the first contact with the health service and the patient is free to make an appointment whenever they feel they need one. In primary care they are met by generalist practitioners who have been trained to recognize and cope with whatever problems come through their door. Primary care is mainly offered by a doctor, the general practitioner (GP), who is part of a primary care team consisting of practice nurses, nurse practitioners, health visitors, midwives and receptionists. In most countries, the primary care doctor would be different to the secondary care doctor, but in the USA and some European countries some doctors are both generalists and specialists. The primary care team deals with a huge range of problems that vary vastly in their severity. For example, they see people with social problems such as housing issues, problems with benefits and those who are struggling with employment or relationships. They see people with chronic illnesses such as diabetes, cancer and heart disease who need weekly management through tests, repeat prescriptions and behaviour modification advice. They see common mild symptoms such as coughs, colds, stomach pain and tiredness and they see potentially serious symptoms (such as coughs, colds, stomach pain and tiredness!). They see people with coughs and colds who really want to talk about contraception or who really have piles but are too embarrassed to ask. The role of the primary care team is to diagnose and manage whatever problems fall within its range of expertise or to refer patients on to the hospital specialists in secondary care for a second opinion and further tests. Those in the primary care team are therefore the gatekeepers into secondary care. This process prevents secondary care being inundated with less serious medical problems, but errors inevitably occur as minor problems are referred on and serious problems are missed.

LEVEL 3: SECONDARY CARE

If referred by their GP, a patient is then permitted to see a specialist in secondary care. In most countries access to secondary care can only occur via a referral letter from the GP, although this is changing as patients are increasingly becoming consumers of health care and demanding their right to see whoever they want. Private practice also changes this division as patients can choose to pay to see secondary care specialists if they have the money or health insurance. Medicine in secondary care is further specialized as health professionals work in teams relating to body systems such as gastroenterology, respiratory medicine, obstetrics and gynaecology, cardiology and ear, nose and throat specialisms. Secondary care tends to be based in a hospital to provide access to beds and operates with an outpatient system (for check-ups, tests and follow-up consultations) and an inpatient system (having an operation, staying overnight).

The role of self-care, primary and secondary care raises some important questions about accessing health care and the care received:

- Why do patients self-care for apparently serious reasons?
- Why do patients attend their doctor's surgery for apparently trivial reasons?

- How do doctors decide upon an appropriate diagnosis?
- How do GPs decide who to refer or who not to refer to secondary care?
- Why do patients not always do as they are told?

These questions will be answered in terms of help-seeking and delay, screening procedures and their uptake, the medical consultation and adherence.

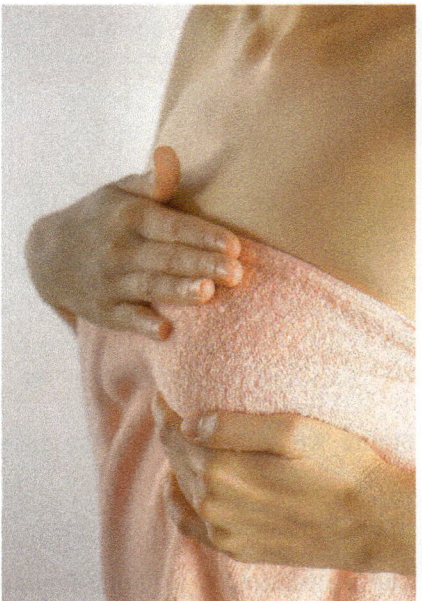

People have to decide whether a symptom is abnormal, or serious before they will seek help

SOURCE: © Shutterstock /BigmanKn

3 | HELP-SEEKING AND DELAY

Help-seeking behaviour is also known as 'illness behaviour' and refers to the process of deciding to get professional help for a health-related problem. According to the medical model perspective, help-seeking relates to two factors:

- *Symptoms:* the patient has a headache, back problem or change in bowel habits that indicates that something is wrong.
- *Signs:* on examination the doctor identifies signs such as raised blood pressure, a lump in the bowel or hears rattling when listening to a patient's chest which indicates that there is a problem.

From this perspective the doctor is a detective and the patient is required to bring them the problem. Help-seeking, however, is not as simple as this, as many people go to the doctor with very minor symptoms (e.g. 'I had a sore throat last week but it's gone now', 'I'm tired but keep going to bed late' or even 'I have a lump at the top of my back' (which is the top vertebrae!)). Furthermore, many patients don't go to their doctor when they have something serious (e.g. 'I have had this breast lump for about five years and it has now come through the skin', 'I have piles but the cream isn't working' (but actually it's anal cancer!)). This is known as the 'clinical iceberg' to reflect the vast number of problems that never reach the doctor. In addition, we all have symptoms all the time such as needing to go to the toilet, an itchy foot, feeling thirsty, feeling tired, coughing or a stiff neck that we do nothing about.

A SERIES OF THRESHOLDS

Help-seeking is therefore much more complex than the detection of symptoms and the identification of signs and can be understood in terms of a number of thresholds that need to be reached. Firstly, the patient needs to take a feeling − 'Ow' − and decide this is a symptom; then they need to decide if this symptom is normal or abnormal; next they need to decide whether it's serious enough to need help and finally they decide whether or not a doctor could help.

These thresholds are as follows:

- *Is it a symptom?* 'I have a pain in my stomach.'
- *Is it normal or abnormal?* 'I have a pain in my stomach and it's not just wind.'
- *Do I need help?* 'I have a pain in my stomach, it's not just wind and it might be cancer.'
- *Could a doctor help?* 'I have a pain in my stomach, it's not just wind and it might be cancer and doctors know about cancer.'

These thresholds can be understood in terms of four processes which have been explored within both psychological and sociological research and are illustrated in Figure 9.8.

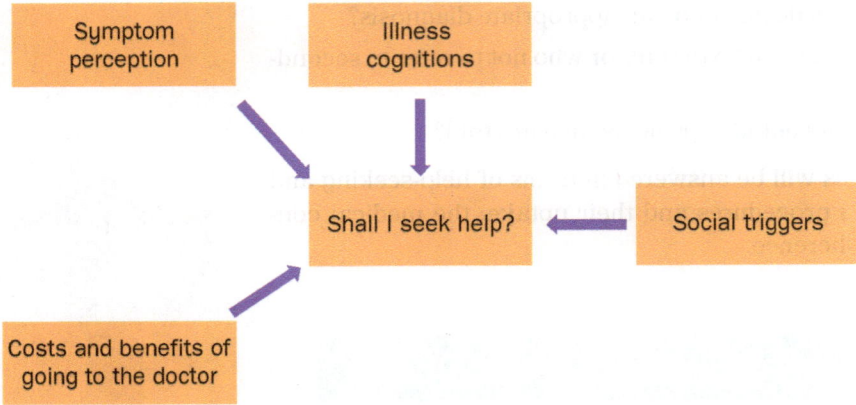

Figure 9.8 Understanding the thresholds of help-seeking

SYMPTOM PERCEPTION

The translation of a vague feeling into the concrete entity of a symptom involves the processes of symptom perception (see Chapter 8 for a detailed description). Research indicates that whether or not we perceive ourselves as having a symptom is influenced by four main sources of information:

- *Bodily data:* Gijsbers van Wijk and Kolk (1997) argued that one influence upon symptom perception is 'data driven' which comes from our bodies. It has also been argued that there is a competition between internal information (our bodies) and external information (our environment) which is why busy working people perceive fewer symptoms (Pennebaker 1982; Rief and Broadbent 2007). Research also indicates that some people show selective attention to their bodily symptoms and are therefore more aware of any changes (Gijsbers van Wijk and Kolk 1997). Symptom perception, however, is not as simple as receiving bodily data and symptom severity can be exacerbated or modified through mood, cognitions and the social context. Symptoms can be generated even in the absence of bodily data (so watching a film of head lice can make people itch, e.g. Ogden and Zoukas 2009).

- *Mood:* stress and anxiety can make symptoms worse whereas relaxation can make them better. For example, a meta-analysis of 244 observational studies of a range of chronic conditions such as irritable bowel syndrome, fibromyalgia and chronic fatigue syndrome showed that higher depression and anxiety were consistently linked with greater symptom perception (Henningsen et al. 2003). Similar results have also been reported for stomach pain, headache and leg pain (Eminson 2007) and IBS symptoms in children (Hollier et al. 2019) and depression and eczema symptoms in adults (Zeiser et al. (2021).

- *Cognitions:* focusing on a symptom makes it worse while distraction makes it better. Therefore many strategies taught to those with chronic pain include encouraging distraction through being busy, talking to friends and staying employed if possible. Likewise, distraction by playing with stress balls or talking to the nurse can reduce pain during conscious surgery for varicose veins (Hudson et al. 2015). Furthermore, during labour women are encouraged to stay distracted as long as possible by keeping active and staying out of hospital in the early stages. In an experimental study, 61 women who had been hospitalized during pre-term labour were randomized to receive either information, distraction or nothing (van Zuuren 1998). The results showed that physical and psychological symptoms were lower in the distraction group.

- *Social context:* symptoms also vary according to social context. For example, 'medical student's disease' describes how medical students often develop the symptoms of whatever condition they are studying (e.g. chest pain, backache, bowel problems) (Mechanic 1962) and research also indicates that smiling, yawning, shivering and itching can be contagious if people watch others experiencing these symptoms (Platek et al. 2005; Schurman et al. 2005).

The processes of symptom perception therefore help to translate a vague experience into a concrete symptom. Before this leads to help-seeking, however, the individual also has to decide whether the symptom is abnormal and whether it requires formal help from a doctor. This is influenced by the development of illness cognitions.

ILLNESS COGNITIONS

Once a symptom has been perceived as such, a person then forms a mental representation of the problem. This has been called their 'illness cognitions' which are described in detail in Chapter 8. Research indicates that illness cognitions often consist of the same dimensions relating to identity ('What is it?'), time line ('How long will it last?'), causes ('What caused it?'), consequences ('Will it have a serious effect on my life?') and control/cure ('Can I manage it or do I need treatment?'). The formation of these cognitions will be helped by social messages from friends, family or the media to decide whether or not a symptom is serious, abnormal or manageable by self-care. It will also be influenced by the individual's own health history and expectations of their own level of health. For example, a patient who has recurring headaches may be less surprised by a new headache whereas someone who is always well may react more strongly to a less serious symptom. This process of *normalization* can pose problems for both the patient and the doctor (once in a consultation) as a heavy smoker may omit to tell the doctor that they are breathless as they always are and have become used to it. Further, if an individual lives in a family where indigestion is normal then chest pain may be more readily labelled 'indigestion' than 'possible heart attack'.

Therefore, illness cognitions take the symptom up to the next threshold as it is deemed to be abnormal (or not) and serious (or not).

SOCIAL TRIGGERS

The process of identifying a problem as abnormal (or not) is also influenced by what Zola (1973) called *social triggers* in his analysis of 'pathways to the doctor'. These triggers relate less to the individual's perception of the symptom itself and more the impact that the symptom will have on their daily lives. From this perspective our state of equilibrium can be disrupted by a symptom if it disturbs our normal life. Help-seeking is therefore a means to re-establish equilibrium. These social triggers are as follows:

- *Perceived interference with work or physical activity:* work and physical activity are core to most people's daily lives. A symptom that disrupts this will be identified as abnormal.
- *Perceived interference with social relations:* similarly, a symptom will also be perceived as abnormal if it interferes with our ability to interact with others.
- *An interpersonal crisis:* people have symptoms all the time that they normalize and habituate to. A sudden crisis such as an argument, divorce, change of job or retirement may trigger increased attention to a long-standing symptom leading to help-seeking for something that the patient appears to have had for a while.
- *Sanctioning:* the notion of sanctioning is similar to social messages as it involves other people encouraging a visit to the doctor so that patients often start a consultation saying, 'Sorry to bother you but my mother insisted I come to see you.'

Together, symptom perception, illness cognitions and social triggers take the individual up the thresholds towards help-seeking for a particular problem. The final set of factors that influence this process are the perceived costs and benefits of going to the doctor.

COSTS AND BENEFITS OF GOING TO THE DOCTOR

The final step before a patient seeks help involves weighing up the costs and benefits of seeing the doctor. These can be classified as follows:

- ***Therapeutic:*** first the patient needs to weigh up the therapeutic costs and benefits. Possible benefits include gaining access to effective treatments and being referred to secondary care for more specialist advice and treatment. Help-seeking also comes with costs, however, such as being given medicines to take for someone who doesn't like taking medicines, having to have a physical and potentially embarrassing examination or having to talk about a personal and embarrassing problem. Further, some patients may believe that medicine has nothing to offer them that they can't offer themselves.
- ***Practical:*** any visit to the doctor involves practical costs as it requires possible time off work, time away from the family, the cost of the fare and the effort of getting to the doctor's surgery.
- ***Emotional:*** many people enjoy visiting their doctor for more emotional reasons. For example, the trip can give a structure to their day, they might meet people to talk to at the surgery and the doctor can be reassuring, interesting, sympathetic and caring. There may, however, also be negative emotions generated by such a visit such as embarrassment or a feeling of being a nuisance to a doctor who is perceived as already too busy and overworked.
- ***The sick role:*** a doctor has the power to turn a person into a patient by legitimizing their symptoms. Therefore, although they may have been complaining of a sore throat, they will get more sympathy if they can say 'my doctor says I have tonsillitis'. Parsons (1951) described the notion of a *sick role* and argued that the doctor can legitimize a patient's experience and admit them into the sick role. According to Parsons, this comes with two benefits and two obligations:
  - ***The benefits:*** the main benefit of a sick role is that it excuses the patient from their normal roles and duties. This can be through a sick note which is used to miss work or simply being able to say 'my doctor says I mustn't lift things'. Therefore once in the sick role patients no longer have to work, do household chores or even have sex if they don't want to. The next benefit is that the sick role means they are no longer responsible for their illness as 'they are ill'. This means that the illness is no longer seen as self-inflicted or even as a punishment but the result of some biological process that has been identified by the doctor.
  - ***The obligations:*** Parsons also argues that once admitted into the sick role patients take on two obligations. The first is that they must want to get well and see the sick role as a temporary status. If the sick role goes on for too long, they will start to be seen as 'putting it on' or 'malingering'. The second obligation is that they will 'cooperate with technically competent help' – that is, adhere to what the doctor says. Adherence is described in detail at the end of this chapter.

Patients therefore weigh up the costs and benefits of going to the doctor in terms of therapeutic, practical and emotional reasons and whether or not they want the benefits and obligations of the sick role.

Overall, help-seeking relates to a number of thresholds whereby an initial sensation ('Ow') is turned into a symptom, which is deemed to be abnormal and serious enough to need professional help and whereby the benefits of seeing the doctor outweigh the costs. This process often means patients visit the doctor with appropriate symptoms at the appropriate time, but sometimes this goes wrong as patients attend with trivial symptoms *or* they delay help-seeking for more serious conditions. These thresholds are illustrated in Figure 9.9.

DELAY

Some patients come to their doctor with symptoms that should have been treated months or even years before. Some don't phone an ambulance and end up having a heart attack at work after days of breathlessness and chest pain. Many treat serious symptoms with over-the-counter medicines or self-care when more effective treatments are needed. Delay in help-seeking presents a problem for health professionals as it undermines their chance to treat patients effectively. Delay can be understood in terms of all the factors described above that relate to help-seeking, but it is not an easy concept to define or measure, which in turn makes research on the predictors of delay problematic. This section will describe definitions of delay, the predictors of delay and interventions to reduce delay.

A series of thresholds

- **Is it a symptom?** *'I have a pain in my stomach'.* (symptom perception)
- **Is it normal or abnormal?** *'I have a pain in my stomach and it's not just wind.* (illness cognitions)
- **Do I need help?** *'I have a pain in my stomach, it's not just wind and it might be cancer'.* (illness cognitions, socail triggers)
- **Could a doctor help:** *'I have a pain in my stomach, it's not just wind and it might be cancer and doctors know about cancer'.* (social triggers, costs and benefits)

Figure 9.9 Help-seeking as a series of thresholds

Definitions of Delay

Patient delay refers to the time between detecting a sign or symptom and the first contact with a health professional. Although this seems quite straightforward given all the factors described above, the notion of delay is more complex. For example, if detecting a symptom involves all the thresholds described above *and* the input of mood, cognitions, social context, illness cognitions and social triggers, then at what point can a symptom be declared 'detected'? It could be at the initial 'Ow' or it could be once the person has decided 'yes this is a symptom that is worth considering'. It is therefore very difficult to measure whether a patient has delayed their help-seeking and, if so, for how long.

Predictors of Delay

Research has identified a number of factors that predict delay which mostly incorporate aspects of symptom perception, illness cognitions, social triggers and the costs and benefits of going to the doctor as described above (see Scott et al. 2007; 2009 for some interesting research on delay for oral cancer). For example, a patient with chest pain would delay help-seeking if the following occurred:

Symptom perception

- 'I am too busy at work to think about my symptoms.'
- 'I am happy and not stressed.'

Illness cognitions

- 'It will go away soon.'
- 'It must be that big meal I ate last night.'

Social triggers

- 'My friends have reassured me that this is normal.'
- 'My chest pain hasn't interfered with my work or relationships.'
- 'People in my family get a lot of indigestion.'

Costs and benefits of going to the doctor

- 'Doctors can't do much for indigestion.'
- 'I don't want to bother a busy doctor with my problems.'

Some research also indicates that men and women may differ in their help-seeking behaviours and tendency to delay (see Chapter 15). In 2015, Yousaf et al. carried out a systematic review of 41 papers investigating the factors associated with delays in medical and psychological help-seeking among men.

The results showed that the most common barriers to help-seeking were reluctance to express emotions or concerns about health, embarrassment, anxiety and fear and poor communication with health care professionals.

Interventions for Delay

Interventions for adherence encourage patients to take their medicines and interventions for behaviour change encourage people to eat more healthily or stop smoking. For such interventions the outcome is clear – do more (or less) of whatever behaviour is being targeted. Interventions for delay, however, are more complicated. Symptoms of serious illnesses are quite often the same as symptoms for minor illnesses (i.e. tiredness, pain, bowel changes etc.). Up to 50 per cent of patients visiting the doctor seem to have 'nothing wrong with them' but have come in with their minor symptoms. If an intervention advised people to seek help whenever they experienced a symptom *and* as soon as this symptom started, then the system would collapse under the weight of demand. A good example of this is ovarian cancer. Ovarian cancer is most feared by women as it has a high mortality rate and presents late in its development. It is often too late to treat once it has been diagnosed. An intervention could therefore encourage women to come earlier to their doctor to give them a better chance of treatment. But ovarian cancer is a relatively silent cancer and the only symptom that women seem to perceive in retrospect is bloatedness. Bloatedness is a very common symptom. If all women came to the doctor when they felt bloated and doctors referred all women with bloatedness for scans, then the financial cost would be huge, the numbers of healthy people put through the inconvenience and potential danger of a scan would be vast and both primary and secondary services would lose resources from other potentially more cost-effective forms of treatment. Interventions to prevent delay therefore need to be extremely specific in terms of the advice they give and who they give it to, and should only intervene if early intervention has been *proven* to be both cost-effective and therapeutically effective.

IN SUMMARY

Help-seeking describes the ways in which an individual detects a symptom and decides to seek help from a health professional. This can be understood in terms of a number of thresholds which involves four processes: symptom perception, illness cognitions, social triggers and evaluating the costs and benefits of going to the doctor. Some people, however, are called into the health care system before they have symptoms. This next section will focus on screening, which aims to detect an illness at an asymptomatic stage of its development.

4 SCREENING

Most people choose to come into contact with health care when they detect a symptom and seek help. This process relies upon two factors. First, patients need to identify that they have a symptom and conclude that health professionals will be able to help. This relates to help-seeking behaviours as described above. Second, this process relies upon an illness having symptoms that can be detected. Many health problems, however, such as cancer, hypertension and genetic disorders are asymptomatic in the early stages but are sometimes too far advanced for successful treatment once symptoms are severe enough to be noticeable. Health care has therefore introduced screening programmes as a means to pick up problems at a time when they cannot be detected by the patient on the premise that early detection leads to better treatment success.

WHAT IS SCREENING?

There are three forms of prevention aimed at improving a nation's health:

1 **Primary prevention** refers to the modification of risk factors (such as smoking, diet, alcohol intake) before illness onset. Health promotion campaigns are a form of primary prevention.

2 **Secondary prevention** refers to interventions aimed at detecting illness at an asymptomatic stage of development so that its progression can be halted or retarded. Screening is a form of secondary prevention.

3 **Tertiary prevention** refers to the rehabilitation of patients or treatment interventions once an illness has manifested itself.

Screening programmes (secondary prevention) take the form of health checks, such as measuring weight, blood pressure, height (particularly in children), urine, carrying out cervical smears and mammograms and offering genetic tests for illnesses such as Huntington's disease, some forms of breast cancer and cystic fibrosis. Until recently, two broad types of screening were defined: *opportunistic screening*, which involves using the time when a patient is involved with the medical services to measure aspects of their health (e.g. when seeing a patient for a sore throat the GP may decide to also check their blood pressure), and *population screening*, which involves setting up services specifically aimed at identifying problems. For example, current programmes involve cervical screening and breast screening. Recently a new form of screening has emerged in the form of *self-screening*. For example, people are encouraged to practise breast and testicular self-examination and it is now possible to buy over-the-counter kits to measure blood pressure, cholesterol and blood sugar levels.

The aim of all screening programmes is to detect a problem at the asymptomatic stage. This results in two outcomes. First, screening can discover a risk of the disease. This is called *primary screening*. For example, cervical screening may detect pre-cancerous cells which place the individual at risk of cervical cancer; genetic screening for cystic fibrosis would give the person an estimate of risk of producing children with cystic fibrosis; and cholesterol screening could place an individual at high risk of developing coronary heart disease (CHD). Second, screening can detect the illness itself. This is called *secondary screening*. For example, a mammogram may discover breast cancer, genetic testing may discover the gene for Huntington's disease and blood pressure assessment may discover hypertension. The recent enthusiasm for screening is reflected in an often-repeated statement by King Edward VII in the early years of the twentieth century: 'If preventable, why not prevented?'.

GUIDELINES FOR SCREENING

As a result of the enthusiasm for screening, sets of criteria have been established. Wilson (1965) outlined the following:

- **The disease**
  - an important problem
  - recognizable at the latent or early symptomatic stage
  - natural history must be understood (including development from latent to symptomatic stage)

- **The screen**
  - suitable test or examination (of reasonable sensitivity and specificity)
  - test should be acceptable by the population being screened
  - screening must be a continuous process

- **Follow-up**
  - facilities must exist for assessment and treatment
  - accepted form of effective treatment
  - agreed policy on whom to treat

- **Economy**
  - cost must be economically balanced in relation to possible expenditure on medical care as a whole

More recently, the criteria have been developed as follows:

- The disease must be sufficiently prevalent and/or sufficiently serious to make early detection appropriate.
- The disease must be sufficiently well defined to permit accurate diagnosis.
- There must be a possibility (or probability) that the disease exists undiagnosed in many cases (i.e. that the disease is not so manifest by symptoms as to make rapid diagnosis almost inevitable).
- There must be a beneficial outcome from early diagnosis in terms of disease treatment or prevention of complications.
- There must be a screening test that has good sensitivity and specificity and a reasonably positive predictive value in the population to be screened.

Research has explored screening in terms of: (1) the predictors of uptake; and (2) the psychological impact of screening.

THE PREDICTORS OF SCREENING UPTAKE

The numbers of individuals who attend different screening programmes vary enormously according to factors such as the country, the illness being screened and the time of the screening programme. For example, uptake for neonatal screening for phenylketonuria is almost 100 per cent. However, whereas up to 99 per cent of pregnant women in Sweden and France undertake HIV testing (Larsson et al. 1990; Moatti et al. 1990), in the UK and North America only a small minority elect to take the test. Marteau (1993) suggested that there are three main factors that influence uptake of screening: patient factors, health professional factors and organizational factors. These are illustrated in Figure 9.10.

1. Patient Factors

Several studies have been carried out to examine which factors predict the uptake of screening. These have included demographic factors, health beliefs, emotional factors and contextual factors.

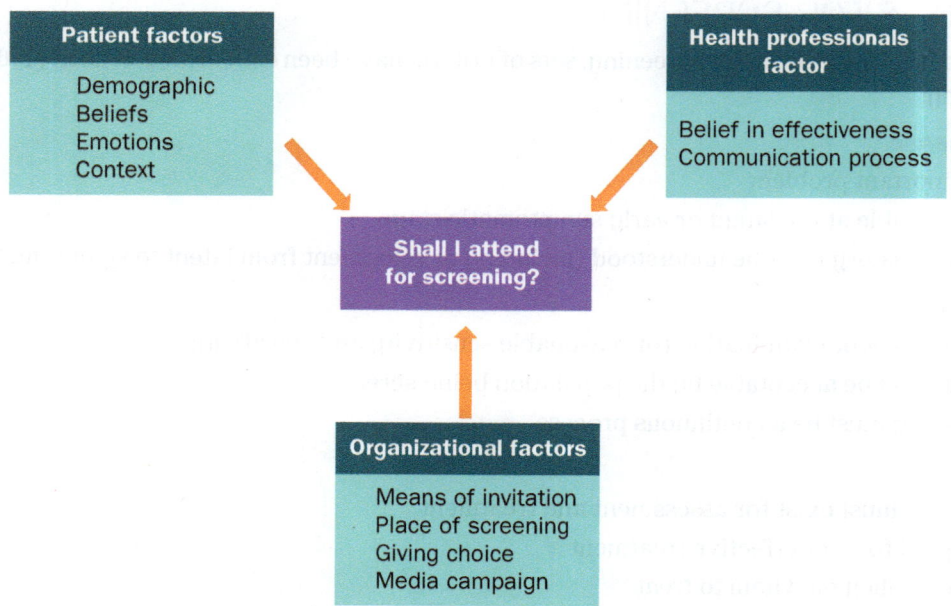

Patient factors

Demographic
Beliefs
Emotions
Context

Health professionals factor

Belief in effectiveness
Communication process

Shall I attend for screening?

Organizational factors

Means of invitation
Place of screening
Giving choice
Media campaign

Figure 9.10 Predicting screening update

Demographic Factors

Simpson et al. (1997) concluded that older women were more likely to attend a worksite screening programme for cardiovascular disease than either younger women or men. In contrast, research shows that women are less likely to attend for lung cancer screening than men, along with those who are older, current smokers and of lower socio-economic status (Ali et al. 2015). In addition, Waller et al. (1990) suggested that those individuals who are the most healthy are more likely to attend for an HIV test, and Sutton et al. (2000) reported that men, home-owners, non-smokers, those who have regular check-ups at the dentist and those with better subjective health were more likely to attend for flexible sigmoidoscopy which screens for colorectal cancer. Bunten et al. (2020) carried out a systematic review of nine studies to assess uptake of NHS Health Checks (NHSHCs). The results showed that older patients and females were more likely to attend although the impact of gender wasn't as consistent as often assumed. They also concluded that the role of ethnicity and deprivation on uptake was mixed across the studies. Similarly, from their review of 18 studies, Moons et al. (2020) concluded that the uptake of screening for colorectal cancer screening prior to colonoscopy was higher in women, although more cancers are diagnosed in men and uptake was lower in those of lower socio-economic status. Mottram et al. (2021) carried out a systematic review and meta-analysis of 66 studies and concluded that breast screening attendance was associated with higher socioeconomic status; higher income; home ownership; being non-immigrant; being married/cohabiting and medium (vs low) level of education and not having had a previous false-positive result. There were no differences by age group or by rural versus urban residence.

Health Beliefs

Health beliefs have also been linked to uptake and have been measured using a number of models (see Chapter 3). For example, Bish et al. (2000) used the health belief model (HBM) and the theory of planned behaviour (TPB) to predict uptake of a routine cervical smear test. The results showed that the TPB was a better predictor of behavioural intentions but that neither model successfully predicted actual uptake at follow-up. Pakenham et al. (2000) also used the HBM in conjunction with knowledge and sociodemographic variables to predict re-attendance for mammography screening. The results showed that although the re-attenders were older and more likely to be married, the HBM variable of perceived benefits of the mammography was a better predictor overall of re-attendance than sociodemographic variables. Likewise, Marmarà et al. (2017) reported that most components of the HBM (perceived barriers; cues to action; self-efficacy) predicted uptake of breast cancer screening in Malta. Similarly, Sutton et al. (2000) also included measures of beliefs and reported that a perception of fewer barriers and more benefits predicted attendance for sigmoidoscopy screening. Over the past few years several reviews of the evidence have been carried out. For example, from studies using the HBM, the best predictors of colorectal cancer screening are: increased perceived susceptibility, benefits and cues to action and reduced perceived barriers (Lau et al. 2020). Likewise, a review of the role of health beliefs in predicting breast cancer screening or self-initiated medical help-seeking showed a key role for: higher perceived barriers to mammography, greater perceived benefits and motivation towards screening, and higher perceived seriousness and susceptibility towards breast cancer (Grimley et al. 2020). Further, Dormandy et al. (2006) explored the predictors of screening for Down's syndrome in pregnant women and showed that although attitudes towards the test predicted both behavioural intentions and uptake of the test, this association was undermined by ambivalence measured by high scores on two items 'For me, having the screening test for Down's syndrome when I am 15 to 16 weeks pregnant will be a bad thing/not a bad thing' and 'For me, having the screening test for Down's syndrome when I am 15 to 16 weeks pregnant will be a good thing/not a good thing'. Some studies have also explored ways to increase uptake of screening through behavioural interventions. For example, Luszczynska et al. (2010) used a stage-matched intervention to encourage participants to focus on the pros of screening for cervical cancer and reported an increase in intentions to participate and Sandberg and Conner (2009) argued that simply completing measures of anticipated regret about not attending cervical screening increased actual attendance by follow-up.

Emotional Factors

Emotional factors such as anxiety, stress, fear, anticipated regret, embarrassment, disgust, uncertainty and feeling indecent have also been shown to relate to uptake. For example, fear has been shown to predict non-uptake of health screening in men (Teo et al. 2016). Morison et al. (2010) explored parental uptake of a school-based vaccination programme for 11–12-year-old girls for the HPV virus that can cause cervical cancer. The results showed that intentions to vaccinate the child were predicted by a number of beliefs but also showed a significant role for anticipated regret if the child did not have the vaccine. Research, also shows that declining a test can result in elevated stress. For example, Almqvist et al. (2003) explored the longer-term consequences of either having or not having a genetic test for Huntington's disease and reported that those who declined the test were the most distressed over a period of 12 months.

Young and Robb (2021) carried out a narrative review of the role of emotions in predicting screening uptake for a range of cancers and concluded that while emotions play a role different aspects of emotions can affect uptake in different ways. In particular they concluded:

- Fear, worry and disgust are more common in those less likely to attend cancer screening.
- Fear can be both a barrier and a facilitator to uptake.
- Fear of cancer can motivate screening attendance.
- Fear of potential embarrassment, discomfort or pain is a barrier to breast, cervical and colorectal screening.
- Worry about cancer is a motivator for breast, cervical and colorectal cancer screening but moderate worry is more motivating than low or high levels or worry.
- Disgust, such as handling stool samples, predicts avoiding colorectal cancer screening.

Some research has also focused on patients' need to reduce their uncertainty and to find 'cognitive closure'. For example, Eiser and Cole (2002) used a quantitative method based upon the stages of change (SOC) model and explored differences between individuals at different stages of attending for a cervical smear in terms of 'cognitive closure' and barriers to screening. The results showed that the pre-contemplators reported most barriers and the least need for closure and to reduce uncertainty. One qualitative study further highlighted the role of emotional factors in the form of feeling indecent. Borrayo and Jenkins (2001) interviewed 34 women of Mexican descent in five focus groups about their beliefs about breast cancer screening and their decision whether or not to take part. The analyses showed that the women reported a fundamental problem with breast screening as it violates a basic cultural standard. Breast screening requires women to touch their own breasts and to expose their breasts to health professionals. Within the cultural norms of respectable female behaviour for these women, this was seen as 'indecent'.

Contextual Factors

Finally, contextual factors have also been shown to predict uptake and can at times be very personal to the individual concerned. For example, Smith et al. (2002) interviewed women who had been offered genetic testing for Huntington's disease. The results showed that the women often showed complex and sometimes contradictory beliefs about their risk status for the disease which related to factors such as prevalence in the family, family size, attempts to make the numbers 'add up' and beliefs about transmission. The results also showed that uptake of the test related not only to the individual's risk perception but also to contextual factors such as family discussion or a key triggering event. For example, one woman described how she had shouted at the cats for going on to the new stair carpet which had been paid for from her father's insurance money after he had died from Huntington's disease. This had made her resolve to have the test.

2. Health Professional Factors

In a study of GPs' attitudes and screening behaviour, a belief in the effectiveness of screening was associated with an organized approach to screening and time spent on screening (Havelock et al. 1988).

Such factors may influence patient uptake. In addition, the means of presenting a test may also influence uptake. For example, uptake rates for HIV testing at antenatal clinics are reported to vary from 3 to 82 per cent (Meadows et al. 1990). These rates may well be related to the way in which these tests were offered by the health professional, which in turn may reflect the health professional's own beliefs about the test. Some research has also focused on the patient/health professional relationship (see later in this chapter for a discussion of the consultation). For example, McLachlan et al. (2018) used a qualitative design and found that the development of a trusting and empathic health professional relationship was critical to screening uptake by patients.

3. Organizational Factors

Many organizational factors may also influence the uptake of screening. Research has examined the effects of the means of invitation on the uptake rate and indicates that if the invitation is issued in person, and if the individual is expected to opt out, not in, the rates of uptake are higher (Mann et al. 1988; Smith et al. 1990). Further, Gidlow et al. (2019) carried out a randomized controlled trial (RCT) to test whether invitation letters personalized to a patient's risk of cardiovascular diseases (CVD), or telephone invitations, could elicit higher uptake for a NHS health check than the current standardized letter. The results showed that a telephone invitation was far more effective (18 per cent more likely to attend) and more effective for younger patients and those with lower CVD risk. The place of the screening programme may also be influential, with more accessible settings promoting higher uptake. In addition, uptake may also be influenced by education and media campaigns. For example, Fernbach (2002) evaluated the impact of a large media campaign designed to influence women's self-efficacy and uptake of cervical screening. The media campaign was called the 'Papscreen Victoria' campaign and took place in Australia. It was evaluated by face-to-face interviews with 1,571 women at baseline and two follow-ups. The results showed that women reported an increase in awareness of cervical screening and rated this as a greater health priority than before the campaign. However, the results were not all positive. The women also stated after the campaign that they would find it more difficult to ring up for test results and reported lowered self-efficacy. Likewise, Durkin et al. (2019) carried out a field experiment to compare an 8-week intensive mass media campaign (eg. 30-second television advertising) versus a less intensive mass media campaign (eg. print materials) on bowel cancer screening uptake using immunochemical faecal occult blood test (iFOBT) kits. The results showed increased return of the kits during and up to 2 months after the intensive media campaign. While more kits were returned after the less intensive campaign, the increase was less pronounced. Finally, time also seems to have an impact. In some countries women can self-check for the HPV virus rather than attend for cervical screening. Bosgraaf et al. (2014) conducted a self-reported questionnaire study with 9,484 women in the Netherlands to explore attendance for HPV screening and the use of a self-sampling device. The results showed that the most common reason for not attending screening was forgetting to make an appointment. The results also showed that the preference for self-sampling over cervical screening at a clinic was simply due to time.

THE PSYCHOLOGICAL IMPACT OF SCREENING

While research indicates positive consequences to the patient of being involved in a screening programme for pancreatic cancer (Cazacu et al. 2019), prenatal screening (Biesecker 2019) and breast cancer screening for those with family histories of breast cancer (Castelo et al. 2021), screening can have several negative consequences. Some of these are practical, such as financial cost and time to the health service and to the patient, and have been described as the 'intangible costs' (Kinlay 1988). Research also indicates that some costs of screening are also experienced by the individuals involved. These psychological consequences can be a result of the various different stages of the screening process:

1 *The receipt of a screening invitation.* Research indicates that sending out invitations to enter into a screening programme may not only influence an individual's behaviour, but also their

psychological state. Fallowfield et al. (1990) carried out a retrospective study of women's responses to receiving a request to attend a breast screening session. Their results showed that 55 per cent reported feeling worried although 93 per cent were pleased. Dean et al. (1984) sent a measure of psychological morbidity to women awaiting breast screening and then followed them up six months later. The results showed no significant increases in psychological morbidity. However, when asked in retrospect 30 per cent said that they had become anxious after receiving the letter of invitation. Therefore receiving a screening invitation may increase anxiety. However, some research suggests that this is not always the case (Cockburn et al. 1994).

2 *The receipt of a negative result.* It may be assumed that receiving a negative result (i.e. not having the condition being tested for) would only decrease an individual's anxiety. Most research suggests that this is the case and that a negative result may create a sense of reassurance (Orton et al. 1991) or no change in anxiety (Sutton et al. 1995). Further, Sutton (1999), in his review of the literature on receiving a negative result following breast cancer screening, concluded that 'anxiety is not a significant problem among women who receive a negative screening result'. However, some research points towards residual levels of anxiety which do not return to baseline (Baillie et al. 2000) and that, even following negative results, some people attend for further tests even though these tests have not been clinically recommended (e.g. Lerman et al. 2000; Michie et al. 2002). Michie et al. (2003) used qualitative methods to explore why negative genetic results can fail to reassure. They interviewed nine people who had received a negative result for familial adenomatous polyposis (FAP) which is a genetic condition and results in polyps in the bowel which can become cancerous if not detected and removed by surgery. They argued that people may not be reassured by a negative result for two reasons. First, they may hold a belief about the cause of the illness that does not directly map onto the cause being tested for. In the case of FAP, people described how they believed that it was caused by genetics but that genetics could change. Therefore, although the test indicated that they did not have the relevant genes, this may not be the case in the future. Second, they may show a lack of faith in the test itself. For FAP, people were sceptical about the ability of a blood test to inform about a disease that occurred in the bowel. Some research has also explored the ways in which a negative result is presented. In the UK in 1997 the policy recommendation for cervical smear results stated that the term 'negative result' could be confusing as women would feel 'positive' to such a 'negative' result and that the term 'normal' smear result should be used instead. Marteau et al. (2006) explored the impact of receiving a result that was either presented as 'normal', or normal and a series of statements of risk, that is, 'you are at low risk of having or developing cervical cancer in the next five years' and a range of numerical presentations of risk. Participants were then asked to describe their levels of perceived risk. The results showed that, when only told that their smear result was 'normal' without any description of risk, women described feeling less at risk than when they received 'normal' and the description of risk. Marteau et al. (2006) argued that a negative smear result still implies a low risk of getting cervical cancer and that the term 'normal' makes people underestimate this risk.

3 *The receipt of a positive result.* As expected, the receipt of a positive result can be associated with a variety of negative emotions ranging from worry to anxiety and shock. For example, an abnormal cervical smear may generate anxiety, morbidity and even terror (Wilkinson et al. 1990; Isaka et al. 2017). Psychological costs have also been reported after screening for CHD (Stoate 1989), breast cancer (Espasa et al. 2012) and genetic diseases (Marteau et al. 2004). However, some research suggests that these psychological changes may only be maintained in the short term and quickly return to baseline levels (Broadstock et al. 2000). This decay in the psychological consequences has been particularly shown with the termination of pregnancy following the detection of foetal abnormalities (Black 1989) and following the receipt of a positive genetic test result (Broadstock et al. 2000). Collins et al. (2011a) carried out a systematic review of screening procedures for a number of health problems and concluded that receiving a positive test result results in a small increase in depression

but that this is short-lasting. Some research has also explored the impact of receiving a positive genetic test result upon individuals' beliefs about their condition and subsequent behaviour. Such an approach is in line with a self-regulatory model (see Chapter 8). For example, Marteau et al. (2004) explored the impact of telling people that they had tested positive for familial hypercholesterolae-mia on their beliefs about the nature of their condition and their behaviour. The results showed that those who were told that they had a genetic mutation reported a lower belief that their cholesterol could be managed by diet. Therefore, being given a medical model of their problem made them less likely to endorse a behavioural solution. No effect was found, however, for perceptions of control, adherence to medication or risk-reducing behaviours. Similarly, two systematic reviews of the impact of communication of personalized genetic risk to patients concluded that such information had no impact upon beliefs about fatalism or perceptions of control and no impact on actual behaviours such as smoking and physical activity (Marteau et al. 2010; Collins et al. 2011b).

4   *The receipt of an inadequate test result.* Although many tests produce either positive or negative results, some produce inadequate results which neither confirm nor disconfirm the presence of the condition. An example of this is cervical screening whereby the test can be 'ruined' due to the presence of pus or the absence of a sufficient number of cervical cells. French et al. (2004, 2006b) explored the immediate and longer-term psychological consequences of receiving either an inadequate test result (n = 180) or a normal test result (n = 226). The results showed that women with an inadequate result reported more anxiety and more concern about their result, perceived themselves to be more at risk of cervical cancer and were less satisfied with the information they had received immediately following the result. By three months' follow-up, the women who had the inadequate results were no longer more anxious. They were, however, more concerned about their test results and less satisfied with the information they had received even after having normal results from subsequent tests. Similarly, Quaife et al. (2021) concluded from their review that the receipt of an indeterminate result following low-dose computed tomography (LDCT) for lung cancer resulted in increased anxiety and lung cancer-specific distress in the short-term but that this appeared to be resolved at long-term follow up.

5   *Being involved in a screening programme.* Most research has explored the relative impact of receiving a positive or negative result from a screening procedure. Collins et al. (2011a) carried out a systematic review to explore the impact of taking part in a screening procedure regardless of the test results. They identified 12 randomized controlled trials for a range of problems including cancer, Type 2 diabetes, CHD and a genetic risk for lung cancer and explored changes in psychological morbidity both before and after four weeks. The results showed no evidence for raised levels of either depression or anxiety or reduced quality of life in the longer term (more than four weeks). Insufficient data were available for an analysis of short-term effects. They argued that their results illustrate a process of self-regulation, with initial negative responses being minimized by one month as people draw upon a number of cognitive strategies to reduce their sense of threat.

6   *The existence of a screening programme.* Marteau (1993) suggested that the existence of screening programmes may influence social beliefs about what is healthy and may change society's attitude towards a screened condition. In a study by Marteau and Riordan (1992), health profession-als were asked to rate their attitudes towards two hypothetical patients, one of whom had attended a screening programme and one who had not. Both patients were described as having developed cervical cancer. The results showed that the health professionals held more negative attitudes towards the patient who had not attended. In terms of the wider effects of screening programmes, it is possible that the existence of such programmes encourages society to see illnesses as prevent-able and the responsibility of the individual, which may lead to victim-blaming of those individuals who still develop these illnesses. This may be relevant to illnesses such as CHD, cervical cancer and breast cancer, which have established screening programmes. In the future, it may also be relevant to genetic disorders which could have been eradicated by terminations.

IN SUMMARY

Screening aims to detect an illness while it is still at an asymptomatic stage as a means to offer early intervention and increase the chances of a positive health outcome. Psychological factors are involved in the uptake of screening and its impact upon the individual. Once then in the health care system, whether through help seeking or screening, patients come into contact with a health care professional in a medical consultation. This will now be explored.

5   THE MEDICAL CONSULTATION

The core component of any interaction with a health care system is the consultation between patient and health professional as this is the context within which key decisions about diagnosis and management strategy are made.

Traditional models of the consultation regarded doctors as having an objective knowledge set that came from their extensive medical education and was communicated to a passive patient who absorbed any suggestions and responded accordingly. Therefore doctors were the experts and patients needed to be educated. Over time this model has evolved towards the notion of the 'expert patient' who has their own beliefs and expectations and doctors who have become more 'human', based upon both personal and professional experience. This shift in perspective is in part a response to an increase in consumerism, patient knowledge and rights, and the availability of medical information through the internet. It is also due to a recognition of the problem of doctor variability and the many factors involved in doctors' decision-making. This section will describe the problem of doctor variability, how doctors make decisions, the role of health professionals' beliefs and the nature of the modern consultation with its focus on patient-centredness and agreement between the health professional and patient.

THE PROBLEM OF DOCTOR VARIABILITY

If doctors were simply the experts who behaved according to their extensive knowledge and training then it could be predicted that doctors with similar levels of knowledge and training would behave in similar ways. Considerable variability has been found, however, among doctors in terms of different aspects of their practice (see Figure 9.11). Some variability is good as research indicates that patients prefer different styles of consultation (Mazzi et al. 2015). Some variability, however, has implications for patient safety. For example, Anderson et al. (1983) reported that doctors differ in their diagnosis of asthma. Mapes (1980) suggested that they vary in terms of their prescribing behaviour, with a variation of 15–90 per cent of patients receiving drugs. Bucknall et al. (1986) reported variation in the methods used by doctors to measure blood pressure, Marteau and Baum (1984) also reported that doctors vary in their treatment of diabetes and Hanbury et al. (2009) indicated that health professionals varied in their adherence to guidelines regarding suicide prevention. Similar variation was also shown in a study of doctor attitudes towards prescribing HAART for patients with HIV infection (Moatti et al. 2000). For example, although a large majority of doctors stated that they would prescribe HAART in line with official recommendations

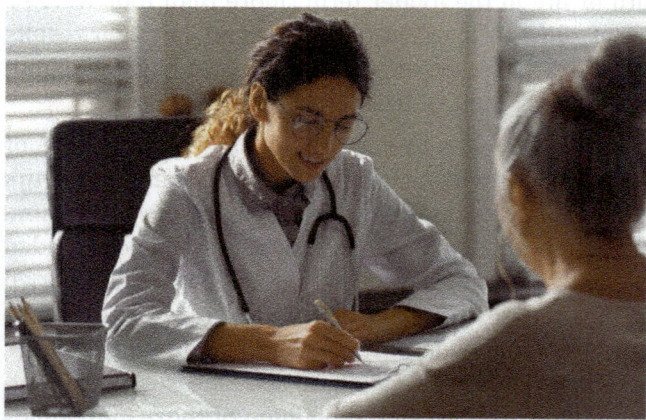

The medical consultation is core to most health care decisions

SOURCE: ©Shutterstock/fizkes

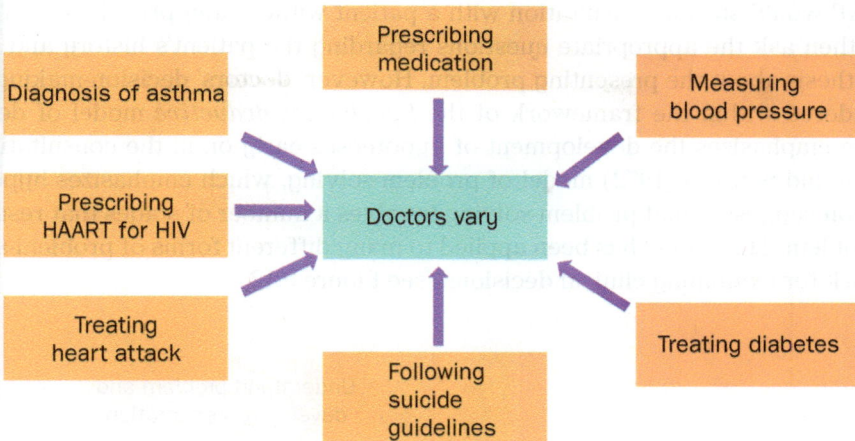

Figure 9.11 The problem of doctor variability

when all patient details were presented, there was much variability in prescribing for patients with less clear histories, indicating that the same patient would receive a different management procedure if they visited more than one doctor. Similar variability can be seen for the treatment of acute myocardial infarction (AMI, heart attack) (Venturini et al. 1999). Although there is clear evidence that AMI should be treated immediately, a study of 1,976 patients from 10 countries showed wide variability with 63.7 per cent being given thrombolysis, 88 per cent being given aspirin and 65.9 per cent being given beta-adrenergic blocking agents. Guidelines indicate that all patients should be given all of these treatments. According to a traditional educational model of doctor – patient communication, this variability could be understood in terms of differing levels of knowledge and expertise. However, this variability can also be understood by examining the other factors involved in the clinical decision-making process.

HOW DOCTORS MAKE DECISIONS

Health professionals are not just confronted with patients with illnesses, diseases or syndromes such as cancer, heart disease or multiple sclerosis: they have patients sitting opposite them with a huge range of vague and often very common symptoms such as headaches, back pain, tiredness and bowel changes, and their role is to decide what these symptoms mean. This involves differentiating between the pain in the chest that means 'indigestion' and the one that means 'heart disease', and the raised temperature that means 'a cold' and the one that means 'meningitis'. Once a problem has been diagnosed, they then have to decide on an appropriate management strategy which could range from 'do nothing, it will go away', to 'prescribe medicine', to 'refer as a non-urgent patient for a second opinion', to 'refer urgently' or 'call the ambulance'. The doctor's role is therefore highly skilled and complex. It is further complicated by the high numbers of people coming through their doors with housing, relationship and benefit issues, symptoms that 'they had last week', patients who come every week with a different symptom and patients who are too embarrassed to describe the real reason for their visit but spend the consultation describing another symptom that is really irrelevant. Therefore, the process of clinical decision-making has to be understood within the framework of problem-solving.

A Model of Problem-Solving

Clinical decision-making processes are a specialized form of problem-solving and have been studied within the context of problem-solving and theories of information processing. It is often assumed that clinical decisions are made by the process of *inductive reasoning*, which involves collecting evidence and data and using these data to develop a conclusion and a hypothesis. For example, within this framework, a GP would start a consultation with a patient without any prior model of their problem. The GP would then ask the appropriate questions regarding the patient's history and symptoms and develop a hypothesis about the presenting problem. However, doctors' decision-making processes are generally considered within the framework of the *hypothetico-deductive* model of decision-making. This perspective emphasizes the development of hypotheses early on in the consultation and is illustrated by Newell and Simon's (1972) model of problem-solving, which emphasizes hypothesis testing. Newell and Simon suggested that problem-solving involves a number of stages that result in a solution to any given problem. This model has been applied to many different forms of problem-solving and is a useful framework for examining clinical decisions (see Figure 9.12).

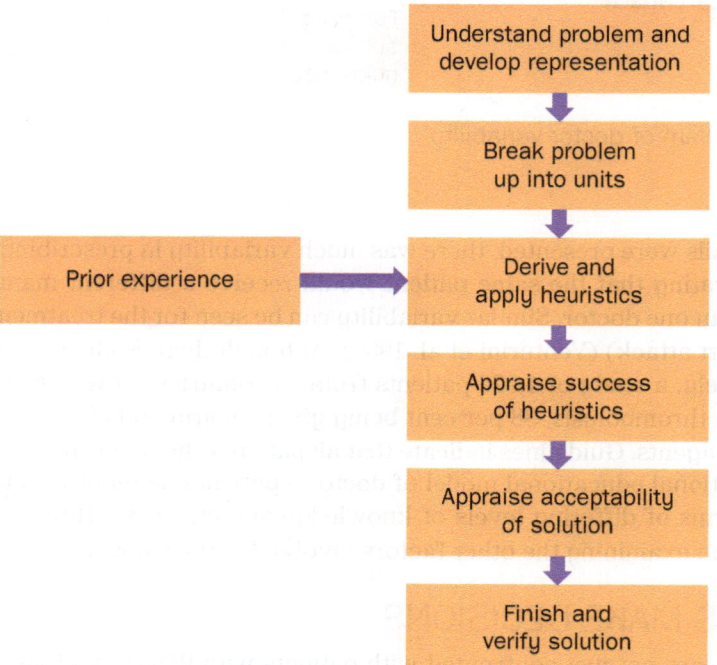

Figure 9.12 A simplified model of problem-solving

The stages involved are as follows:

1 *Understand the nature of the problem and develop an internal representation.* At this stage, the individual needs to formulate an internal representation of the problem. This process involves understanding the goal of the problem, evaluating any given conditions and assessing the nature of the available data.

2 *Develop a plan of action for solving the problem.* Newell and Simon differentiated between two types of plan: heuristics and algorithms. An algorithm is a set of rules that will provide a correct solution if applied correctly (e.g. addition, multiplication, etc. involve algorithms). However, most human problem-solving involves heuristics, which are 'rules of thumb'. Heuristics are less definite and specific but provide guidance and direction for the problem-solver. Heuristics may involve developing parallels between the present problem and previous similar ones.

3 *Apply heuristics.* Once developed, the plans are then applied to the given situation.

4 *Determine whether heuristics have been fruitful.* The individual then decides whether the heuristics have been successful in the attempt to solve the given problem. If they are considered unsuccessful, the individual may need to develop a new approach to the problem.

5 *Determine whether an acceptable solution has been obtained.*

6 *Finish and verify the solution.* The end-point of the problem-solving process involves the individual deciding that an acceptable solution to the problem has been reached and that this solution provides a suitable outcome.

According to Newell and Simon's model of problem-solving, hypotheses about the causes and solutions to the problem are developed very early on in the process. They regarded this process as dynamic and ever-changing and suggested that at each stage the individual applies a 'means end analysis', whereby they assess the value of the hypothesis, which is either accepted or rejected according to the evidence. This type of model involves information processing whereby the individual develops hypotheses to convert an open problem, which may be unmanageable with no obvious end-point, to one that can be closed and tested by a series of hypotheses.

Clinical Decisions as Problem-Solving

Clinical decisions can be conceptualized as a form of problem-solving and involve the development of hypotheses early on in the consultation process. These hypotheses are subsequently tested by the doctor's selection of questions. Models of problem-solving have been applied to clinical decision-making by several authors (e.g. MacWhinney 1973), who have argued that the process of formulating a clinical decision involves the stages shown in Figure 9.13.

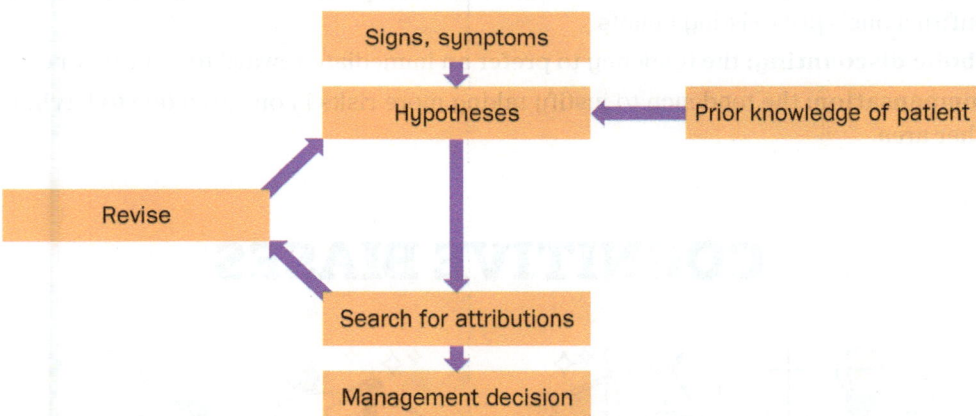

Figure 9.13 Diagnosis as a form of problem-solving

1 *Accessing information about the patient's symptoms.* The initial questions in any consultation from the health professional to the patient will enable the health professional to understand the nature of the problem and to form an internal representation of the type of problem.

2 *Developing hypotheses.* Early on in the problem-solving process, the health professional develops hypotheses about the possible causes and solutions to the problem.

3 *Search for attributes.* The health professional then proceeds to test the hypotheses by searching for factors either to confirm or to refute them. Research into the hypothesis-testing process has indicated that although doctors aim to either confirm or refute their hypothesis by asking balanced questions, most of their questioning is biased towards confirmation of their *original* hypothesis. Therefore an initial hypothesis that a patient has a psychological problem may cause the doctor to focus on the patient's psychological state and ignore the patient's attempt to talk about their physical symptoms. Studies have shown that doctors' clinical information collected subsequent to the development of a hypothesis may be systematically distorted to support the original hypothesis (Wallsten 1978). Furthermore, the type of hypothesis has been shown to bias the collection and interpretation of any information received during the consultation (Wason 1974).

4 *Making a management decision.* The outcome of the clinical decision-making process involves the health professional deciding on the way forward. The outcome of a consultation and a diagnosis, however, is not an absolute entity, but is itself a hypothesis and an informed guess that will be either confirmed or refuted by future events.

The role of cognitive bias

As with all decision-making, clinical decision-making is influenced by a wide range of cognitive biases which influence all aspects of the decision-making process from the questions asked to access the patients' symptoms, how the original hypothesis is developed and what this hypothesis is, which attributes are searched for and what answered are listened and then which management decision is finally settled upon. The classic work by Kahneman and Tversky (eg. 1972; 1983; 1996) described how decision-making is underpinned by two systems, namely a fast one which is driven by heuristics and a slower one which involves a more rational and considered approach. They also described range of cognitive biases which influence decision-making. These are illustrated in Figure 9.14 and include:

- **The availability bias:** the tendency to overestimate the likelihood of an event due to greater 'availability' in memory (e.g. more recent, more emotional, more unusual).
- **The anchoring bias:** the tendency to rely too heavily on one piece of information (usually the first piece of information acquired).
- **The confirmation bias:** the tendency to search for, interpret, focus on and remember information that confirms one's pre-existing beliefs.
- **Hyperbolic discounting:** the tendency to prefer an immediate reward to a future one.
- **Risk compensation:** the tendency to justify taking more risks in one area due to having been safer in another area.

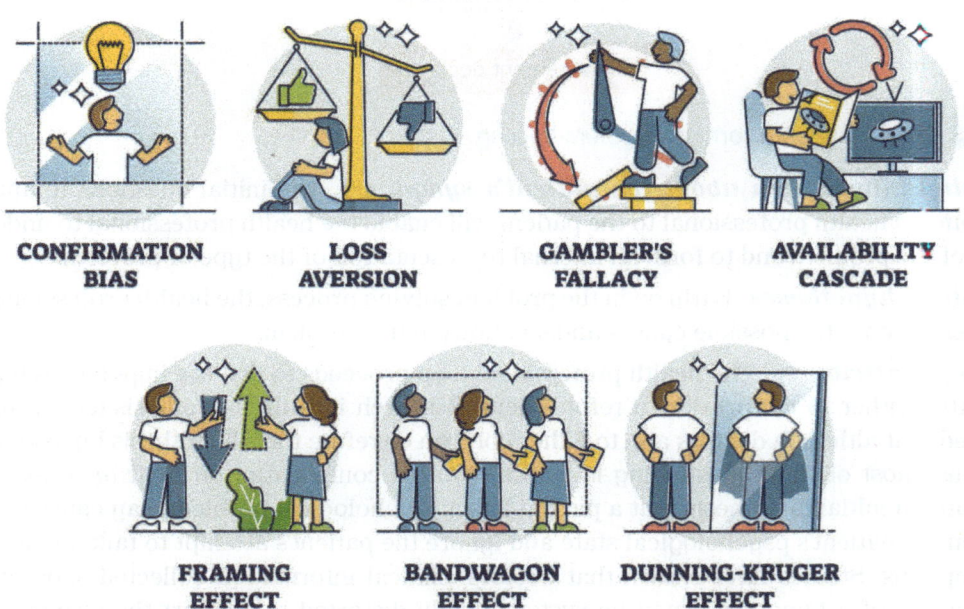

Figure 9.14: Cognitive bias

SOURCE: ©Shutterstock/VectorMine

Featherston et al. (2020) carried out a scoping review (n = 149) and identified 27 biases that influenced decisions made by allied healthcare professionals and concluded that confirmation bias (n = 12) was one of the most frequently tested cognitive biases. Elston (2020) wrote an interesting analysis of the role of biases in decision-making and argued that while healthcare professionals are hard wired for confirmation bias, techniques can be used to counterbalance these tendencies such as attempting to disprove the favoured diagnosis or performing balanced testing. He also summed this up nicely and said, 'When you hear hoofbeats, think of horses but don't forget to consider zebras and always keep in mind that your favoured diagnosis could be wrong'.

Explaining Variability

Variability in the behaviour of health professionals can therefore be understood in terms of the processes involved in clinical decisions. For example, health professionals may:

- access different information about the patient's symptoms
- develop different hypotheses
- access different attributes either to confirm or to refute their hypotheses
- have differing degrees of a bias towards confirmation
- consequently reach different management decisions.

This variability will be influenced by a range of cognitive biases. It is also influenced by the health professional's own beliefs.

HEALTH PROFESSIONALS' HEALTH BELIEFS

Patients are described as having lay beliefs, which are individual and variable. Health professionals are usually described as having professional beliefs, which are often assumed to be consistent and predictable. However, the many stages of clinical decision-making from the development of the original hypothesis to the management decision involves the health professional's own health beliefs, which may vary as much as those of the patient (see Chapters 2 and 8). Components of models such as the HBM, protection motivation theory (PMT) together with their illness beliefs have been developed to examine health professionals' beliefs. The beliefs involved in decision-making can be categorized as follows:

1 *The health professional's own beliefs about the nature of clinical problems.* Health professionals have their own beliefs about health and illness. This pre-existing factor will influence their choice of hypothesis. For example, if a health professional believes that health and illness are determined by biomedical factors (e.g. lesions, bacteria, viruses) then they will develop a hypothesis about the patient's problem that reflects this perspective (e.g. a patient who reports feeling tired all the time may be anaemic). However, a health professional who views health and illness as relating to psychosocial factors may develop hypotheses reflecting this perspective (e.g. a patient who reports feeling tired all the time may be under stress).

2 *The health professional's estimate of the probability of the hypothesis and disease.* Health professionals will have pre-existing beliefs about the prevalence and incidence of any given health problem that will influence the process of developing a hypothesis. For example, some doctors may regard childhood asthma as a common complaint and hypothesize that a child presenting with a cough has asthma, whereas others may believe that childhood asthma is rare and so will not consider this hypothesis.

3 *The seriousness and treatability of the disease.* Health professionals are motivated to consider the 'payoff' involved in reaching a correct diagnosis and that this will influence their choice of hypothesis. This payoff is related to their beliefs about the seriousness and treatability of an illness. For example, a child presenting with abdominal pain may result in an original hypothesis of appendicitis as this is both a serious and treatable condition, and the benefits of arriving at the correct diagnosis for this condition far outweigh the costs involved (such as time-wasting) if this hypothesis is refuted.

4 *Personal knowledge of the patient.* The original hypothesis will also be related to the health professional's existing knowledge of the patient. This may include the patient's medical history, knowledge about their psychological state, an understanding of their psychosocial environment and a belief about why the patient uses medical services.

5 *The health professional's stereotypes.* Stereotypes are sometimes seen as problematic and as confounding the decision-making process. However, most meetings between health professionals and patients are time-limited and consequently stereotypes play a central role in developing and testing a hypothesis and reaching a management decision. Stereotypes reflect the process of 'cognitive economy' and may be developed according to a multitude of factors such as how the patient looks/talks/walks or whether they remind the health professional of previous patients. Without stereotypes, consultations between health professionals and patients would be extremely time-consuming.

Other factors that may influence the development of the original hypothesis include the following:

1 *The health professional's mood.* The health professional's mood may influence the choice of hypotheses and the subsequent process of testing this hypothesis. Isen et al. (1991) manipulated mood in a group of medical students and evaluated the effect of induced positive affect on their decision-making processes. Positive affect was induced by informing subjects in this group that they had performed in the top 3 per cent of all graduate students nationwide in an anagram task. All subjects were then given a set of hypothetical patients and asked to decide which one was most likely to have lung cancer. The results showed that those subjects in the positive affect group spent less time to reach the correct decision and showed greater interest in the case histories by going beyond the assigned task. The authors therefore concluded that mood influenced the subjects' decision-making processes. Research has also explored the role of the health care professional's own emotions when working with seriously ill and dying patients (Childers and Arnold 2019) and when managing angry patients in emergency settings (Isbell et al. 2020) and highlights how there can often be a tension between personal emotion and what is a seen as a professional role and how this can impact upon the decisions made, the quality of care provided to the patient and the well-being of the health care professional.

2 *The profile characteristics of the health professional.* Factors such as age, sex, weight, geographical location, previous experience and the health professional's own behaviour may also affect the decision-making process. For example, smoking doctors have been shown to spend more time counselling about smoking than their non-smoking counterparts (Stokes and Rigotti 1988). Further, thinner practice nurses have been shown to have different beliefs about obesity and offer different advice to obese patients than overweight practice nurses (Hoppe and Ogden 1997). Likewise, Rajiah and Venaktaraman (2019) reported that pharmacists who were older, more experienced and working in urban areas reported fewer ethical dilemmas in their practice and Brechbiel and Keeley (2019) reported that clinicians with more years of experience and slower response times had higher rates of diagnostic accuracy.

In summary, variability in health professionals' behaviour can be understood in terms of the factors involved in the decision-making process. In particular, many factors pre-dating the development of the original hypothesis such as cognitive biases and the health professional's own beliefs, mood and demographics may contribute to this variability.

COMMUNICATING BELIEFS TO PATIENTS

If health professionals hold their own cognitive biases and health-related beliefs, these may be communicated to their patients. This has particularly been studied in the domain of risk communication. A study by McNeil et al. (1982) examined the effects of health professionals' language on the patients' choice of hypothetical treatment. They assessed the effect of offering surgery either if it would 'increase the probability of survival' or would 'decrease the probability of death'. The results showed that patients are more likely to choose surgery if they believed it increased the probability of survival rather than if it decreased the probability of death. The phrasing of such a question would very much reflect the individual beliefs of the doctor, which in turn influence the choices of the patients. Similarly, Senior et al. (2000) explored the impact of framing risk for heart disease or arthritis as either genetic or unspecified using hypothetical scenarios. The results showed that how risk was presented influenced both the participants' ratings of how preventable the illness was and their beliefs about causes. In a similar vein, Misselbrook and Armstrong (2000) asked patients whether they would accept treatment to prevent stroke and presented the effectiveness of this treatment in four different ways. The results showed that although all the forms of presentation were actually the same, 92 per cent of the patients said they would accept the treatment if it reduced their chances of stroke by 45 per cent (relative risk); 75 per cent said they would accept the treatment if it reduced their risk from 1 in 400 to 1 in 700 (absolute risk); 71 per cent said they would accept it if the doctor had to treat 35 patients for 25 years to prevent one stroke (number needed to treat); and only 44 per cent said they would accept it if the treatment had a 3 per cent chance of doing them good and a 97 per cent chance of doing no good or not being needed (personal probability of benefit). Therefore, although the actual risk of the treatment was the same in all four conditions, the ways of presenting the risk varied and this resulted in a variation in patient uptake. Harris and Smith (2005) carried out a similar study but compared absolute risk (high versus low risk) with comparative risk (above average versus below average). They asked participants to read information about deep-vein thrombosis (DVT) and to rate a range of beliefs. Participants were then told to imagine their risk of DVT in either absolute or comparative terms. The results showed that the US sample were more disturbed by absolute risk. A detailed analysis of risk communication can be found in Berry (2004).

However, doctors not only have beliefs about risk but also about illness, which could be communicated to patients. Over recent years there has been much interest in the notion of weight bias and the negative views people often have about those who are obese (Pearl and Puhl 2018; see Chapter 13). In 2015, Phelan et al. carried out a review of the evidence and concluded not only that weight bias was common amongst health professionals but that it can also influence how they interact with patients and deliver health care through their interpersonal behaviour within consultations, judgments and medical decision-making. At times beliefs can also be communicated through the language used by the health professional. To assess the specific impact of language, Ogden et al. (2003) used an experimental design to explore the impact of type of diagnosis on patients' beliefs about common problems. Patients were asked to read a vignette in which a person was told either that they had a problem using a medical diagnostic term (tonsillitis/gastroenteritis) or using a lay term (sore throat/stomach upset). The results showed that, although doctors are often being told to use lay language when speaking to patients, patients actually preferred the medical labels as it made the symptoms seem more legitimate and gave the patient more confidence in the doctor. In contrast the lay terms made the patients feel more to blame for the problem. Recently, Ogden and Bridge (2022) also explored the impact of language on patients with Poly Cystic Ovary Syndrome (PCOS). Patients with PCOS were asked to recall the words used when they received their first diagnosis and showed that lower communication comfort during the diagnostic consultation and greater use of the word 'raised' predicted poorer current body esteem and poorer quality of life, greater use of the word 'irregular' predicted greater current concerns about fertility and greater focus on appearance predicted greater current concerns about hirsutism. Therefore, if a doctor holds particular beliefs about risk or the nature of an illness, and chooses language that reflects these beliefs, then these beliefs may be communicated to the patient in a way that may then influence the patient's own beliefs and their subsequent behaviour.

THE MODERN CONSULTATION

The explanations of variability in health professionals' behaviour presented so far have focused on the health professional in isolation. This explanation, however, ignores another important factor, namely the patient, as any variability in health professionals' behaviour exists in the context of both the health professional and the patient. Therefore, in order to understand any variability in the outcome of the consultation, both the patient and health professional should be considered as a dyad. The modern consultation therefore involves two individuals and a communication process that exists between them. This reflects a shift from a traditional model of health care in which the doctor was the expert and the patient a grateful recipient of this expertise, towards a more modern model emphasizing interaction which is reflected in the notions patient-centredness and agreement between the health professional and patient.

Patient-Centredness

First developed by Byrne and Long in 1976, the concept of patient-centredness has become increasingly in vogue over recent years. The prescriptive literature has recommended patient-centredness as the preferred style of doctor–patient communication as a means to improve patient outcomes (Pendleton et al. 1984; Neighbour 1987; McWhinney 1995). Further, empirical research has explored both the extent to which consultations can be deemed to be patient-centred. For example, in one classic study Tuckett et al. (1985) analysed recorded consultations and described the interaction between doctor and patient as a 'meeting between experts'. Research has also addressed whether patient-centredness is predictive of outcomes such as patient satisfaction, compliance and health status (Savage and Armstrong 1990). Such research has raised questions concerning both the definition of patient-centredness and its assessment, which has resulted in a range of methodological approaches. For example, some studies have used coding frames such as the Stiles Verbal Response Mode System (Stiles 1978) or the Roter Index (Roter et al. 1997) as a means to code whether a particular doctor is behaving in a patient-centred fashion. In contrast, other studies have used interviews with patients and doctors (Tuckett at al. 1985) while some have used behavioural checklists (Byrne and Long 1976). Complicating the matter further, research studies exploring the doctor – patient interaction and the literature proposing a particular form of interaction have used a wide range of different but related terms such as 'shared decision-making' (Elwyn et al. 1999), 'patient participation' (Guadagnoli and Ward 1998) and 'patient partnership' (Coulter 1999).

In general, patient-centredness is considered to consist of three central components:

- A receptiveness by the doctor to the patient's opinions and expectations, and an effort to see the illness through the patient's eyes.
- Patient involvement in the decision-making and planning of treatment.
- An attention to the affective content of the consultation in terms of the emotions of both the patient and the doctor.

This framework is comparable to the six interactive components described by Levenstein et al. (1986) and is apparent in the five key dimensions described by Mead and Bower (2000) in their comprehensive review of the patient-centred literature. Finally, it is explicitly described by Winefield et al. (1996) in their work comparing the effectiveness of different measures. In a systematic review of 40 articles exploring the relationship between patient-centred care and patient outcomes, Rathert et al. (2013) found mixed results for the impact of patient-centred care on clinical outcomes but stronger evidence for its impact on patient satisfaction and self-management. Patient-centredness is now the way in which consultations are supposed to be managed. It emphasizes negotiation between doctor and patient and places the interaction between the two as central. In line with this approach, research has explored the relationship between health professional and patient with an emphasis not on either the health professional or the patient but on the interaction between the two in terms of the level of agreement between health professional and patient and the impact of this agreement on patient outcome.

Agreement between Health Professional and Patient

If health professional–patient communication is seen as an interaction between two individuals, then it is important to understand the extent to which these two individuals speak the same language, share the same beliefs and agree as to the desired content and outcome of any consultation. This is of particular relevance to general practice consultations where patient and health professional perspectives are most likely to coincide. For example, as noted, Tuckett et al. (1985) argued that the consultation should be conceptualized as a 'meeting between experts' and emphasized the importance of the patient's and doctor's potentially different views of the problem. Recent research has examined levels of agreement between GPs' and patients' beliefs about different health problems. Ogden et al. (1999) explored GPs' and patients' models of depression in terms of symptoms (mood and somatic), causes (psychological, medical, external) and treatments (medical and non-medical). The results showed that GPs and patients agreed about the importance of mood-related symptoms, psychological causes and non-medical treatments. However, the GPs reported greater support for somatic symptoms, medical causes and medical treatments. Therefore the results indicated that GPs hold a more medical model of depression than patients. From a similar perspective, Ogden et al. (2001b) explored GPs' and patients' beliefs about obesity. The results showed that the GPs and patients reported similar beliefs for most psychological, behavioural and social causes of obesity. However, they differed consistently in their beliefs about medical causes. In particular, the patients rated a gland/hormone problem, slow metabolism and overall medical causes more highly than did the GPs. For the treatment of obesity, a similar pattern emerged with the two groups reporting similar beliefs for a range of methods, but showing different beliefs about who (GP or patient) was most helpful. Whereas the patients rated the GP as more helpful, the GPs rated the obese patients themselves more highly. Therefore, although GPs seem to have a more medical model of depression, they have a less medical model of obesity. Research has also shown that doctors and patients differ in their beliefs about the role of the doctor (Ogden et al. 1997), about the value of patient-centred consultations (Ogden et al. 2002), about the very nature of health (Ogden et al. 2001a), about chronic disease and the role of stress (Heijmans et al. 2001) and in terms of what it is important to know about medicines (Berry et al. 1997). If health professional – patient communication is seen as an interaction, then these studies suggest that it may well be an interaction between two individuals with very different perspectives. Do these different perspectives influence patient outcomes?

The Role of Agreement in Patient Outcomes

If doctors and patients have different beliefs about illness, different beliefs about the role of the doctor and about medicines, does this lack of agreement relate to patient outcomes? It is possible that such disagreement may result in poor compliance to medication ('Why should I take antidepressants if I am not depressed?'), poor compliance to any recommended changes in behaviour ('Why should I eat less if obesity is caused by hormones?') or low satisfaction with the consultation ('I wanted emotional support and the GP gave me a prescription'). To date, little research has explored these possibilities. One study did, however examine the extent to which a patient's expectations of a GP consultation were met by the GP and whether this predicted patient satisfaction. Williams et al. (1995) asked 504 general practice patients to complete a measure of their expectations of the consultation with their GP prior to it taking place and a measure of whether their expectations were actually met afterwards. The results showed that having more expectations met was related to a higher level of satisfaction with the consultation. However, this study did not explore compliance, nor did it examine whether the GP and patient had a shared belief about the nature of the consultation.

IN SUMMARY

The medical consultation is at the heart of most interactions between the patient and the health care system. Traditional models of the consultation regarded the doctor as the expert and the patient as a passive recipient of this expertise who simply responded to what the doctor said. Doctors, however, vary in their decisions and behaviours more than this model would allow for, suggesting a role for other factors in their decision-making processes. Research has therefore explored clinical decision-making as a form of problem-solving and has highlighted a role for health professionals' own beliefs, behaviours, past experiences and mood. Nowadays the modern consultation is seen much more as a meeting between experts and the emphasis is on patient-centred care, shared decision-making and a level of agreement between doctor and patient. The consultation has therefore changed enormously in the past 100 years. But one issue that still remains a problem for the medical world is that of adherence. However much medical advances improve the effectiveness of medical care, it cannot work if patients don't behave in ways that doctors would like. This will now be considered.

6   ADHERENCE

In 1987, HIV was a terrifying, acute and fatal illness and many people who were infected died within a couple of years. Nowadays, in the West, it is regarded as a chronic illness and people have survived for over 20 years. In the main, this is due to medical advances and the development of HAART (see p. 375). In Africa the picture is completely different as people do not always have the same access to treatment that we do (see Figures 9.1 and 9.2, in Chapter 9, section 1: A brief history of health care) and many are still desperate for medicines. Yet people in the West who are prescribed their treatment don't always take it. From the outside this non-adherence seems inexplicable. Why would people not take a drug that can stop them from dying? But this is the very essence of research on adherence. Medicine invents treatments that research shows can prevent illness, manage illness and cure illness, yet the people with the illnesses do not take the medicines as prescribed. This section explores definitions of adherence, measuring adherence, why adherence is important, models of adherence, predictors of adherence and how adherence can be changed.

DEFINING ADHERENCE

The concept of adherence used to be referred to as 'compliance', which was defined by Haynes et al. (1979) as 'the extent to which the patient's behaviour (in terms of taking medications, following diets or other lifestyle changes) coincides with medical or health advice'. Compliance excited an enormous amount of clinical and academic interest and it was calculated that 3,200 articles on compliance in English were listed between 1979 and 1985 (Trostle 1988). The term 'compliance', however, was deemed too paternalistic and was seen to relate to a more traditional model of the consultation with the doctor as expert and the patient as a passive recipient of this expertise who wasn't doing as they were told. The term 'adherence' was therefore introduced in the 1990s as a means to encapsulate a more active and empowered patient and most research nowadays uses this term. Adherence has been defined as the extent to which a patient's behaviour matches agreed recommendations from their health professional (Horne 2006; NICE 2009). Although this appears similar to the notion of compliance the terms 'agreed', and 'recommendations' illustrate a shift in perspective away from a paternalistic doctor towards one who negotiates and agrees management plans with their patient. This is in line with ideas of patient-centredness and shared decision-making. Adherence is mostly explored in the context of medication-taking and the extent to which patients take their drugs as recommended. It also, however, relates to other behaviours such as smoking, dietary change and exercise, if these are what the doctor has recommended. As a means to understand why people do not adhere, researchers have further defined non-adherence as being either 'unintentional non-adherence' which occurs when an individual simply forgets or has misunderstood the instructions and 'intentional non-adherence' which describes those times when a patient chooses not to take their medicine or engage in a risk-reducing behaviour. As mentioned in Chapters 8 and 13, an obesity drug called orlistat causes unpleasant side-effects (anal leakage and oily stools) if taken with fatty foods. People therefore often have 'drug holidays' to enable them to have a meal out every now and again. This is a form of intentional non-adherence.

MEASURING ADHERENCE

Before any construct can be measured it needs to be clearly operationalized and adherence is particularly difficult for two key reasons. First, self-reported adherence may be inaccurate due to issues such as memory, social desirability and the wish to be prescribed further medicines in the future ('I can't remember whether I took my pills last Wednesday', 'If I tell them I didn't take my medication as I wanted a break, then they might not give me any more'). Second, the behaviour itself can be highly complex. For example, recommended medication-taking may involve instructions about time of day, amount, whether with or with out food, number of days or legitimate reasons for not taking the medication such as illness or side-effects. Deciding whether or not a patient has been adherent therefore requires a decision on whether they need to meet all, some or most of these recommended criteria. For example, a patient could be told to take two pills, four times a day for seven days. But if they miss a day and then take them all the next day is this adherence or not? Measures of adherence are broadly objective or subjective with each having their strengths and weaknesses. Horne and Clatworthy (2010) provide a detailed analysis of measurement which is summarized as follows:

Objective measures

- *Observation:* researchers/clinicians can directly observe how many pills a patient takes. This is accurate but time-consuming and not always feasible.
- *Blood or urine samples:* these can be taken to assess blood levels of the drug. This is objective but costly, time-consuming and varies according to how drugs are metabolized by different individuals.
- *Pill counting:* patients are asked to bring their remaining pills in to be counted. This requires face-to-face meetings which are time-consuming and inconvenient and patients may throw away pills in order to appear adherent.
- *Electronic monitors:* pill bottles can contain a computer chip to record each time the bottle is opened. This can provide detailed information about drug-taking. But it assumes that a pill is taken each time the bottle is opened and is expensive.
- *Assessing prescriptions:* records can be made of when patients ask for new prescriptions. This assumes that patients have taken the used pills and that they ask for a new prescription exactly when they have run out.

Subjective measures

- *Self-report:* patients can rate their own adherence either during an interview or using a questionnaire. This is inexpensive and simple but may be contaminated by recall problems and social desirability. It is possible to 'normalize' non-adherence as a means to reduce social desirability but this may in fact promote non-adherence. A commonly used self-report measure is the Medication Adherence Report Scale (MAARS, Horne and Weinman 2002).

WHY IS ADHERENCE IMPORTANT?

Adherence is considered to be important primarily because following the recommendations of health professionals is believed essential to patient recovery. For example, DiMatteo et al. (2002) reviewed 63 studies of adherence to a wide range of recommendations (e.g. medication, diet, physical activity) and concluded that the odds of having a good treatment were three times higher in those that showed good adherence. Similarly, Simpson et al. (2006) reported that the odds of dying were halved if people took their medication. Interestingly they also showed an adherence effect whereby adherence, regardless of whether it was to an active drug or a placebo, also halved the odds of dying. This is discussed further in the section on placebos in Chapter 11. Likewise, George and Bender (2019) concluded from their review that adherence to asthma or COPD medication was associated with better symptom control, reduced asthma-related mortality, reduced COPD-related mortality, lower health care costs and a lower risk of an intensive care unit stay. Further, Evans et al. (2022) concluded from their systematic review that adherence to antidiabetic medication in people with Type 2 diabetes was associated with greater reductions in glycated haemoglobin levels, fewer microvascular and/or macrovascular outcomes, being less likely to be hospitalized or to have emergency department visits/admissions and spending fewer days in hospital. Adherence is therefore related to health outcomes. Yet studies estimate that about half of the patients with chronic illnesses, such as diabetes and hypertension, are non-adherent with their medication regimens and that even adherence for a behaviour as apparently simple as using an inhaler for asthma is poor (e.g. Dekker et al. 1992). In addition, the WHO (2003) estimated that about a third of all prescribed drugs are not taken as directed. This also has cost implications as money is wasted when drugs are prescribed, prescriptions are cashed, but the drugs not taken. In the UK this has been estimated at about £4 billion per year (NICE 2009).

MODELS OF ADHERENCE

Researchers have developed models as a means to understand, predict and possibly change adherence.

Cognitive Hypothesis Model

An early model of adherence was developed by Ley (1989) who described a cognitive hypothesis model of compliance (as it was then). This model is illustrated in Figure 9.15.

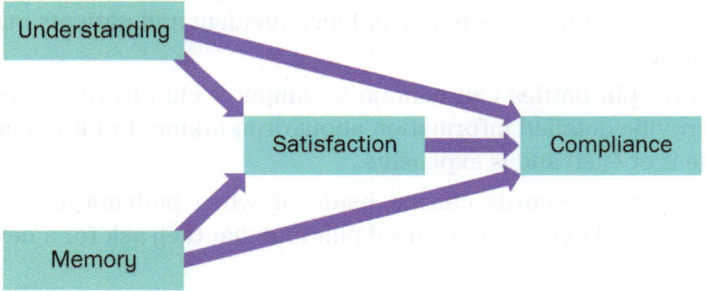

Figure 9.15 Ley's cognitive hypothesis model of compliance

From this model it was predicted that a patient would adhere to their doctor's recommendations if they understood these recommendations, could recall the instructions and were satisfied with the consultation.

The Perceptions and Practicalities Approach

From a different perspective Horne (2001) developed a model of adherence that emphasized perceptions and practicalities of adherence and focused on the predictors of unintentional non-adherence and intentional non-adherence. From this perspective adherence is seen as relating to motivation ('I want to get well') and resources ('I have access to my pills') and perceptual barriers ('My medicine isn't really necessary') and practical barriers ('I can't get to the pharmacist') are deemed to prevent adherence from happening. This model is shown in Figure 9.16.

These two models provide a different structure for understanding adherence. However, there are several similarities in terms of the constructs used. These will now be explored in terms of the predictors of adherence.

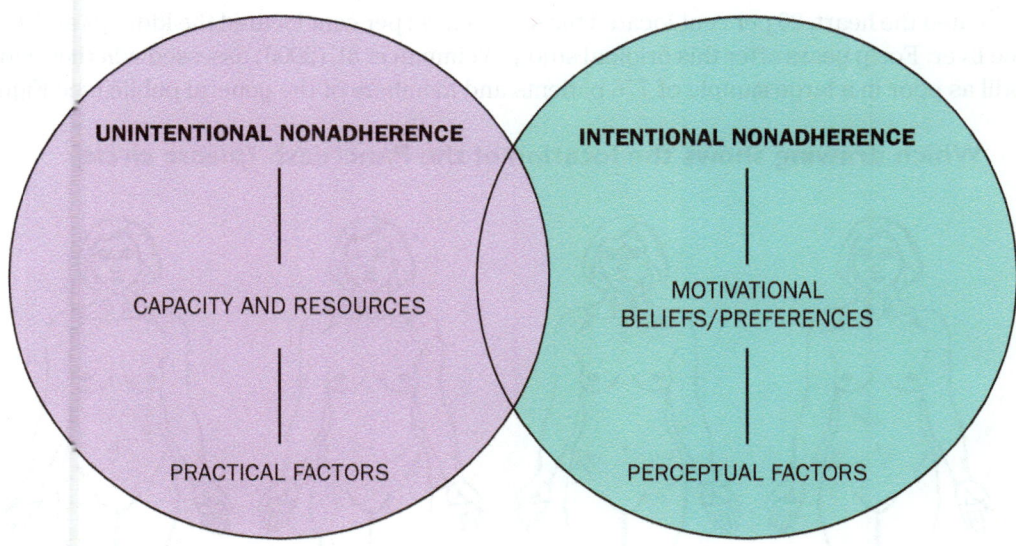

Figure 9.16 The perceptions and practicalities approach
SOURCE: Horne (2001)

PREDICTORS OF ADHERENCE

The models described above highlight a number of factors that may predict adherence. Some of these remain to be tested explicitly whereas others are more evidence-based.

Patient Satisfaction

Ley (1988) examined the extent of patient satisfaction with the consultation. He reviewed 21 studies of hospital patients and found that 41 per cent of patients were dissatisfied with their treatment and that 28 per cent of general practice patients were also dissatisfied. Ley also reported that satisfaction is determined by the content of the consultation and that patients want to know as much information as possible, even if this is bad news. For example, in studies looking at cancer diagnosis, patients showed improved satisfaction if they were given a diagnosis of cancer rather than if they were protected from this information. Berry et al. (2003) explored the impact on satisfaction of making information more personal to the patient. Participants were asked to read some information about medication and then to rate their satisfaction. Some were given personalized information, such as 'If you take this medicine, there is a substantial chance of you getting one or more of its side-effects', whereas some were given non-personalized information, such as 'A substantial proportion of people who take this medication get one or more of its side-effects'. The results showed that a more personalized style was related to greater satisfaction, lower ratings of the risks of side-effects and lower ratings of the risk to health. Sala et al. (2002) explored the relationship between humour in consultations and patient satisfaction. The authors coded recorded consultations for their humour content and for the type of humour used. They then looked for differences between high and low satisfaction-rated consultations. The results showed that high satisfaction was related to the use of more light humour, more humour that relieved tension, more self-effacing humour and more positive-function humour. Patient satisfaction therefore relates to a range of professional and patient variables and is increasingly used in health care assessment as an indirect measure of health outcome based on the assumption that a satisfied patient will be a healthier patient. It is possible that in line with Ley's model, increased satisfaction may predict increased adherence.

Patient Understanding

Several studies have also examined the extent to which patients understand the content of the consultation. Boyle (1970) examined patients' beliefs about the location of organs and found that only 44 per cent correctly located the heart, 20 per cent located the stomach. 42 per cent located the kidneys and 49 per cent located the liver. Forty years after this original study, Weinman et al. (2009) assessed whether understanding was still as poor in a large sample of 776 patients and members of the general public (see Figure 9.17).

Which drawing shows the location of the Pancreas? *(please circle)*

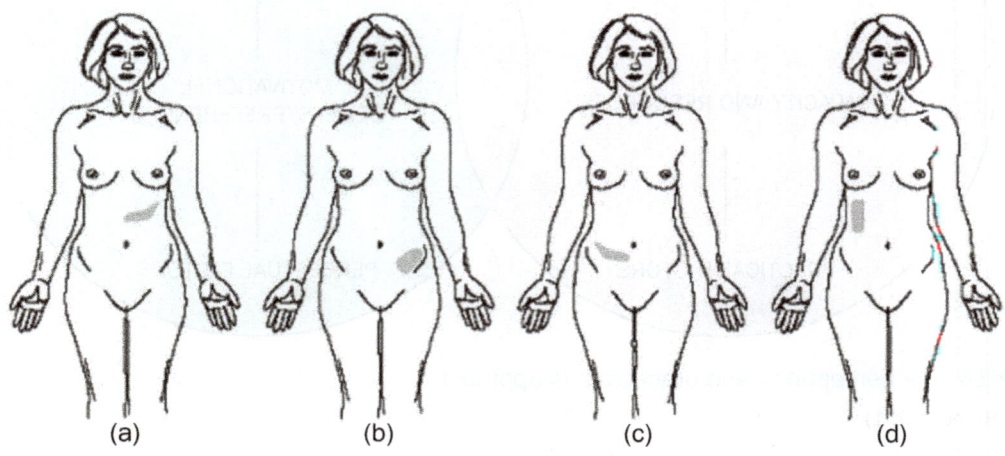

(a)   (b)   (c)   (d)

Which drawing shows the location of the Kidneys? *(please circle)*

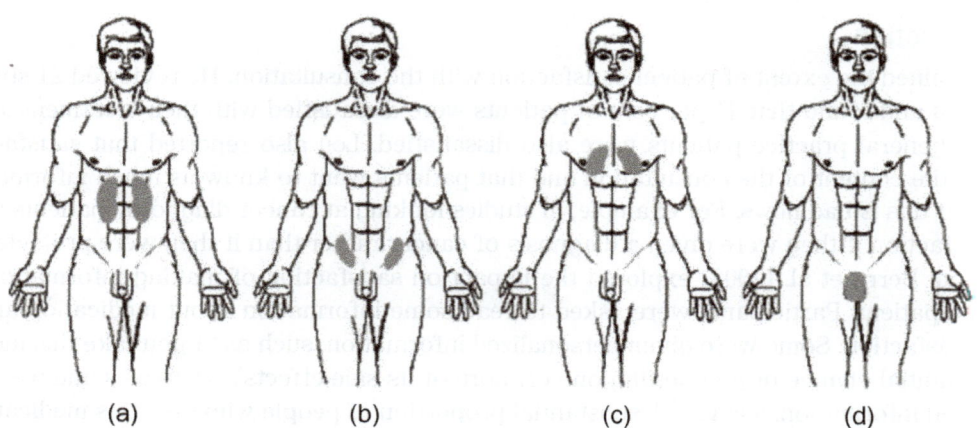

(a)   (b)   (c)   (d)

Figure 9.17 Assessing anatomical knowledge
SOURCE: Weinman et al. (2009)

The results showed no significant improvements since the earlier study and that knowledge got worse the older the participant. If the doctor gives advice to the patient or suggests that they follow a particular treatment programme and the patient does not understand the causes of their illness, the correct location of the relevant organ or the processes involved in the treatment, then this lack of understanding is likely to affect their compliance with the advice.

Patients' Recall

Researchers have also examined the process of recall of the information given during the consultation. Bain (1977) examined the recall from a sample of patients who had attended a GP consultation and found that 37 per cent could not recall the name of the drug, 23 per cent could not recall the frequency of the dose and 25 per cent could not recall the duration of the treatment. Likewise, Crichton et al. (1978)

found that 22 per cent of patients had forgotten the treatment regime recommended by their doctors. Further, Linn et al. (2013) explored medication adherence in a sample of 68 patients with inflammatory bowel disease and found that patients could only recall about half of the information presented to them in consultations and that recall was significantly associated with adherence. In a meta-analysis of the research into recall of consultation information, Ley (1989) found that recall is influenced by a multitude of factors. For example, Ley argued that the greater the anxiety, medical knowledge, intellectual level, importance of the statement, primacy effect and number of statements all increase recall. However, he concluded that recall is not influenced by the age of the patient, which is contrary to some predictions of the effect of ageing on memory and some of the myths and counter-myths of the ageing process. Recalling information after the consultation may be related to compliance.

Beliefs About the Illness

Research shows that patients hold beliefs about their illness and that these consistently relate to key dimensions of cause, consequences, time line, control and identity (see Chapter 8 for a discussion of illness cognitions). In addition, research indicates that these beliefs predict adherence. For example, Halm et al. (2006) explored 198 asthmatics' beliefs about their problem, their perception of symptoms and their adherence to medication. The results showed that those who believed they only had asthma when they had symptoms (the 'acute asthma belief') showed lower levels of adherence. Similarly, Brewer et al. (2002) examined the relationship between illness cognitions and adherence to medication in patients with hypercholesterolaemia (involving very high cholesterol). The results showed that a belief that the illness has serious consequences was related to medication adherence.

Beliefs About the Behaviour

People also hold beliefs about their health-related behaviours and within the framework of social cognition models adherence can be predicted by beliefs about the costs and benefits of taking medication, perceptions of risk for illness, self-efficacy for taking drugs, the norms of those around the patient and their attitudes to medication. Norman et al. (2003) used PMT to predict children's adherence to wearing an eye patch. Parents of children diagnosed with eye problems completed a baseline questionnaire concerning their beliefs and described their child's adherence after 2 months. The results showed that higher adherence was predicted by greater perceived susceptibility and lower response costs.

Beliefs About Medication

One area of research that has received much attention over the past few years is the specific beliefs that people have about their medication. Horne (1997) identified two key sets of beliefs labelled 'necessity' beliefs ('How much do I need this medicine?') and 'concerns' beliefs ('I worry about side-effects'). This has been called the necessity/concerns framework (NCF) (Horne 1997; Horne and Weinman 2002) and research indicates that beliefs about necessity and concerns are good predictors of adherence in the context of illnesses such as asthma (Horne and Weinman 2002); diabetes, cancer and CHD (Horne and Weinman 1999; Świątoniowska-Lonc et al. 2021); HIV/AIDS (Horne et al. 2007), multiple sclerosis (Neter et al. 2021) and rheumatoid arthritis (Neame and Hammond 2005). In 2013, Horne et al. conducted a meta-analysis of the role of these beliefs in predicting medication adherence for long-term conditions. They found that in 94 studies (n = 25,072), stronger necessity beliefs and lower concerns beliefs were associated with higher adherence.

Adherence to medication may therefore be predicted by a number of variables. Some of these, such as patient satisfaction, recall and understanding, are central to Ley's cognitive hypothesis model and others find reflection in Horne's perceptions and practicalities approach and research on health and illness beliefs. In the main adherence to medication is predicted by a wide range of factors. For example, Świątoniowska-Lonc et al. (2021) carried out a review of 36 studies to explore the predictors of adherence in patients with Type 2 diabetes. Their analysis indicated that poorer adherence was predicted by anxiety, diabetes distress, older age, poor communication with physicians, stress, concerns about medicines and cognitive impairment on aspects of self-care and medication taking whereas self-efficacy, social and family support, and acceptance of illness had a beneficial effect on adherence. Understanding the predictors of adherence is a step towards improving adherence.

HOW CAN ADHERENCE BE IMPROVED?

Adherence is considered essential to patient well-being. Studies have therefore explored how adherence can be improved with a focus on information-giving to improve recall and changing cognitions and emotions.

The Role of Information

Researchers have examined the role and the type of information used to improve patient adherence. Using a meta-analysis, Mullen et al. (1985) found that 64 per cent of patients were more adherent when using instructional and educational information. Haynes (1982) reported that information could improve adherence from 52 to 66 per cent. Information-giving could improve adherence in the following ways.

Oral Information

Ley (1989) suggested that oral information can improve adherence in the following ways by facilitating understanding and recall:

- Primacy effect – patients have a tendency to remember the first thing they are told.
- Stressing the importance of adherence.
- Simplifying the information.
- Using repetition.
- Being specific.
- Following up the consultation with additional interviews.

Written Information

Researchers also looked at the use of written information in improving adherence. Ley and Morris (1984) examined the effect of written information about medication and found that it increased knowledge in 90 per cent of the studies, increased compliance in 60 per cent of the studies and improved outcome in 57 per cent of the studies. Interventions have therefore explored the role of information-giving in improving adherence and suggestions have been made to make information clearer and easier to remember. However, Haynes et al. (2002) concluded from their review of the literature that although information-based interventions can improve adherence for short-term regimens (less or equal to two weeks), more complex interventions are needed for longer-term medication taking. Similarly, Kripalini et al. (2007) carried out a systematic review of interventions to improve medication adherence in chronic conditions and concluded that although good information is important, it is not sufficient to improve adherence.

Changing Beliefs and Emotions

Because knowledge is not enough to improve adherence, research has turned its focus onto changing cognitions and emotions. This is in line with the interventions to change other health-related behaviours described in Chapter 7. It can involve behavioural strategies such as reinforcement, incentives or modelling, social cognition theory-based interventions such as implementation intentions, the use of stage models and motivational interviewing, changing affect or drawing upon integrated models such as the COM-B and the role of BCTS. Safren et al. (2012) carried a trial to evaluate the use of CBT for adherence and depression in a sample of 89 HIV positive drug users. The results showed improvements in both depression and adherence immediately after the intervention but whereas changes in depression were sustained over time improvements in adherence were not. Similarly, Harne-Britner et al. (2011)

evaluated the impact of a reinforcement system (i.e. stickers) on adherence to hand hygiene in health care workers and found that although the intervention resulted in a 15.5 per cent increase in hand hygiene during the first month, this effect was not sustained. Haynes et al. (2002) carried out a review of 33 randomized controlled trials designed to improve medication adherence for a range of psychiatric (e.g. depression, psychosis) or chronic medical conditions (e.g. hypertension, asthma, HIV/AIDs). The interventions included counselling, education, family systems therapy, self-monitoring, face-to-face consultations, group sessions and behaviour therapy. Although their review included a diverse number of problems and interventions, they concluded that 49 per cent of the studies reported significant improvements in medication adherence and that the most effective used the most complex interventions involving a combination of all forms of behaviour modification strategy. However, even the most effective still showed modest results.

Improved Communication between HCP and Patient

There is therefore a role for a number of strategies to improve adherence. In essence, however, most of these strategies involve improving communication between health care professional and patient whether through oral or written information or the way in which HCPs explain why medication needs to be taken and how to take it. In line with this, George and Bender (2019) concluded from their review of asthma and COPD that the best ways to improve adherence were shared decision-making, smart technology to provide feedback, individualized counselling and regular phone contact to discuss any concerns. Likewise, Guraya et al. (2021) concluded that the best ways to improve adherence to psoriasis treatments was through a well-written prescription, shared decision-making, having frequent follow-ups and reframing any side effects of medication. (See the previous section on the The Medical Consultation for further information on communication.)

IN SUMMARY

Adherence is important as appropriate medicine-taking is believed to be a core part of effective treatment and non-adherence has both health and cost implications. Over the past few decades the term 'compliance' has been replaced with 'adherence' as a means to reflect a more empowered model of the patient and a less paternalistic model of the doctor. In line with most behaviours, adherence is difficult to measure due to problems of social desirability and recall for subjective measures and cost and time for more objective measures. Research, however, has identified possible predictors of adherence with a focus on patient satisfaction, understanding, recall and beliefs relating to behaviour, illness and a patient's treatment regimen. Research has also explored ways in which adherence can be improved, drawing upon a range of intervention strategies, often relying upon improved communication between HCP and patient, although, in line with all attempts at behaviour change, short-term changes seem easier to create compared to changes in the longer term.

BOX 9.1
Critical Approaches to Health Psychology

Research and theories relating to accessing health care highlights some of the bigger issues in health psychology as follows:

The individual vs the social vs the political: Accessing health care clearly exists within a social and political context. People can only attend for screening if screening programmes exist; can only go their doctor if it is free or they can afford to pay and can only take their medication if they can afford the prescription. We may measure these variables as constructs such as 'opportunity', 'social context' or 'social norms' or just demographics but this cannot capture the complexity of this wider context in which beliefs and behaviours exist.

Individual differences: Much research in this area explores differences by demographics such as gender, age or ethnicity and tells us that men are more likely to delay seeking help, that women are more likely to turn up for health checks or that older people go to the doctor more. These grouping variables are useful for analysis and managing data but impose false dichotomies and miss the complexity of who people are.

The role of culture: Most research within our discipline is written in English, published in English speaking journals and presented at English speaking conferences. The meaning of health and the management of illness is hugely impacted upon by culture in terms of the role of human agency vs fate, the structure of different health care systems and whether or not these are free at the point of access and whether the patient can chose which specialist to see or require a referral by a GP. If research is carried out in different cultures and published in non-English speaking journals, this can get missed by the rest of the world. We can therefore minimize the role of culture as we never read anything to contradict our own perspectives.

7 THINKING CRITICALLY ABOUT ACCESS TO HEALTH CARE

There are several problems with research exploring how and when people access health care which should be considered (see Ogden, 2016c for a discussion of the potential harms of accessing health care).

SOME CRITICAL QUESTIONS

When thinking about research in this area ask yourself the following questions:

- Is more access to health care always a good thing?
- When we promote help-seeking, screening or adherence what should we use as our outcome variable? Should it be help-seeking, screening or adherence OR patient health?
- Does a more patient-centred approach reflect what patients really want?
- Why is studying the consultation so difficult?

SOME PROBLEMS WITH. . .

These are several problems with research in this area as follows:

Help-Seeking Research

Help-seeking research makes the assumption that early help-seeking is beneficial for patient health outcomes and that early detection leads to longer life expectancy. There are some problems with this assumption as follows:

Lead times: Patients live longer if they present earlier. But they may only live longer from the time of diagnosis rather than longer in real time. Early help-seeking may therefore not only make people 'live longer', it may also make them 'be ill for longer' rather than extending life in any meaningful way.

Health anxiety: Encouraging help-seeking through symptom vigilance may create health anxiety and hypochondriasis. Symptoms are a precept rather than a sensation influenced by a range of psychological factors including focus. Encouraging people to focus on their symptoms may exacerbate or even create symptoms and also generate unnecessary worry and concern.

Increased consultation rates: Early help-seeking and increased symptom focus may increase consultation rates, overwhelming an already over-stretched health service. This means that health professionals spend more with the worried well and less time with the elderly and ill. It may also change clinical decision-making.

Clinical decision-making: Clinical judgement is influenced by beliefs about risk and probability and a balance between the likelihood of false positives versus false negatives. Clinicians also draw upon heuristics. Therefore following one patient with a heart attack, subsequent patients with indigestion are more likely to be seen as at risk of a heart attack as the clinician's perception of risk will have changed. Likewise, the more consultations consist of health anxious rather than 'real' symptoms, the more a doctor's perception of risk will lead them to expect more benign problems. Therefore, a higher ratio of worried well versus ill patients may increase the chances of false negatives compared to false positives and real illness will be missed.

Unnecessary treatments and false hope: Medicine cannot treat or cure all illnesses. By seeking help patients may expect to have treatment, or even get treatment but still die because no treatment can cure their illness. The help-seeking literature encourages the view that medicine has a cure for everything.

Quantity vs quality of life: Sometimes the emphasis is on promoting longer life through medical intervention rather than having quality of life. Seeking help may promote more quantity of life but it may well reduce quality of life.

Screening Research

Screening research is based upon the premise that identifying an illness at an asymptomatic stage will lead to improved outcomes. There are several problems with this assumption as follows:

Conflicting outcomes: Evaluating the impact of screening can involve measuring both psychological (e.g. fear, anxiety) and medical (e.g. health status, detection) outcomes. Sometimes these outcomes occur in opposite directions (it may make a person anxious but benefit their health status). Combining these contradictory outcomes and deciding upon the right way forward can be a complex and difficult process.

Patient autonomy: Screening may detect an illness at an early stage. Some people, however, may not wish to know that they have something wrong with them. This can present researchers and clinicians with a dilemma as medicine also emphasizes truth-telling, openness and patient autonomy. Balancing the different ethical positions and perspectives of medicine can prove difficult.

Do more harm than good: Screening programmes are delivered in order to promote health outcomes. There is emerging evidence, however, that some screening programmes may do more harm than good. For example, although they may pick up some conditions, such as breast cancer, early, they also subject many people to unnecessary treatments through the high number of false positives they also detect. Evaluating the effectiveness of a screening programme therefore needs an assessment of lives saved (compared to those not in a screening programme) together with the false positives (those given treatment when they didn't need it), the harms of the intervention (i.e. x-rays from the scans) and the false negatives (those missed by the screening programme).

Costs to the health service: Any health service has a limited budget. Therefore money spent on one resource cannot be spent on another. Nationwide screening programmes are extremely expensive. An evaluation of any screening programme needs to take into account not only the harm versus the benefit, but also the cost of delivering the programme, compared to what else the money could be spent on.

Politics: Screening programmes are often delivered by the health service with the support of a government. This is seen by the public as a 'good thing' and part of appropriate patient care.

If research evidence were to show that the screening programme was ineffective, harmful and costing unnecessary money it would be very hard for a government to remove the programme due to political reasons.

Consultation Research

There are also some problems with research on the consultation:

A clash of ideology: The current emphasis within clinical care is on patient-centredness, shared decision-making and informed decisions. This emphasizes respecting the patient's perspective and understanding the patient's beliefs. However, health professionals also have training and expertise which encourages them to feel they know what is the correct mode of management and the correct way forward. At times these two perspectives can clash. For example, a patient with epilepsy may believe that they can manage their problem through self-care and the use of alternative medicines. The doctor may disagree and feel that anti-epileptic drugs are the safest option. How these two perspectives can sit alongside each other while enabling the doctor to be both patient-centred and safe is unclear. Sometimes the literature appears to be trying to have it all ways.

Understanding what happens between people: Research exploring the interaction between health professional and patient uses a variety of methods. Some studies ask each party about the interaction, some record the interaction, some code the interaction and some observe the interaction. All these methods involve a level of interpretation (by the researcher, the health professional or the patient). Trying to access what 'really' goes on in a consulting room is not really possible.

Adherence Research

Research on medication adherence encourages people to take their medicines and provides explanations as to why they do not as a means to develop intervention to promote adherence. There are some problems with assumptions behind this perspective as follows:

Financial cost: Drugs cost money – the estimates indicate that the drug budget costs most health care systems millions of pound/euros/dollars (etc.) per year. This is money that will then not be spent on staff, surgery or machinery.

Side effects: All drugs have side effects including nausea, tiredness, stomach upset, heart attack or cancer. Researchers can estimate the level of harm a drug causes known as the NNH (Number Needed to Harm) which describes how many people need to be treated with a drug for one person to be harmed.

Not effective: The effectiveness of drugs is calculated from trials which show that one drug is more effective than either nothing or another drug. This does not mean the drug is effective for all the people all of the time. Researchers calculate the effectiveness of drugs using a NNT (Number Needed to Treat) which describes how many people need to be treated for one person to benefit.

Weighing up risk: Each drug therefore has a NNH and a NNT. It is possible to weigh up the risk of harm against the risk of benefit. Research exploring medication adherence encourages people to take their medication and explores intervention to improve adherence rates. This is often done without a consideration of whether the drug in question should actually be taken.

Optimism bias: People show an optimism bias and tend to focus on the benefits rather than the costs. When promoting medication adherence researchers are often showing this bias as they believe that it is better to take a chance of getting the benefit of a drug regardless of the potential harm. This is also the bias patients show when they decide to take a drug 'just in case' it works for them, even though it could well do harm.

Immortality: Researchers often seem to believe that if we seek help early and take medicine then we can live forever. We seem to have forgotten that we are all mortal and that death is an inherent part of life. This view is also sometimes adopted by patients and also by charities trying to solve their particular medical problem. This can lead to an emphasis on quantity rather than quality of life and a shift away from living in the moment and making the most of what life we have.

TO CONCLUDE

Accessing health care involves a number of different pathways to the doctor. The patient then encounters a health professional, usually within primary care, who makes a diagnosis and decides how to manage their problem. The patient can then choose whether or not to follow this advice. This chapter has explored this process in terms of help-seeking and delay whereby the patient is responsible for their first point of contact with health care, or screening, which involves the patient being asked to attend. The chapter then described the medical consultation in terms of the changing nature of interaction with health professionals, how doctors make decisions and the role of their health beliefs and the issue of adherence and how this can be predicted or improved. Finally the chapter outlined how to think critically about research in this area with a focus on some of the harms caused by accessing health care.

QUESTIONS

1 Why do some people seek help for seemingly minor problems?
2 Why do some people delay seeking help for serious problems?
3 What are the costs and benefits of a screening programme?
4 To what extent is a medical diagnosis based upon knowledge and expertise?
5 Discuss the role of health professionals' beliefs in the communication process.
6 Health professionals should attempt to respect and share the beliefs of their patients. Discuss.
7 Patients should be made to adhere to their medication regimen. Discuss.
8 What factors influence whether or not a patient takes their medicine?
9 Is medication adherence always a good thing?
10 Should patients be encouraged to seek help earlier?

FOR DISCUSSION

Consider the last time you had contact with a health professional (e.g. doctor, dentist, nurse, etc.). Discuss why you went to the doctor and how the health professional's health beliefs may have influenced how they decided to manage you.

FURTHER READING

Berry, D. (2004) *Risk, Communication and Health Psychology*. Maidenhead: Open University Press.
The communication of risk is a central part of many consultations. This book provides a comprehensive overview of research on risk communication.

Marteau, T.M. and Johnston, M. (1990) Health professionals: a source of variance in health outcomes, *Psychology and Health*, **5**: 47–58.

This is quite an old paper now but it set the scene for much psychological research in the area of health professional behaviour. It examines the different models of health professionals' behaviour and emphasizes the role of health professionals' health beliefs.

Ogden, J. (2019) Do no harm: balancing the costs and benefits of patient outcomes in health psychology research and practice. *Journal of Health Psychology*, 24; 25–37. doi: 10.1177/1359105316648760

This is my paper that I wrote following a talk at our annual conference. It highlights some of the potential harms of research, exploring help-seeking, screening, medication adherence and behaviour change. It is useful for generating debate in a seminar or discussion group.

Tuckett, D., Boulton, M., Olson, C. and Williams, A. (1985) *Meetings Between Experts*. London: Tavistock.

This is a classic book which describes a study involving consultation analysis. It set the scene for much subsequent research and shifted the emphasis from doctor as expert to seeing the consultation as an interaction.

10
Stress and Illness

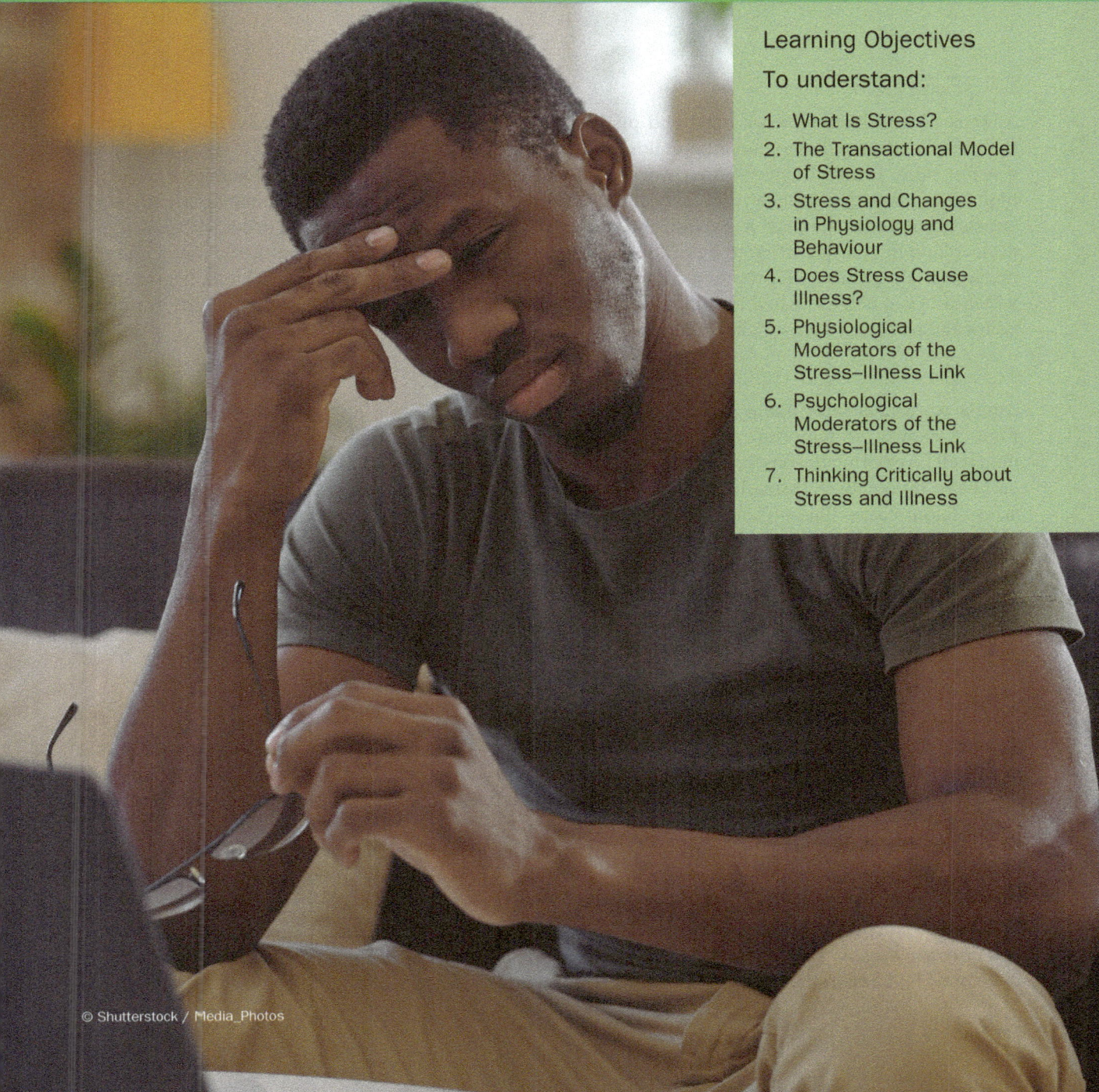

Learning Objectives

To understand:

1. What Is Stress?
2. The Transactional Model of Stress
3. Stress and Changes in Physiology and Behaviour
4. Does Stress Cause Illness?
5. Physiological Moderators of the Stress–Illness Link
6. Psychological Moderators of the Stress–Illness Link
7. Thinking Critically about Stress and Illness

CHAPTER OVERVIEW

This chapter examines definitions of stress and looks at the early models of stress. It then describes the concept of appraisal and Lazarus's transactional model of stress which emphasizes psychology as central to eliciting a stress response. The chapter then describes the impact of stress on changes in physiological factors, such as arousal and cortisol production, and behaviours, such as smoking and diet. Next the chapter assesses whether stress causes illness and explores both the direct/indirect pathways approach and the chronic and acute model of the stress–illness link. The chapter then explores physiological and psychological moderators of the stress–illness link. Finally, it describes how to think critically about research in this area.

CASE STUDY

Amir is 25 and likes to work hard and play hard. He and his friends love to take risks and spend their weekends sky diving, mountain biking, cliff jumping or just going to the local theme park for the scariest rides. During the week Amir works in the City as a banker and has tight deadlines to work to, high financial targets to meet, high expectations from his boss and he works very long hours. His job is stressful but mostly he finds it exciting and rewarding and he often goes out for a drink with colleagues after a long day in the office to let off steam. They probably drink too much but he is young and can manage it. He hasn't really worried about his health until recently when his father had a heart attack, which was a shock as he had always seemed quite fit. His father had also worked in the City for many years and had risen very quickly through the system to a top job.

Through the Eyes of Health Psychology. . .

Amir's story illustrates many aspects of the literature on stress and how it can be linked to illness. First, it shows the importance of appraisal in the stress response; what is stressful to one person may well be exciting to someone else (sky diving, cliff jumping). Second, it shows the impact that stress can have on our lives through changing health behaviours (drinking too much). Next, it shows how stress might cause illness (his father's heart attack). The research shows that the stress–illness link can be via behaviour change and changes in physiology. Finally, it illustrates the role of psychological factors such as social support (his friends, his father) and sense making (not worrying about his own health; being shocked by his father's heart attack) on how a person responds to stress and whether stress impacts upon their health status. These issues are the focus of this chapter.

1   WHAT IS STRESS?

The term 'stress' means many things to many different people. A layperson may define stress in terms of pressure, tension, unpleasant external forces or an emotional response. Psychologists have defined stress in a variety of different ways. Contemporary definitions regard stress from the external environmental as a *stressor* (e.g. problems at work), the response to the stressor as *stress* or *distress* (e.g. the feeling of tension), and the concept of *stress* as something that involves biochemical, physiological, behavioural and psychological changes. Researchers have also differentiated between stress that is harmful and damaging (*distress*) and stress that is positive and beneficial (*eustress*). In addition, researchers differentiate between *acute stress,* such as an exam or having to give a public talk, and *chronic stress,* such as job stress and poverty. The most commonly used definition of stress was developed by Lazarus and Launier (1978), who regarded stress as a transaction between people and the environment and described stress in terms of 'person–environment fit'. If a person is faced with a potentially difficult stressor, such as an exam or having to give a public talk, the degree of stress they experience is determined first by their appraisal of the event ('Is it stressful?') and second by their appraisal of their own personal resources ('Will I cope?). A good person–environment fit results in no or low stress and a poor fit results in higher stress. The speed of the appraisal process varies from person to person and between different situations.

MEASURING STRESS

Given the different definitions of stress, stress has been measured both in the laboratory and in a naturalistic setting, and using both physiological measures and those involving self-report.

Stress involves a person–environment fit: What is stressful to one person may not be to another

Laboratory Setting

Many stress researchers use an acute stress paradigm to assess stress reactivity and the stress response. This involves taking people into the laboratory and asking them either to complete a stressful task such as an intelligence test, a mathematical task, giving a public talk or watching a horror film, or exposing them to an unpleasant event such as a loud noise, white light or a puff of air in the eye. The acute stress paradigm has enabled researchers to study gender differences in stress reactivity, the interrelationship between acute and chronic stress, the role of personality in the stress response and the impact of exercise on mediating stress-related changes.

Naturalistic Setting

Some researchers study stress in a more naturalistic environment. This includes measuring stress responses to specific events such as a public performance, before and after an examination, during a job interview or while undergoing physical activity. Naturalistic research also examines the impact of ongoing stressors such as work-related stress, normal 'daily hassles', poverty or marriage conflicts. These types of study have provided important information on how people react to both acute and chronic stress in their everyday lives.

Costs and Benefits of Different Settings

Both laboratory and naturalistic settings have their costs and benefits:

1 The degree of stressor delivered in the laboratory setting can be controlled so that differences in stress response can be attributed to aspects of the individual rather than to the stressor itself.

2 Researchers can artificially manipulate aspects of the stressor in the laboratory to examine corresponding changes in physiological and psychological measures.

3 Laboratory researchers can artificially manipulate mediating variables such as control and the presence or absence of social support to assess their impact on the stress response.

4 The laboratory is an artificial environment which may produce a stress response that does not reflect that triggered by a more natural environment. It may also produce associations between variables (i.e. control and stress) which might be an artefact of the laboratory.

5 Naturalistic settings allow researchers to study real life stress and how people really cope with it.

6 However, there are many other uncontrolled variables which may contribute to the stress response that the researcher needs to measure in order to control for it in the analysis.

Physiological Measures

Physiological measures are mostly used in the laboratory as they involve participants being attached to monitors or having fluid samples taken. However, some ambulatory machines have been developed which can be attached to people as they carry on with their normal activities. To assess stress reactivity from a physiological perspective, researchers can use a polygraph to measure heart rate, respiration rate, blood pressure and the galvanic skin response (GSR), which is effected by sweating. They can also take blood, urine or saliva samples to test for changes in catecholamine and cortisol production.

Self-Report Measures

Researchers use a range of self-report measures to assess both chronic and acute stress. Some of these focus on life events and include the original Social Readjustment Rating Scale (SRRS) (Holmes and Rahe 1967) which asks about events such as 'death of a spouse', 'changing to a different line of work' and 'change of residence'. Other measures focus more on an individual's own perception of stress. The Perceived Stress Scale (PSS) (Cohen et al. 1983) is the most commonly used scale to assess self-perceived stress and asks questions such as 'In the last month how often have you been upset because of something that happened unexpectedly?', and 'In the last month how often have you felt nervous or stressed?' Some researchers also assess minor stressors in the form of 'daily hassles'. Kanner et al. (1981) developed the Hassles Scale which asks participants to rate how severe a range of hassles have been over the past month including 'misplacing or losing things', 'health of a family member' and 'concerns about owing money'. Johnston et al. (2006) used a small hand-held computer called a personal digital assistant (PDA) which participants carry around with them and which prompts them at pre-set intervals to complete a diary entry describing their level of stress. Self-report measures have been used to describe the impact of environmental factors on stress whereby stress is seen as the outcome variable (i.e. 'a poor working environment causes high stress'). They have also been used to explore the impact of stress on the individual's health status whereby stress is seen as the input variable (i.e. 'high stress causes poor health').

Costs and Benefits of Different Measures

Physiological and self-report measures of stress are used in the main to complement each other. The former reflect a more physiological emphasis and the latter a more psychological perspective. A researcher who has a greater interest in physiology might argue that physiological measures are more central to stress research, while another researcher who believes that experience is more important might favour self-report. Most stress researchers measure both physiological and psychological aspects of stress and study how these two components interact. However, in general the different types of measures have the following costs and benefits:

1 Physiological measures are more objective and less affected by the participant's wish to give a desirable response or the researcher's wish to see a particular result.

2 Self-report measures reflect the individual's experience of stress rather than just what their body is doing.

3 Self-report measures can be influenced by problems with recall, social desirability, and different participants interpreting the questions in different ways.

4 Self-report measures are based upon the life events or hassles that have been chosen by the author of the questionnaire. One person's hassle, such as 'troublesome neighbours' which appears on the Hassles Scale, may not be a hassle for another, whereas worries about a child's school might be, which doesn't appear on this scale.

EARLY STRESS MODELS

Stress models vary in terms of their definition of stress, their differing emphasis on physiological and psychological factors, and their description of the relationship between individuals and their environment.

Cannon's Fight-or-Flight Model

One of the earliest models of stress was developed by Cannon (1932) who took a more biomedical model approach to stress. His approach was called the fight-or-flight model of stress, which suggested that external threats elicited the fight-or-flight response involving an increased activity rate and increased arousal. He suggested that these physiological changes enabled the individual to either escape from the source of stress or fight. Within Cannon's model, stress was defined as a response to external stressors, which was predominantly seen as physiological. Cannon considered stress to be an adaptive response as it enabled the individual to manage a stressful event. However, he also recognized that prolonged stress could result in medical problems.

Selye's General Adaptation Syndrome

Selye's general adaptation syndrome (GAS) was developed in 1956 and described three stages in the stress process (Selye 1956). The initial stage was called the 'alarm' stage, which described an increase in activity, and occurred as soon as the individual was exposed to a stressful situation. The second stage was called 'resistance', which involved coping and attempts to reverse the effects of the alarm stage. The third stage was called 'exhaustion', which was reached when the individual had been repeatedly exposed to the stressful situation and was incapable of showing further resistance. This model is shown in Figure 10.1.

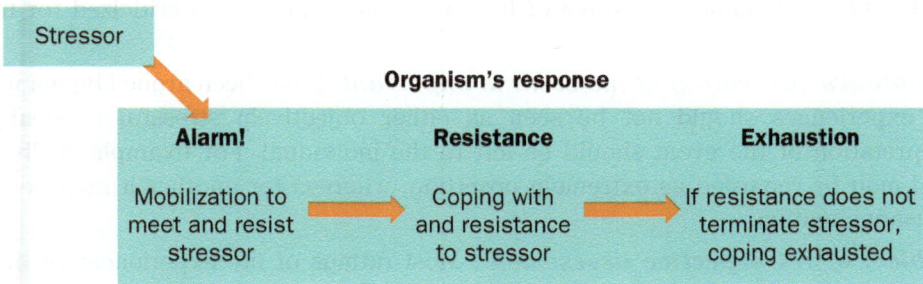

Figure 10.1 Selye's (1956) three-stage general adaptation syndrome (GAS)

Problems with the Cannon and Selye Models

Cannon's early fight/flight model and Selye's GAS laid important foundations for stress research. However, there are problems with them:

1 Both regarded the individual as automatically responding to an external stressor and described stress within a straightforward stimulus–response framework. They therefore did not address the issue of individual variability and psychological factors were given only a minimal role. For example, while an exam could be seen as stressful for one person, it might be seen as an opportunity to shine for another.

2 Both also described the physiological response to stress as consistent. This response is seen as non-specific in that the changes in physiology are the same regardless of the nature of the stressor. This is reflected in the use of the term 'arousal' which has been criticized by more recent researchers. Therefore these two models described individuals as passive and as responding automatically to their external world.

Life Events Theory

In an attempt to depart from both the Selye and Cannon models of stress, which emphasized physiological changes, life events theory was developed to examine stress and stress-related changes as a response to life experiences. Holmes and Rahe (1967) developed the Schedule of Recent Experiences (SRE), which provided respondents with an extensive list of possible life changes or life events. These ranged in supposed objective severity from events such as 'death of a spouse', 'death of a close family member' and 'jail term', to more moderate events such as 'son or daughter leaving home' and 'pregnancy', to minor events such as 'vacation', 'change in eating habits', 'change in sleeping habits' and 'change in number of family get-togethers'. Originally the SRE was scored by simply counting the number of actual recent experiences. For example, someone who had experienced both the death of a spouse and the death of a close family member would receive the same score as someone who had recently had two holidays. It was assumed that this score reflected an indication of their level of stress. Early research using the SRE in this way showed some links between individuals' SRE score and their health status. However, this obviously crude method of measurement was later replaced by a variety of others, including a weighting system whereby each potential life event was weighted by a panel, creating a degree of differentiation between the different life experiences. A longitudinal study explored the impact of life events on mortality at 17 years follow-up (Phillips et al. 2008). Participants were 968 Scottish men and women aged 56 years old who completed measures of stressful life events for the preceding 2 years at baseline, then after 8 or 9 years and then at 11/13 years. By 17 years, 266 participants had died. The results showed that when sex, occupational status, smoking, body mass index (BMI) and systolic blood pressure were controlled for the number of health-related life events, the stress load they imposed (not health *un*related life events) was strongly predictive of mortality.

Problems with Life Events Theory

The use of the SRE and similar measures of life experiences have been criticized for the following reasons:

1 *The individual's own rating of the event is important.* It has been argued by many researchers that life experiences should not be seen as either objectively stressful or benign, but that this interpretation of the event should be left to the individual. For example, a divorce for one individual may be regarded as extremely upsetting, whereas for another it may be a relief from an unpleasant situation.

2 *The problem of retrospective assessment.* Most ratings of life experiences or life events are completed retrospectively, at the time when the individual has become ill or has come into contact with the health profession. This has obvious implications for understanding the causal link between life events and subsequent stress and stress-related illnesses. For example, if an individual has developed cancer and is asked to rate their life experiences over the last year, their present state of mind will influence their recollection of that year.

3 *Life experiences may interact with each other.* When individuals are asked to complete a checklist of their recent life experiences, these experiences are regarded as independent of each other. For example, a divorce, a change of job and a marriage would be regarded as an accumulation of life events that together would contribute to a stressful period of time. However, one event may counter the effects of another and cancel out any negative stressful consequences. For example, moving house may be stressful but could be ameliorated by making new friends in a new community. Evaluating the potential effects of life experiences should include an assessment of any interactions between events.

4 *Stressors may be short term or ongoing.* Traditionally, assessments of life experiences have conceptualized such life events as acute short-term experiences. However, many events may be ongoing and chronic.

2   THE TRANSACTIONAL MODEL OF STRESS

The most commonly used model of stress is the transactional model of stress which emphasizes the key role of appraisal.

THE ROLE OF APPRAISAL

In the 1970s, Lazarus's work on stress introduced psychology to understanding the stress response (Lazarus and Cohen 1973; Lazarus 1975; Lazarus and Folkman 1987). This role for psychology took the form of his concept of *appraisal.* Lazarus argued that stress involved a transaction between the individual and their external world, and that a stress response was elicited if the individual appraised a potentially stressful event as actually being stressful. Lazarus's model therefore described individuals as psychological beings who appraised the outside world, rather than simply passively responding to it. Lazarus defined two forms of appraisal: primary and secondary. According to Lazarus, the individual initially appraises the event itself – defined as *primary appraisal.* There are four possible ways that the event can be appraised: (1) irrelevant; (2) benign and positive; (3) harmful and a threat; (4) harmful and a challenge. Lazarus then described *secondary appraisal,* which involves the individual evaluating the pros and cons of their different coping strategies. Therefore primary appraisal involves an appraisal of the outside world and secondary appraisal involves an appraisal of the individual themselves. This model is shown in Figure 10.2. The form of the primary and secondary appraisals determines whether the individual shows a stress response or not. According to Lazarus's model this stress response can take different forms: (1) direct action; (2) seeking information; (3) doing nothing; or (4) developing a means of coping with the stress in terms of relaxation or defence mechanisms.

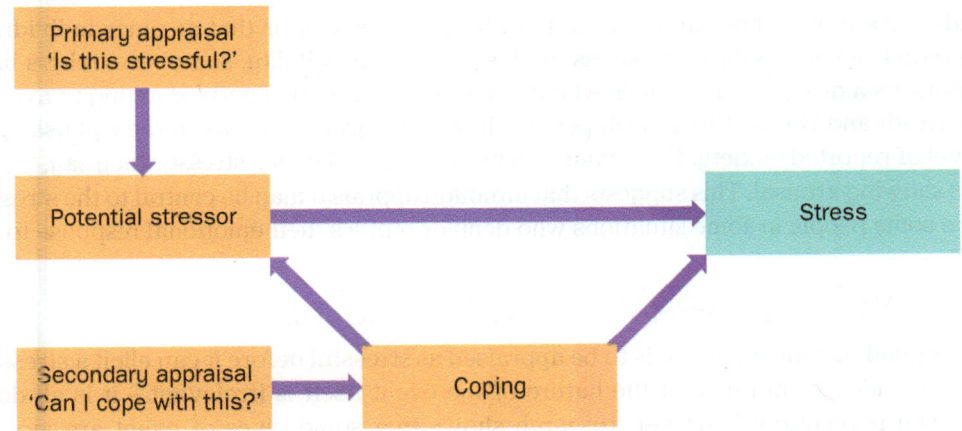

Figure 10.2 The role of appraisal in stress

Lazarus's model of appraisal and the transaction between the individual and the environment indicated a novel way of looking at the stress response – the individual no longer passively responded to their external world, but interacted with it.

DOES APPRAISAL INFLUENCE THE STRESS RESPONSE?

Several studies have examined the effect of appraisal on stress and have evaluated the role of the psychological state of the individual on their stress response. In an early study by Speisman et al. (1964), subjects were shown a film depicting an initiation ceremony involving unpleasant genital surgery. The film was shown with three different soundtracks. In condition 1, the trauma condition, the soundtrack emphasized the pain and the mutilation. In condition 2, the denial condition, the soundtrack showed

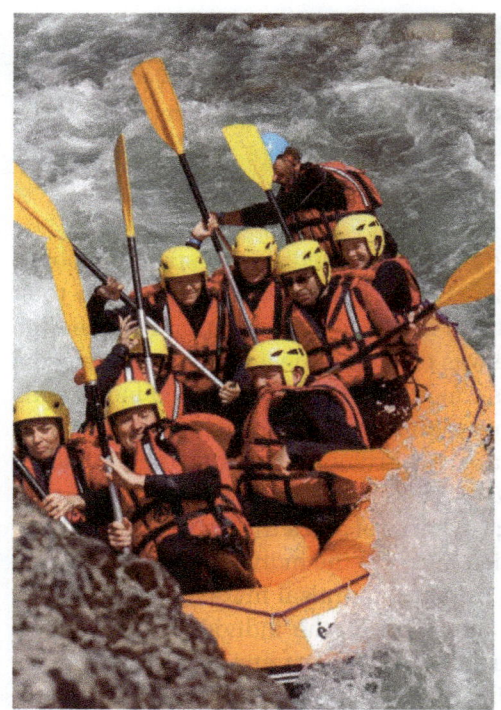

An event needs to be appraised as stressful to elicit a stress response

the participants as being willing and happy. In condition 3, the intellectualization condition, the soundtrack gave an anthropological interpretation of the ceremony. The study therefore manipulated the subjects' appraisal of the situation and evaluated the effect of the type of appraisal on their stress response. The results showed that subjects reported that the trauma condition was most stressful. This suggests that it is not the events themselves that elicit stress, but the individuals' interpretation or appraisal of those events. Similarly, Mason (1975) argued that the stress response needed a degree of awareness of the stressful situation and reported that dying patients who were unconscious showed less signs of physiological stress than those who were conscious. He suggested that the conscious patients were able to appraise their situation whereas the unconscious ones were not. These studies therefore suggest that appraisal is related to the stress response. However, in contrast, some research indicates that appraisal may not always be necessary. For example, Repetti (1993) assessed the objective stressors (e.g. weather conditions, congestion) and subjective stressors (e.g. perceived stress) experienced by air traffic controllers and reported that both objective and subjective stressors independently predicted both minor illnesses and psychological distress.

This could indicate that either appraisal is not always necessary or that at times individuals do not acknowledge their level of subjective stress. In line with this possibility, some researchers have identified 'repressors' as a group of individuals who use selective inattention and forgetting to avoid stressful information (Roth and Cohen 1986). Such people show incongruence between their physiological state and their level of reported anxiety. For example, when confronted with a stressor they say, 'I am fine' but their body is showing arousal. This suggests that although appraisal may be central to the stress response there may be some people in some situations who deny or repress their emotional response to a stressor.

WHICH EVENTS ARE APPRAISED AS STRESSFUL?

Lazarus has argued that an event needs to be appraised as stressful before it can elicit a stress response. It could be concluded from this that the nature of the event itself is irrelevant – it is all down to the individual's own perception. However, research shows that some types of event are more likely to result in a stress response than others.

- *Salient events.* People often function in many different domains such as work, family and friends. For one person, work might be more salient, while for another their family life might be more important. Swindle and Moos (1992) argued that stressors in salient domains of life are more stressful than those in more peripheral domains.

- *Overload.* Multitasking seems to result in more stress than the chance to focus on fewer tasks at any one time (Lazarus and Folkman 1987). Therefore a single stressor which adds to a background of other stressors will be appraised as more stressful than when the same stressor occurs in isolation – commonly known as the 'straw that broke the camel's back'.

- *Ambiguous events.* If an event is clearly defined, then the person can efficiently develop a coping strategy. If, however, the event is ambiguous and unclear, then the person first has to spend time and energy considering which coping strategy is best. This is reflected in the work stress literature which illustrates that poor job control and role ambiguity in the workplace often result in a stress response (e.g. Karasek and Theorell 1990).

- *Uncontrollable events.* If a stressor can be predicted and controlled, then it is usually appraised as less stressful than a more random uncontrollable event. For example, experimental studies show that unpredictable loud bursts of noise are more stressful than predictable ones (Glass and Singer 1972).

In summary, most current stress researchers consider stress as the result of a person–environment fit and emphasize the role of primary appraisal ('Is the event stressful?') and secondary appraisal ('Can I cope?'). Psychological factors are seen as a central component to the stress response. However, they are always regarded as co-occurring with physiological changes.

3 | STRESS AND CHANGES IN PHYSIOLOGY AND BEHAVIOUR

Stress causes changes in physiology and behaviour which in turn can have an impact upon health and illness.

CHANGES IN PHYSIOLOGY

The physiological consequences of stress have been studied extensively, mostly in the laboratory using the acute stress paradigm which involves bringing individuals into a controlled environment, putting them into a stressful situation such as counting backwards, completing an intelligence task or giving an unprepared speech, and then recording any changes. This research has highlighted two main groups of physiological changes (see Figure 10.3):

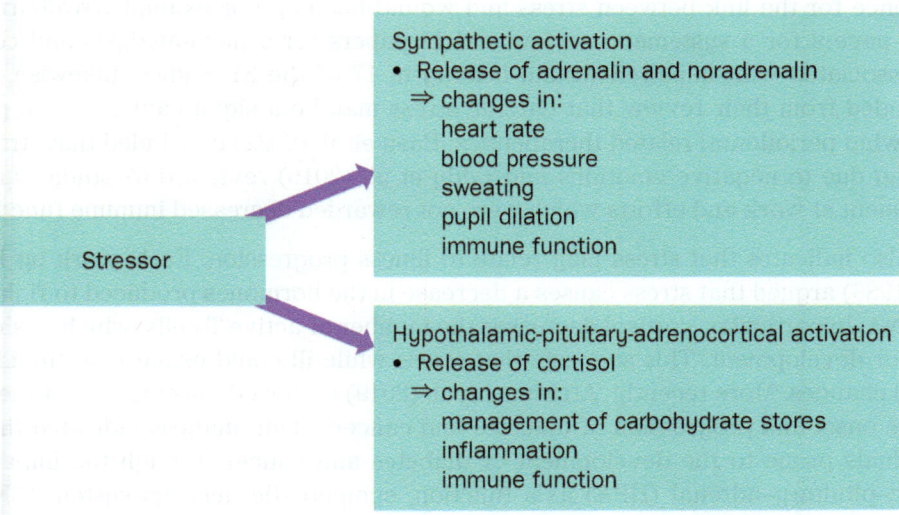

Figure 10.3 Stress and changes in physiology

1. *Sympathetic activation:* when an event has been appraised as stressful it triggers responses in the sympathetic nervous system. This results in the production of stress hormones known as catecholamines (adrenalin and noradrenalin, also known as epinephrine and norepinephrine) which cause changes in factors such as blood pressure, heart rate, sweating and pupil dilation. This is experienced as a feeling of **arousal.** This process is similar to the fight-or-flight response described by Cannon (1932). Catecholamines also have an effect on a range of the body's tissues and can lead to changes in immune function.

2 *Hypothalamic-pituitary-adrenocortical (HPA) activation:* in addition to sympathetic activation, stress also triggers changes in the HPA system. This results in the production of increased levels of corticosteroids, the most important of which is **cortisol,** which results in more diffuse changes, such as the management of carbohydrate stores and inflammation. These changes constitute the background effect of stress and cannot be detected by the individual. They are similar to the alarm, resistance and exhaustion stages of stress described by Selye (1956). In addition, raised levels of the brain opioids beta endorphin and enkephalin have been found following stress, and these are involved in immune-related problems.

Stress therefore causes physiological changes through both sympathetic and HPA activation. These two systems are not as discrete as often described, however, as prolonged sympathetic activation can lead to HPA activation and the release of cortisol. In turn both these forms of activation can lead to illnesses such as coronary heart disease (CHD) (see later in this chapter and Chapter 13).

Stress has also been shown to cause changes in the immune system. Early research on rats showed that stressors such as tail pinching, a loud noise and electric shocks could produce immunosuppression (Moynihan and Ader 1996). Research in humans shows a similar picture. One area of research which has received much attention relates to the impact of stress on wound healing. Kiecolt-Glaser et al. (1995) explored differences in wound healing between people who were caring for a person with Alzheimer's disease and a control group. Using a punch biopsy, which involves removing a small area of skin and tissue, they explored the relationship between caregiver stress and the wound healing process. The results showed that wound healing was slower in the caregivers than the control group. The wound healing paradigm has also been used to show links between stress and slower healing in students during an exam period (Marucha et al. 1998) and slower healing using high resolution ultrasound scanning, which is more accurate than the more traditional measurement strategies involving photography (Ebrecht et al. 2004). Over recent years there have been several reviews assessing the evidence for the link between stress and wound healing. For example, Walburn et al. (2009) identified 21 papers for a systematic review and 11 papers for a meta-analysis and concluded that stress was associated with impaired wound healing in 17 of the 21 studies. Likewise, Decker et al. (2021) concluded from their review that chronic stress may be a significant factor in poorer wound healing following periodontal-related therapeutics, Basu et al. (2022) concluded that stress may delay wound healing due to negative emotions and Eddy et al. (2016) reviewed 57 studies and found that over-commitment at work and efforts which were not rewarded decreased immune functioning.

Research also indicates that stress may relate to illness progression. Early work by Kiecolt-Glaser and Glaser (1986) argued that stress causes a decrease in the hormones produced to fight carcinogens and repair DNA. In particular, cortisol decreases the number of active T cells, which could increase the rate of tumour development. This suggests that stress while ill could exacerbate the illness through physiological changes. More recently, Afrisham et al. (2019) reviewed the evidence of the link between stress and the onset and progression of diabetes and cancer. Their analysis indicated that stress may make individuals prone to the development of diabetes and cancer through the impairment of the hypothalamic–pituitary–adrenal (HPA) axis function, sympathetic nervous system (SNS) and cytokines balance. Further, diabetes onset may be facilitated through the renin-angiotensin system (RAS) and insulin signalling pathway and decreased levels of oxytocin and dopamine may increase the risk of cancer. In line with this, Antoni and Dhabhar (2019) also provided evidence from their review of a link between stress and cancer progression and growth in those once diagnosed. Such stress may occur independently of the illness. However, stress may also be a result of the illness itself, such as relationship breakdown, changes in occupation or simply the distress from a diagnosis. Therefore, if the illness is appraised as being stressful, this itself may be damaging to the chances of recovery. The impact of stress on immune function and the role of psychoneuroimmunology (PNI) is discussed further in Chapter 12 with a focus on HIV and AIDS.

CHANGES IN BEHAVIOUR

Stress also causes changes in behaviour which in turn are linked with health (see Chapters 3–8). In line with this, some research has examined the effect of stress on specific health-related behaviours.

Smoking

Research suggests a link between stress and smoking behaviour in terms of smoking initiation, relapse and the amount smoked. Wills (1985) reported that smoking initiation in adolescents was related to the amount of stress in their lives. In addition, there has been some support for the prediction that children who experience the stressor of changing schools may be more likely to start smoking than those who stay at the same school throughout their secondary education (Santi et al. 1991). In terms of relapse, Lichtenstein et al. (1986) and Carey et al. (1993) reported that people who experience high levels of stress are more likely to start smoking again after a period of abstinence than those who experience less stress. Similarly, Metcalfe et al. (2003) used the Reeder Stress Inventory to relate stress to health behaviours and concluded that higher levels of stress were associated with smoking more cigarettes. This association was also found in one large-scale study of over 6,000 Scottish men and women which showed that higher levels of perceived stress were linked to smoking more (Heslop et al. 2001). Stress has also been shown to relate to smoking during pregnancy (Damron 2017).

Alcohol

Research has also examined the relationship between stress and alcohol consumption. The tension-reduction theory suggests that people drink alcohol for its tension-reducing properties (Cappell and Greeley 1987). This theory has been supported by some evidence of the relationship between negative mood and drinking behaviour (Violanti et al. 1983), suggesting that people are more likely to drink when they are feeling depressed or anxious. Similarly, both Metcalfe et al. (2003) and Heslop et al. (2001) reported an association between perceived stress and drinking more alcohol (if a drinker). Sacco et al. (2014) conducted a large-scale national survey in the USA with 4,360 participants and found that stressful life events were associated with alcohol use disorder in both men and women. However, whereas greater perceived stress was associated with lower alcohol consumption among women it was associated with increased chances of alcohol use disorder in men.

Eating

Greeno and Wing (1994) proposed two hypotheses concerning the link between stress and eating: (1) the *general effect model*, which predicts that stress changes food intake generally; and (2) the *individual difference model*, which predicts that stress only causes changes in eating in vulnerable groups of individuals. Most research has focused on the individual difference model and has examined whether either naturally occurring stress or laboratory-induced stress causes changes in eating in specific individuals. For example, Michaud et al. (1990) reported that exam stress was related to an increase in eating in girls but not in boys; Baucom and Aiken (1981) reported that stress increased eating in both the overweight and dieters and Cools et al. (1992) reported that stress was related to eating in dieters only. Furthermore, O'Conner et al. (2008) concluded from their study that the snacking–stress relationship was stronger in those with higher levels of dietary restraint, more emotional eating, greater disinhibition, higher levels of external eating, women and obese participants. Likewise, Darling et al. (2017) found that first-year university students showed stress eating and weight increase and that this was moderated by social support particularly in men. There are, however, several inconsistencies in the literature which have been described by Stone and Brownell (1994) as the 'stress eating paradox' to explain how at times stress causes overeating and at others it causes undereating without any clear pattern emerging.

Exercise

Research indicates that stress may reduce exercise (e.g. Heslop et al. 2001; Metcalfe et al. 2003) whereas stress management, which focuses on increasing exercise, has been shown to result in some improvements in coronary health. This has been described as the bi-directional relationship between stress and exercise with stress reducing exercise and exercise reducing stress (Burg et al. 2017). One study explored the impact of gardening on relief following experimentally induced stress (Van den Berg and Custers 2011). For this study, 30 allotment gardeners performed a stressful Stroop task and were then randomly allocated to outdoor gardening or indoor reading on their allotment plot. The results showed that although both groups showed a decrease in salivary cortisol, this was greater in the gardening group. It is not clear, however, whether this is due to gardening as a form of exercise, gardening as a form of creativity or whether simply being outdoors created this effect.

Accidents

Accidents are a very common and rarely studied cause of injury or mortality. Barkhordari et al. (2019) carried out a survey of 450 participants in Iran and concluded that occupational stress had a positive direct effect on accident proneness. Similarly, research suggests that individuals who experience high levels of stress show a greater tendency to perform behaviours that increase their chances of becoming injured (Wiebe and McCallum 1986). Further, Johnston (2002) has also suggested that stress increases accidents at home, at work and in the car. Leung et al. (2015) conducted a survey of construction workers to investigate the relationship between stress and accidents. They found that support from supervisors and reduced physical stress predicted safety behaviour in construction workers and that safety behaviour in turn predicted fewer accidents happening at work. Further, Lööw and Nygren (2019) analysed safety in the Swedish mining industry over a 30-year period, from the 1980s to the 2010s, and argued that understanding stress at work was key to accident prevention as when they are stressed people can make work choices that can be detrimental to their safety.

STRESS, COVID AND BEHAVIOUR CHANGE

The COVID pandemic started in January 2020, causing disruption, lockdown, distress and stress and since this time much research exploring the impact of stress on behaviour change has focused on the impact of COVID-related stress. In general, it is clear that COVID has resulted in an increase in most unhealthy behaviours.

Smoking: Grogan et al. (2022) conducted an online survey with 132 smokers in the UK during lockdown and analysed the written accounts using thematic analysis. The results showed that some participants smoked more as a coping mechanism to reduce perceived stress due to COVID-19. As one 27-year-old woman wrote: 'I already suffer from depression and anxiety, but it has been exacerbated by the pandemic. I smoke more now, as I feel more anxious.' Likewise, Stanton et al.'s (2020) survey of 1491 Australian adults showed that an increase in stress following the social isolation rules was associated with increases in smoking. In contrast, however, Bommelé et al. (2020) examined the relationship between COVID-19 stress and smoking in Dutch smokers and reported that while some smokers increased their smoking (18.9 per cent) due to reasons such as boredom (48.6 per cent), others decreased their smoking (14.1 per cent) due to reasons such as living a healthier life (32.3 per cent).

Alcohol intake: For alcohol intake, the pattern of change is more clear cut than smoking, with studies showing a fairly consistent increase in alcohol intake during the pandemic. For example, Schmidt et al. (2021) carried out a systematic review of 53 studies assessing changes in prevalence, incidence and severity of alcohol use during COVID and reported an association between stress and increased alcohol use. This is further reflected in the findings by Stanton et al. (2020) who explored the link between COVID-induced stress and alcohol in Australia and in a further review by Acuff et al. (2022).

Diet: Diet also seems to have been negatively impacted by COVID. For example, Bennett et al. (2021) conducted a scoping review of 23 studies and concluded that the stress induced by COVID was associated with unhealthier dietary habits, such as increased snacking and the intake of 'comfort foods'. Likewise, Chang et al. (2021) concluded from their systematic review that COVID-19 lockdowns had resulted in increased body weight and unhealthier eating patterns in children and adolescents.

Exercise: Exercise also changed during the COVID pandemic but results are mixed. Chew and Lopez carried out a scoping review in 2021 of 14 studies on physical activity in a wide range of countries (e.g. Poland, Brazil, China, US, Italy, Spain, UK, Croatia) exploring walking, jogging, swimming, cycling, sports, weight lifting, and leisure-time activities and sedentary behaviours including increased sitting time, TV watching, using electronics and social media. Whilst four studies reported that more respondents increased rather than decreased their physical activity, seven studies reported the majority decreasing their activity levels. Further, four studies reported a significant increase in sedentary behaviours.

4   DOES STRESS CAUSE ILLNESS?

One of the reasons that stress has been studied so consistently is because of its potential effect on the health of the individual. Research shows that hypertension rates are more common in those with high-stress jobs such as air traffic controllers (Cobb and Rose 1973) than in less stressed occupations such as nuns (Timio et al. 1988) and that higher life stress is associated with greater reporting of physical symptoms (Cropley and Steptoe 2005). Both cross-sectional and longitudinal studies also show that stressful occupations are associated with an increased risk of coronary heart disease (CHD) (Karasek et al. 1981; Kivimaki et al. 2002). Further, Phillips et al. (2008) reported from their longitudinal study of 968 men and women aged 56 that the number of health-related life events at baseline and their stress load predicted mortality by 17 years (266 participants had died). In addition Appels et al. (2002) indicated that 'vital exhaustion' is common in the year preceding a heart attack. In one classic study people were given nasal drops either containing viruses responsible for the common cold or placebo saline drops. Their level of stress was then assessed in terms of life events during the past year (Cohen et al. 1991). The results showed that not everyone who was given the virus contracted the virus and not everyone who did contract the virus actually exhibited cold symptoms and became ill. Stress was shown to predict, first, who contracted the virus, and second, who developed symptoms. However, these studies involved a cross-sectional, prospective or retrospective design which raises the problem of causality as it is unclear whether stress causes illness or illness causes stress (or stress ratings). To solve this problem some research has used an experimental design which involves inducing stress and assessing subsequent changes in health. Because of the ethical problems with such a design most experimental work has been done using animals. A classic series of animal studies by Manuck, Kaplan and colleagues (e.g. Kaplan et al. 1983; Manuck et al. 1986) experimentally manipulated the social groupings of Bowman Gray monkeys who have a strong social hierarchy. The results showed that the monkeys illustrated not only behavioural signs of stress but also a marked increase in the disease of their coronary arteries. In addition, stress management, which involves experimentally reducing stress, has had some success in reducing CHD (Johnston 1989, 1992) and in reducing recurrent cold and flu in children (Hewson-Bower and Drummond 2001).

HOW DOES STRESS CAUSE ILLNESS?

Researchers have identified two approaches to understanding the link between stress and illness. The first highlights the direct and indirect pathways and reflects the impact of stress on changes in physiology and behaviour. The second approach reflects the differential effects of chronic and acute stress. These two models will now be described. The modification of stress through stress management interventions is discussed in Chapter 13 in the context of coronary heart disease (CHD).

The Direct/Indirect Pathways

Stress can cause illness through either a direct pathway (via changes in physiology) or an indirect pathway (via changes in behaviour). This can create illnesses such as cancer, CHD and general physical symptoms such as tiredness, headaches and bowel problems. It can also lead to accidents. The direct and indirect pathways are shown in Figure 10.4 and reflects the model of health psychology described in Chapter 1.

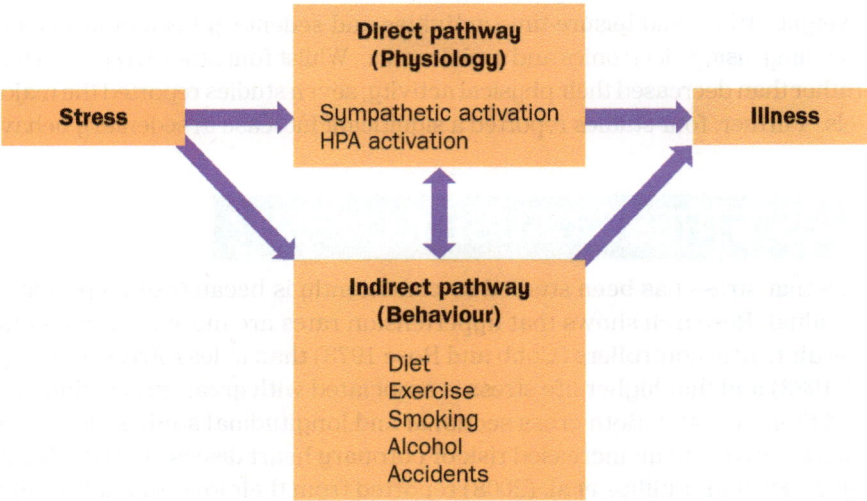

Figure 10.4 The direct / indirect pathways of stress and illness

The Direct Pathway

The direct pathway reflect changes in physiology. Stress causes changes in **sympathetic activation** (e.g. heart rate, sweating, blood pressure) via the production of stress hormones (i.e. the catecholamines adrenalin and noradrenalin) and causes the experience of arousal. This can result in blood clot formation, increased blood pressure, increased heart rate, irregular heart beats, fat deposits, plaque formation and immunosuppression. These changes may increase the chances of heart disease and kidney disease and leave the body open to infection. Stress also causes changes in **hypothalamic-pituitary-adrenocortical (HPA) activation** via the production of cortisol. The prolonged production of cortisol can result in decreased immune function and damage to neurons in the hippocampus. These changes may increase the chances of infection, psychiatric problems and losses in memory and concentration. A recent systematic review of 47 papers exploring stress and illness (Turner et al. 2020) concluded that exaggerated and blunted sympatho-adrenal medullary system and HPA axis stress reactivity predicted distinct physical and mental health and disease outcomes over time. Likewise, Afrisham et al.'s (2019) review concluded that psychological stress was related to the onset and progression of diabetes and cancer and identified a number of physiological mechanisms including HPA axis, SNS function, and cytokines balance. Recently, following the COVID pandemic in 2020, research has also explored the link between stress and COVID infections. For example, using an observational cohort study of 1087 UK adults, Ayling et al. (2022) concluded that psychological distress (operationalized as stress, anxiety and depression, and low levels of positive mood) during the early phase of the pandemic was significantly associated with subsequent self-reported SARS-CoV-2 infection, as well as the experience of a greater number and more severe symptoms. In line with this, Peters et al. (2021) concluded from their review of the evidence that stress-associated neuroendocrine-immune mechanisms could contribute to increases in both the susceptibility to the virus and its progression.

The Indirect Pathway

The indirect pathway reflects changes in behaviours which in turn can cause illness (see Chapters 2–7). For example, stress may increase smoking and alcohol intake, reduce exercise levels, change someone's diet to make them prefer high fat snack foods rather than meals, make them forget to take their medication, not practise safer sex or encourage them to take risks such as driving too fast, not wearing a cycle helmet or undertaking dangerous activities which could increase the chances of an accident. These behaviours can all contribute to conditions such as cancer, CHD or obesity or reduce life expectancy and are discussed in the previous section (eg. Stanton et al. 2020; Bommelé et al. 2020; Schmidt et al. 2021) .

Inter-related Pathways

Stress can therefore influence health and illness by changing behaviour or by directly impacting upon an individual's physiology. These two pathways also inter-relate. For example, stress may cause changes in behaviours such as smoking and diet, which impact upon health by changing the individual's physiology. Likewise, stress may cause physiological changes such as raised blood pressure but this is often most apparent in those who also exhibit particularly unhealthy behaviours (Johnston 1989). Therefore, in reality, stress is linked to illness via a complex interaction between behavioural and physiological factors. Further, Johnston (1989) argued that these factors are multiplicative, indicating that the more factors that are changed by stress, the greater the chance that stress will lead to illness.

The Chronic/Acute Stress Model

Johnston (2002) argued that the stress-illness link can also be understood in terms of the chronic and acute model. Chronic stress is more likely to involve **hypothalamic-pituitary-adrenocortical (HPA) activation** and the release of cortisol. This results in ongoing wear and tear and the slower process of atherosclerosis and damage to the cardiovascular system. Acute stress operates primarily through changes in **sympathetic activation** with changes in heart rate and blood pressure. This can contribute to atherosclerosis and kidney disease but is also related to sudden changes such as heart attacks. These processes may also be inter-related and are shown in Figure 10.5.

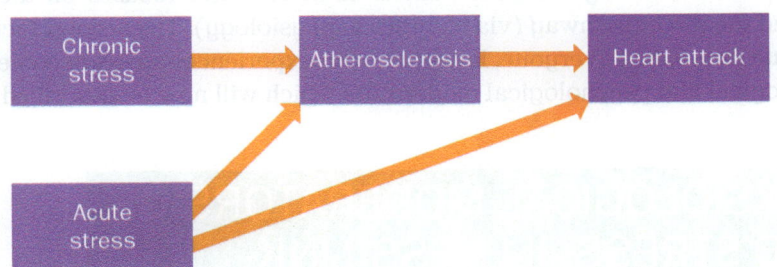

Figure 10.5 Chronic/acute model of stress–illness link

The Chronic Process

The most commonly held view of the link between stress and illness suggests that stress leads to disease due to a prolonged interaction of physiological, behavioural and psychological factors. For example, chronic work stress may cause changes in physiology and changes in behaviour which over time lead to damage to the cardiovascular system. In particular, chronic stress is associated with atherosclerosis, which is a slow process of arterial damage that limits the supply of blood to the heart. Further, this damage might be greater in those individuals with a particular genetic tendency. This chronic process is supported by research indicating links between job stress and cardiovascular disease (Karasek et al. 1981; Kivimaki et al. 2002). Further, a review by Dhabhar (2014) found that whereas short-term stress (from minutes to hours) enhanced adaptive immune responses, long-term stress suppressed these immune responses.

However, there are several problems with a purely chronic model of the stress–illness link:

1 Exercise protects against the wear and tear of stress with more active individuals being less likely to die from cardiovascular disease than more sedentary individuals (Kivimaki et al. 2002). However, exercise can also immediately precede a heart attack.

2 The wear and tear caused by stress can explain the accumulative damage to the cardiovascular system, but this chronic model does not explain why coronary events occur when they do.

In the light of these problems, Johnston (2002) also argues for an acute model.

The Acute Process

Heart attacks are more likely to occur following exercise, following anger, upon wakening, during changes in heart rate and during changes in blood pressure (e.g. Muller et al. 1994; Moller et al. 1999). They are acute events and involve a sudden rupture and thrombogenesis. Johnston (2002) argues that this reflects an acute model of the link between stress and illness with acute stress triggering a sudden cardiac problem. This explains how exercise can be protective in the longer term but a danger for an at-risk individual. It also explains why and when a heart attack occurs.

Links between the Acute and Chronic Processes

The acute and chronic processes are intrinsically interlinked. Chronic stress may simply be the frequent occurrence of acute stress; acute stress may be more likely to trigger a cardiac event in someone who has experienced chronic stress; and acute stress may also contribute to the wear and tear on the cardiovascular system. Therefore, although the acute and chronic process are described as discrete they are clearly inter-related.

IN SUMMARY

Stress, therefore, has been shown to cause illness and is linked to problems such as colds, flu, cancer, heart attacks, hypertension and physical symptoms such as tiredness and headaches. There are two approaches to understanding the stress–illness link. The first focuses on the indirect pathway (via behaviour) and the direct pathway (via changes in physiology). The second focuses on the impact of chronic and acute stress. Not everyone, however, who experiences stress becomes ill. This points to the role of physiological and psychological moderators which will now be described.

5 | PHYSIOLOGICAL MODERATORS OF THE STRESS–ILLNESS LINK

Not everyone who experiences stress becomes ill. Research indicates that some of this variability is due to individual differences in physiological factors such as stress reactivity, stress recovery, the allostatic load and stress resistance. The moderating effect of these physiological factors is shown in Figure 10.6.

STRESS REACTIVITY

Some individuals show a stronger physiological response to stress than others, which is known as their level of 'cardiovascular reactivity' or 'stress reactivity'. This means that when given the same level of stressor and regardless of their self-perceived stress, some people show greater sympathetic activation than others (e.g. Vitaliano et al. 1993). Research suggests that greater stress reactivity may make people more susceptible to stress-related illnesses. For example, individuals with both hypertension and heart disease have higher levels of stress reactivity (e.g. Frederickson et al. 1991, 2000).

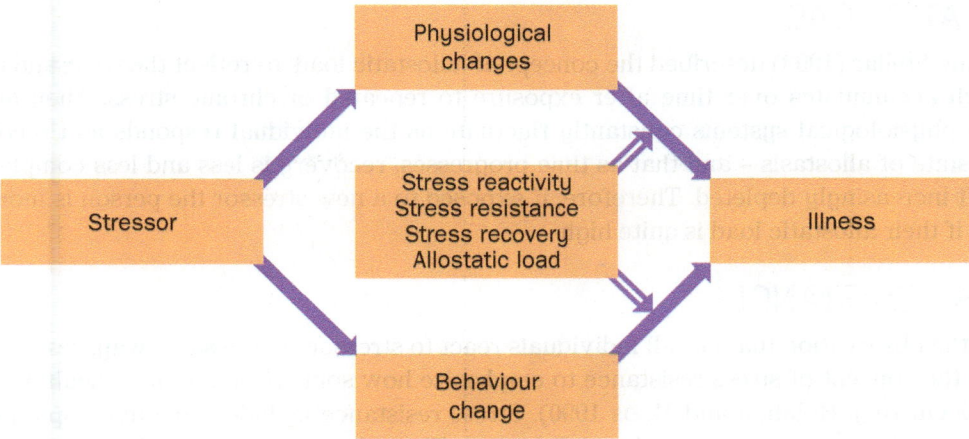

Figure 10.6 The stress–illness link: physiological moderators

However, these studies used a cross-sectional design which raises the problem of causality. Some research has therefore used a prospective design. For example, in an early study Keys et al. (1971) assessed baseline blood pressure reaction to a cold pressor test and found that higher reactivity predicted heart disease at follow-up 23 years later. Similarly, Boyce et al. (1995) measured baseline levels of stress reactivity in children following a stressful task and then rated the number of family stressors and illness rates over the subsequent 12 weeks. The results showed that stress and illness were not linked in the children with low reactivity but that those with higher reactivity showed more illness if they had experienced more stress. Everson and colleagues (1997) also assessed baseline stress reactivity and explored cardiac health using echo cardiography at follow-up. The results showed that higher stress reactivity at baseline was predictive of arterial deterioration after four years. In addition, stress reactivity has been suggested as the physiological mechanism behind the impact of coronary-prone behaviours on the heart (Suarez et al. 1991). This doesn't mean that individuals who show greater responses to stress are more likely to become ill. It means that they are more likely to become ill *if subjected to stress,* particularly if this pattern of responding to stress is maintained over a long period of time.

Over recent years there has also been an interest in blunted stress reactivity. In particular, some studies show that while some individuals show high levels of stress reactivity when under stress, those who have experienced a lifetime of ongoing and chronic stress, or childhood trauma or abuse may show a blunted reaction to stress, showing lower than expected arousal and reduced production of cortisol (Carpenter et al. 2007, 2009, 2011). The impact of blunted stress reactivity on health is unclear but there is some evidence that it may be linked to substance abuse and depression (Carroll et al. 2009; Heim et al. 2008). Recently, Turner et al.'s (2020) systematic review of 47 papers assessed the relationship between stress reactivity and future health outcomes and concluded that both exaggerated and blunted stress reactivity predicted poorer physical and mental health over time.

STRESS RECOVERY

After reacting to stress the body recovers and levels of sympathetic and HPA activation return to baseline. However, some people recover more quickly than others and some research indicates that this rate of recovery may relate to a susceptibility to stress-related illness. This is reflected in Selye's (1956) notion of 'exhaustion' and the general wear and tear caused by stress. Some research has focused particularly on changes in cortisol production, suggesting that slower recovery from raised cortisol levels could be related to immune function and a susceptibility to infection and illness (e.g. Perna and McDowell 1995).

ALLOSTATIC LOAD

McEwan and Stellar (1993) described the concept of 'allostatic load' to reflect the wear and tear on the body which accumulates over time after exposure to repeated or chronic stress. They argued that the body's physiological systems constantly fluctuate as the individual responds and recovers from stress – a state of allostasis – and that as time progresses, recovery is less and less complete and the body is left increasingly depleted. Therefore, if exposed to a new stressor the person is more likely to become ill if their allostatic load is quite high.

STRESS RESISTANCE

To reflect the observation that not all individuals react to stressors in the same way, researchers have developed the concept of stress resistance to emphasize how some people remain healthy even when stressors occur (e.g. Holahan and Moos 1990). Stress resistance includes adaptive coping strategies, certain personality characteristics and social support. These factors are dealt with in detail later on as they reflect psychological moderators.

6 | PSYCHOLOGICAL MODERATORS OF THE STRESS–ILLNESS LINK

There is also evidence that psychological factors moderate the link between stress and illness. These factors are as follows:

- *Health behaviours.* Exercise, smoking, alcohol intake and eating can also cause a reduction in stress (see Chapters 3–5).
- *Coping styles.* The individual's type of coping style may well mediate the stress–illness link and determine the extent of the effect of the stressful event on their health status (see Chapter 8 for a discussion of coping with illness).
- *Social support.* Increased social support has been related to a decreased stress response and a subsequent reduction in illness.

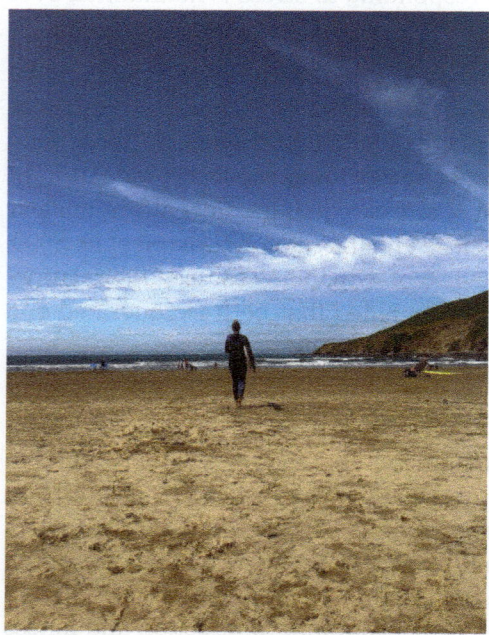

Exercise can help alleviate stress

- *Personality.* It has been suggested that personality may influence the individual's response to a stressful situation and the effect of this response on health. This has been studied with a focus on type A behaviour and personality and the role of hostility (see Chapter 13 for details in the context of CHD).
- *Actual or perceived control.* Control over the stressor may decrease the effects of stress on the individual's health status.
- The role of coping, social support, personality and control as psychological moderators of stress is shown in Figure 10.7. These will now be considered in more detail.

COPING

Over the past few years the literature on coping has grown enormously and has explored different types of coping styles, the links between coping and a range of health outcomes and the nature of coping itself (de Ridder 1997; de Ridder and Schreurs 2001; de Ridder et al. 2008).

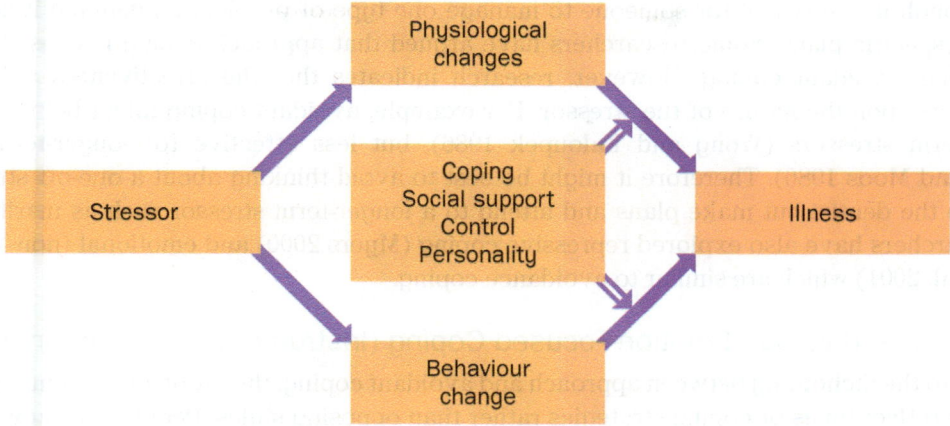

Figure 10.7 The stress–illness link: psychological moderators

How individuals cope with illness was described in Chapter 9 with a focus on crisis theory, cognitive adaptation theory and benefit-finding. This section will describe how coping relates to the stress–illness link.

What is Coping?

Coping has been defined by Lazarus and colleagues as the process of managing stressors that have been appraised as taxing or exceeding a person's resources and as the 'efforts to manage . . . environmental and internal demands' (Lazarus and Launier 1978). In the context of stress, coping therefore reflects the ways in which individuals interact with stressors in an attempt to return to some sort of normal functioning. This might involve correcting or removing the problem, or it might involve changing the way a person thinks about the problem or learning to tolerate and accept it. For example, coping with relationship conflict could involve leaving the relationship or developing strategies to make the relationship better. In contrast, it could involve lowering one's expectations of what a relationship should be like. Lazarus and Folkman (1987) emphasized the dynamic nature of coping which involves appraisal and reappraisal, evaluation and re-evaluation. Lazarus's model of stress emphasized the interaction between the person and their environment. Likewise, coping is also seen as a similar interaction between the person and the stressor. Further, in the same way that Lazarus and colleagues described responses to stress as involving primary appraisal of the external stressor and secondary appraisal of the person's internal resources, coping is seen to involve regulation of the external stressor and regulation of the internal emotional response. Cohen and Lazarus (1979) defined the goals of coping as:

1 To reduce stressful environmental conditions and maximize the chance of recovery.
2 To adjust or tolerate negative events.
3 To maintain a positive self-image.
4 To maintain emotional equilibrium.
5 To continue satisfying relationships with others.

   Researchers have described different types of coping. Some differentiate between approach and avoidance coping, while others describe emotion-focused and problem-focused coping.

Approach versus Avoidance

Roth and Cohen (1986) defined two basic modes of coping: approach and avoidance. *Approach coping* involves confronting the problem, gathering information and taking direct action. In contrast, *avoidant coping* involves minimizing the importance of the event. People tend to show one form of coping or the other, although it is possible for someone to manage one type of problem by denying it and another by making specific plans. Some researchers have argued that approach coping is consistently more adaptive than avoidant coping. However, research indicates that the effectiveness of the coping style depends upon the nature of the stressor. For example, avoidant coping might be more effective for short-term stressors (Wong and Kaloupek 1986), but less effective for longer-term stressors (Holahan and Moos 1986). Therefore it might be best to avoid thinking about a one-off stressor such as going to the dentist but make plans and attend to a longer-term stressor such as marital conflict. Some researchers have also explored repressive coping (Myers 2000) and emotional (non-)expression (Solano et al. 2001) which are similar to avoidance coping.

Problem-Focused versus Emotion-Focused Coping (Instrumentality–Emotionality)

In contrast to the dichotomy between approach and avoidant coping, the problem- and emotion-focused dimensions reflect types of coping strategies rather than opposing styles. People can show both problem-focused coping and emotion-focused coping when facing a stressful event. For example, Tennen et al. (2000) examined daily coping in people with rheumatoid arthritis and showed that problem-focused and emotion-focused coping usually occurred together and that emotion-focused coping was 4.4 times more likely to occur on a day when problem-focused coping had occurred than when it had not.

Problem-Focused Coping

This involves attempts to take action to either reduce the demands of the stressor or to increase the resources available to manage it. Examples include devising a revision plan and sticking to it, setting an agenda for a busy day, studying for extra qualifications to enable a career change and organizing counselling for a failing relationship.

Emotion-Focused Coping

This involves attempts to manage the emotions evoked by the stressful event. People use both behavioural and cognitive strategies to regulate their emotions. Examples include talking to friends about a problem, turning to drink or smoking more, or getting distracted by shopping or watching a film. Examples of cognitive strategies include denying the importance of the problem and trying to think about the problem in a positive way.

Several factors have been shown to influence which coping strategy is used:

- *Type of problem.* Work problems seem to evoke more problem-focused coping whereas health and relationship problems tend to evoke emotion-focused coping (Vitaliano et al. 1990).

- *Age.* Children tend to use more problem-focused coping strategies whereas emotion-focused strategies seem to develop in adolescence (Compas et al. 1991). Folkman et al. (1987) reported that middle-aged men and women tended to use problem-focused coping whereas the elderly used emotion-focused coping.

- *Gender.* It is generally believed that women use more emotion-focused coping and that men are more problem-focused. Some research supports this belief. For example, Stone and Neale (1984) considered coping with daily events and reported that men were more likely to use direct action than women. However, Folkman and Lazarus (1980) found no gender differences.

- *Controllability.* People tend to use problem-focused coping if they believe that the problem itself can be changed. In contrast, they use more emotion-focused coping if the problem is perceived as being out of their control (Lazarus and Folkman 1987).

- *Available resources.* Coping is influenced by external resources such as time, money, children, family and education (Terry 1994). Poor resources may make people feel that the stressor is less controllable by them, resulting in a tendency not to use problem-focused coping.

- *Coping training.* Kaluza (2000) evaluated an intervention designed to change the coping profiles of 82 healthy working men and women. The intervention lasted for 12 weeks and focused on assertiveness, cognitive restructuring, time management, relaxation, physical activities and the scheduling of pleasant activities. Changes were compared to a control group who received no intervention. The results showed significant improvements in emotion-focused coping and problem-focused coping which were related to the individual's original coping profiles. In particular, those who were originally more problem-focused became more emotion-focused and those who were more avoidant copers became more problem-focused. The authors suggest that the intervention changed unbalanced coping profiles. In addition, these changes were related to improvements in aspects of well-being.

Coping and the Stress–Illness Link

Some research indicates that coping styles may moderate the association between stress and illness. For some studies the outcome variable has been more psychological in its emphasis and has taken the form of well-being, psychological distress or adjustment. For example, Kneebone and Martin (2003) critically reviewed the research exploring coping in carers of persons with dementia. They examined both cross-sectional and longitudinal studies and concluded that problem-solving and acceptance styles of coping seemed to be more effective at reducing stress and distress. In a similar vein, research exploring coping with rheumatoid arthritis suggests that active and problem-solving coping are associated with better outcomes whereas passive avoidant coping is associated with poorer outcomes (e.g. Newman et al. 1996). For patients with chronic obstructive pulmonary disease (COPD), wishful thinking and emotion-focused coping were least effective (Buchi et al. 1997). Similarly, research exploring stress and psoriasis shows that avoidant coping is the least useful (e.g. Leary et al. 1998). Other studies have focused on more illness-associated variables. For example, Holahan and Moos (1986) examined the relationship between the use of avoidance coping, stress and symptoms such as stomach-ache and headaches. The results after one year showed that, of those who had experienced stress, those who used avoidance coping had more symptoms than those who used more approach coping strategies. Likewise, Yi-Frazier et al. (2015) explored coping in adolescents with Type 1 diabetes and found that maladaptive coping strategies predicted low resilience which in turn was linked with poorer glycaemic control.

Coping and Positive Outcomes

Over recent years there has been an increasing recognition that stressful events such as life events and illness may not only result in negative outcomes but may also lead to some positive changes in people's lives. This phenomenon has been given a range of names including *stress-related growth* (Park et al. 1996), *benefit-finding* (Tennen and Affleck 1999), *meaning-making* (Park and Folkman 1997), *growth-orientated functioning* and *crisis growth* (Holahan et al. 1996). This finds reflection in Taylor's (1983) cognitive adaptation theory and is in line with a new movement called 'positive psychology' (Seligman and Csikszentmihalyi 2000). Though a new field of study, research indicates that coping processes that involve finding meaning in the stressful event, positive reappraisal and problem-focused coping are associated with positive outcomes (Folkman and Moskowitz 2000). (See Chapter 8 for further discussion of benefit-finding following illness.)

SOCIAL SUPPORT

What Is Social Support?

The term 'social support' is generally used to refer to the perceived comfort, caring, esteem or help one individual receives from others (e.g. Wallston et al. 1983). Initially, it was defined according to the number of friends that were available to the individual. However, this has been developed

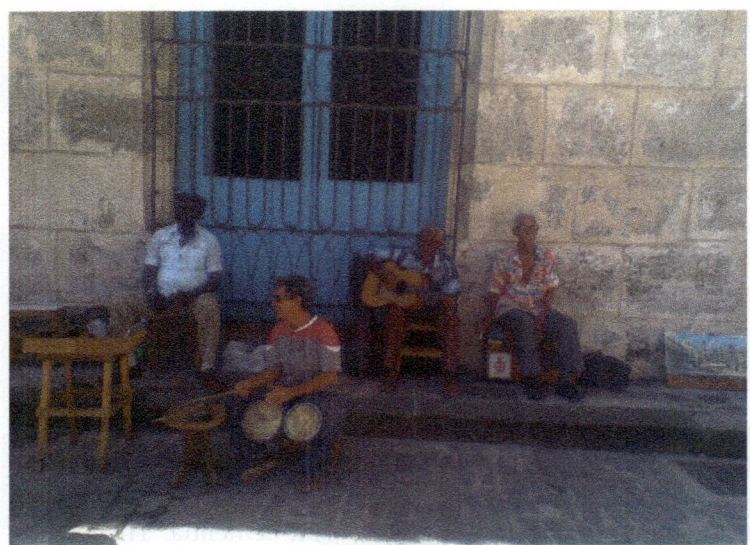

Some communities are high on social capital which can reduce stress

to include not only the number of friends supplying social support, but the satisfaction with this support (Sarason et al. 1983). Wills (1985) has defined several types of social support:

- *Esteem support:* whereby other people increase one's own self-esteem.
- *Support:* whereby other people are available to offer advice.
- *Companionship:* which involves support through activities.
- *Instrumental support:* which involves physical help.

Lett et al. (2005) also put forward a definition of social support that differentiates between two types:

- *Structural support (or network support):* which refers to the type, size, density and frequency of contact with the network of people available to any individual.
- *Functional support:* which refers to the perceived benefit provided by this structure. This has also been classified into *available functional support* (i.e. potential access to support) and *enacted functional support* (i.e. actual support received) (Tardy 1985).

Taking a broader view, Bavik et al. (2020) synthesized findings from more than 4,500 studies across a number of disciplines. They argued that social support can be considered in terms of **six characteristics:** quantity and quality, utilization, source, content, format and consistency; and in terms of **four dynamic roles:** a positivity catalyst, a positivity enhancer, a negativity buffer and a negativity exacerbator.

Since the 1990s researchers have also explored the notion of 'social capital' which has been shown to have an impact on health (e.g. Putnam 1993; Veenstra 2000; Almedon 2005). Social capital is a broad construct that incorporates trust, social networks, social participation, successful cooperation and reciprocity. Therefore, rather than a person having social capital, it could be argued that a town or village is high on social capital if there is a strong sense of community and mutual support. Social capital is hard to measure as it contains components at both the individual (i.e. trust) and group (i.e. social networks) levels. Within psychology, therefore, the focus has tended to be upon social support from a more individualistic perspective, although Abbott and Freeth (2008) argued that social capital, particularly the elements of trust and reciprocity, could be useful in understanding ways to reduce stress.

Does Social Support Affect Health?

A number of studies have examined whether social support influences the health status of the individual. For example, Lynch (1977) reported that widowed, divorced or single individuals have higher mortality rates from heart disease than married people and suggested that heart disease and mortality are related to lower levels of social support. However, problems with this study include the absence of a direct measure of social support and the implicit assumption that marriage is an effective source of social support.

Berkman and Syme (1979) reported the results of a prospective study whereby they measured social support in 4,700 men and women aged 30–69, whom they followed up for nine years. They found that increased social support predicted a decrease in mortality rate indicating a role for social support in health. Research has also indicated that birth complications are lower in women who have high levels of social support, again suggesting a link between social support and health status (Oakley 1992). Research has also explored the impact of social support on health behaviours. Graven and Grant (2014) conducted a review of 13 studies of people with heart failure and found that increased social support

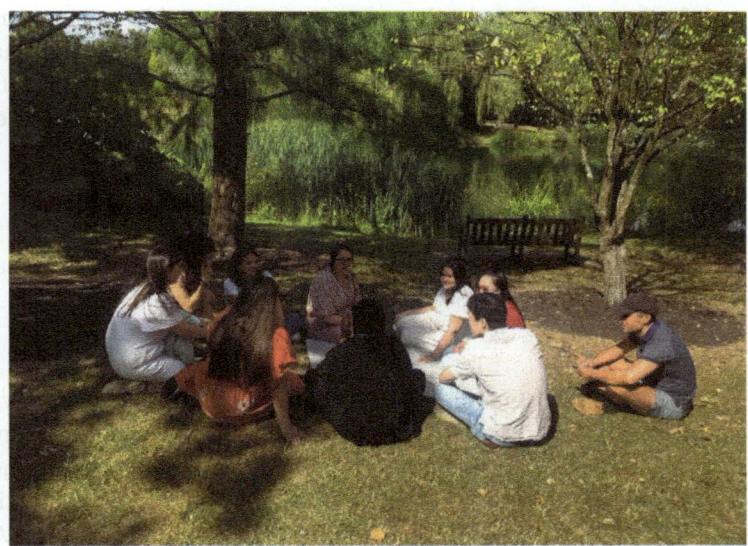

Social support can help moderate stress for students if they study together

increased heart failure self-care behaviours with a key role for patients' families helping individuals to maintain these behaviours. Social support has also been shown to have an impact on immune functioning and consequently health. For example, Cohen et al. (2015) investigated whether hugging as a means of social support can buffer against interpersonal stress-induced susceptibility to infectious disease. They exposed 406 healthy adults to a virus for the common cold and found that more frequent hugging and greater perceived social support predicted less severe illness signs in those who were infected by the virus. Likewise, Lee and Waters (2021) examined self-reported racial discrimination toward 410 Asians and Asian-Americans living in the United States and concluded that social support significantly buffered the effect of discrimination on depressive symptoms and marginally buffered the effect on physical symptoms. Following the pandemic in 2020, much research has also addressed the impact of social support on health outcomes related to COVID. In line with this, d'Ettorre et al. (2021) carried out a systematic review of 16 studies and reported that lack of social support was a predictor of post-traumatic stress symptoms in healthcare workers during the COVID-19 pandemic.

How Does Social Support Influence Health?

If social support does influence or mediate the stress–illness link, then what are the possible mechanisms? Two theories have been developed to explain the role of social support in health status:

1 The *main effect hypothesis* suggests that social support itself is beneficial and that the absence of social support is itself stressful. This suggests that social support mediates the stress–illness link, with its very presence reducing the effect of the stressor and its absence acting as a stressor (e.g. Wills 1985).

2 The *stress buffering hypothesis* suggests that social support helps individuals to cope with stress, therefore mediating the stress–illness link by buffering the individual from the stressor; social support influences the individual's appraisal of the potential stressor (Wills 1985). This process, which has been described using *social comparison theory*, suggests that the existence of other people enables individuals exposed to a stressor to select an appropriate coping strategy by comparing themselves with others. For example, if an individual was going through a stressful life event, such as divorce, and existed in a social group where other people had dealt with divorces, the experiences

of others would help them to choose a suitable coping strategy. The stress buffering hypothesis has also been described using *role theory*. This suggests that social support enables individuals to change their role or identity according to the demands of the stressor. Role theory emphasizes an individual's role and suggests that the existence of other people offers choices as to which role or identity to adopt as a result of the stressful event.

PERSONALITY

The role of personality on health has focused on Type A behaviour, conscientiousness, hostility and the Big 5 personality types in general.

Type A

Friedman and Rosenman (1959) initially defined type A behaviour in terms of excessive competitiveness, impatience, hostility and vigorous speech. Using a semi-structured interview, three types of type A behaviour were identified. Type A1 reflected vigour, energy, alertness, confidence, loud speaking, rapid speaking, tense clipped speech, impatience, hostility, interrupting, frequent use of the word 'never' and frequent use of the word 'absolutely'. Type A2 was defined as being similar to type A1, but not as extreme, and type B was regarded as relaxed, showing no interruptions and quieter (e.g. Rosenman 1978). The Jenkins Activity Survey was developed in 1971 to further define type A behaviour. Support for a relationship between type A behaviour and CHD using the Jenkins Activity Survey has been reported by a number of studies (Rosenman et al. 1975; Haynes et al. 1980). However, research has also reported no relationship between type A behaviour and CHD. For example, Johnston et al. (1987) used Bortner's (1969) questionnaire to predict heart attacks in 5,936 men aged 40–59 years, who were randomly selected from British general practice lists. All subjects were examined at the start of the study for the presence of heart disease and completed the Bortner questionnaire. They were then followed up for morbidity and mortality from heart attack and for sudden cardiac death for an average of 6.2 years. The results showed that non-manual workers had higher type A scores than manual workers and that type A score decreased with age. However, at follow-up the results showed no relationship between type A behaviour and heart disease.

Conscientiousness

O'Connor et al. (2009) explored the role of conscientiousness on moderating the link between daily hassles and changes in health behaviours. Using a prospective design, 422 employees completed ratings of daily hassles and health behaviours over a four-week period. The results showed that greater daily hassles were linked to a higher intake of high fat snacks, a greater consumption of caffeinated drinks, higher levels of smoking but lower intakes of alcohol, vegetables and less exercise. Furthermore, the results indicated that these associations were influenced by conscientiousness.

Hostility

Hostility is most frequently measured using the Cook Medley Hostility Scale (Cook and Medley 1954) which asks people to rate statements such as 'I have often met people who were supposed to be experts who were no better than I', 'It is safer to trust nobody', and 'My way of doing things is apt to be misunderstood by others'. Agreement with such statements is an indication of high hostility. Hostility has also been classified according to cynical hostility and neurotic hostility. Hostility is higher in men than women (Matthews et al. 1992), higher in those of lower socioeconomic status (e.g. Siegman et al. 2000) and seems to run in families (Weidner et al. 2000). It seems to be more common in people whose parents were punitive, abusive or interfering and where there was a lot of conflict (Matthews et al. 1996), and Houston and Vavak (1991) have argued that it relates to feelings of insecurity and negative feelings about others.

 Much research has shown an association between hostility and CHD. In particular, researchers have argued that hostility is not only an important risk factor for the development of heart disease (e.g. Miller et al. 1996) but is also a trigger for cardiac events such as heart attacks (Moller et al. 1999; Rafenelli et al, 2016) particularly the expression of hostility as anger (Ramsay et al. 2001; McDermott et al. 2001; Siegman and Snow 1997). In 2013, Silton et al. investigated correlates of subjective health status in 1,629 adults in the USA. The results showed that increased hostility was associated with poorer health whereas forgiveness had a positive effect on health. The link between hostility and heart disease illustrates a role for three pathways. First, hostility may impact upon the physiological pathway and is associated with heightened stress reactivity and larger and longer-lasting changes in blood pressure leading to cardiac damage (Guyll and Contrada 1998; Fredrickson et al. 2000). Second, hostility is linked to unhealthy behaviours such as smoking, alcohol intake, caffeine consumption and poorer diet (e.g. Lipkus et al. 1994) and third, hostility may be associated with other moderating factors. For example, hostile individuals may avoid social support and refuse to draw upon any help when under stress. In fact, this is implicit within some of the measures of hostility with responses to statements such as 'No one cares much what happens to me'. Hostility may also relate to coping as believing that 'It is safer to trust nobody' could be seen to reflect an avoidant coping style.

The Big 5 Personality Types

The Big 5 personality types are extraversion, agreeableness, openness, conscientiousness and neuroticism. Over the years, many papers have been written about the link between the Big 5 and health. Strickhouser et al. (2017) conducted a meta-synthesis to investigate whether personality could predict health and well-being; 36 meta-analyses were included in the synthesis which provided data from over 500,000 participants. The results showed that when entered simultaneously, the Big 5 traits were moderately associated with overall health; however, personality-health relationships were stronger for mental health than physical health outcomes.

CONTROL

The final potential mediator of the stress–illness link is control. The effect of control on the stress–illness link has also been extensively studied.

What is Control?

Control has been studied within a variety of different psychological theories.

1 *Attributions and control.* Kelley's (1967) attributional theory examines control in terms of attributions for causality (see Chapter 2 for a discussion of attribution theory). If applied to a stressor, the cause of a stressful event would be understood in terms of whether the cause was controllable by the individual or not. For example, failure to get a job could be understood in terms of a controllable cause (e.g. 'I didn't perform as well as I could in the interview', 'I should have prepared better') or an uncontrollable cause (e.g. 'I am stupid', 'The interviewer was biased').

2 *Self-efficacy and control.* Control has also been discussed by Bandura (1977) in his self-efficacy theory. Self-efficacy refers to an individual's confidence to carry out a particular behaviour. Control is implicit in this concept.

3 *Categories of control.* Five different types of control have been defined by Thompson (1986): behavioural control (e.g. avoidance); cognitive control (e.g. reappraisal of coping strategies); decisional control (e.g. choice over possible outcome); informational control (e.g. the ability to access information about the stressor); and retrospective control (e.g. 'Could I have prevented that event from happening?').

4 *The reality of control.* Control has also been subdivided into perceived control (e.g. 'I *believe* that I can control the outcome of a job interview') and actual control (e.g. 'I *can* control the outcome of a job interview'). The discrepancy between these two factors has been referred to as *illusory control* (e.g. 'I control whether the plane crashes by counting throughout the journey'). However, within psychological theory, most control relates to perceived control.

Does Control Affect the Stress Response?

Research has examined the extent to which the controllability of the stressor influences the stress response to this stressor, both in terms of the subjective experience of stress and the accompanying physiological changes.

1 *Subjective experience.* Corah and Boffa (1970) examined the relationship between the controllability of the stressor and the subjective experience of stress. Subjects were exposed to a loud noise (the experimental stressor) and were either told about the noise (the stressor was predictable) or not (an unpredictable stressor). The results indicated that if the noise was predictable, there was a decrease in subjective experiences of stress. The authors argued that predictability enables the subject to feel that they have control over the stressor, and that this perceived control reduces the stress response. Baum et al. (1981) further suggested that if a stressor is predicted, there is a decrease in the stress response, and reported that predictability or an expectation of the stress enables the individual to prepare their coping strategies.

2 *Physiological changes.* Research has also examined the effect of control on the physiological response to stress. For example, Meyer et al. (1985) reported that if a stressor is regarded as uncontrollable, the release of corticosteroids is increased.

Does Control Affect Health?

If control influences the stress response, does control also influence the effect of stress on health and illness? This question has been examined by looking at both animal and human models.

Animal Research

Seligman and Visintainer (1985) reported the results of a study whereby rats were injected with live tumour cells and exposed to either controllable or uncontrollable shocks. The results indicated that the uncontrollable shocks resulted in promotion of the tumour growth. This suggests that controllability may influence the stress response, which may then promote illness. In a further study, the relationship between control and CHD was studied in monkeys (Manuck et al. 1986). Some breeds of monkey exist in social hierarchies with clearly delineated roles. The monkeys are categorized as either dominant or submissive and this hierarchy is usually stable. However, the authors introduced new members to the groups to create an unstable environment. They argued that the dominant monkeys showed higher rates of CHD in the unstable condition than the dominant monkeys in the stable condition, or the submissive monkeys in the stable condition. It was suggested that the dominant monkeys had high expectations of control, and were used to experiencing high levels of control. However, in the unstable condition, there was a conflict between their expectations of control and the reality which, the authors argued, resulted in an increase in CHD. These animal models are obviously problematic in that many assumptions are made about the similarities between the animals' experience of control and that of humans. However, the results indicate an association between control and health in the predicted direction.

Human Research

Human models have also been used to examine the effect of control on the stress–illness link. For example, the job strain model was developed to examine the effects of control on CHD (e.g. Karasek and Theorell 1990). The three factors involved in the model are (1) psychological demands of the job in terms of workload; (2) the autonomy of the job, reflecting control; and (3) the satisfaction with the job. This model has been used to predict CHD in the USA (Karasek et al. 1988), and in Sweden (Karasek et al. 1981). The results of these studies suggest that a combination of high workload (i.e. high demand), low satisfaction and low control are the best predictors of CHD. Research also indicates that an external locus of control is associated with greater disease severity in those with Parkinson's disease (Rizza et al. 2017) although this was a cross-sectional study limiting conclusions about causality.

How Does Control Mediate the Stress–Illness Link?

A number of theories have been developed to explain how control influences health and mediates the stress–illness link:

- *Control and preventive behaviour.* It has been suggested that high control enables the individual to maintain a healthy lifestyle by believing that 'I can do something to prevent illness'.
- *Control and behaviour following illness.* It has also been suggested that high control enables the individual to change behaviour after illness. For example, even though the individual may have low health status following an illness, if they believe there is something they can do about their health, they will change their behaviour.
- *Control and physiology.* It has been suggested that control directly influences health via physiological changes.
- *Control and personal responsibility.* It is possible that high control can lead to a feeling of personal responsibility and consequently personal blame and learned helplessness. These feelings could lead either to no behaviour change or to unhealthy behaviours resulting in illness.

STRESS AS A COMPLEX PSYCHO-PHYSIOLOGICAL PROCESS

This chapter has illustrated the ways in which stress and its impact on illness reflect an interaction between **psychological processes** (e.g. appraisal, behaviour, coping, social support, personality, control) and **physiological processes** (i.e. sympathetic activation, HPA activation, immune response, stress reactivity, allostatic load, stress recovery, stress resistance). This is reflected in a complex **psycho-physiological model** of stress shown in Figure 10.8.

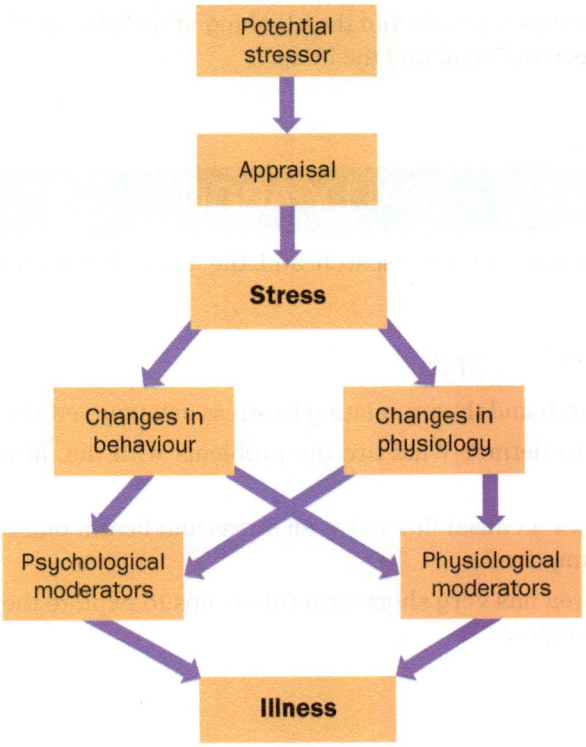

Figure 10.8 A psycho-physiological model of stress

BOX 10.1
Critical Approaches to Health Psychology

Research and theories relating to stress and illness highlight some of the bigger issues in health psychology as follows:

The individual vs social vs political: Stress research focuses on how an individual reacts to a stressor, whether they way they cope helps and how then then behave. Research then explores whether this response to the stressor influences their health. But stressors exist within a social and political context and focusing only on appraisal can neglect the importance of this external world. At times it can also push the responsibility for change from the outside world onto the individual. So if a person is stressed because they are overworked, health psychology interventions would help them to re-appraise the stressor, adopt different coping mechanisms and utilize appropriate and health behaviours. It doesn't involve telling the managers at work to reduce their workload! Likewise, if children are stressed because of all the exams they have to do we teach them stress management skills rather than questioning whether they need to be assessed this much. By focusing on the individual and their psychology, the social and political world can often be neglected.

Individual differences: Research often focuses on differences in the stress response by occupation, by age, by personality or by gender. For example, we know that certain occupations create more stress than others and we know there are differences between men and women or between those with hostile personality in their stress reactivity. This helps with data analysis but is an over-simplification of who we are and the many factors that determine how we respond to the world around us.

The mind–body split: Stress research illustrates the ways in which how we think (i.e. appraise or cope) influences our body (i.e. whether we get ill). This shows the interaction between mind and body but by defining them as separate and then looking at their interaction we are still recreating a false dichotomy between the mind and the body.

7   THINKING CRITICALLY ABOUT STRESS AND ILLNESS

There are some problems with stress research and the ways in which stress links to illness that should be considered.

SOME CRITICAL QUESTIONS

When thinking about research and theory relating to stress ask yourself the following questions:

- Why is stress difficult to define? What are the problems with the different ways of defining and measuring stress?
- Research often concludes a causal link between stress and health outcomes. What are some of the problems with this assumption?
- Much research in this area has very short-term follow-ups to explore the impact of stress. What are the problems with this method?

- Research also uses longitudinal data to explore changes over time. There are also some problems with this method. What might they be?
- Stress illustrates the link between psychological and biological processes. What are the problems with making these links?

SOME PROBLEMS WITH. . .

Below are some of the problems with research and theory in this area.

Definitions: Defining stress can be difficult as it depends upon the focus of the researcher involved. Therefore, from a more physiological perspective stress is defined as arousal and the production of cortisol whereas from a more psychological perspective it is defined as the experience of stress.

Measuring stress: Stress can be assessed using either self-report or physiological changes which both have their problems. Self-report can be open to bias and a desire to appear more or less stressed depending upon the person and the situation. Physiological measures may be intrusive and actually create stress and may change the way in which a person responds to their environment. The measurement of stress very much depends upon the definition being used.

Appraisal processes are not discrete: The appraisal model suggests that people appraise the stressor and then appraise their coping mechanisms. This conceptualizes these two processes as separate and discrete. However, it is likely that they are completely interdependent as a stressor is only really stressful in the context of whether the individual feels they can or cannot cope with it.

Changes are not discrete: Stress is considered to be made up of both psychological and physiological changes. However, how these two sets of changes interact is unclear as it is possible to perceive stress without showing physiological changes or to show a physiological reaction without labelling it as stress.

Causal links: The models tend to describe causal links between stress and changes in behaviour or stress and changes in physiology. Further, they also describe links between stress and illness. In reality, however, all these processes probably exist in an iterative dynamic with everything causing and changing everything else.

Methodological issues: If we want to know whether, and if, stress causes illness then we would need to experimentally induce stress in a random selection of people, compare to a randomly assigned control group and then follow up for a very long period of time. This isn't feasible or ethical. Therefore, much stress research is short term, cross sectional or longitudinal, with many confounding variables that cannot be controlled for. This makes drawing conclusions about the links between stress and illness problematic.

The mind–body split: Although much stress research examines how the mind may influence the body (e.g. appraisal relates to the release of stress hormones; coping reduces the risk of illness) these relationships may suggest an interaction between the mind and the body but they still define them as separate entities which influence each other, not as the same entity. Health psychology emphasizes a holistic approach to the mind and body but often these two factors are defined as separate to each other, maintaining the mind–body split.

TO CONCLUDE

This chapter has explored what stress is, how it is defined and measured. It has then described the transactional model of stress with its focus on appraisal which emphasizes a key role for psychology in the stress response. Once appraised as a stressor, the chapter then addressed changes in physiology including arousal (sympathetic activation) and the release of cortisol (HPA activation) and changes in behaviour (e.g. smoking, diet, exercise). Much research shows a link between stress and illness and this chapter next explored mechanisms for this link in terms of the direct and indirect pathways and the chronic and acute model. Not all people who experience stress become ill, however, and the chapter then explored the role of physiological moderators (e.g. stress reactivity, allostatic load) and psychological moderators (e.g. coping, social support, personality and control). Stress can therefore be understood as a complex interplay between psychological and physiological factors, which is illustrated in the psycho-physiological model. Finally, the chapter outlined some of the problems with research in this area including problems with definition and measurement, problems caused by the overlap between different constructs and processes and methodological issues.

QUESTIONS

1 Discuss the role of appraisal in the stress response.
2 How does stress cause changes in physiology?
3 Which behaviours might change when you are under stress?
4 Evaluate the evidence that stress causes illness.
5 To what extent might the acute and chronic pathways of stress interact?
6 To what extent could the indirect and direct pathways of stress interact?
7 Discuss the possible physiological factors that might moderate the stress–illness link.
8 Discuss the psychological factors that might moderate the stress–illness link.
9 What are the methodological problems with research exploring the impact of stress on illness?

FOR DISCUSSION

Think of the last time you felt stressed. What factors made this experience either better or worse? Discuss the extent stress may have impacted upon your health.

FURTHER READING

Cropley, M. (2015) *The Off Switch: Leave Work on Time, Relax Your Mind But Still Get More Done*. London: Random House.
This is an easy-to-read and accessible book using theories of stress and rumination to show how we can and should switch off from work.

Jones, F., Burke, R.J. and Westmen, M. (eds) (2006) *Work–Life Balance: A Psychological Perspective.* Hove: Psychology Press.

This book is an edited collection of chapters which describe and explore different aspects of the work–life balance including the changing nature of work, the legal and policy context of work, managing home and work, managing family and work and recovery after work.

Lazarus, R.S. (2000) Towards better research on stress and coping, *American Psychologist,* **55:** 665–73.

This paper is part of a special issue on stress and coping, and reflects Lazarus's own comments on developments and critiques of the stress literature.

Taris, T.W (2018) *The Psychology of Working Life.* London: Routledge.

This little book explores the psychological aspects of work–life balance and the stressors and strains of working life in an accessible way.

Vedhara, K. (2012) Psychoneuroimmunology: The Whole And The Sum Of Its Parts, *Brain, Behavior, and Immunity,* **26**(2): 210–11.

This review provides an excellent overview of the research on PNI and covers key concepts, research and methods.

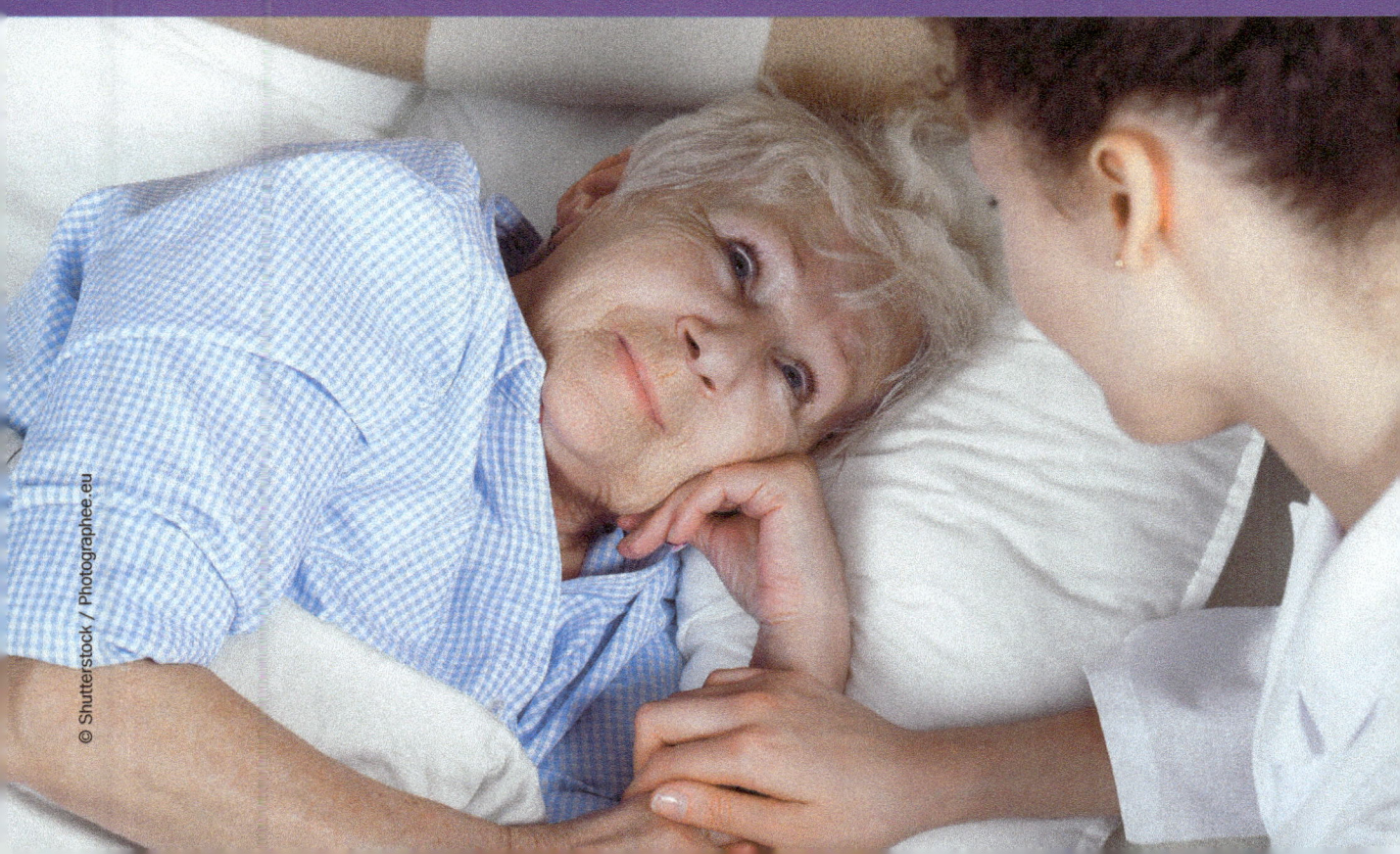

11

Pain and the Placebo Effect

CHAPTER OVERVIEW

This chapter examines early models of pain and their description of pain as a sensation. It then examines the increasing emphasis on a role for psychology in pain, the shift towards the notion of pain perception and the development of the gate control theory. The chapter then describes the role of psychosocial factors in pain perception with a focus on learning, affect, cognition and behaviour. Next, the role of psychology in treating and managing pain is discussed. The chapter then explores the placebo effect, the impact that expectations can have on physical symptoms including pain and the role of placebos across the breadth of health psychology. Finally, the chapter describes how to think critically about research on pain and the placebo effect.

CASE STUDY

Tamsin is 45 and suffers from chronic back pain. She used to work in marketing and had a stressful desk job but she has been on sick leave for the past six months as she finds it painful to drive and sitting at her desk seems to make it worse. Her sick pay is coming to an end but fortunately her partner has a good job so she is thinking of taking redundancy and staying at home full time. To help her back, she spends many hours a day lying down and watches films to keep herself entertained. She is quite scared of making the pain worse, as at times it has been dreadful, so over the past six months she has done less and less each day and now very rarely goes out. She is lucky though, as her friends live near by and sometimes visit to bring her a coffee and have lunch with her. Fortunately her back seems to feel better in the middle of the day so it is good that her friends come at this time. She is hoping that her partner will be able to take early retirement so that they can spend more time together but she says that her work want her to stay on as long as possible.

Through the Eyes of Health Psychology. . .

Research indicates that pain is best understood as a perception influenced by many psychological issues. Tamsin's story illustrates some of the issues described in this chapter including the role of reinforcement (watching films), focus (stopping work, staying at home), distraction (friends coming for lunch), pain behaviour (lying down, not going out), secondary gains (not having to work, encouraging her partner to retire early) and fear avoidance (doing less and less). This chapter describes the theories and research relating to pain and its treatment. It also addresses the placebo effect and how expectations can make symptoms (including pain) get better or worse.

1   WHAT IS PAIN?

Pain seems to have an obvious function. It provides constant feedback about the body, enabling us to make adjustments to how we sit or sleep and stops us from burning or cutting ourselves as we go about our daily lives. Pain is also a warning sign that something is wrong and results in protective behaviour, such as avoiding moving in a particular way or lifting heavy objects. Pain triggers help-seeking behaviour and is a common reason for patients visiting their doctor. From an evolutionary perspective, therefore, pain is a sign that action is needed. It functions to generate change either in the form of seeking help or avoiding activity.

But pain is not that simple. Some pain seems to have no underlying cause and functions to hinder rather than to help a person carry on with their life. Researchers differentiate between acute pain and chronic pain. Acute pain is defined as pain that lasts for six months or less. It usually has a definable cause and is mostly treated with painkillers. A broken leg or a surgical wound is an example of acute pain. In contrast, chronic pain lasts for longer than six months and can be either benign, in that it varies in severity, or progressive, in that it gets gradually worse. Chronic low back pain is often described as chronic benign pain whereas illnesses such as rheumatoid arthritis result in chronic progressive pain. Most of the research described in this chapter is concerned with chronic pain which shows an important role for psychological factors. But even acute pain is influenced by psychology.

Imagine a small child falling over. They look up at you and you have a split second to turn their experience into 'nothing' or 'pain'. So if you say, 'Never mind, up you get' and smile enthusiastically, chances are they will get up and carry on playing. But if you look frightened and say, 'Oh, that must have hurt, give me a cuddle,' then they will cry. In that split second all the psychological factors that influence the pain experience come into play and translate the signals being sent to the brain into something that hurts or something that is OK. Without these factors pain would be considered a *sensation*. But this example illustrates why pain is considered a *perception* and not a sensation (if their arm is hanging off, they will cry regardless of what you do!).

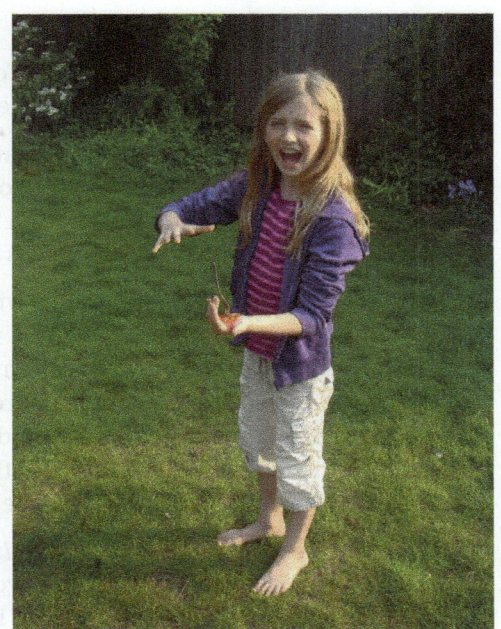

Giving a child's pain meaning illustrates the role of psychological factors in pain perception

EARLY PAIN THEORIES: PAIN AS A SENSATION

Early models described pain within a biomedical framework as an automatic response to an external factor. Descartes, perhaps the earliest writer on pain, regarded it as a response to a painful stimulus. He described a direct pathway from the source of pain (e.g. a burnt finger) to an area of the brain that detected the painful sensation. Von Frey (1895) developed the *specificity theory of pain,* which again reflected this very simple stimulus–response model. He suggested that there were specific sensory receptors which transmit touch, warmth and pain, and that each receptor was sensitive to specific stimulation. This model was similar to that described by Descartes in that the link between the cause of pain and the brain was seen as direct and automatic. In a similar vein, Goldschneider (1920) developed a further model of pain called the *pattern theory*. He suggested that nerve impulse patterns determined the degree of pain and that messages from the damaged area were sent directly to the brain via these nerve impulses. These three models of pain describe pain as a sensation as follows:

- Tissue damage causes the sensation of pain.
- Psychology is involved in these models of pain only as a consequence of pain (e.g. anxiety, fear, depression). Psychology has no causal influence.
- Pain is an automatic response to an external stimulus. There is no place for interpretation or moderation.
- The pain sensation has a single cause.
- Pain was categorized into being either *psychogenic pain* or *organic pain*. Psychogenic pain was considered to be 'all in the patient's mind' and was a label given to pain when no organic basis could be found. Organic pain was regarded as being 'real pain' and was the label given to pain when some clear injury could be seen.

INCLUDING PSYCHOLOGY IN THEORIES OF PAIN

These early models of pain had no role for psychology. However, psychology came to play an important part in understanding pain during the twentieth century. This was based on several observations.

First, it was observed that medical treatments for pain (e.g. drugs, surgery) were mostly only useful for treating *acute* pain (i.e. pain with a short duration). Such treatments were fairly ineffective for treating *chronic* pain (i.e. pain that lasts for a long time). This suggested that there must be something else involved in the pain sensation which was not included in the simple stimulus–response models.

It was also observed that individuals with the same degree of tissue damage differed in their reports of the painful sensation and/or painful responses. Beecher (1956) observed soldiers' and civilians' requests for pain relief in a hospital during the Second World War. He reported that although soldiers and civilians often showed the same degree of injury, 80 per cent of the civilians requested medication, whereas only 25 per cent of the soldiers did. He suggested that this reflected a role for the meaning of the injury in the experience of pain; for the soldiers, the injury had a positive meaning as it indicated that their war was over. This meaning mediated the pain experience.

The third observation was *phantom limb pain*. The majority of amputees tend to feel pain in an absent limb. This pain can actually get worse after the amputation, and continues even after complete healing. Sometimes the pain can feel as if it is spreading and is often described as a hand being clenched with the nails digging into the palm (when the hand is missing) or the bottom of the foot being forced into the ankle (when the foot is missing). Phantom limb pain has no peripheral physical basis because the limb is obviously missing. In addition, not everybody feels phantom limb pain and for those who do, they do not experience it to the same extent. Further, even individuals who are born with missing limbs sometimes report phantom limb pain.

These observations indicate variation between individuals. This variation indicates a role for psychology.

MEASURING PAIN

Whether it is to examine the causes or consequences of pain or to evaluate the effectiveness of a treatment for pain, pain needs to be measured. This has raised several questions and problems. For example, 'Are we interested in the individual's own experience of the pain?' (i.e. what someone says is all important), 'What about denial or self-image?' (i.e. someone might be in agony but deny it to themselves and to others), 'Are we interested in a more objective assessment?' (i.e. can we get over the problem of denial by asking someone else to rate their pain?) and 'Do we need to assess a physiological basis to pain?' These questions have resulted in three different perspectives on pain measurement: self-reports, observational assessments and physiological assessments, which are very similar to the different ways of measuring health status (see Chapter 14). In addition, these different perspectives reflect the different theories of pain.

Self-Reports

Self-report scales of pain rely on the individual's own subjective view of their pain level. They take the form of visual analogue scales (e.g. 'How severe is your pain?' Rated from 'not at all' (0) to 'extremely' (100)), verbal scales (e.g. 'Describe your pain: no pain, mild pain, moderate pain, severe pain, worst pain') and descriptive questionnaires (e.g. the McGill Pain Questionnaire (MPQ); Melzack 1975). The MPQ attempts to access the more complex nature of pain and asks individuals to rate their pain in terms of three dimensions: sensory (e.g. flickering, pulsing, beating), affective (e.g. punishing, cruel, killing) and evaluative (e.g. annoying, miserable, intense). Some self-report measures also attempt to access the impact that the pain is having upon the individual's level of functioning and ask whether the pain influences their ability to do daily tasks such as walking, sitting and climbing stairs. Similarly, pain is often assessed within the context of quality of life scales which include a pain component (e.g. see Chapter 14 for a discussion of quality of life scales).

Observational Assessment

Observational assessments attempt to make a more objective assessment of pain and are used when the patient's own self-reports are considered unreliable or when they are unable to provide them. For example, observational measures would be used for children, some stroke sufferers and some terminally ill patients. In addition, they can provide an objective validation of self-report measures. Observational measures include an assessment of the pain relief requested and used, pain behaviours (such as limping, grimacing and muscle tension) and time spent sleeping and/or resting.

Physiological Measures

Both self-report measures and observational measures are sometimes regarded as unreliable if a supposedly 'objective' measure of pain is required. In particular, self-report measures are open to the bias of the individual in pain and observational measures are open to errors made by the observer. Therefore physiological measures are sometimes used as an index of pain intensity. Such measures include an assessment of inflammation and measures of sweating, heart rate and skin temperature. However, the relationship between physiological measures and both observational and self-report measures is often contradictory, raising the question, 'Are the individual and the rater mistaken or are the physiological measurements not measuring pain?'

2 | PAIN AS A PERCEPTION

Early models of pain emphasized pain as a sensation with a minimal role for psychology. Nowadays, researchers consider pain to be a perception with a key role for psychological factors. This is illustrated by the gate control theory of pain and the psychosocial model of pain perception.

THE GATE CONTROL THEORY OF PAIN

In 1965, Melzack and Wall developed the gate control theory of pain (GCT), which represented an attempt to introduce psychology into the understanding of pain. This model is illustrated in Figure 11.1. It suggested that although pain could still be understood in terms of a stimulus–response pathway, this pathway was complex and mediated by a network of interacting processes. The GCT therefore integrated psychology into the traditional biomedical model of pain and not only described a role for physiological causes and interventions, but also allowed for psychological causes and interventions (see Melzack and Katz 2004 for a more recent discussion of the GCT).

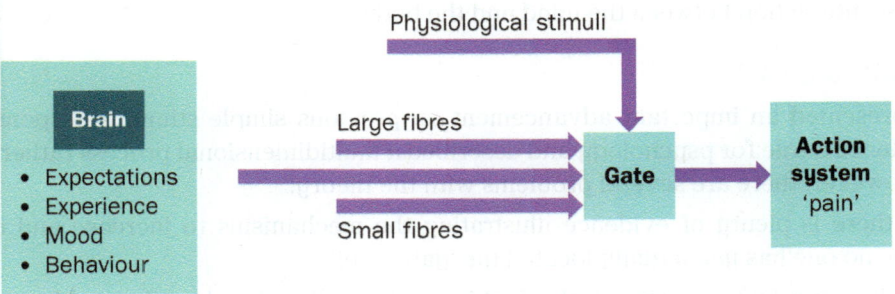

Figure 11.1 The gate control theory (GCT) of pain

SOURCE: Adapted from Melzack and Wall (1965)

Input to the Gate

Melzack and Wall suggested that a gate existed at the spinal cord level, which received input from the following sources:

- *Peripheral nerve fibres.* The site of injury (e.g. the hand) sends information about pain, pressure or heat to the gate.

- *Descending central influences from the brain.* The brain sends information related to the psychological state of the individual to the gate. This may reflect the individual's behavioural state (e.g. attention, focus on the source of the pain); emotional state (e.g. anxiety, fear, depression); and previous experiences or self-efficacy (e.g. 'I have experienced this pain before and know that it will go away') in terms of dealing with the pain.

- *Large and small fibres.* These fibres constitute part of the physiological input to pain perception.

Output from the Gate

They then described how the gate integrates all of the information from these different sources and produces an output. This output from the gate sends information to an action system, which results in the perception of pain.

How Does the GCT Differ from Earlier Models of Pain?

The GCT differs from earlier models in a number of fundamental ways:

- *Pain as a perception.* According to the GCT, pain is a perception and an experience rather than a sensation. This change in terminology reflects the role of the individual in the degree of pain experienced. In the same way that psychologists regard vision as a perception, rather than a direct mirror image, pain is described as involving an active interpretation of the painful stimuli.

- *The individual as active, not passive.* According to the GCT, pain is determined by central and peripheral fibres. Pain is seen as an active process as opposed to a passive one. The individual no longer just responds passively to painful stimuli, but actively interprets and appraises painful stimuli.

- *The role of individual variability.* Individual variability is no longer a problem in understanding pain but central to the GCT. Variation in pain perception is understood in terms of the degree of opening or closing of the gate.

- *The role for multiple causes.* The GCT suggests that many factors are involved in pain perception, not just a singular physical cause.

- *Is pain ever organic?* The GCT describes most pain as a combination of physical and psychological. It could, therefore, be argued that within this model pain is never totally either organic or psychogenic.

- *Pain and dualism.* The GCT attempts to depart from traditional dualistic models of the body and suggests an interaction between the mind and the body.

Problems with the GCT

The GCT represented an important advancement on previous simple stimulus–response theories of pain. It introduced a role for psychology and described a multidimensional process rather than a simple linear one. However, there are several problems with the theory:

- Although there is plenty of evidence illustrating the mechanisms to increase and decrease pain perception, no one has yet actually located the 'gate' itself.

- Although the input from the site of physical injury is mediated and moderated by experience and other psychological factors, the model still assumes an organic basis for pain. This integration of physiological and psychological factors can explain individual variability and phantom limb pain to an extent, but because the model still assumes some organic basis it is still based on a simple stimulus–response process.

- The GCT attempted to depart from traditional dualistic models of health by its integration of the mind and the body. However, although the GCT suggests some integration or interaction between mind and body, it still sees them as separate processes. The model suggests that physical processes are influenced by the psychological processes, but that these two sets of processes are distinct.

A PSYCHOSOCIAL MODEL OF PAIN PERCEPTION

The GCT was a development from previous theories in that it allowed for the existence of mediating variables, and emphasized active perception rather than passive sensation. In recent years this approach has been developed and elaborated upon to create a psychosocial model of pain perception. This involves physiological processes together with a role for learning, affect, cognition and behaviour. These processes are illustrated in Figure 11.2 and are described in more detail in the following section.

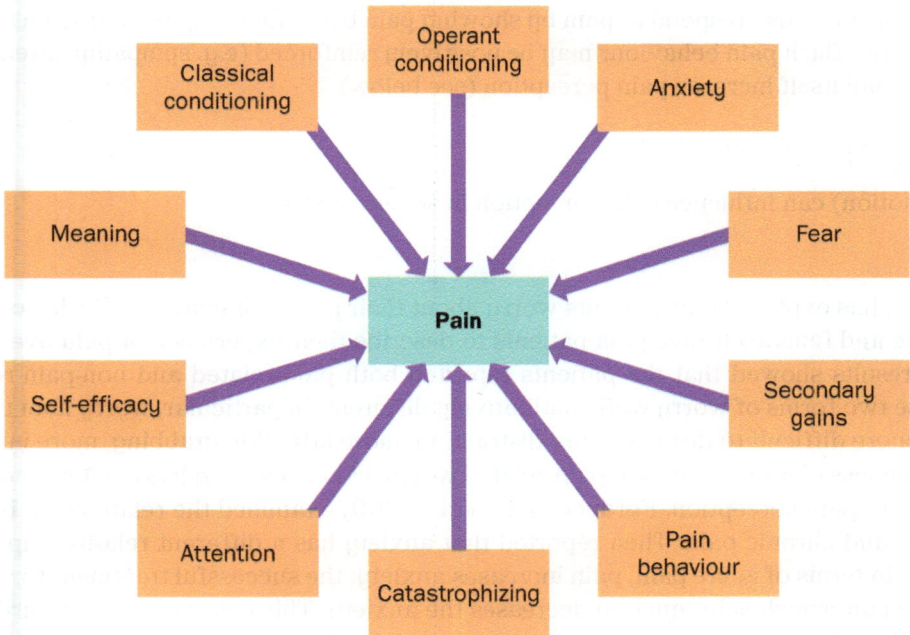

Figure 11.2 Psychosocial aspects of pain

THE ROLE OF LEARNING

Pain perception is clearly influenced by learning.

Classical Conditioning

Research suggests that *classical conditioning* may have an effect on the perception of pain. As described by theories of associative learning, an individual may associate a particular environment with the experience of pain. For example, if an individual associates the dentist with pain due to past experience, the pain perception may be enhanced when attending the dentist due to this expectation. In addition, because of the association between these two factors, the individual may experience increased anxiety when attending the dentist, which may also increase pain. Jamner and Tursky (1987) examined the effect of presenting migraine sufferers with words associated with pain. They found that this presentation increased both anxiety and pain perception and concluded that the words caused a change in mood, which caused a change in the subject's perception of pain. Likewise, Madden et al. (2016) conducted a study to investigate whether human pain thresholds can be changed using classical conditioning and found that after conditioning participants reported the paired stimulus as painful more often, as more intense, and as more unpleasant. Zhang et al. (2019) carried out a review of the evidence for the impact of conditioning on increased pain (conditioned hyperalgesia) or decreased pain (conditioned hypoalgesia) and concluded that classical conditioning profoundly changes the pain experience and relates to both the onset and maintenance of chronic pain.

Operant Conditioning

Research suggests that there is also a role for *operant conditioning* in pain perception and this can be moderated through positive or negative reinforcement. Adamczyk et al. (2019) carried out a systematic review and meta-analysis of research on the hyperalgesic effect (i.e. an exaggerated pain experience to a normally painful stimulus) and the allodynic effect (i.e. pain triggered by a stimulus that does not normally elicit pain). Their analysis showed that both hyperalgesic and allodynic effects can be induced in healthy humans through reinforcement and that this might illustrate a pathway from acute to chronic pain. Individuals may also respond to pain by showing pain behaviour (e.g. resting, grimacing, limping, staying off work). Such pain behaviour may be positively reinforced (e.g. sympathy, attention, time off work), which may itself increase pain perception (see below).

THE ROLE OF AFFECT

Affect (or emotion) can influence pain perception in several ways.

Anxiety

Some research has explored how patients worry about their pain. For example, Eccleston et al. (2001) asked 34 male and female chronic pain patients to describe their experience of pain over a seven-day period. The results showed that the patients reported both pain-related and non-pain-related worry and that these two forms of worry were qualitatively different. In particular, worry about chronic pain was seen as more difficult to dismiss, more distracting, more attention grabbing, more intrusive, more distressing and less pleasant than non-pain-related worry. Other research has explored how worry and anxiety relate to pain perception. Fordyce and Steger (1979) examined the relationship between anxiety and acute and chronic pain. They reported that anxiety has a different relationship to these two types of pain. In terms of acute pain, pain increases anxiety; the successful treatment for the pain then decreases the pain which subsequently decreases the anxiety. This can then cause a further decrease in the pain. Therefore, because of the relative ease with which acute pain can be treated, anxiety relates to this pain perception in terms of a cycle of pain *reduction*. However, the pattern is different for chronic pain. Because treatment has very little effect on chronic pain, this increases anxiety, which can further increase pain. Therefore, in terms of the relationship between anxiety and chronic pain, there is a cycle of pain *increase*. Research has also shown a direct correlation between high anxiety levels and increased pain perception in children with migraines and sufferers of back pain and pelvic pain (Feuerstein et al. 1987; McGowan et al. 1998). In an experimental study, participants took part in the cold pressor test which involves placing the hand and arm in icy water as a means to induce pain. Their trait anxiety was assessed and some were actively distracted from thinking about their pain (James and Hardardottir 2002). The results showed that both distraction and low anxiety reduced the pain experience. Further, research indicates that anxiety pre-surgery can increase pain perception after surgery when in recovery (Sommer et al. 2010). Recently, Ma et al. (2018) experimentally manipulated uncertainty as a way to induce anxiety and explored the impact on pain perception. Participants were told that they would receive four types of electric shocks: low-intensity shock, high-intensity shock, 50–50 chance of low-intensity or high-intensity shock, and no shock. They found that being uncertain (50–50 chance) about the type of shock led to increased anxiety, which in turn resulted in higher pain once the shock was received. From their review of the literature, Girão et al. (2019) concluded that anxiety can be expressed somatically as different forms of pain including gastrointestinal pain, precordial chest pain, dental pain or migraine headaches. They also concluded that anxiety can exacerbate dental pain and migraines and can facilitate the transition from acute to chronic pain for back pain and migraines.

Fear

Junge et al. (2018) used a longitudinal design to explain the impact of women's fear of childbirth on the pain experienced during the actual birth. In this large-scale study, 1,649 women rated their fear at 17–19 weeks, and 32 weeks of pregnancy, and then again 8 weeks post-partum. They found that women with a severe fear of childbirth reported a significantly higher perception of pain during birth than those without a severe fear of childbirth. Some research also suggests that fear may be involved in exacerbating existing pain and turning acute pain into chronic pain. For example, Crombez et al. (1999) explored the interrelationship between attention to pain and fear. They argued that pain functions by demanding attention, which results in a lowered ability to focus on other activities. Their results indicated that pain-related fear increased this attentional interference, suggesting that fear about pain increased the amount of attention demanded by the pain. They concluded that pain-related fear can create a hypervigilance towards pain which could contribute to the progression from acute to chronic pain.

Many patients with pain also have extensive fear of increased pain or of the pain reoccurring which can result in them avoiding a whole range of activities that they perceive to be high risk. For example, patients can avoid moving in particular ways and exerting themselves to any extent. However, these patients often do not describe their experiences in terms of fear but rather in terms of what they can and cannot do. Therefore they do not report being frightened of making the pain worse by lifting a heavy object, but they state that they can no longer lift heavy objects. Fear of pain and fear avoidance beliefs have been shown to be linked with the pain experience in terms of triggering pain in the first place. For example, Linton et al. (2000) measured fear avoidance beliefs in a large community sample of people who reported no spinal pain in the preceding year. The participants were then followed up after one year and the occurrence of a pain episode and their physical functioning were assessed. The results showed that 19 per cent of the sample reported an episode of back pain at follow-up and that those with higher baseline scores of fear avoidance were twice as likely to report back pain and had a 1.7 times higher risk of lowered physical functioning. The authors argued that fear avoidance may relate to the early onset of pain. These conclusions were further supported by a comprehensive review of the research. This indicates that treatment that exposes patients to the very situations they are afraid of, such as going out and being in crowds, can reduce fear avoidance beliefs and modify their pain experience (Vlaeyen and Linton 2000). Over the past few years, several systematic reviews and meta analysis provide consistent support for the link between fear and pain outcomes for a range of pain-related conditions such as pain onset, pain maintenance, pain sensitivity, pain severity and the transition from acute to chronic pain (e.g. Martinez-Calderon et al. 2019; Markfelder and Pauli 2020; Panhale et al. 2021). One mechanism for this process may be through a vicious cycle whereby fear causes a reduction in physical activity and work leading to disability (Panhale et al. 2021) and another maybe through excessive fear generalization (Meulders 2019).

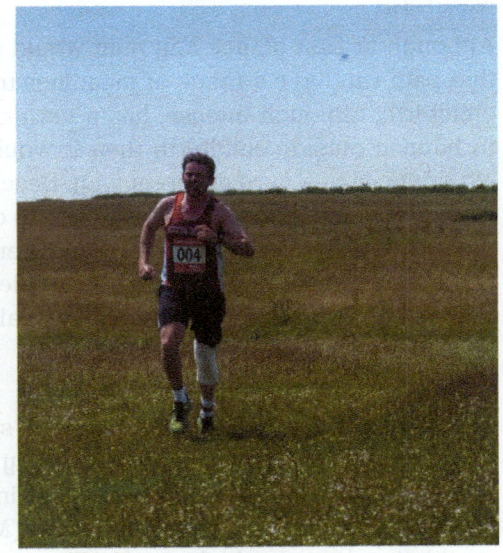

Fear of Pain can make prople avoid activity. Some people decide to push on through!

THE ROLE OF COGNITION

An individual's cognitive state also influences their pain experience.

Catastrophizing

Patients with pain, particularly chronic pain, often show *catastrophizing*. Keefe et al. (2000) described catastrophizing as involving three components: (1) rumination – a focus on threatening information, both internal and external ('I can feel my neck click whenever I move'); (2) magnification – over-estimating the extent of the threat ('The bones are crumbling and I will become paralysed'); and (3) helplessness – underestimating personal and broader resources that might mitigate the danger and disastrous consequences ('Nobody understands how to fix the problem and I just can't bear any more pain'). Catastrophizing has been linked to both the onset of pain and the development of longer-term pain problems (Sullivan et al. 2001). For example, in the prospective study described earlier by Linton et al. (2000), the authors measured baseline levels of pain catastrophizing. The results showed some small associations between this and the onset of back pain by follow-up. Crombez et al. (2003) developed a new measure of catastrophizing to assess this aspect of pain in children which consisted of three subscales reflecting the dimensions of catastrophizing – namely rumination, magnification and helplessness. They then used this measure to explore the relationship between catastrophizing and pain intensity in a clinical sample of 43 boys and girls aged between 8 and 16. The results indicated that catastrophizing independently predicted both pain intensity and disability regardless of age and gender. The authors argued that catastrophizing functions by facilitating the escape from pain and by communicating distress to others. Pain catastrophizing has also been shown to be linked to increased pain perception after surgery (Pavlin et al. 2005), increased pain in those with burns (Van Loey et al. 2018), oral facial pain (Dinan et al. 2021) and chronic low back pain (Meints et al. 2019). Due to the possible bi-directional relationship between pain catastrophizing and pain intensity (i.e. which comes first?), Crawford et al. (2021) carried out a longitudinal study of women with interstitial cystitis/bladder pain syndrome (IC/BPS) who were followed up at 6 and 12 months. The results showed that earlier changes in pain catastrophizing predicted later changes in pain intensity but that earlier changes in pain did not predict later changes in pain catastrophizing. This suggests that pain catastrophizing drives increases in pain, but not vice versa.

Meaning

Although at first glance any pain would seem to be only negative in its meaning, research indicates that pain can have a range of meanings to different people. For example, the pain experienced during childbirth, although intense, has a very clear cause and consequence. If the same kind of pain were to happen outside childbirth then it would have a totally different meaning and would probably be experienced in a very different way. Beecher (1956), in his study of soldiers' and civilians' requests for medication, was one of the first people to examine this and asked the question, 'What does pain mean to the individual?' Beecher argued that differences in pain perception were related to the meaning of pain for the individual. In this study, the soldiers benefited from their pain. This has also been described in terms of *secondary gains* whereby the pain may have a positive reward for the individual.

Self-Efficacy

Some research has emphasized the role of self-efficacy in pain perception and reduction. Turk et al. (1983) suggested that increased pain self-efficacy may be an important factor in determining the degree of pain perception. In addition, the concept of pain *locus of control* has been developed to emphasize the role of individual cognitions in pain perception (Manning and Wright 1983). Recent reviews show a consistent association between higher self-efficacy and reduced pain perception for patients with rheumatoid arthritis (Martinez-Calderon et al. 2020) and chronic musculoskeletal pain (Hayward and Stynes 2021).

Attention

There has also been much research exploring the impact of attention on pain and much work shows that attention to the pain can exacerbate it whereas distraction can reduce the pain experience. Eccleston and Crombez have carried out much work in this area which they reviewed in the *Psychological Bulletin* in 1999. They illustrated how patients who attend to their pain experience more pain than those who are distracted. This association explains why patients suffering from back pain who take to their beds and therefore focus on their pain take longer to recover than those who carry on working and engaging with their lives. This associa-

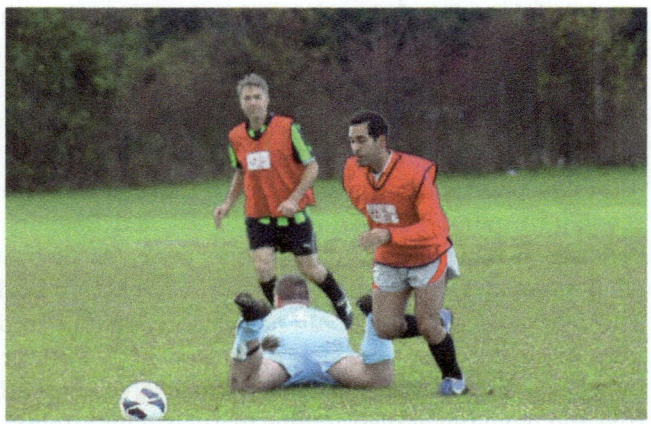

Pain is reduced when it means winning a game or when you are distracted by fun

tion is also reflected in relatively recent changes in the general management approach to back pain problems — bed rest is no longer the main treatment option. In addition, Eccleston and Crombez provide a model of how pain and attention are related (Eccleston 1994; Eccleston and Crombez 1999). They argue that pain interrupts and demands attention and that this interruption depends upon pain-related characteristics such as the threat value of the pain and environmental demands such as emotional arousal. They argue that pain causes a shift in attention towards the pain as a way to encourage escape and action. The result of this shift in attention is a reduced ability to focus on other tasks, resulting in attentional interference and disruption. This disruption has been shown in a series of experimental studies indicating that patients with high pain perform less well on difficult tasks that involve the greatest demand of their limited resources (e.g. Eccleston 1994; Crombez et al. 1998a, 1999). In addition, research shows that distractions such as comforting words (Shenefelt 2013), chatting to the nurse during conscious surgery (Hudson et al. 2015), music (Bradt et al. 2013), audio-visual stimuli (Man and Yap 2003), touch (Chanif et al. 2013) and playing with stress balls (Hudson et al. 2015) can reduce both pain and anxiety when used before, during or after surgery.

BEHAVIOURAL PROCESSES

Research also shows a role for behaviour in pain perception.

Pain Behaviour

The way in which an individual responds to pain can itself increase or decrease the pain perception. In particular, research has looked at pain behaviours which have been defined by Turk et al. (1985) as facial or audible expression (e.g. clenched teeth and moaning), distorted posture or movement (e.g. limping, protecting the pain area), negative affect (e.g. irritability, depression) or avoidance of activity (e.g. not going to work, lying down). It has been suggested that pain behaviours are reinforced through attention, the acknowledgement they receive, and through secondary gains, such as not having to go to work. Positively reinforcing pain behaviour may increase pain perception. Pain behaviour can also cause a lack of activity and muscle wastage, no social contact and no distraction leading to a sick role, which can also increase pain perception. Williams (2002) provides an evolutionary analysis of facial expressions of pain and argues that if the function of pain is to prioritize escape, recovery and healing, facial expressions are a means to communicate pain and to elicit help from others to achieve these goals. Further, she argues that people often assume that individuals have more control over the extent of their pain-induced facial expressions than they actually do and are more likely to offer help or sympathy when expressions are mild. Stronger forms of expression are interpreted as amplified and as indications of malingering.

Secondary Gains

Although pain is clearly unpleasant, there is also evidence that pain can have some benefits called secondary gains. For example, Leknes and Bastian (2014) reviewed the evidence for the possible benefits of pain and concluded that pain can distract us from other more unpleasant experiences, elicit sympathy, motivate us to seek medical and social support, and can also reduce guilt following self-indulgence. Further, pain may also enable us to delegate our roles and responsibilities to others, miss work and adopt the sick role (see Chapter 10 for a discussion of help-seeking and the sick role). In turn, these secondary gains may themselves exacerbate the pain experience if people adopt the sick role and have fewer distractions to avert their attention away from their pain.

The Interaction Between these Different Processes

This psychosocial model describes the separate components that influence pain perception. These different components, however, are not discrete but interact and are at times interchangeable. For example, emotional factors may influence an individual's physiology and cognitive factors may influence an individual's behaviour. Further, association may increase pain in terms of learning but this might be due to changes in anxiety and focus, with places and experiences that have previously been associated with pain resulting in increased anxiety and increased attention to pain, therefore increasing the pain experience. Likewise, pain behaviours may exacerbate pain by limiting physical movement. But it is also likely that they operate by increasing focus and anxiety – staying in bed leaves the individual with nothing to do other than think and worry about their pain. Research also indicates that fear influences attention, that fear interacts with catastrophizing and that catastrophizing influences attentional interference (Crombez et al. 1998a, 1998b, 1999; Van Damme et al. 2002). The psychosocial model offers a framework for mapping out the different factors that influence pain. However, this categorization is probably best seen as a framework only, with the different components being interrelated rather than discrete categories of discrete factors.

THE EXPERIENCE OF PAIN

So far this chapter has explored the kinds of factors that contribute to why people feel pain and theories that can explain pain onset, maintenance and the translation of acute pain into chronic pain. What is missing in this research, however, is how pain is *experienced*. Some of the measures of pain capture these experiences by asking people whether their pain can be described by words such as 'flickering', 'punishing', 'cruel', 'killing' or 'annoying' (see 'Measuring pain' in previous section What is pain? for a discussion of pain measures). Qualitative research has further explored the pain experience. For example, Osborn and Smith (1998) interviewed nine women who experienced chronic back pain and analysed the transcripts using interpretative phenomenological analysis (IPA) (Smith and Osborn 2003). The results showed that the patients experienced their pain in a range of ways which were conceptualized into four main themes. First, they showed a strong motivation to understand and explain their situation and to know why they had developed chronic pain. Second, they showed a process of social comparison and compared themselves with others and with themselves in the past and future. Third, they described how they were often not believed by others as they had no visible signs to support their suffering or disability. Finally, they described how their pain had resulted in them withdrawing from public view as they felt a burden to others and felt that when in public they had to hide their pain and appear healthy and mobile. For these sufferers, chronic back pain seemed to have a profound effect on their lives, impacting on how they felt about themselves and how they interacted with others.

In a further qualitative study, McGowan et al. (2007) asked 32 women with chronic pelvic pain to write stories about their illness trajectories. The data were analysed using a narrative approach to explore why women disengaged from their treatment and often become dissatisfied with the care they received. The results showed that the women wanted validation and recognition of their experiences and therefore engaged with the process of finding a diagnosis. But they often felt that they were not listened to and opted out of this process, leaving them with a sense of disempowerment and being in limbo. Much of this failure was attributed to the medical consultation and its dualistic model of the mind and body being separate.

Some research has also used visual imagery to provide insights into the pain experience. For example, Phillips et al. (2015) asked 90 patients from a pain clinic to draw their pain. The results showed that the majority were able to provide an image (n = 54) which was analysed using critical visual analysis. Image content was described using three main themes; pain as an attacker; the nature of pain (i.e., pain sensations, timeline, pain location); and the impact of pain (i.e., pain as a barrier, being trapped by pain and the future with pain). The images provided a novel and in-depth insight into the pain experience and could be used in pain management either just as part of discussions about the patient's pain experience or for a re-scripting process to change the patient's meaning of pain. These images are shown in Figure 11.3.

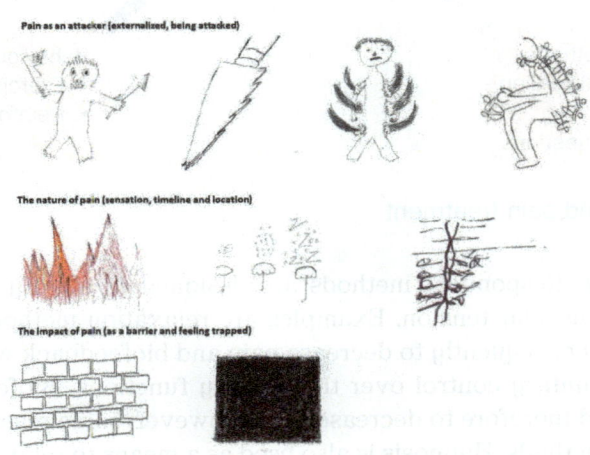

Figure 11.3 Patients' images of their pain
SOURCE: Phillips et al. (2015)

Acute pain is mostly treated with pharmacological interventions. Chronic pain has proved to be more resistant to such approaches and recently pain clinics have been set up that adopt a multidisciplinary approach to pain treatment. The goals set by such clinics include the following:

- *Improving physical and lifestyle functioning.* This involves improving muscle tone, self-esteem, self-efficacy and distraction, and decreasing boredom, pain behaviour and secondary gains.

- *Decreasing reliance on drugs and medical services.* This involves improving personal control, decreasing the sick role and increasing self-efficacy.

- *Increasing social support and family life.* This aims to increase optimism and distraction and decrease boredom, anxiety, sick role behaviour and secondary gains.

Current treatment philosophy also emphasizes early intervention to prevent the transition of acute pain to chronic pain.

Research shows that psychology is involved in the perception of pain in terms of factors such as learning, anxiety, worry, fear, catastrophizing, meaning and attention. Multidisciplinary pain clinics increasingly place psychological interventions at their core. There are several methods of pain treatment, which reflect an interaction between psychology and physiological factors. These methods can be categorized as respondent, cognitive and behavioural methods and are illustrated in Figure 11.4.

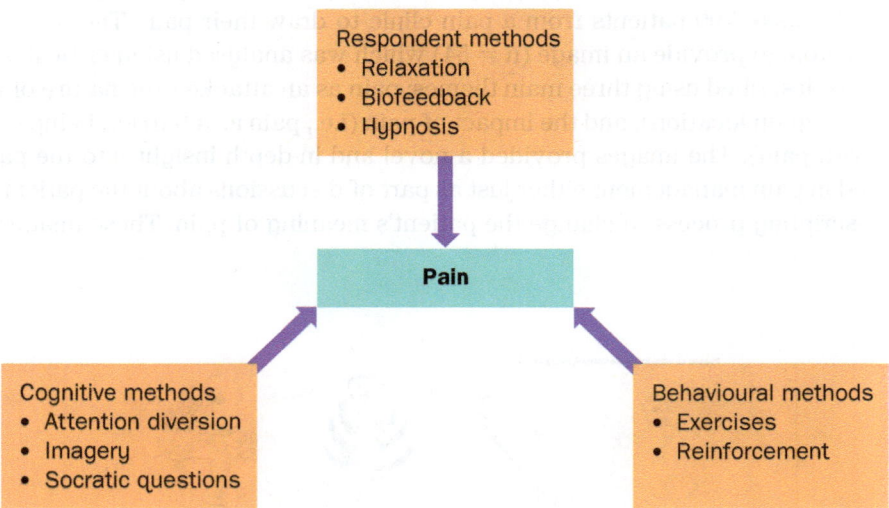

Figure 11.4 Psychology and pain treatment

- *Respondent methods.* Respondent methods are designed to modify the physiological system directly by reducing muscular tension. Examples are relaxation methods which aim to decrease anxiety and stress and consequently to decrease pain and biofeedback which is used to enable the individual to exert voluntary control over their bodily functions. Biofeedback aims to decrease anxiety and tension and therefore to decrease pain. However, some research indicates that it adds nothing to relaxation methods. Hypnosis is also used as a means to relax the individual. It seems to be of most use for acute pain and for repeated painful procedures such as burn dressing.

- *Cognitive methods.* A cognitive approach to pain treatment focuses on the individual's thoughts about pain and aims to modify cognitions that may be exacerbating their pain experience. Techniques used include attention diversion (i.e. encouraging the individual not to focus on the pain), imagery (i.e. encouraging the individual to have positive, pleasant thoughts) and the modification of maladaptive thoughts by the use of Socratic questions. Socratic questions challenge the individual to try to understand their automatic thoughts and involve questions such as, 'What evidence do you have to support your thoughts?' and 'How would someone else view this situation?' The therapist can use role play and role reversal (see Chapter 7 for a discussion of cognitive behavioural therapy — CBT — and Socratic questions).

- *Behavioural methods.* Some treatment approaches draw upon the basic principles of operant conditioning and use reinforcement to encourage the individual to change their behaviour. For example, if a chronic pain patient has stopped activities that they believe may exacerbate their pain, the therapist will incrementally encourage them to become increasingly more active. Each change in behaviour will be rewarded by the therapist and new exercises will be developed and agreed to encourage the patient to move towards their pre-set goal.

The three components of psychological therapy are often integrated into a cognitive behavioural treatment package (see Chapter 7 for a discussion of CBT in the context of behaviour change).

COGNITIVE BEHAVIOURAL THERAPY

CBT is increasingly used with chronic pain patients and is based upon the premise that pain is influenced by four sources of information: cognitive sources such as the meaning of the pain ('it will prevent me from working'); emotional sources such as the emotions associated with the pain ('I am anxious that it will never go away'); physiological sources such as the impulses sent from the site of physical damage; and behavioural sources such as pain behaviour that may either increase the pain (such as not doing any exercise) or decrease the pain (such as doing sufficient exercise). CBT focuses on these aspects of pain perception and uses a range of psychological strategies to enable people to unlearn unhelpful practices and learn new ways of thinking and behaviours. CBT draws upon the three treatment approaches described earlier, namely respondent methods such as relaxation and biofeedback, cognitive methods such as attention diversion and Socratic questioning, and behavioural methods involving graded exercises and reinforcement. Several individual studies have been carried out to explore the relative effectiveness of CBT compared to other forms of intervention and/or waiting list controls. Recently, systematic reviews have been published which have synthesized these studies in terms of CBT for adults and for children and adolescents.

CBT and Adults

Van Tulder et al. (2000) carried out a systematic review of randomized controlled trials which had used behavioural therapy for chronic non-specific low back pain in adults. Their analysis of six studies showed that behavioural treatments effectively reduced pain intensity, increased functional status (e.g. return to work) and improved behavioural outcomes (e.g. activity level). In a similar vein, Eccleston et al. (2009b) carried out a systematic review of trials of CBT and behaviour therapy for chronic pain in 4,781 adults excluding headache. Their analysis of 40 trials showed that behaviour therapy was effective at reducing pain but only immediately following treatment when compared to treatment as usual. The results for CBT were more positive but the effects were small, showing improvements in pain, disability, depression and anxiety. In addition, some of these improvements were maintained at six-month follow-up. The authors concluded that psychological therapies that include CBT seem to be an effective way to reduce aspects of chronic pain but that the effects are often small. In line with the increasing use of online interventions (see Chapter 7) Eccleston et al. (2014) also conducted a review of CBT-style interventions delivered over the internet. They included 15 studies with a total of 2012 participants. The results showed a reduction in pain for those with headaches but no change in their anxiety or depression whereas those with non-headache conditions showed less pain and a reduction in their anxiety and depression. In a recent review of the use of CBT across a range of chronic conditions, Urits et al. (2019) concluded that CBT improved pain for headaches, fibromyalgia, arthritis, cancer, non-specific chronic low back pain and functional gastrointestinal disorders.

Children and Adolescents

Children with chronic and/or recurrent pain are also increasingly offered some form of psychological intervention. At times this takes the form of CBT. However, it also takes the form of individual components such as relaxation, coping skills training, biofeedback and hypnosis. Eccleston et al. (2009a) carried out a systematic review of 29 trials using psychological therapies for the management of chronic and recurrent pain in children and adolescents. The problems included were chronic or recurrent headache, abdominal pain, musculoskeletal pain, sickle-cell pain and fibromyalgia and involved 1,432 patients, with about half receiving the psychological treatment, which was mostly relaxation or CBT. The control groups received standard medical care, placebo or were waiting list controls. The results of their analysis showed that psychological therapies were very effective at reducing headache pain, musculoskeletal pain and recurrent abdominal pain in children and adolescents. The results also showed that these effects persisted by six-month follow-up. There were no significant effects for mood or disability. Likewise, Lonergan (2016) carried out a meta-analysis of nine trials exploring the effectiveness of CBT for pain in childhood and adolescence. It was found that CBT had a large effect on pain intensity for recurrent abdominal pain, a medium effect on fibromyalgia and a small effect on headaches. CBT generally had a medium effect on pain duration. In 2022, Fisher et al. carried out a WHO systematic review and meta-analysis of 63 studies of pharmacological, physical and psychological therapies for children with chronic pain conditions and concluded that there was most evidence for the effectiveness of CBT.

Psychological factors can therefore exacerbate pain perception. Research indicates that they are also important in the treatment and management of pain.

A ROLE FOR PAIN ACCEPTANCE?

The psychological treatment of pain includes respondent, cognitive and behavioural methods. These are mostly used in conjunction with pharmacological treatments involving analgesics or anaesthetics. The outcome of such interventions has traditionally been assessed in terms of a reduction in pain intensity and pain perception. Recently, however, some researchers have been calling for a shift in focus towards pain acceptance. Risdon et al. (2003) asked 30 participants to describe their pain using a Q factor analysis. This methodology encourages the participant to describe their experiences in a way that enables the researcher to derive a factor structure. From their analysis the authors argued that the acceptance of pain involves eight factors. These were: taking control, living day-by-day, acknowledging limitations, empowerment, accepting loss of self, a belief that there's more to life than pain, a philosophy of not fighting battles that can't be won and spiritual strength. In addition, the authors suggest that these factors reflect three underlying beliefs: (1) the acknowledgement that a cure for pain is unlikely; (2) a shift of focus away from pain to non-pain aspects of life; and (3) a resistance to any suggestion that pain is a sign of personal weakness. In a further study, McCracken and Eccleston (2003) showed that pain acceptance was a better predictor than coping of pain intensity, disability, depression and anxiety and better work status. Similarly, Samwel et al. (2009) concluded from their study of 220 participants, half of whom attended a chronic pain multidisciplinary clinic, that pain acceptance at baseline predicted greater reduction in pain intensity in the intervention but not the control group. In line with this focus on acceptance, some researchers have explored the use of Acceptance Commitment Therapy (ACT) with pain patients (Hayes et al. 2006; McCracken and Eccleston 2006). ACT stems from behavioural therapy and CBT and is an action-oriented approach which encourages patients to stop avoiding and struggling with their inner emotions (or pain) and accept that they can be appropriate responses to certain situations that should not get in the way of them living their lives. Scott et al. (2016) explored whether pain acceptance could be improved using ACT for chronic pain and found that nine months after ACT, patients reported less pain, greater functioning, less depression and greater pain acceptance. Galvez-Sánchez et al. (2021) carried out a systematic review of 21 studies exploring the effectiveness of ACT in patients with central pain sensitization syndromes (e.g. fibromyalgia syndrome, irritable bowel syndrome and migraine). They concluded that ACT reduced anxiety, depression, pain and quality of life and that this effect might be mediated by pain acceptance, psychological flexibility, optimism, self-efficacy or adherence to values. Further, ACT showed better results in comparison to waiting list controls, pharmacological and psychoeducational interventions. It has been argued that the extent of pain acceptance may relate to changes in an individual's sense of self and how their pain has been incorporated into their self-identity. It is also argued that pain acceptance may be an important way forward for pain research, particularly given the nature of chronic pain.

IN SUMMARY

Whereas early models described pain as a sensation, pain is now considered to be a perception that is influenced by a multitude of psychological factors. The psychosocial model of pain perception illustrates these factors and highlights the role of learning, cognition, affect and behaviour. Further, these factors are also key to pain treatment and are incorporated into the work of pain clinics which often use CBT or ACT to help their patients towards pain acceptance.

4 | THE PLACEBO EFFECT

Placebos are used in randomized control trials to compare an active drug with the effects of simply taking 'something'. They have also, however been shown to have an independent effect on a multitude of conditions including pain relief, asthma, diabetes and smoking (for reviews, see Haas et al. 1959; Colloca et al. 2013). Interestingly, a recent and controversial review of the published and the unpublished clinical trial data for the effectiveness of anti-depressant medication for the reduction of depression and anxiety concluded that most (if not all) of the benefits of anti-depressants were due to the placebo response, that the differences found between drug and placebo were not clinically meaningful and that any differences may be due to the patients and/or clinicians being unblinded to their arm of the trial (Kirsch 2019). Placebos will now be explored in terms of their definition, a brief history of inert treatments, how placebos work and their implications for health psychology.

WHAT IS A PLACEBO?

Placebos have been defined as follows:

- Inert substances that cause symptom relief (e.g. 'My headache went away after having a sugar pill').
- Substances that cause changes in a symptom not directly attributable to specific or real pharmacological actions of a drug or operation (e.g. 'After I had my hip operation I stopped getting headaches').
- Any therapy that is deliberately used for its non-specific psychological or physiological effects (e.g. 'I had a bath and my headache went away').

These definitions illustrate some of the problems with understanding placebos. For example:

- What are specific/real versus non-specific/unreal effects? For example, 'My headaches went after the operation': is this an unreal effect (it was not predicted) or a real effect (it definitely happened)?
- Why are psychological effects non-specific? (e.g. 'I feel more relaxed after my operation': is this a non-specific effect?).
- Are there placebo effects in psychological treatments? For example, 'I specifically went for cognitive restructuring therapy and ended up simply feeling less tired': is this a placebo effect or a real effect?

The problems inherent in the distinctions between specific versus non-specific effects and physiological versus psychological effects are illustrated by examining the history of apparently medically inert treatments.

A HISTORY OF INERT TREATMENTS

For centuries, individuals (including doctors and psychologists) from many different cultural backgrounds have used (and still use) apparently inert treatments for various different conditions. For example, medicines such as wild animal faeces and the blood of a gladiator were supposed to increase strength, and part of a dolphin's penis was supposed to increase virility. These so-called 'medicines' have been used at different times in different cultures but have no apparent medical (active) properties. In addition, treatments such as bleeding by leeches to decrease fever or travelling to religious sites such as Lourdes in order to alleviate symptoms have also continued across the years without any obvious understanding of the processes involved. Faith healers are another example of inert treatments, including Jesus Christ, Buddha and Krishna. The tradition of faith healers has persisted, although our understanding of the processes involved is very poor.

Such apparently inert interventions, and the traditions involved with these practices, have lasted over thousands of years. In addition, the people involved in these practices have become famous and have gained a degree of credibility. Furthermore, many of the treatments are still believed in. Perhaps the maintenance of faith, both in these interventions and in the people carrying out the treatments, suggests that they were actually successful, giving the treatments themselves some validity. Why were they successful? It is possible that there are medically active substances in some of these traditional treatments that were not understood in the past and are still not understood now (e.g. gladiators' blood may actually contain some still unknown active chemical). It is also possible that the effectiveness of some of these treatments can be understood in terms of modern-day placebo effects.

MODERN-DAY PLACEBOS

Placebos are now studied in their own right and have been found to have a multitude of effects. For example, Haas et al. (1959) listed a whole series of areas where placebos have been shown to have some effect, such as allergies, asthma, cancer, diabetes, enuresis, epilepsy, multiple sclerosis, insomnia, ulcers, obesity, acne, smoking and dementia.

Perhaps one of the most studied areas in relation to placebo effects is pain (see Colloca et al. 2013 for a review). Beecher (1955), in an early study of the specific effects of placebos in pain reduction, suggested that 30 per cent of chronic pain sufferers show relief from a placebo when using both subjective (e.g. 'I feel less pain') and objective (e.g. 'You are more mobile') measures of pain. In the 1960s, Diamond et al. (1960) carried out several sham operations to examine the effect of placebos on pain relief. A sham heart bypass operation involved the individual believing that they were going to have a proper operation, being prepared for surgery, being given a general anaesthetic, cut open and then sewed up again without any actual bypass being carried out. The individual therefore believed that they had had an operation and had the scars to prove it. This procedure obviously has serious ethical problems. However, the results suggested that angina pain can actually be reduced by a sham operation by comparable levels to an actual operation for angina. This indicates how a placebo procedure can have its own independent impact on patient outcomes.

PLACEBOS: TO BE TAKEN OUT OF AN UNDERSTANDING OF HEALTH?

Since the 1940s, research into the effectiveness of drugs has used randomized controlled trials and placebos to assess the real effects of a drug versus the unreal effects. Placebos were seen as something to take out of the health equation. However, if placebos have a multitude of effects as described above rather than being taken out, perhaps they should be seen as central to health. For this reason it is interesting to examine how placebos work.

5   HOW DO PLACEBOS WORK?

If placebos have a multiple number of possible effects, what factors actually mediate these changes? In 2015, Colagiuri et al. reviewed the evidence for the mechanisms of placebos and highlighted factors ranging from individual expectancies to neurons to genes. Several theories have been developed to

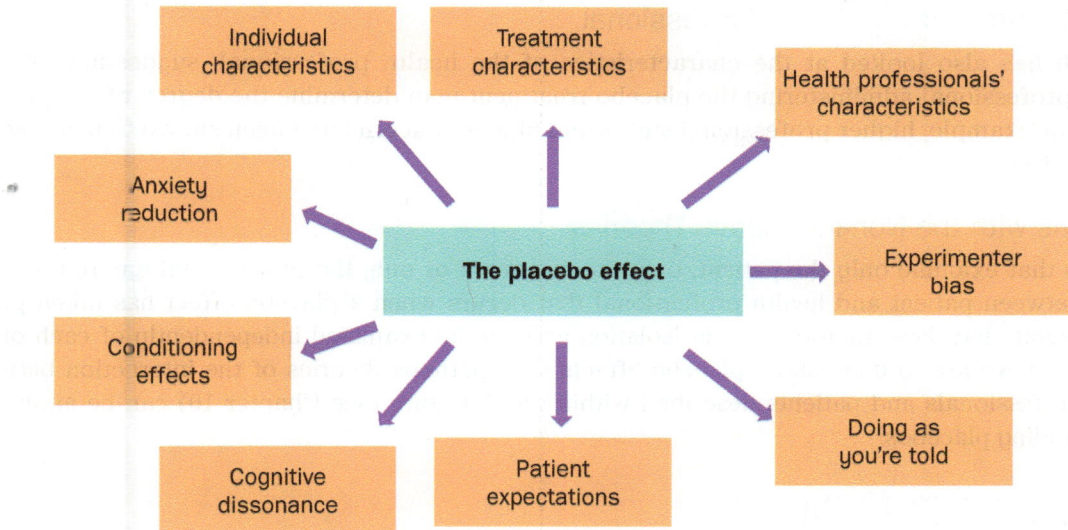

Figure 11.5 The placebo effect

try to understand the process of placebo effects. These can be described as *non-interactive* theories in that they examine individual characteristics, characteristics of the treatment and characteristics of the health professional, or *interactive* theories in that they involve an examination of the processes involved in the interactions between patients, the treatment and the health professional. These mechanisms are illustrated in Figure 11.5.

NON-INTERACTIVE THEORIES

Characteristics of the Individual

Individual trait theories suggest that certain individuals have characteristics that make them susceptible to placebo effects. Such characteristics have been described as emotional dependency, extroversion, neurosis and being highly suggestible. However, many of the characteristics described are conflicting and there is little evidence to support consistent traits as predictive of placebo responsiveness.

Characteristics of the Treatment

Other researchers have focused on treatment characteristics and have suggested that the characteristics of the actual process involved in the placebo treatment relate to the effectiveness or degree of the placebo effect. For example, if a treatment is perceived by the individual as being serious, the placebo effect will be greater. Accordingly, surgery, which is likely to be perceived as very serious, has the greatest placebo effect, followed by an injection, followed by having two pills versus one pill. Research has also looked at the size of the pill and suggests that larger pills are more effective than small pills in eliciting a change.

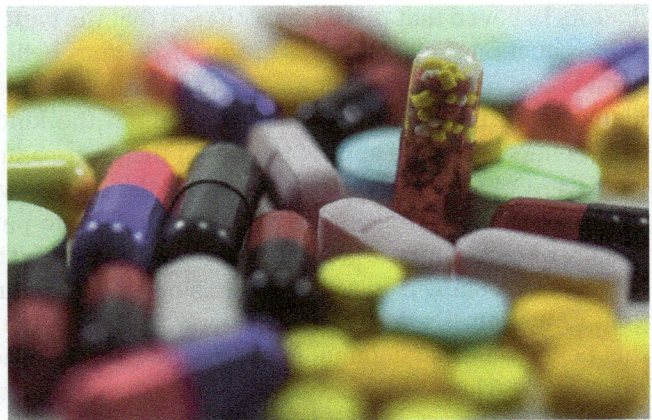

The placebo effect: which pill do you think would be more effective?

SOURCE: © Phongphan Phongphan / Alamy Stock Photo

Characteristics of the Health Professional

Research has also looked at the characteristics of the health professional, suggesting that the kind of professional administering the placebo treatment may determine the degree of the placebo effect. For example, higher professional status and higher concern have been shown to increase the placebo effect.

Problems with the Non-Interactive Theories

Theories that examine only the patient, only the treatment or only the professional ignore the interaction between patient and health professional that occurs when a placebo effect has taken place. They assume that these factors exist in isolation and can be examined independently of each other. However, if we are to understand placebo effects then perhaps theories of the interaction between health professionals and patients described within the literature (see Chapter 10) can be applied to understanding placebos.

INTERACTIVE THEORIES

It is therefore necessary to understand the process of placebo effects as an interactive process, which involves patient, treatment and health professional variables. Many of these mechanisms are similar to the factors highlighted in the psychosocial model of pain perception described above.

Experimenter Bias

Experimenter bias refers to the impact that the experimenter's expectations can have on the outcome of a study. For example, if an experimenter were carrying out a study to examine the effect of seeing an aggressive film on a child's aggressive behaviour (a classic social psychology study), then the experimenter's expectations may themselves be responsible for changing the child's behaviour (by their own interaction with the child), not the film. This phenomenon has been used to explain placebo effects. For example, Gracely et al. (1985) examined the impact of doctors' beliefs about the treatment on the patients' experience of placebo-induced pain reduction. Subjects were allocated to one of three conditions and were given either an analgesic (a painkiller), a placebo or naloxone (an opiate antagonist, which increases the pain experience). The patients were therefore told that this treatment would either reduce, have no effect or increase their pain. The doctors giving the drugs were themselves allocated to one of two conditions. They believed that either the patients would receive one of three of these substances (a chance of receiving a pain killer), or that the patient would receive either a placebo or naloxone (no chance of receiving a pain killer). Therefore one group of doctors believed that there was a chance that the patient would be given an analgesic and would show pain reduction, and the other group of doctors believed that there was no chance that the patient would receive some form of analgesia. In fact, all subjects were given a placebo. This study, therefore, manipulated both the patients' beliefs about the kind of treatment they had received and the doctors' beliefs about the kind of treatment they were administering. The results showed that the subjects who were given the drug treatment by the doctor who believed they had a chance to receive the analgesic showed a decrease in pain whereas the patients whose doctor believed that they had no chance of receiving the painkiller showed no effect. This suggests that if the doctors believed that the subjects may show pain reduction, this belief was communicated to the subjects who actually reported pain reduction. However, if the doctors believed that the subjects would not show pain reduction, this belief was also communicated to the subjects who accordingly reported no change in their pain experience. This study highlights a role for an interaction between the doctor and the patient and is similar to the effect described as 'experimenter bias' within social psychology. Experimenter bias suggests that the experimenter is capable of communicating their expectations to the subjects who respond in accordance with these expectations. Therefore, if applied to placebo effects, subjects show improvement because the health professionals expect them to improve.

Patient Expectations

Research has also looked at expectancy effects and focused on the expectations of the patient. Ross and Olson (1981) examined the effects of patients' expectations on recovery following a placebo. They suggested that most patients experience spontaneous recovery following illness as most illnesses go through periods of spontaneous change and patients attribute these changes to the treatment. Therefore, even if the treatment is a placebo, any change will be understood in terms of the effectiveness of this treatment. This suggests that because patients want to get better and expect to get better, any changes that they experience are attributed to the drugs they have taken. Sanders et al. (2020) further explored the impact of patient expectations as part of a double-blind, placebo-controlled, randomized clinical trial with 200 adults with temporomandibular disorder–associated myalgia (jaw pain). Patients rated their expectations of pain relief and were then randomly allocated to receive either placebo or propranolol. The results showed that propranolol was superior to placebo, but only in those who showed modest expectations of pain relief. In those with high expectations of pain relief, no differences were found between propranolol and placebo. This indicates that expecting to improve can create actual improvement. This effect, however, also seems to work if patients are told they are receiving a placebo. For example, Park and Covi (1965) gave sugar pills to a group of neurotic patients and actually told the patients that the pills were sugar pills and would therefore have no effect. The results showed that the patients still showed some reduction in their neuroticism. It could be argued that in this case, even though the patients did not expect the treatment to work, they still responded to the placebo. Likewise, Schafer et al. (2015) showed that placebo analgesics still reduced pain in 54 participants even when the true nature of the placebo treatment was revealed to participants. However, it could also be argued that these patients would still have some expectations that they would get better otherwise they would not have bothered to take the pills.

Conditioning Effects

Traditional conditioning theories have also been used to explain placebo effects (Wickramasekera 1980). It is suggested that patients associate certain factors with recovery and an improvement in their symptoms. For example, the presence of doctors, white coats, pills, injections and surgery are associated with improvement, recovery and effective treatment. According to conditioning theory, the unconditioned stimulus (treatment) would usually be associated with an unconditioned response (recovery). However, if this unconditioned stimulus (treatment) is paired with a conditioned stimulus (e.g. hospital, a white coat), the conditioned stimulus can itself elicit a conditioned response (recovery, the placebo effect). The conditioned stimulus might be comprised of a number of factors, including the appearance of the doctor, the environment, the actual site of the treatment or simply taking a pill. This stimulus may then elicit placebo recovery. For example, people often comment that they feel better as soon as they get into a doctor's waiting room, that their headache gets better before they have had time to digest a pill and that symptoms disappear when a doctor appears. According to conditioning theory, these changes would be examples of placebo recovery. Several reports provide support for conditioning theory. For example, research suggests that taking a placebo drug is more effective in a hospital setting when given by a doctor than if taken at home and given by someone who is not associated with the medical profession. This suggests that placebo effects require an interaction between the patient and their environment. In addition, placebo pain reduction is more effective with clinical and real pain than with experimentally created pain. This suggests that experimentally created pain does not elicit the association with the treatment environment, whereas the real pain has the effect of eliciting memories of previous experiences of treatment, making it more responsive to placebo intervention.

Anxiety Reduction

Placebos have also been explained in terms of anxiety reduction. Downing and Rickels (1983) argued that placebos decrease anxiety, thus helping the patient to recover. For example, according to gate control theory, anxiety reduction may close the gate and reduce pain, whereas increased anxiety may open the gate and increase pain (see p. 344). Placebos may decrease anxiety by empowering the individual and encouraging them to feel that they are in control of their pain. This improved sense of control may lead to decreased anxiety, which itself reduces the pain experience. Placebos may be particularly effective in chronic pain by breaking the anxiety–pain cycle (see earlier in this chapter).

Doing as You're Told

One classic study shows the importance of adherence to medical recommendations and how this may also illustrate a mechanism of the placebo effect (Horwitz et al. 1990). In 1982, a large-scale study showed that beta blockers reduced the risk of death by heart attack at follow up compared to placebo (Beta-blocker Heart Attack Trial Research Group 1982). Horwitz and colleagues decided to reanalyse this data to see whether adherence to *any* medication could also predict mortality. They therefore analysed data from 1,082 men in the experimental condition (who had received the beta-blocker) and 1,094 men in the placebo condition. Follow-up data were analysed for 12 months. The results showed that those with poor adherence were twice as likely to have died by one year compared to patients with good adherence. Therefore, regardless of what the drug was (whether a beta-blocker or a placebo), taking it as recommended halved the subjects' chances of dying. These results persisted even when factors such as smoking, medical history, stress and marital status were controlled for. Doing as you are told and taking medication (regardless of what it is) seems to impact upon mortality.

THE CENTRAL ROLE OF PATIENT EXPECTATIONS

Galen is reported to have said about the physician, 'He cures most in whom most are confident'. In accordance with this, all the theories of placebo effects described so far involve the patient *expecting* to get better. *Experimenter bias* describes the expectation of the doctor, which is communicated to the patient, changing the patient's expectation. *Expectancy effects* describe directly the patients' expectations derived from previous experience of successful treatment and the misattribution of any spontaneous changes. Further, *conditioning theory* requires the individual to expect the conditioned stimuli to be associated with successful intervention, *anxiety-reduction theory* describes the individual as feeling less anxious after a placebo treatment because of the belief that the treatment will be effective and *doing as you're told* suggests that by being adherent patients expect to get better. The central role of patient expectations is illustrated in Figure 11.6.

Ross and Olson (1981) summarize the placebo effects as follows:

- The direction of placebo effects parallels the effects of the drug under study.
- The strength of the placebo effect is proportional to that of the active drug.
- The reported side-effects of the placebo drug and the active drug are often similar.
- The time needed for both the placebo and the active drug to become active are often similar.

As a result, they conclude that 'most studies find that an administered placebo will alter the recipient's condition (or in some instances self-report of the condition) in accordance with the placebo's expected effects' (1981: 419). Therefore, according to the above theories, placebos work because the patient and the health professionals expect them to work. This emphasizes the role of expectations and regards placebo effects as an interaction between individuals and between individuals and their environment.

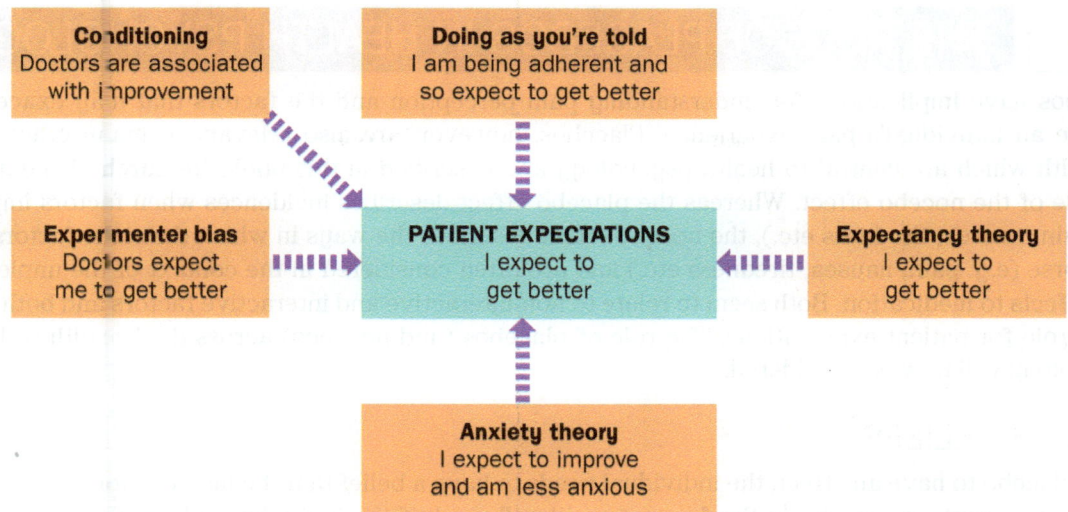

Figure 11.6 The central role of patient expectations in placebo effects

COGNITIVE DISSONANCE THEORY

The theories of placebos described so far emphasize patient expectations. The *cognitive dissonance theory* of placebos developed by Totman (1987) attempted to remove patient expectations from the placebo equation and emphasized justification and dissonance. Totman placed his cognitive dissonance theory of placebos in the following context: 'Why did faith healing last for such a long time?' and 'Why are many of the homeopathic medicines, which have no medically active content, still used?' He argued that faith healing has lasted and homeopathic medicines are still used because they work. In answer to his question why this might be, Totman suggested that the one factor that all of these medically inert treatments have in common is that they require an investment by the individual in terms of money, dedication, pain, time or inconvenience. He argued that if medically inactive drugs were freely available, they would not be effective and that if an individual lived around the corner to Lourdes then a trip to Lourdes would have no effect on their health status.

The Effect of Investment

Totman (1987) suggested that investment results in the individual having to go through two processes: (1) the individual needs to justify their behaviour; and (2) the individual needs to see themselves as rational and in control. If these two factors are in line with each other (e.g. 'I spent money on a treatment and it worked'), then the individual experiences low dissonance. If, however, there is a conflict between these two factors (e.g. 'I spent money on a treatment and I do not feel any better'), the individual experiences a state of high dissonance. Totman argued that high justification (it worked) results in low guilt and low dissonance (e.g. 'I can justify my behaviour, I am rational and in control'). However, low justification (e.g. 'it didn't work') results in high guilt and high dissonance (e.g. 'I cannot justify my behaviour, I am not rational or in control'). The best way to resolve this dissonance, according to Totman, is for there to be an outcome that enables the individual to be able to justify their behaviour and to see themselves as rational and in control. Accordingly, Totman argued that when in a state of high dissonance, unconscious regulating mechanisms are activated which may cause physical changes that improve the health of the individual, which in turn enables the individual to justify their behaviour and this resolves the dissonance. Totman therefore suggested that for a placebo effect to occur, the individual does not require an expectation that they will get better, but a need to find justification for their behaviour and a state of cognitive dissonance to set this up.

6 THE ROLE OF PLACEBOS IN HEALTH PSYCHOLOGY

Placebos have implications for understanding pain perception and the factors that may exacerbate or ease an individual's pain experience. Placebos, however, are also relevant to many other areas of health which are central to health psychology and described in this book. Research also explores the role of the nocebo effect. Whereas the placebo effect describes incidences when factors improve (i.e .pain, nausea, tiredness etc.), the nocebo effect describes the ways in which the same factors may get worse (e.g. pain, nausea, tiredness etc.) and are often considered in the context of the unpleasant side effects to medication. Both seem to relate to non-interactive and interactive factors and both show a key role for patient expectations. The role of placebos (and nocebos) across the breadth of health psychology will now be considered.

HEALTH BELIEFS

For a placebo to have an effect, the individual needs to have a belief that the intervention will be effective. For example, a placebo in the form of a pill will work if the individual subscribes to a medical model of health and illness and believes that traditional medical interventions are effective. A placebo in the form of herbal tea may only be effective if the individual believes in alternative medicines and is open to non-traditional forms of intervention. Furthermore, the conditioning effects, reporting error and misattribution process may only occur if the individual believes that health professionals in white coats can treat illness, that hospitals are where people get better and that medical interventions should produce positive results.

ILLNESS COGNITIONS

For a placebo to have an effect, the individual needs to hold particular beliefs about their illness. For example, if an illness is seen as long-lasting without episodes of remission, times of spontaneous recovery may not happen, which therefore cannot be explained in terms of the effectiveness of the treatment. Likewise, if an individual believes that their illness has a medical cause, then a placebo in the form of a pill would be effective. However, if the individual believes that their illness is caused by their lifestyle, a pill placebo may not be effective.

HEALTH PROFESSIONALS' HEALTH BELIEFS

Placebos may also be related to the beliefs of the health professional. For example, a doctor may need to believe in the intervention for it to have an effect. If the doctor believes that an illness is the result of lifestyle, and can be cured by changes in that lifestyle, then a placebo in the form of a medical intervention may not work, as the doctor's expectation of failure may be communicated to the patient.

HEALTH-RELATED BEHAVIOURS

A placebo may function via changes in health-related behaviour. If an individual believes that they have taken something or behaved in a way that may promote good health, they may also change other health-related behaviours (e.g. smoking, drinking, exercise), which may also improve their health.

STRESS

Placebos also have implications for understanding responses to stress. If placebos have an effect either directly (physiological change) or indirectly (behaviour change), then this is in parallel with theories of stress. In addition, placebos may function by reducing any stress caused by illness. The belief that an individual has taken control of their illness (perceived control) may reduce the stress response, reducing any effects this stress may have on the illness.

CHRONIC ILLNESS

Health psychology explores the role of psychology across the spectrum from health to illness and throughout the different stages of chronic illness including obesity, CHD, cancer and HIV. The placebo and nocebo effects are relevant to all these different stages. For example, the expectations of negative side effects of health behaviours such as withdrawal (for giving up smoking), hunger (for eating less), tiredness (for exercise) or loss of pleasure (for condom use) may prevent healthier lifestyles, so increasing the risk of illness onset. In contrast, more positive expectancies could promote health behaviours. Likewise, expectations of treatments may create either positive or negative changes in symptoms such as nausea (for cancer treatment), hunger (for obesity treatment) or tiredness (for rehabilitation for CHD). This in turn could influence adherence to treatment, health outcomes and subsequent longevity.

BOX 11.1:
Critical Approaches to Health Psychology

Research and theories relating to pain and placebos highlight some of the bigger issues in health psychology as follows:

The role of culture: The pain experience very much varies by culture and we know that different cultures respond in different ways to universal problems such as childbirth, illness and death. We also know that different languages have different ways of describing and making sense of pain. Much of our research in health psychology is written in English and published in English-speaking journals. Therefore while we acknowledge these cultural differences we can never fully comprehend them as we do not access research from other cultures and, even when we do, the research has been translated into English so any cultural subtleties will have been removed.

Individual differences: Research explores differences in pain perception by individual variables such as gender, age or personality. This process can create false dichotomies and underestimates the complexity of these variables and the role they play in our experience.

Mind–body split: Pain is the perfect example of mind–body interaction with the way we think about pain influencing our experience of pain. From this perspective we emphasize how the mind and body are not discrete but by using different words to describe them (the mind vs the body), and by measuring them separately, we still perpetuate the belief that they are separate.

7 | THINKING CRITICALLY ABOUT PAIN AND PLACEBO RESEARCH

There are several problems with research exploring pain and the placebo effect.

SOME CRITICAL QUESTIONS

When thinking about research in this area ask yourself the following questions.

- Why is pain so difficult to measure?
- What are the implications of these measurement issues for synthesizing across different studies?

- Pain illustrates the interaction between psychological and physiological processes. Is this distinction useful or even appropriate?
- The placebo effect illustrates the impact of expectations on health outcomes. Is it possible to carry out research without changing expectations?

SOME PROBLEMS WITH. . .

The are several problems with pain and placebo research that need to be considered:

Measurement: Pain cannot be observed and is a subjective experience. Therefore measuring pain is problematic. Self-report measures are reliant upon the individual attempting to give an accurate description of how they feel which may well be influenced by how they want other people to believe that they feel and the ability of the existing measures to describe their experience. More objective measures, such as the observation of pain behaviour or medication use, may miss the subjective nature of the pain experience.

Discrete processes: Pain research highlights the interaction between biological and psychological processes. This is particularly apparent in the GCT and the role of affect and cognitions in mediating the pain experience. However, how these different processes actually interact remains unclear. Why is it that focusing on pain actually makes it hurt more?

Pain onset: Pain research emphasizes the role of psychological factors in promoting chronic pain and exacerbating acute pain. Little, however, is known about pain onset. Why do some people get headaches while others do not? Why is there such cultural variation in where and when people experience pain? (see Chapter 9 for a discussion of symptom onset).

Research synthesis: Pain is difficult to measure, difficult to define and treatment studies often use different protocols, different outcomes and different time points. This makes synthesizing evidence across studies difficult. This is discussed in detail in Eccleston et al. (2010) and Moore et al. (2010).

The impact of measurement: Central to understanding the placebo effect is the role of expectations, with people seeming to feel pain or get better if they expect to do so. But how can the role of expectations be tested, as taking part in any study or being offered any medication will ultimately change an individual's expectations? It is not really possible therefore to 'placebo' the placebo effect.

Like magic: Placebo research suggests that expecting to get better, even just in the form of adhering to medication, seems to make people better. However, it is not clear how this process actually works. How does a placebo effect make a wound heal faster, a pain go away or lungs function better?

Mind–body interactions: Placebos illustrate a direct relationship between a person's mind and their body. This is central to health psychology. We still, however, do not know how this works – it seems to have a magical feel to it, which remains unexplained.

> **TO CONCLUDE**
>
> Early models suggested that pain was a sensation with no causal role for psychology. The GCT was then developed in the 1960s which included psychological factors and emphasized pain as a perception. The psychosocial model of pain provides a more detailed account of pain as a perception and highlights the impact of learning, affect, cognitions and behaviour. This chapter has described these factors and then explored the role of psychology in pain management. The chapter also explored the role of placebo effects which are central not only to understanding pain and its management but also have implications for all other areas of health psychology. Finally, this chapter described some of the problems with research in this area.

QUESTIONS

1 Pain is a response to painful stimuli. Discuss.
2 To what extent does gate control theory depart from earlier models of pain?
3 Pain is a perception. Discuss.
4 How might psychological factors exacerbate pain perception?
5 To what extent can psychological factors be used to reduce pain perception?
6 Self-report is the only true way of measuring pain. Discuss.
7 Placebos are all in the mind. Discuss.
8 Discuss the role of patient expectations in improvements in health.
9 To what extent does pain research inform our understanding of how the mind and body interact?
10 Discuss the measurement issues with exploring both pain and the placebo effect.

FOR DISCUSSION

Consider the last time you experienced pain (e.g. period pain, headache, sports injury) and discuss the potential role of learning, affect, cognition and behaviour pain in making your pain either worse or better.

FURTHER READING

Dekker, J., Lundberg, U. and Williams, A. (eds) (2001) *Behavioural Factors and Interventions in Pain and Musculoskeletal Disorders: A Special Issue of the International Journal of Behavioural Medicine.* Mahwah, NJ: Lawrence Erlbaum Associates.
This provides a detailed analysis of the psychosocial factors involved in the development of chronic pain.

Eccleston, C. (2015) *Embodied: The Psychology of Physical Sensation.* Oxford: Oxford University Press.
This is a novel book that covers how and why we experience symptoms such as pain, itch, breathing, fatigue and temperature. This is a great book based upon interviews with those suffering from extremes of these symptoms and concludes with a theoretical analysis of their experiences.

Main, C.J. and Spanswick, C.C. (eds) (2000) *Pain Management: An Interdisciplinary Approach.* Edinburgh: Churchill Livingstone.
This edited collection provides a detailed account of contemporary approaches to treating pain.

Simpson, S.H., Eurich, D.T., Majumdar, S.R. et al. (2006) A meta-analysis of the association between adherence to drug therapy and mortality, *British Medical Journal,* **333:** 15.
This is an excellent review of the literature exploring how simply adhering to medication has a powerful placebo effect which is linked with improved mortality.

Totman, R.G. (1987) *The Social Causes of Illness*. London: Souvenir Press.
This is an old book now but it inspired me many years ago and provides an interesting perspective on placebos and the interrelationship between beliefs, behaviours and health.

Wainwright, E. and Eccleston, C. (eds) (2019) *Work and Pain. A Lifespan Developmental Approach*. Oxford: Oxford University Press.
This edited book explores the relationship between occupation and pain, from being a child at school to experiencing pain in the workplace. It covers theories of pain and pain perception and describes interventions for all ages.

12
Chronic Illness: HIV and Cancer

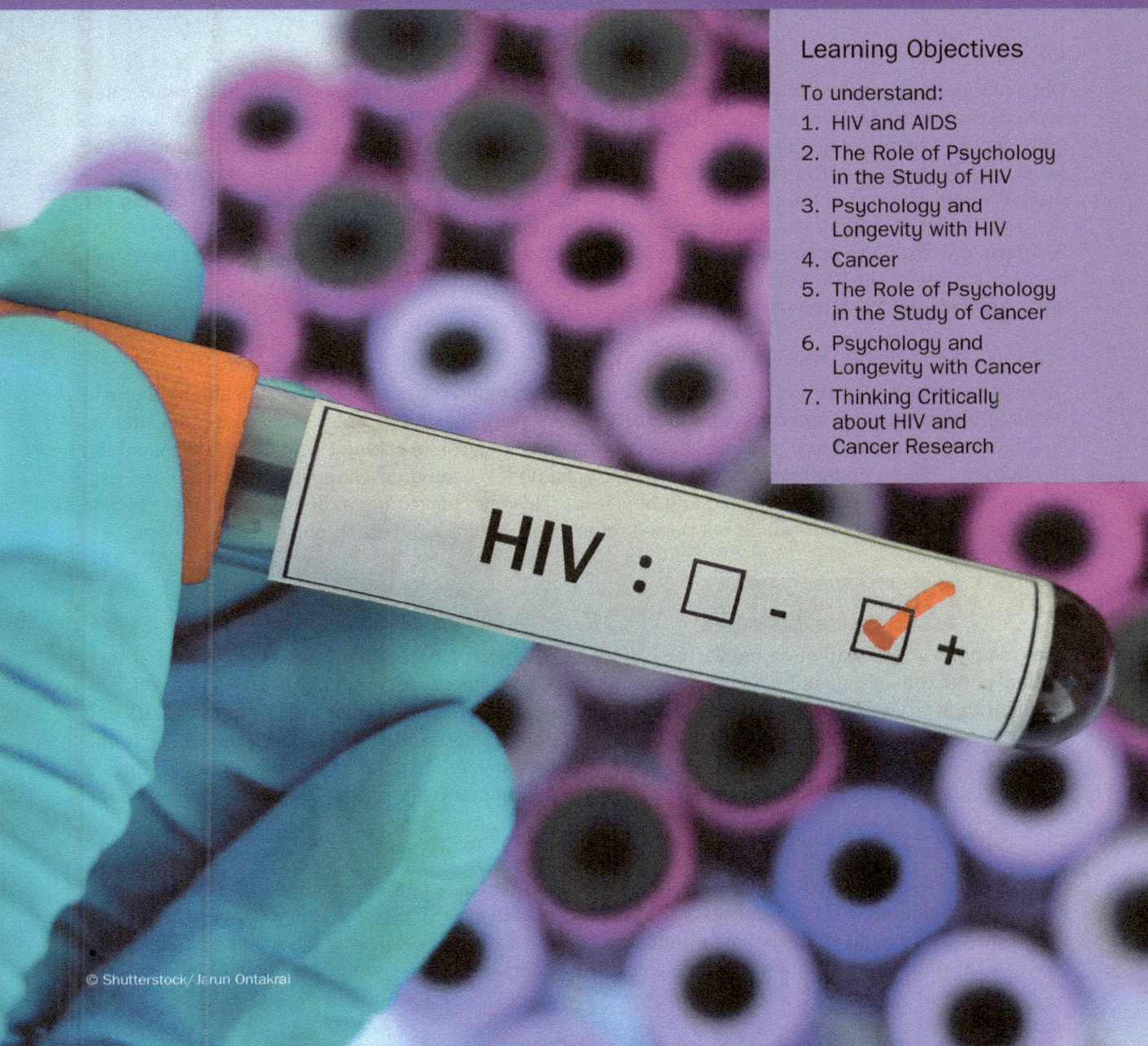

Learning Objectives

To understand:

1. HIV and AIDS
2. The Role of Psychology in the Study of HIV
3. Psychology and Longevity with HIV
4. Cancer
5. The Role of Psychology in the Study of Cancer
6. Psychology and Longevity with Cancer
7. Thinking Critically about HIV and Cancer Research

CHAPTER OVERVIEW

This chapter and the next examine the role that psychology plays at each stage of a chronic illness, from illness onset, through the adaptation to illness, its progression, the psychological consequences and longevity. They do not aim to be comprehensive overviews of the immense literature on illness, but to illustrate the possible varied role of psychology in illness. This chapter uses the examples of HIV and cancer and Chapter 13 focuses on obesity and coronary heart disease (CHD). These psychological factors, however, are also relevant to a multitude of other common or less common chronic and acute illnesses including multiple sclerosis, fibromyalgia, rheumatoid arthritis, asthma, chronic fatigue syndrome and chronic pain. These are illustrated throughout this chapter and the next with case examples. Rather than being seen as a passive response to biomedical factors, such chronic illnesses are better understood in terms of a complex interplay of physiological, psychological and social processes.

CASE STUDY

Obi is 68 and has smoked for most of his life. He has recently been diagnosed with lung cancer and started treatment a few weeks ago. Although he has always known that smoking is dangerous he is still quite shocked by the diagnosis and is struggling to come to terms with what it means for himself and his family. He is also starting to suffer side effects of the chemotherapy and feels sick and extremely tired after his sessions at the hospital. The doctor has told him to stop smoking but he can't really see the point as he feels that 'the damage has been done' and is feeling quite hopeless about the future. His partner is trying to encourage him to eat well, rest and generally look after himself but he spends his days staring at the TV and feeling very sad. It doesn't seem fair as he knows plenty of people who have smoked and drank too much and they are all fine.

Through the Eyes of Health Psychology. . .

Chronic illnesses illustrate a role for psychological factors along the continuum from health to illness in terms of illness onset, progression and longevity. Obi's story illustrates many of these factors such as health behaviours (smoking), health beliefs (smoking is dangerous), coping ('why me?'), sense making (its not fair), illness cognitions (the damage has been done), behaviour change (eating well) and psychological consequences (feeling sad and hopeless). This chapter explores the psychology of chronic illness focusing on HIV and cancer but these factors are relevant to all other long-term conditions.

1   HIV AND AIDS

The first part of this chapter examines the history of HIV, what HIV is and how it is transmitted. It then evaluates the role of psychology in understanding HIV in terms of susceptibility to HIV and AIDS, progression from HIV to AIDS and longevity. A detailed discussion of condom use in the context of HIV and AIDS can be found in Chapter 6 and a detailed description of stress and illness progression can be found in Chapter 10. Chapter 7 also provides a description of behaviour change interventions. Chapter 2 describes the role of beliefs in predicting behaviour and Chapter 9 describes adherence to medication.

THE HISTORY OF HIV

AIDS (acquired immune deficiency syndrome) was identified as a new syndrome in 1981. At that time, it was regarded as specific to homosexuality and was known as GRIDS (gay-related immune deficiency syndrome). As a result of this belief, a number of theories were developed to try to explain the occurrence of this new illness among homosexuals. These ranged from the suggestion that AIDS may be a response to the over-use of recreational drugs such as 'poppers' or to over-exposure to semen, and focused on the perceived lifestyles of the homosexual population. In 1982, however, AIDS occurred in people with haemophilia. As haemophiliacs were seen not to have lifestyles comparable with the homosexual population, scientists started to reform their theories about AIDS and suggested, for the first time, that perhaps it was caused by a virus. Such a virus could reach haemophiliacs through their use of Factor VIII, a donated blood-clotting agent.

The HIV virus was first isolated in 1983 although there is debate as to whether this was achieved by Gallo in the USA or/and Montagnier in France. Both these researchers were looking for a retrovirus, having examined a cat retrovirus that caused leukaemia and appeared to be very similar to what they thought was causing this new illness. In 1984, the human immunodeficiency virus type 1 (HIV 1) was identified and, in 1985, HIV 2 was identified in Africa.

WHAT IS HIV?

The Structure of HIV

The HIV virus is a *retrovirus*, a type of virus containing RNA. There are three types of retrovirus: oncogenic retroviruses which cause cancer, foamy retroviruses which have no effect at all on the health status of the individual, and lentiviruses, or slow viruses, which have slow long-term effects. HIV is a lentivirus.

The HIV virus is structured with an outer coat and an inner core. The RNA is situated in the core and contains eight viral genes, which encode the proteins of the envelope and the core, and also contains enzymes, which are essential for replication.

The Transmission of HIV

In order to be transmitted from one individual to the next, the HIV virus generally needs to come into contact with cells that have CD4 molecules on their surface. Such cells are found within the immune system and are called T-helper cells. The process of transmission of the HIV virus involves the following stages:

1 HIV binds to the CD4 molecule of the T-helper cell.

2 HIV virus is internalized into the cytoplasm of the cell.

3 The cell itself generates a pro-viral DNA, which is a copy of the host cell.

4 This pro-virus enters the nucleus of the host cell.

5 The host cell produces new viral particles, which it reads off from the viral code of the viral DNA.

6 These viral particles bud off and infect new cells.

7 Eventually, after much replication, the host T-helper cell dies.

THE PROGRESSION FROM HIV TO AIDS

The progression from HIV to HIV disease and AIDS varies in time. AIDS reflects a reduction in T-helper cells and specifically those that are CD4-positive T-cells. This causes immune deficiency and the appearance of opportunistic infections. The progression from initial HIV seroconversion through to AIDS tends to go through the following stages:

1 The initial viral seroconversion illness.

2 An asymptomatic stage.

3 Enlargement of the lymph nodes, onset of opportunistic infections.

4 AIDS-related complex (ARC).

5 AIDS.

THE PREVALENCE OF HIV AND AIDS

In 2015 there were an estimated 36.7 million people worldwide infected with the HIV virus. Generally, the incidence of HIV peaked in the late 1990s and has now mostly stabilized. However, the numbers of people living with HIV has increased due to population growth as have the numbers of people now taking antiretroviral therapy which has significantly improved the life expectancy of those infected with the HIV virus (see Figures 9.1 and 9.2 in Chapter 9 for the impact of HIV medication on life expectancy).

Although much western interest has been on the incidence of HIV within the gay populations of the western world, the epicentre of the global epidemic is in sub-Saharan Africa. For example, in Swaziland, Lesotha and Botswana more than 20 per cent of the population are HIV-positive. Although marginally lower, rates in countries such as South Africa, Nambia, Zimbabwe and Monzambique are between 10 and 20 per cent. Rates are also very high in parts of Asia, particularly India and China, whereas countries including Australia, Malta, Russia, the Netherlands and Sweden have much lower rates between 0.1 and 0.2 per cent. The rate in the USA is 0.3 per cent and in Canada it is 0.4 per cent. In the UK, the current rate is 0.16 per cent and it is estimated that within London 1 in 7 gay/bisexual men are living with HIV. In terms of changing rates of HIV, there was a decline in new cases across the USA and Europe in the 1990s although there is some evidence of a resurgent epidemic in men who have sex with men in the USA and some European countries. There has also been a recent increase in the UK, mostly due to heterosexual transmission with an increasing number of women accounting for the rise in numbers, although some of this increase may also relate to a sense of immunity in gay men and the increasing prevalence of 'barebacking' (e.g. Flowers et al. 1998; Ridge 2004; see Chapter 6). There have been declines in rates in some parts of sub-Saharan Africa (Kenya and Zimbabwe), declines in some parts of India (Tamil Nadu) but no signs of decline in most of southern Africa, and increases in China, Indonesia, Papua New Guinea, Bangladesh and Pakistan. Worldwide deaths from HIV-related illness in 2016 are shown in Figure 12.1 which reveals that the highest death rates are in Africa, North, Central and South America and South East Asia. Figure 12.2 shows the estimated number of adults living with HIV (both diagnosed and undiagnosed) in the UK in 2017. The data from this graph indicate

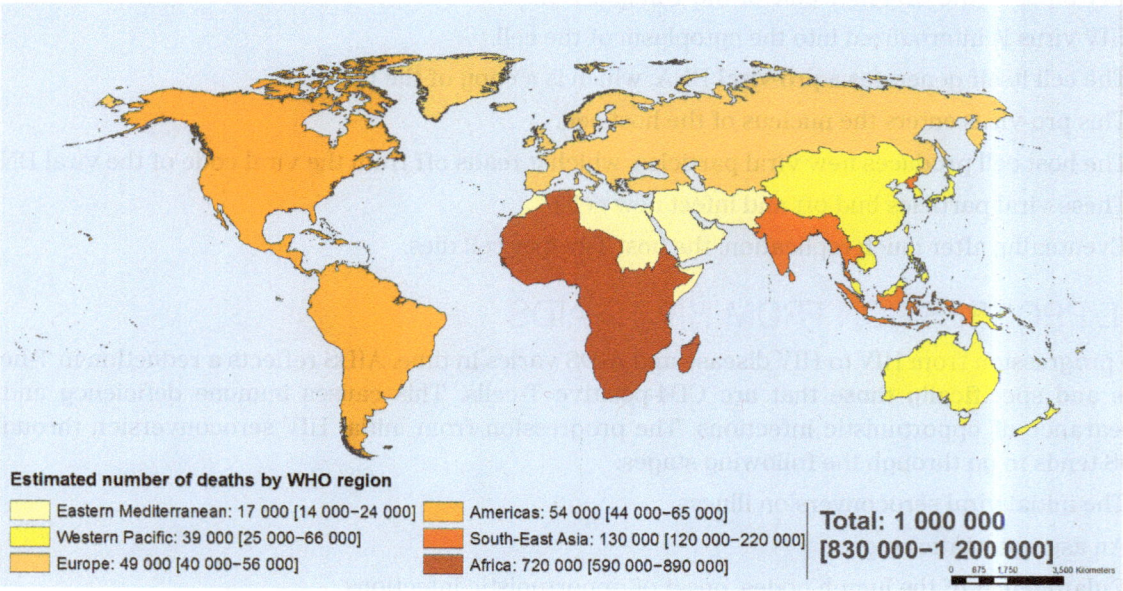

Estimated number of deaths by WHO region

Eastern Mediterranean: 17 000 [14 000–24 000]
Western Pacific: 39 000 [25 000–66 000]
Europe: 49 000 [40 000–56 000]
Americas: 54 000 [44 000–65 000]
South-East Asia: 130 000 [120 000–220 000]
Africa: 720 000 [590 000–890 000]

Total: 1 000 000
[830 000–1 200 000]

Figure 12.1 Worldwide death from HIV-related causes in 2016

SOURCE: WHO (2017)

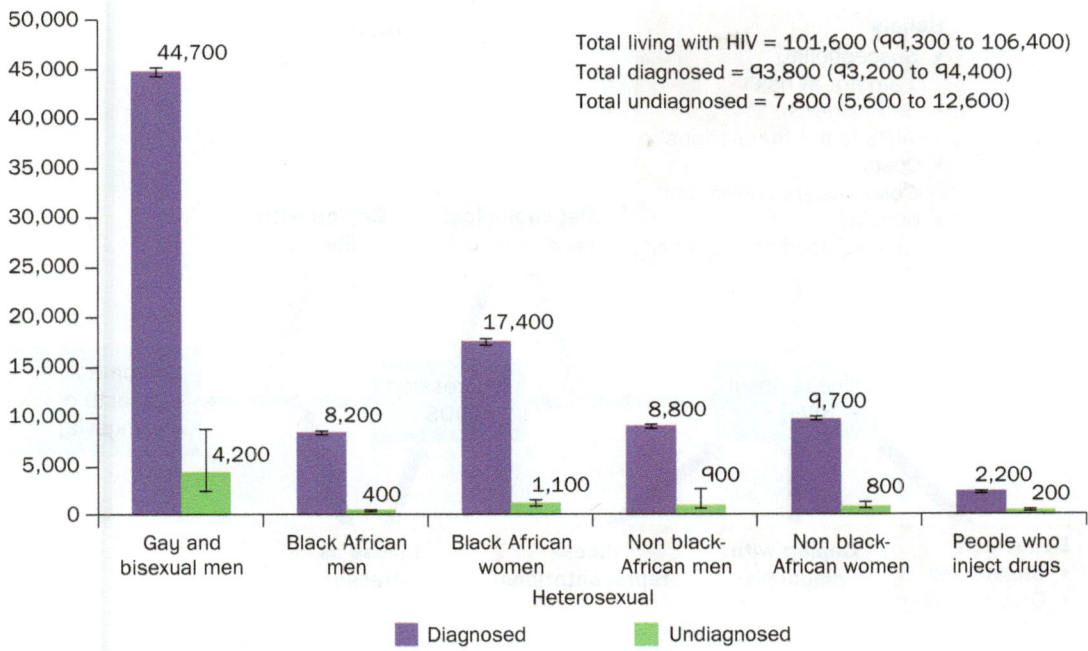

Figure 12.2 Number of adults living with HIV (both diagnosed and undiagnosed) in the UK, 2017
SOURCE: Public Health England (2018)

that the highest rates of HIV in the UK are in gay and bisexual men followed by heterosexual women born in Africa.

2 THE ROLE OF PSYCHOLOGY IN THE STUDY OF HIV

Some HIV transmission is through blood transfusions or from mother to child during birth. Most transmission, however, is through human behaviour involving sexual intercourse or shared needle use. Health psychology has studied HIV in terms of attitudes to HIV and safe sex, changing these attitudes, examining predictors of behaviour and the development of interventions to change behaviour. Chapters 2–9 provide insights into aspects of health beliefs, illness cognitions, health behaviours, medication adherence, help-seeking and behaviour change interventions which are all relevant to understanding the role of psychology in HIV and AIDS.

The potential role of psychological factors in understanding HIV and AIDS is shown in Figure 12.3.

The following observations suggest that psychology has an additional role to play in HIV:

- *Not everyone exposed to the HIV virus becomes HIV-positive.* This suggests that psychological factors may influence an individual's susceptibility to the HIV virus.
- *The time for progression from HIV to AIDS is variable.* Psychological factors may have a role in promoting the replication of the HIV virus and the progression from being HIV-positive to having AIDS.
- *Not everyone with HIV dies from AIDS.* Psychological factors have a role to play in determining the longevity of the individual.

This chapter will focus on the role of psychology in AIDS in terms of susceptibility to AIDS, progression from HIV to AIDS and longevity.

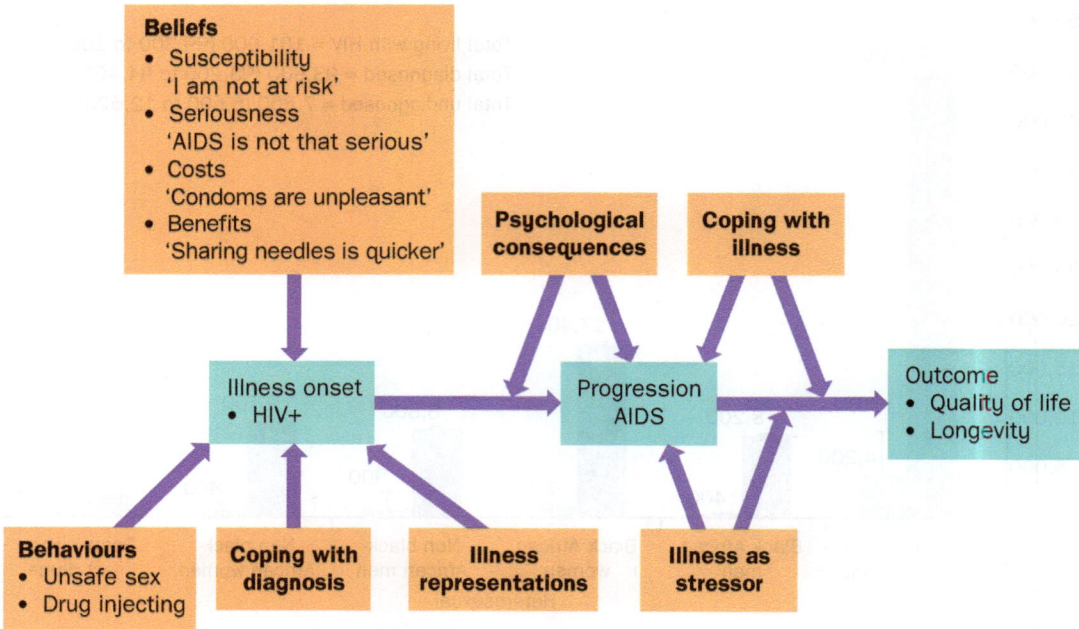

Figure 12.3 The potential role of psychology in HIV

PSYCHOLOGY AND SUSCEPTIBILITY TO THE HIV VIRUS

Research described in Chapters 2 and 6 illustrates a number of factors that influence whether people practise safer sex or carry out risky behaviours, In the context of HIV, Card et al. (2018) conducted a self-report study of 719 predominantly white gay and bisexual men and found that although alcohol use was not associated with risky sexual behaviours, depressive symptoms and polysubstance use led to an increase in risky sexual behaviours leading to an increased risk of contracting HIV. Remien et al. (2019) also concluded from their review that mental health problems are more common among people vulnerable to acquiring HIV and people living with HIV, compared with the general population and suggest that mental health impairments increase risk for HIV acquisition. Not all those individuals who come into contact with HIV become HIV-positive, however, and research also suggests that psychology may also have a role to play in the susceptibility to the virus. One train of thought argues that the lifestyle of an individual may increase their chances of contracting HIV once exposed to the virus. Van Griensven et al. (1986) suggested that the use of other drugs, such as nitrates and cannabis, increases the chance of contracting HIV once exposed to the virus. Lifson et al. (1989) also argued that the existence of other viruses, such as herpes simplex and cytomegalovirus (CMV), in the bloodstream may increase the chances of contracting HIV. These viruses are also thought to be associated with unsafe sex and injecting drugs. Therefore unhealthy behaviours may not only be related to exposure to the HIV virus but also to the likelihood that an individual will become HIV-positive once exposed.

PSYCHOLOGY AND THE PROGRESSION FROM HIV TO AIDS

Research has also examined the role of psychology in the progression from HIV to AIDS (Taylor et al. 1998). This research points to roles for minority stress, adherence to medication, comorbidities, lifestyle, cognitive adjustment and type C coping style.

Minority Stress and Stigma

In many parts of the world homosexuality remains illegal which results in prejudice and stigma. Such prejudice and stigma is also common across countries where homosexuality is legal.

Furthermore, HIV and AIDS remain stigmatized conditions. As a result, those who are gay *and* those with HIV/AIDS experience prejudice and stigma which has been explored within the framework of minority stress and has implications for health in general as well as in the context of HIV. For example, Frost et al. (2015) explored the relationship between minority stress and physical health among 396 lesbian, gay and bisexual individuals using baseline interviews and follow-ups after 1 year. The results showed that the odds of experiencing a physical health problem at follow-up were significantly higher among those who experienced an externally rated prejudiced event, suggesting that minority stress reduced health status. In terms of HIV, Sanjuán et al. (2013) explored the relationships between stigma perception, coping and well-being in a sample of 133 people living with HIV. They found that stigma perception and using avoidant coping strategies were both associated with poorer well-being, whereas active coping resulted in increased well-being. Furthermore, perceived stigma has also been associated with adherence to medication for HIV (Katz et al. 2013 see below).

Adherence to Medication

Over recent years the life expectancy and quality of life of those with HIV have improved dramatically (e.g. Mocroft et al. 1998). Much of this has been attributed to the success of highly active anti-retroviral therapy (HAART) and HIV is often now described as a chronic illness rather than a terminal one. Many people who are offered HAART, however, do not take the treatment. For example, Steinberg (2001) reported that only 75 per cent of those eligible for treatment received treatment. Of those who did not receive treatment, 58 per cent had declined the offer. Research has therefore explored the reasons behind adherence and non-adherence to medication (see Chapter 9 for a discussion of adherence). Before HAART, the most common medication was AZT monotherapy. Early research by Siegel et al. (1992) reported that reasons for non-adherence included lack of trust in doctors, feelings of well-being, negative beliefs about medical treatments, the belief that AZT would make the person worse and the belief that taking AZT would reduce treatment options in future. In a similar vein, Cooper et al. (2002) explored people's beliefs about HAART. They interviewed 26 gay men about their views about HAART shortly after it had been recommended by their doctor. The results showed that the men held beliefs about the necessity of their medication in terms of whether they felt it could control their HIV or whether they were inclined to let their condition take its natural course; they described their concerns about taking the drugs in terms of side-effects, the difficulties of the drug regimen and its effectiveness; and they described feelings about their control over the decision to take the medication. In an associated study, Gellaitry et al. (2005) further examined beliefs about HAART and linked them with adherence. These results showed that concerns about the adverse effects of HAART were related to declining treatment. Likewise, in a longitudinal study, Viswanathan et al. (2015) reported that adherence to HAART in a sample of men who have sex with men (MSM) was predicted by older age, non-black race and no alcohol, cigarette or recreational drug use. Katz et al. (2013) conducted a systematic review and meta-synthesis of 75 studies on 14,854 HIV-positive people across 32 countries to investigate the impact of HIV-related stigma on treatment adherence. They found that experiencing HIV-related stigma reduced adherence to medication by compromising general psychological processes such as social support and adaptive coping.

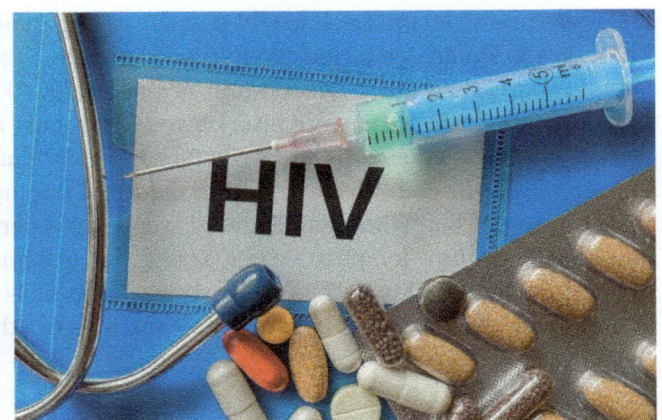

The treatment regimen for AIDs can be complex and can lead to non-adherence

SOURCE: © Shutterstock/vchal

Comorbidities

Given that HIV is a disease of the immune system it has been suggested that general health status and the existence of other illnesses could promote the progression from HIV to AIDS. Chepchirchir et al. (2018) explored the relationship between hypertension and AIDS progression in 297 participants. They found that the majority of those with HIV also had hypertension, which can progress HIV due to the relationship between CD4 counts and creatinine which exacerbates problems with underlying immunosuppression (see later for a discussion of PNI). There is also some evidence for the role of mental health problems in the progression to AIDS. For example, Remien et al. (2019) concluded from their review that mental health impairments increase risk for negative health outcomes at each step in the HIV care continuum and Yousuf et al. (2019) concluded from their review that psychosocial, neurohormonal and virologic factors associated with depression promote the progression of HIV to AIDS.

Lifestyle

It has been suggested that injecting drugs further stimulates the immune system, which may well influence replication, and thereby points to a role for drug use not only in contracting the virus but also for its replication. In addition, research has indicated that replication of the HIV virus may be influenced by further exposure to the virus, suggesting a role for unsafe sex and drug use in its progression. Furthermore, it has been suggested that contact with drugs, which may have an immunosuppressive effect, or other viruses, such as herpes complex and CMV, may also be related to an increase in replication. Edelman et al. (2015) conducted a longitudinal study on 77 Russian participants with HIV and found that those with persistent heroin use had a significant increase in CD4 count, whereas those with intermittent to no use had a significant decrease in CD4 count. They argue that heroin withdrawal may relate to disease progression.

Cognitive Adjustment

Research from the Multi Center AIDS Cohort Study (MACS) in the USA has suggested a role for forms of cognitive adjustment to bereavement and illness progression (Bower et al. 1998; Reed et al. 1999). In the first part of this study, 72 men who were HIV-positive, asymptomatic and half of whom had recently experienced the death of a close friend or primary partner, completed measures of their psychosocial state (HIV-specific expectancies, mood state and hopelessness) and had the number of their CD4 T-helper cells recorded. They were then followed up over a six-year period. The results showed that about half the sample showed symptoms over the follow-up period. However, the rate and extent of the disease progression were not consistent for everyone. In particular, the results showed that symptom development was predicted by baseline HIV-specific expectancies, particularly in those who had been bereaved. Therefore it would seem that having more negative expectancies of HIV progression is predictive of actual progression. In the second part of this study, 40 HIV-positive men who had recently lost a close friend or partner to AIDS were interviewed about how they made sense of this death. These interviews were then classified according to whether the individual had managed to find meaning in the death in line with Taylor's cognitive adaptation theory of coping (Taylor 1983) (see Chapter 8). An example of meaning would be: 'What his death did was snap a certain value into my behaviour, which is "Listen, you don't know how long you've got. You've just lost another one. Spend more time with the people that mean something to you".' The results showed that those who had managed to find meaning maintained their levels of CD4 T-helper cells at follow-up, whereas those who did not find meaning showed a decline.

Type C Coping Style

Research has also explored the link between how people cope with HIV and the progression of their disease with a focus on type C coping style which reflects emotional inexpression and a decreased recognition of needs and feelings. For example, Solano et al. (2001, 2002) used CD4 cells as a measure of disease status, assessed baseline coping and followed 200 patients up after 6 and 12 months.

The results showed that type C coping style predicted progression at follow-up, suggesting that a form of coping that relies upon a lack of emotional expression may exacerbate the course of HIV disease. However, the results also showed that very high levels of emotional expression were also detrimental. The authors conclude that working through emotions rather than just releasing them may be the most protective coping strategy for people diagnosed as HIV-positive.

3   PSYCHOLOGY AND LONGEVITY WITH HIV

In the 1980s HIV/AIDS was an acute terminal illness with life expectancy post diagnosis ranging from days up to about 18 months. Nowadays, fortunately, in most countries it is seen as a chronic condition with the life expectancy of those who are HIV positive almost matching those who are not. For example, the numbers of deaths from HIV/AIDS declined by 62 per cent in the USA between 2001 and 2012. This dramatic decline in death rate is shown in Figure 12.4 (FDA 1997).

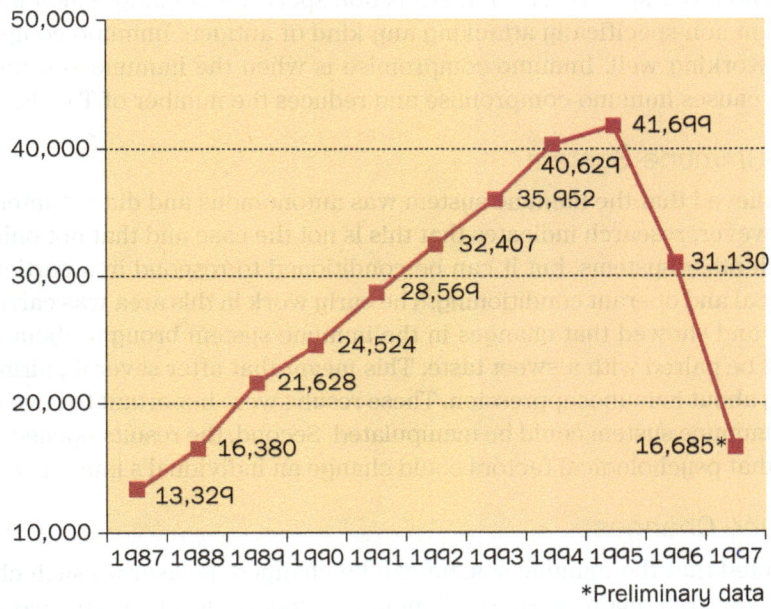

Figure 12.4 Decrease in deaths from HIV in the US 1987–1997

SOURCE: FDA (1997)

Much of this change in longevity can be accounted for by the development of anti-retroviral therapy (HAART) and research has explored the reasons why people do or do not adhere to their medication (see Chapter 9 and the previous section). Some research, however, has explored the more direct relationship between psychological factors and longevity for those with HIV and has drawn upon the study of psychoneuroimmunology (PNI).

PSYCHONEUROIMMUNOLOGY (PNI)

PNI is based on the prediction that an individual's psychological state can influence their immune system via the nervous system. This perspective provides a scientific basis for the 'mind over matter', 'think yourself well' and 'positive thinking, positive health' approaches to life. PNI and its role in HIV can be understood in terms of: (1) what is the immune system; (2) conditioning the immune system; (3) measuring immune changes; (4) psychological state and immunity. A good review of this area can be found in Vedhara (2012).

What is the Immune System?

The role of the immune system is to distinguish between the body and its invaders and to attack and protect the body from anything that is considered foreign. These invaders are called 'antigens'. When the immune system works well, the body is protected and infections and illnesses are kept at bay. If the immune system overreacts then this can lead to allergies. If the immune system mistakes the body itself for an invader then this can form the basis of autoimmune disorders. The main organs of the immune system are the lymphoid organs which are distributed throughout the body and include the bone marrow, lymph nodes and vessels, the spleen and thymus. These organs produce a range of 'soldiers' which are involved in identifying foreign bodies and disabling them. There are three levels of immune system activity. The first two are called specific immune processes and are 'cell mediated immunity' and 'humoral mediated immunity'. Cell mediated immunity involves a set of lymphocytes called T cells (killer T cells, memory T cells, delayed hypersensitivity T cells, helper T cells and suppressor T cells). These operate within the cells of the body and are made within the thymus (hence 'T'). Humoral mediated immunity involves B cells and antibodies and takes place in the body's fluids before the antigens have entered any cells. Third, there is non-specific immunity which involves phagocytes which are involved in non-specifically attacking any kind of antigen. Immuno-competence is when the immune system is working well. Immuno-compromise is when the immune system is failing in some way. The HIV virus causes immuno-compromise and reduces the number of T cells.

Conditioning the Immune System

Originally it was believed that the immune system was autonomous and did not interact with any other bodily systems. However, research indicates that this is not the case and that not only does the immune system interact with other systems, but it can be conditioned to respond in a particular way using the basic rules of classical and operant conditioning. The early work in this area was carried out by Ader and Cohen (1975, 1981) and showed that changes in the immune system brought about by an immunosuppressive drug could be paired with a sweet taste. This meant that after several pairings, the sweet taste itself began to bring about immunosuppression. These results were important for two reasons. First, they confirmed that the immune system could be manipulated. Second, the results opened up the area for PNI and the possibility that psychological factors could change an individual's immune response.

Measuring Immune Changes

Although it is accepted that the immune system can be changed, measuring such changes has proved to be problematic. The four main markers of immune function used to date have been as follows: (1) tumour growth, which is mainly used in animal research; (2) wound healing, which can be used in human research by way of a removal of a small section of the skin and can be monitored to follow the healing process; (3) secretory immunoglobulin A (sIgA), which is found in saliva and can be accessed easily and without pain or discomfort to the subject; and (4) natural killer cell cytoxicity (NKCC), T lymphocytes and T helper lymphocytes, which are found in the blood.

Psychological State and Immunity

Research has focused on the capacity of psychological factors to change immune functioning. In particular, it has examined the role of mood, beliefs, emotional expression and stress.

Mood: Studies indicate that positive mood is associated with better immune functioning (as measured by sIgA), that negative mood is associated with poorer functioning.

Beliefs: It has also been suggested that beliefs may themselves have a direct effect on the immune system. In particular, some research has explored the impact of how pessimism, attributional style, fighting spirit, hopelessness and helplessness may all impact upon immune function.

Emotional expression: Some evidence also suggests that certain coping styles and the ways in which emotions are expressed may change immune function. In particular, research highlights that suppression, denial, Type C coping and repressive coping may be harmful for health. There is also evidence that encouraging emotional expression through writing or disclosure groups may be beneficial. This work has been particularly pioneered by Pennebaker (e.g.1993, 1997; Pennebaker and Smyth 2016) using his basic writing paradigm which involves writing for three to five consecutive days for 15 to 30 minutes each day. The experimental group is asked to 'write about your very deepest thoughts and feelings about an extremely emotional issue that has affected you and your life. In your writing I'd really like you to let go and explore your very deepest emotions and thoughts. . .'. The writing paradigm has been shown to impact upon a range of outcome measures including visits to the doctor, re-employment following job loss, absenteeism from work, reduction in self-reported physical symptoms, pain reduction in patients with rheumatoid arthritis and changes in negative mood and wound healing after a small punch biopsy (see Pennebaker and Smyth 2016 for a review). Therefore this simple intervention provides support for the PNI model, suggesting a link between an individual's psychological state and their immune system.

PNI AND HIV LONGEVITY

The HIV virus causes immuno-compromise and renders people open to other conditions such as TB and rare cancers. Research indicates that psychological factors might influence the degree of immuno-compromise which in turn impacts upon the health status of the individual. This is the focus of PNI. In terms of HIV and longevity, research has focused on stress, stress management, emotional expression, beliefs and coping.

Stress: Women who are HIV-positive are more at risk from cervical intraepithelial neoplasia (CIN) and cervical cancer. Pereira et al. (2003) explored the relationship between the likelihood of developing the lesions associated with CIN and life stress. The results showed that higher life stress increased the odds of developing lesions by sevenfold over a one-year period. Life stress therefore seemed to link with illness progression. This is similar to the impact of stigma and minority stress (e.g. Frost et al. 2015; Katz et al. 2013).

Stress management: Antoni et al. (2006) randomized 130 gay men who were HIV-positive to receive either a cognitive behavioural stress management intervention (CBSM) and anti-retroviral medication adherence training (MAT), or to receive MAT alone. The men were then followed up after 9 and 15 months in terms of viral load. The results showed no differences overall between the two groups. When only those men who already showed detectable viral loads at baseline were included (i.e. those with a lot of virus in the blood already), differences were found. In particular, for these men, those who received the stress management showed a reduction in their viral load over the 15-month period even when medication adherence was controlled for. The authors conclude that for HIV-positive men who already show a detectable viral load, stress management may enhance the beneficial effects of their anti-retroviral treatment. In a similar study, the mechanisms behind the impact of stress management were explored (Antoni et al. 2005). For this study, 25 HIV-positive men were randomized to receive stress management or a waiting list control. Urine samples were taken before and after the intervention period. The results again showed that stress management was effective and that this effect was related to reduction in cortisol and depressed mood. The authors conclude that stress management works by reducing the stress induced by being ill with a disease such as HIV. Therefore, whereas stress can exacerbate illness stress management can aid the effectiveness of treatment and reduce the consequences of the stress resulting from being ill.

Emotional expression: In light of the evidence that emotional expression through expressive writing can have a range of positive affects on health outcomes (Pennebaker and Smyth 2016) some research has explored its impact on HIV progression and longevity. For example, Ironson et al. (2020) carried out a longitudinal study of individuals (n = 169) who at baseline were HIV-positive in the mid-range of disease with no AIDS-defining symptoms. At baseline, participants wrote an essay about the most traumatic event in their life (56 per cent wrote about HIV diagnosis, 10.1 per cent wrote about HIV disclosure, 8.9 per cent wrote about HIV-related stress, 8.9 per cent wrote about death of a loved one and 4.7 per cent wrote about relationship issues). This essay was then coded for the number of positive and negative emotional words. The results showed more positive words, more negative words and greater overall emotional expression predicted survival at 17 years follow up. The results also showed that those in the top third of total emotional expression had 3.83 times the survival rate compared to those in the bottom third.

Beliefs and coping: Research has also examined the role of psychological factors in longevity following infection with HIV. In particular, this has looked at the direct effects of beliefs and behaviour on the state of immunosuppression of the individual. In 1987, Solomon et al. studied 21 AIDS patients and examined their health status and the relationship of this health status to predictive baseline psychological variables. At follow-up, they found that survival was predicted by their general health status at baseline, their health behaviours, hardiness, social support, type C behaviour (self-sacrificing, self-blaming, not emotionally expressive) and coping strategies. In a further study, Solomon and Temoshok (1987) reported an additional follow-up of AIDS patients. They argued that a positive outcome was predicted by perceived control over illness at baseline, social support, problem-solving, help-seeking behaviour, low social desirability and the expression of anger and hostility. This study indicated that type C behaviour was not related to longevity.

Reed et al. (1994) also examined the psychological state of 78 gay men who had been diagnosed with AIDS in terms of their self-reported health status, psychological adjustment and psychological responses to HIV, well-being, self-esteem and levels of hopelessness. In addition, they completed measures of 'realistic acceptance', which reflected statements such as 'I tried to accept what might happen', 'I prepare for the worst' and 'I go over in my mind what I say or do about this problem'. At follow-up, the results showed that two-thirds of the men had died. However, survival was predicted by 'realistic acceptance' at baseline, with those who showed greater acceptance of their own death dying earlier. Therefore psychological state may also relate to longevity.

IN SUMMARY

The study of HIV and AIDS illustrates the role of psychology at different stages of an illness. Psychological factors are important not only for beliefs about HIV, health behaviour and medication adherence (see Chapters 2–9), but may also be involved in an individual's susceptibility to contracting the virus, the replication of the virus once it has been contracted and the individual's subsequent longevity.

> ### BOX 12.1
> ### Less common chronic conditions: Spinal cord injury (SCI)
>
> Spinal Cord Injury (SCI) is any damage to the spinal cord that changes its function and can be either temporary or permanent. This can result in loss of muscle function or loss of sensation or function in the parts of the body below the level of the injury and may include bowel and bladder incontinence and paralysis. SCI can either be complete, resulting in a total loss of sensation and muscle function, or incomplete, so that some nervous signals can still travel past the injured area of the cord. Long-term outcomes vary widely, from full recovery to permanent paralysis. Complications can include muscle atrophy, loss of voluntary motor control, spasticity, pressure sores, infections and breathing problems. The most common causes of SCI are due to physical trauma such as car accidents, gunshot wounds, falls or sports injuries, but sometimes SCI is the result of infection, insufficient blood flow and tumours.
>
> The sudden and traumatic occurrence of SCI is clearly life changing for everyone as life has to be re-evaluated and any life aspirations or goals may become irrelevant, unimportant or impossible (Hammell 2007; Buunk et al. 2006; Galvin and Godfrey 2001). Health psychology research has therefore explored how people with SCI adjust to their new life circumstances and indicates

that, while they may show psychological distress and reduced quality of life, many end up showing positive adjustment in the form of benefit finding, post-traumatic growth and response shift (Buckelew et al. 1990; Kennedy et al. 2003; Van Leeuwen et al. 2012).

In one study, Dibb et al. (2014) interviewed 21 people with SCI in four focus groups to explore how they made sense of their condition and had adjusted to their new life circumstances. The participants were recruited from four spinal centres in the UK. The majority were male (n = 19), aged 31–67 years (mean age 49) with most SCIs caused by a trauma (n = 20). The mean time since injury was 14 years (ranged from 1 to 37 years). Types of injuries were incomplete tetraplegia (n = 5), complete tetraplegia (n = 5), incomplete paraplegia (n = 6) and complete paraplegia (n = 5).

The results showed how participants used a range of strategies to adjust to SCI. These included setting realistic goals and managing expectations to avoid disappointment as participants felt that they would rather aim low and not be faced with failure. Social comparison was also key. They described engaging in both upward and downward social comparisons with regard to their level of injury, physical function and success at rehabilitation. Generally these comments were positive and participants compared aspects where they felt they were better-off as a means of coping with their situation. They also described avoiding situations that brought about negative comparisons and some said they avoided meeting people who reminded them of themselves. Participants also sought out positive comparisons with people without SCI. While this could be potentially threatening, these comparisons were also positive as they chose a dimension for which the other person was worse-off. Further, positive comparisons tended to occur on dimensions over which the participant had control. Participants also talked about feeling useful, with comments made about occupation and helping others, and participants also described the importance of not blaming others for their situation.

Overall, therefore, people with SCI seem to manage to adjust to their new situation and find some level of acceptance of their condition. This is primarily through setting reasonable expectation and goals, making social comparisons that enable a level of gratitude and positivity. People's experiences of this less common and life-changing condition reflect aspects of illness cognitions, coping, cognitive adaptation theory and sense making described in Chapter 8 and response shift described in Chapter 14 and reflect the ways in which health psychology can help to frame a person's experience of illness.

4 CANCER

The second part of this chapter examines what cancer is, looks at its prevalence and then assesses the role of psychology in understanding cancer in terms of its initiation and promotion, its psychological consequences, dealing with the symptoms of cancer, longevity and the promotion of a disease-free interval. Chapters 2–10 provide detailed descriptions of health and illness beliefs, coping, health behaviour, screening and adherence to medication which are all relevant to understanding cancer in terms of its onset and impact upon the individual.

WHAT IS CANCER?

Cancer is defined as an uncontrolled growth of abnormal cells, which produces tumours called neoplasms. There are two types of tumour: *benign* tumours, which do not spread throughout the body, and *malignant* tumours, which show metastasis (the process of cells breaking off from the tumour and moving elsewhere). There are three types of cancer cell: *carcinomas*, which constitute 90 per cent of all cancer cells and which originate in tissue cells; *sarcomas*, which originate in connective tissue; and *leukaemias*, which originate in the blood.

THE PREVALENCE OF CANCER

In 2015, cancer was responsible for 8.8 million deaths globally. It was the leading cause of death and nearly 1 in 6 deaths was due to cancer. The most common causes of cancer death are: lung cancer (1.69 million deaths); liver cancer (788,000 deaths); colorectal cancer (774,000 deaths); stomach cancer (754,000 deaths) and breast cancer (571,000 deaths). Deaths from cancer worldwide are projected to continue to rise to over 11 million in 2030. In 2012, the highest cancer rates were found in Denmark, France, Australia, Belgium, Norway and the USA, with the lowest rates reported in Japan, Argentina and Puerto Rico. In the UK, in 2015, 53 per cent of all new cancer cases were breast, prostate, lung and bowel cancers, although the greatest increase in incidence was for thyroid and liver cancers, while stomach cancers have shown the fastest decrease.

The incidence of newly diagnosed cancer in the UK in 2015 is shown in Figure 12.5, which shows that the most commonly diagnosed cancers in men are prostate cancer, lung cancer and bowel cancer and in women are breast cancer, lung cancer and bowel cancer.

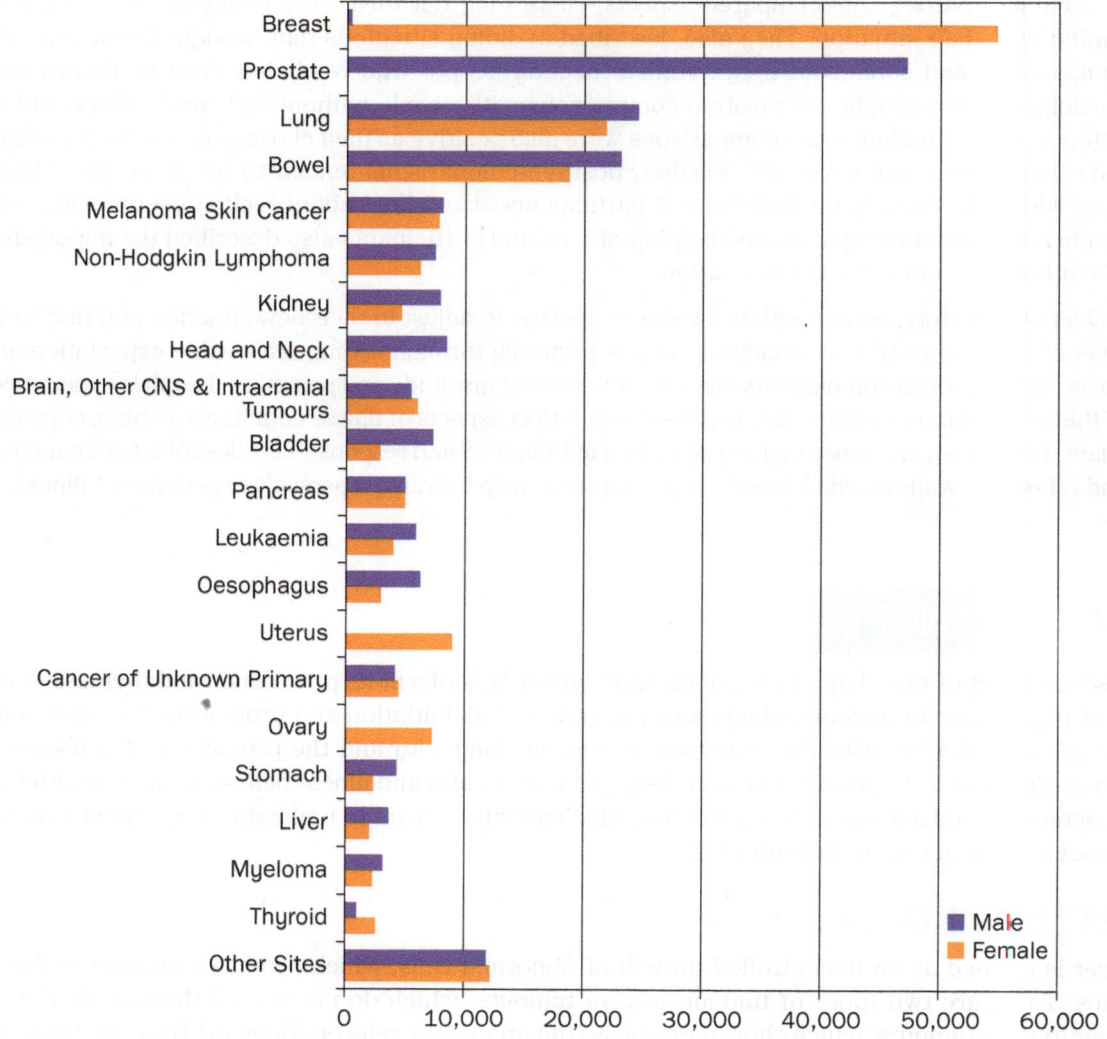

Figure 12.5 UK incidence of newly diagnosed cancers for men and women

SOURCE: Cancer Research UK (2015)

5 | THE ROLE OF PSYCHOLOGY IN THE STUDY OF CANCER

A role for psychology in cancer was first suggested by Galen in AD 200–300, who argued for an association between melancholia and cancer, and also by Gedman in 1701, who suggested that cancer might be related to life disasters. In addition, more than 30 per cent of cancer deaths are thought to be preventable. Psychology therefore plays a role in cancer in a number of ways. First, psychological factors are important in terms of cancer onset and a discussion of health and illness beliefs, health behaviours and behaviour change interventions can be found in Chapters 2–7. Second, psychology is involved in factors such as screening, help-seeking, delay and adherence, which are described in Chapter 9. Further, sufferers of cancer report psychological consequences, which have implications for coping, adjustment, pain and a person's quality of life (see Chapters 8, 11 and 14).

The potential role of psychology in understanding cancer is shown in Figure 12.6.

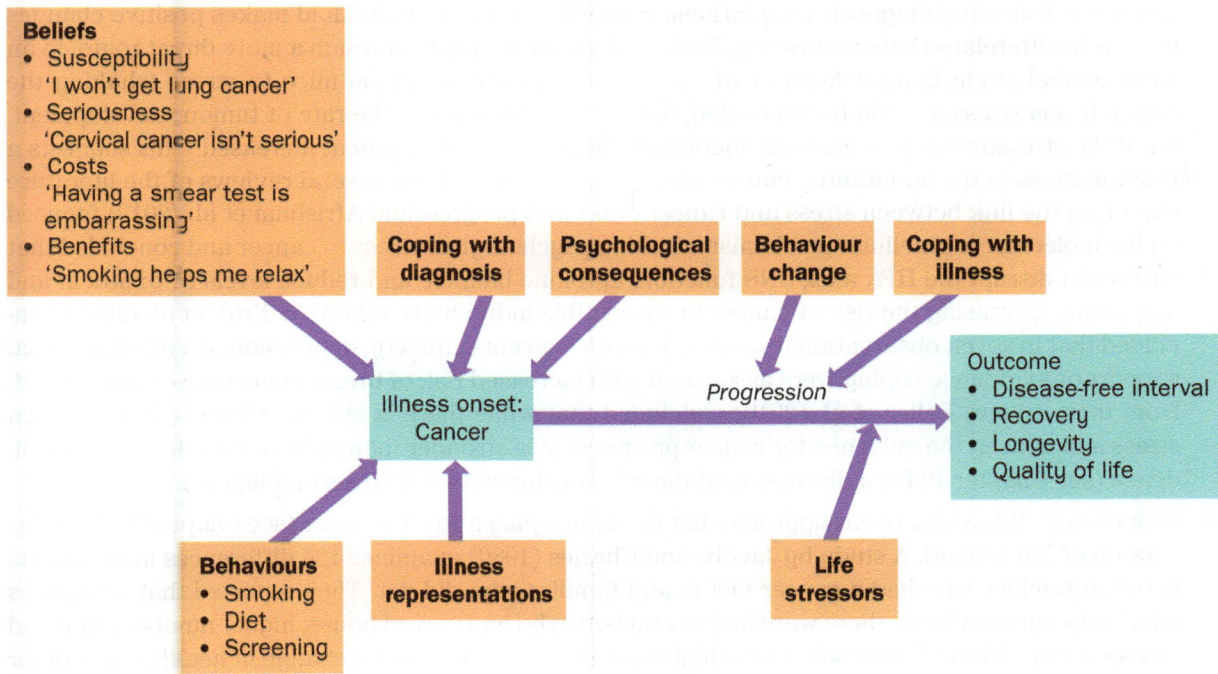

Figure 12.6 The potential role of psychology in cancer

The role of psychology in cancer is also illustrated by the following observations:

- *Cancer cells are present in most people but not everybody gets cancer.* In addition, although research suggests a link between smoking and lung cancer, not all heavy smokers get lung cancer. Perhaps psychology is involved in the susceptibility to cancer.
- *All those who have cancer do not always show progression towards death at the same rate.* Perhaps psychology has a role to play in the progression of cancer.
- *Not all cancer sufferers die of cancer.* Perhaps psychology has a role to play in longevity.

The role of psychology in cancer will now be examined in terms of: (1) the initiation and promotion of cancer; (2) the psychological consequences of cancer; (3) dealing with the symptoms of cancer; and (4) longevity and promoting a disease-free interval.

PSYCHOLOGY AND THE INITIATION AND PROMOTION OF CANCER

1 *Behavioural factors.* Behavioural factors have been shown to play a role in the initiation and promotion of cancer with research indicating that up to 75 per cent of all cancers are linked to behaviours such as smoking, poor diet, alcohol and sexual behaviour (e.g. Doll and Peto 1981; Mokdad et al. 2004; Khaw et al. 2008). These behaviours can be predicted by examining individual health beliefs (see Chapters 2–6). They can also be modified using behaviour change interventions (see Chapter 7). In addition, screening, help-seeking behaviour and symptom perception all influence early detection which may influence health outcomes (see Chapter 9). For example, Mason and White (2008) concluded that the components of the theory of planned behaviour (TPB) could predict breast self-examination in young women, Hale et al. (2007) identified a number of barriers to seeking help in men with prostate disease and Fang et al. (2006) highlighted the role of perceptions of control and coping in predicting screening uptake for ovarian cancer. Further, Ali et al. (2015) found that being female, older, a current smoker, from a lower socioeconomic group and having higher risk perception was associated with non-uptake of lung cancer screening among high risk individuals.

2 *Stress.* Stress has also been shown to have a role to play in cancer. This could be through behaviour and stress following diagnosis may influence whether or not an individual makes positive changes to their health-related behaviours (e.g. Park et al. 2008). It may be through a more direct route. In an early animal study Laudenslager et al. (1983) exposed cancer-prone mice to stress (shaking the cage). If this stressor could be controlled, there was a decrease in the rate of tumour development, but if the stressor was perceived as uncontrollable, tumour development increased. This suggests a role for stress in the initiation of cancer. Recently, there have been several reviews of the literature exploring the link between stress and cancer onset and progression. Afrisham et al. (2019) focused on the molecular and cellular mechanisms linking psychological stress to cancer and concluded that stress can disrupt the HPA axis, SNS function, cytokine balance and reduce levels of oxytocin and dopamine, increasing the risk of cancer in susceptible individuals. Likewise, Kruk et al. (2019) concluded that in seven observational studies, severe life events, anxiety, depression, insufficient social support or avoidance coping were associated with increased risk of breast cancer onset. In contrast, from their review, Feller et al. (2019) concluded that while there is evidence for the link between stress and cancer, the evidence for cancer progression is stronger than the evidence for cancer incidence (see Chapter 10 for a discussion of the relationship between stress and illness).

3 *Life events.* It has also been suggested that life events play a role in cancer (see Chapter 10 for a discussion of life events). A study by Jacobs and Charles (1980) examined the differences in life events between families who had a cancer victim and families who did not. They reported that in families who had a cancer victim, there were higher numbers who had moved house, higher numbers who had changed some form of their behaviour, higher numbers who had had a change in health status other than the cancer person and higher numbers of divorces, indicating that life events may well be a factor contributing to the onset of cancer. However, the results from a meta-analysis by Petticrew et al. (1999) do not support this suggestion. They identified 29 studies, from 1966 to 1997, which met their inclusion criteria (adult women with breast cancer, group of cancer-free controls, measure of stressful life events) and concluded that although several individual studies report a relationship between life events and breast cancer, when methodological problems are taken into account and when the data across the different studies are merged, 'the research shows no good evidence of a relationship between stressful life events and breast cancer'. In contrast, Bahri et al. (2019) concluded from their systematic review and meta-analysis of 11 studies that a history of stressful life events slightly increases the risk of breast cancer which was supported by the review by Kruk et al. (2019).

4 *Control.* Control also seems to play a role in the initiation and promotion of cancer and it has been argued that control over stressors and control over environmental factors may be related to an increase in the onset of cancer (see Chapters 8 and 10 for a discussion of control and the stress–illness link).

5 *Coping styles.* Coping styles are also important. If an individual is subjected to stress, then the methods they use to cope with this stress may well be related to the onset of cancer. For example, maladaptive, disengagement coping strategies, such as smoking and alcohol, may have a relationship with an increase in cancer. (see Chapters 8 and 10 for a discussion of coping).

6 *Depression.* Bieliauskas (1980) highlighted a relationship between depression and cancer and suggested that chronic mild depression, but not clinical depression, may be related to cancer. This was part supported by a recent systematic review and meta analysis of 51 studies by Wang et al. (2020) which concluded that both depression and anxiety (assessed by diagnostic criteria and symptom scales) are associated with cancer incidence and cancer-specific mortality.

7 *Personality.* Some research has also explored the relationship between personality and cancer. Temoshok and Fox (1984) argued that individuals who develop cancer have a 'type C personality', which is described as passive, appeasing, helpless, 'other focused' and unexpressive of emotion. Eysenck (1990) described 'a cancer-prone personality', and suggested that this is characteristic of individuals who react to stress with helplessness and hopelessness, and individuals who repress emotional reactions to life events. An early study by Kissen (1966) supported this relationship between personality and cancer and reported that heavy smokers who develop lung cancer have a poorly developed outlet for their emotions, perhaps suggesting type C personality. In 2014, Weston et al. conducted a study on 6,904 participants from the longitudinal Health and Retirement study to investigate the relationships between personality traits and the onset of new disease. They measured the Big 5 personality traits at baseline (conscientiousness, neuroticism, openness, extraversion, agreeableness) and after 4 years assessed the onset of the following diseases: high blood pressure or hypertension, diabetes, cancer, lung disease, heart disease, stroke and arthritis. Although the results showed some links between personality, stroke, heart disease and arthritis, no associations between personality and cancer were found.

PSYCHOLOGICAL CONSEQUENCES OF CANCER

Psychology also has a role to play in cancer in terms of how people respond to their diagnosis.

Lowered Mood

Up to 20 per cent of cancer patients may show severe depression, grief, lack of control, personality change, anger and anxiety. Depression seems to be particularly high in those with head and neck cancer (Humphris and Ozakinci 2008). Some patients also report a sense of hopelessness (Abbey et al. 2006) and Nanton et al. (2009) highlighted feelings of uncertainty in men with prostate cancer. Pinder et al. (1993) examined the emotional responses of women with operable breast cancer and reported that these can differ widely from little disruption of mood to clinical states of depression and anxiety. Maass et al. (2015) conducted a systematic review of 17 articles exploring the prevalence of mood changes after breast cancer treatment and found that the prevalence of depression varied between 9.4 and 66.1 per cent and anxiety 17.9 and 33.3 per cent. They also noted that these symptoms changed over time and that although there was an increase in depression one year post diagnosis, this decreased over the ensuing years. Likewise, Riedl and Schuessler (2021) concluded from their review that rates of clinical depression varied from 7.9 per cent to 32.4 per cent, (mean 21.2 per cent) across a range of different cancers. The emotional state of breast cancer sufferers appears to be unrelated to the type of surgery they have (Kiebert et al. 1991), whether or not they have radiotherapy (Hughson et al. 1987) and is only affected by chemotherapy in the medium term (Hughson et al. 1986). However, persistent deterioration in mood does seem to be related to previous psychiatric history (Dean 1987), lack of social support (Bloom 1983), age and lack of an intimate relationship (Pinder et al. 1993). Pinder et al. also reported that in sufferers with advanced cancer, psychological morbidity was related to functional status (how well the patient functioned physically) and suggested that lowered functional status was associated with higher levels of depression, which was also related to lower social class.

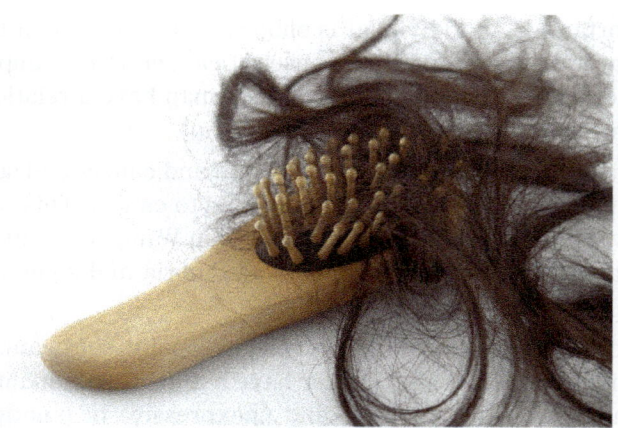

Hair loss from chemotherapy can be damaging to a patient's body image and self-esteem

SOURCE: © Shutterstock/szefei

Body Image

Lowered mood is not the only emotional consequence of cancer. Women with breast cancer often report changes in their sense of femininity, attractiveness and body image. This has been shown to be greater in women who have radical mastectomies rather than lumpectomies (e.g. Moyer 1997) and to occur across a range of ethnic groups (e.g. Petronis et al. 2003). Harcourt and Frith (2008) carried out a qualitative interview study with 19 women having chemotherapy for breast cancer, focusing on how the treatment could alter their physical appearance. The results indicated that the women were anxious that the treatment would make them identifiable as a 'person with cancer' which would change their interactions with others. In a similar vein, Frith et al. (2007) particularly focused on the impact of hair loss and identified a number of ways in which women actively anticipate and manage their hair loss and use both affective and behavioural rehearsal strategies even before they have lost their hair as a means to feel more in control. Tollow et al. (2020) also explored how people with incurable cancer felt about the role of appearance on their well-being. Thematic analysis of 24 interviews indicated that appearance was felt to be an important part of their identity, which was often dominated by cancer. In addition, changes in their appearance influenced how they communicated with others, sometimes forcing discussions about their diagnosis and resulting in them having to manage the emotional impact on loved ones, and also challenged their ability to maintain a sense of normality. As one woman said: 'I'm not a vain person. I'm not one of these sort of make-up on people every day and everything like that. I'm not that at all but [. . .] I feel that when you lose your hair you lose your identity. You become a cancer patient. . . if you see what I mean?' And as one man said: 'I'm okay with people knowing I have cancer and, um, and I don't mind having that conversation, but I want to be in charge of when we have it.' Some research has also explored the impact of reconstructive surgery after breast cancer surgery with a focus on timing. For example, Teo et al. (2016) found that women waiting to initiate delayed reconstruction appear at particular risk for reduced body image and emotional distress.

Cognitive Adaptation

Taylor (1983) examined the cognitive adaptation of 78 women with breast cancer. She reported that these women responded to their cancer in three ways. First, they made a search for meaning, whereby the cancer patients attempted to understand why they had developed cancer. Meanings that were reported included stress, hereditary factors, ingested carcinogens such as birth control pills, environmental carcinogens such as chemical waste, diet and a blow to the breast. Second, they also attempted to gain a sense of mastery by believing that they could control their cancer and any relapses. Such attempts at control included meditation, positive thinking and a belief that the original cause was no longer in effect. Third, the women began a process of self-enhancement. This involved social comparison, whereby they tended to analyse their condition in terms of others they knew. Taylor argued that they showed 'downward comparison', which involved comparing themselves to others worse off, thus improving their beliefs about their own situation. According to Taylor's theory of cognitive adaptation, the combination of meaning, mastery and self-enhancement creates illusions which are a central component of attempts to cope. This theory is discussed in more detail in Chapter 8. In a similar vein, Jim and Andersen (2007) also explored meaning-making in cancer survivors but focused on a patient's meaning of life rather than the meaning of cancer. In this study, cancer survivors completed measures of social and physical functioning, distress and the meaning of their lives. The authors concluded that the negative social and physical consequences of cancer cause distress but that this association is mediated through the ways in which cancer disrupts a person's meaning of life. In 2016, Winger et al. conducted a meta-analysis of 62 papers and found that having both a stronger meaning in life and a sense of coherence was related to reduced distress in cancer patients.

Benefit-finding

Not all consequences of cancer are negative and many patients report finding benefit in their illness. This has been explored within the frameworks of stress-related growth, post-traumatic growth, benefit-finding, meaning-making and existential growth (see Chapter 8 for details). In terms of cancer, research indicates that positive shifts are common following diagnosis and treatment and that greater benefit-finding is predicted by factors such as spirituality, talking and assigning meaning to the illness, financial stability, being a woman, greater optimism, high intrusive thinking and high social support (Cordova et al. 2001; Cole et al. 2008; Dunn et al. 2011). Interestingly, one study also highlighted how 76 per cent of their participants engaged in pre-emptive benefit finding while waiting for the results of a breast biopsy (Rankin et al. 2020). In particular they identified possible self and other focused benefits including health benefits, personal growth, appreciation for life, physical change, strengthening relationships, spreading awareness, supporting others and role modelling. Benefit finding therefore seems to begin even before the bad news has arrived. Some research has also focused on the notion of gratitude and interventions have been developed to promote gratitude across a wide number of patient groups which involves 'counting your blessings' (see Emmons and McCullough 2003). Ruini and Vescovelli (2013) explored gratitude in patients with breast cancer and found that gratitude was strongly related to post-traumatic growth, reduced distress and an increase in positive emotions but not with increased psychological well-being.

DEALING WITH THE SYMPTOMS OF CANCER

Psychology has a role to play in the alleviation of symptoms of cancer, and in promoting quality of life (see Chapter 14 for a discussion of quality of life theory and measurement). Cartwright et al. (1973) described the experiences of cancer sufferers, which included very distressing pain, breathing difficulties, vomiting, sleeplessness, loss of bowel and bladder control, loss of appetite and mental confusion. Psychosocial interventions have therefore been used to attempt to alleviate some of the symptoms of the cancer sufferer and to improve their quality of life:

1 *Pain management.* One of the main roles of psychology is in terms of pain management, and this has taken place through a variety of different pain management techniques (see Chapter 11). For example, biofeedback and hypnosis have been shown to decrease pain. Syrjala et al. (2014) conducted a review of the evidence for psychological and behavioural approaches to cancer pain management. The results showed that patients use many strategies to manage pain and that whereas catastrophizing is associated with increased pain, self-efficacy is associated with reduced pain reports. They also concluded that the most effective pain management methods were education (with coping skills training), hypnosis, cognitive behavioural approaches and relaxation with imagery.

2 *Social support interventions.* Social support interventions have also been used through the provision of support groups, which emphasize control and meaningful activities and aim to reduce denial and promote hope. It has been suggested that although this intervention may not have any effect on longevity, it may improve the meaningfulness of the cancer patient's life. In line with this, Holland and Holahan (2003) explored the relationship between social support, coping and positive adaptation to breast cancer in 56 women. The results showed that higher levels of perceived social support and approach-coping strategies were related to positive adjustment.

3 *Treating nausea and vomiting.* Psychology has also been involved in treating the nausea and vomiting experienced by cancer patients. Patients are often offered chemotherapy as a treatment for their cancer, which can cause anticipatory nausea, vomiting and anxiety. Respondent conditioning and visual imagery, relaxation, hypnosis and desensitization have been shown to decrease nausea and anxiety in cancer patients. Redd (1982) and Burish et al. (1987) suggested that 25–33 per cent of cancer patients show conditioned vomiting and 60 per cent show anticipatory anxiety. It is reported that relaxation and guided imagery may decrease these problems. Some patients are also offered integrative therapeutic approaches including acupuncture/acupressure, aromatherapy, herbal supplements and hypnosis. From their systematic review, Momani et al. (2017) concluded that there is little evidence of the effectiveness of these approaches for reducing chemotherapy-induced nausea in children.

4 *Body image counselling.* The quality of life of cancer patients may also be improved through altered body image counselling, particularly following the loss of a breast and, more generally, in dealing with the grief at loss of various parts of the body.

5 *Sense-making strategies.* Research also suggests that quality of life may be improved using sense-making strategies. Taylor (1983) used cognitive adaptation strategies to improve patients' self-worth, their ability to be close to others and the meaningfulness of their lives. Such methods have been suggested to involve self-transcendence and this has again been related to improvement in well-being and decrease in illness-related distresses. Some research has also focused on acceptance as an outcome. For example, Nipp et al. (2016) found that most patients in their study receiving palliative care used emotional support coping (77.0 per cent), whereas fewer reported acceptance (44.8 per cent), self-blame (37.9 per cent), and denial (28.2 per cent). The results showed that whereas acceptance was associated with better quality of life and mood, denial and self-blame were associated with poorer quality of life and mood. Teo et al. (2019) carried out a systematic review of 68 studies and concluded that there was strong evidence for the use of meaning-centred psychotherapy to improve meaning and quality of life.

6 *Fear reduction.* Many patients experience enduring fear that their cancer will return which can impact upon their adjustment and ability to plan for the future. Humphris and Ozakinci (2008) developed a programme called AFTER (Adjustment for the Fear, Threat or Expectation of Recurrence) to help patients with head and neck cancer manage their fear of recurrence. The intervention targets fears, inappropriate checking behaviour and beliefs about cancer and is based upon Leventhal's self-regulatory model (see Chapter 8). Preliminary evidence indicates that it is acceptable and may be of use to patients with a number of different cancers. Likewise, Dieng et al. (2016) evaluated the effectiveness of a psycho-educational intervention to reduce fear of cancer recurrence in patients with a high risk of developing another primary melanoma. The intervention involved a newly developed psycho-educational resource and three telephone-based psycho-therapeutic sessions over a one-month period. The results showed reduced fear by 6 months in those who received the intervention compared to the control group.

Adjuvant Psychological Therapy

Evidence suggests that a substantial minority of cancer patients show psychological ill health, particularly in terms of depression and anxiety. As a result, a number of psychotherapeutic procedures have been developed to improve cancer patients' emotional well-being. These are sometimes known as adjuvant psychological therapy (APT). However, evaluating the effectiveness of such procedures raises several ethical and methodological problems. Greer et al. (1992) outlined these problems as follows: (1) the ethical considerations of having a control group (can patients suffering from psychological distress not be given therapy?); (2) the specificity of any psychological intervention (terms such as 'counselling' and 'psychotherapy' are vague and any procedure being evaluated should be clarified); and (3) the outcome measures chosen (many measures of psychological state include items that are not appropriate for cancer patients, such as weight loss and fatigue, which may change as a result of the cancer, not the individual's psychological state). Greer et al. (1992) carried out a RCT to compare changes in measures of quality of life in patients receiving APT with those receiving no therapy. APT is a cognitive behavioural treatment developed specifically for cancer patients. Therapy involved approximately eight one-hour weekly sessions with individual patients and their spouses (if appropriate). The therapy focused on the personal meaning of the cancer for the patient, examined their coping strategies and emphasized the current problems defined jointly by the therapist and the patient. The results showed that, at 8 weeks, the patients receiving the APT had significantly higher scores on fighting spirit and significantly lower scores on helplessness, anxious preoccupation, fatalism, anxiety, psychological symptoms and orientation towards health care than the control patients. At 4 months, patients receiving the APT had significantly lower scores than the controls on anxiety, psychological symptoms and psychological distress. The authors concluded that APT improves the psychological well-being of cancer patients who show increased psychological problems and that some of these improvements persist for up to 4 months. They suggested that APT relates to 'improvement in the psychological dimension of the quality of life of cancer patients'. These results are supported by a pilot study by Louro et al. (2016) who found that a positive emotion-based APT including an Enhancing Positive Emotions Procedure (EPEP) resulted in reduced insomnia and improved positive affect, global health status, physical, role and social functioning in patients with colorectal cancer. Over recent years there has been a move to deliver interventions to cancer patients online. Willems et al. (2020) concluded from their systematic review that while there was some support for a reduction in psychological distress and depression following online interventions, the evidence for reducing anxiety was less convincing.

6 PSYCHOLOGY AND LONGEVITY WITH CANCER

The final question about the role of psychology in cancer is its relationship to longevity: do psychosocial factors influence longevity?

COGNITIVE RESPONSES AND LONGEVITY

Greer et al. (1979) carried out a prospective study in which they examined the relationship between cognitive responses to a breast cancer diagnosis and disease-free intervals. Using semi-structured interviews, they defined three types of responder: those with 'fighting spirit', those who showed denial of the implications of their disease and those who showed a hopeless/helpless response. The authors reported that the groups who showed either 'fighting spirit' or 'denial' had a longer disease-free interval than the other group. In addition, at a further 15-year follow-up, both a fighting spirit and denial approach also predicted longevity. However, there were problems with this study. At baseline the authors did not measure several important physiological prognostic indicators, such as lymph node involvement, as these measures were not available at the time. These physiological factors may have contributed to both the disease-free interval and the survival of the patients. More recently, Svensson et al. (2016) conducted a prospective study on 55,130 participants aged 50–79 who had no history of cancer diagnosis to investigate the relationship between coping strategies and cancer outcomes. At 10 years follow-up the results showed that whereas approach coping strategies and positive reappraisal behaviours were associated with a reduced risk of cancer mortality, avoidance coping strategies were associated with increased cancer incidence but only after excluding events occurring in the first 3 years of follow-up.

LIFE STRESS AND DISEASE-FREE INTERVAL

In a case control study, Ramirez et al. (1989) examined the relationship between life stress and relapse in operable breast cancer. The life events and difficulties occurring during the disease-free interval were recorded in 50 women who had developed their first recurrence of breast cancer and 50 women who were in remission. The two subject groups were matched for the main physical and pathological factors believed to be associated with prognosis and for the sociodemographic variables believed to be related to life events and difficulties. The results showed that life events rated as severe were related to first recurrence of breast cancer. However, the study was cross-sectional in nature, which has implications for determining causality.

THERE IS NO RELATIONSHIP BETWEEN PSYCHOLOGICAL FACTORS AND LONGEVITY

Not all research has pointed to an association between psychological factors and longevity. Barraclough et al. (1992) measured severe life events, social difficulties and depression at baseline in a group of breast cancer patients, and followed them up after 42 months. Of a total of 204 subjects, 26 died and 23 per cent relapsed. However, the results showed no relationship between these outcomes and the psychosocial factors measured at baseline. These results caused debate in the light of earlier studies and it has been suggested that the absence of a relationship between life events and outcome may be due to the older age of the women in Barraclough's study, the short follow-up period used and the unreported use of chemotherapy (Ramirez et al. 1992).

Over the years there has also been much interest in the role of personality in predicting cancer incidence and longevity which has led to the term 'Type C personality' or cancer prone personality. In 2015, Weston et al. conducted a study on 6,904 participants from the longitudinal Health and Retirement study and found no associations between the Big 5 personality traits and cancer onset. Likewise, in 2014, Jokela et al. conducted a meta-analysis of data from six prospective cohort studies including 42,843 cancer-free men and women at baseline to investigate whether personality traits from the Big 5 model were associated with cancer incidence and mortality. The results showed no evidence for the relationship between personality traits and either cancer incidence or mortality.

IN SUMMARY

Psychology has many roles to play in cancer in terms of illness onset through behaviours such as smoking and diet, the ways in which people adjust and cope with their illness, illness progression and ultimate health outcomes. This part of the chapter has particularly focused on beliefs and behaviours, which may be related to the onset of cancer, psychological consequences such as lowered mood, altered body image, cognitive adaptation and benefit-finding, the treatment of symptoms through pain relief, relaxation or fear management and improving quality of life, disease-free intervals and longevity.

BOX 12.2

Less common chronic conditions: Fibromyalgia

Fibromyalgia syndrome (FMS) affects up to 11 per cent of the general population and is a chronic condition characterized by persistent widespread pain (for 43 months) and self-reported pain in 11 of 18 tender points on digital palpitation (with the amount of pressure sufficient to blanch a finger nail). It tends to affect more women than men and the usual age of onset is between 55 and 65 years. It is also associated with fatigue, cognitive dysfunction, such as difficulty concentrating and word retrieval, and sleep disturbance. It can have a profound impact on people's lives, with many people having to reduce their working hours or leave work completely. To date, the causes of FMS are unknown although possible theories include a disruption to the neurotransmitters in the central nervous system and/or dysregulation of the sympathetic nervous system. Treatment is also fairly ineffective and outcomes from standard medical care indicate that over half of patients show only slight improvement, no change or a deterioration by three years. Evidence indicates that up to 99 per cent of sufferers of FMS experience serious sleep disturbance (Osorio et al. 2006). In light of this, some research in health psychology has explored how people cope with FMS with a focus on sleep, the predictors of quality of life and the role of mind–body therapies in improving health outcomes.

In a qualitative study, Theadom and Cropley (2010) interviewed 16 people with FMS about all aspects of their sleep experience and how this influenced their day-to-day lives. The interviews were analysed using interpretative phenomenological analysis (IPA; Smith et al. 2009) and high-lighted the extent to which poor sleep dominated participants' lives. In particular, they described how it affected their levels of pain and fatigue, disrupted their ability to engage in daily activities and undermined their ability to cope. Participants also described having blocks of sleep and dif-ficulty getting back to sleep after a night time of being awake. This all culminated in them feeling very out of control of their sleep difficulties and many resorted to daytime napping as a useful coping strategy for relieving daytime sleepiness and feelings of fatigue.

In line with this emphasis on daytime napping, Theadom et al. (2015a) carried out a cross-sectional online survey to explore the association between sleep patterns and symptom severity. Adults (n = 1044) diagnosed with FMS by a clinician completed an online questionnaire. The results showed that daytime napping was associated with increased pain, depression, anxiety, fatigue, memory difficulties and sleep problems. Further, those who napped for more than 30 minutes had higher memory difficulties and depression than those who napped for shorter periods. In support of this, Theadom et al. (2007) carried out an additional survey with 101 people with FMS and concluded that poor sleep quality predicted pain, fatigue, and poor social functioning in patients with FMS. While these both used cross-sectional designs, the findings suggest that poor sleep may exacerbate symptoms of FMS and that although daytime napping may feel like a positive coping strategy for those with FMS it may not be helpful and may even do harm.

Researchers have therefore drawn upon a number of therapeutic interventions as a means to improve health outcomes in those with FMS including psychological therapies, biofeedback, mindfulness, movement therapies and relaxation strategies. Theadom et al. (2015b) carried out a systematic review of 74 studies to assess the costs and benefits of a range of mind-body thera-pies compared either standard care or attention placebo control groups for adults with FMS. Overall, the researchers concluded that quality of evidence was low but that psychological intervention therapies may improve physical functioning, pain and low mood for adults with fibromyalgia in comparison to usual care. There was some evidence that biofeedback improved physical functioning, pain and mood, that movement therapies improved pain and mood and that relaxation improved physical functioning and pain. Mindfulness showed no advantage over usual care. They also concluded, however, that the impact of biofeedback, mindfulness, move-ment therapies and relaxation-based therapies was less clear as the quality of evidence for these therapies was very low.

FMS is a debilitating condition causing pain and sleep problems. Research from a health psy-chology perspective illustrates how people cope with this condition and how one consequence of the problem (i.e. sleep difficulties) can exacerbate other related symptoms. It also illustrates how people with FMS may feel that they have identified a suitable coping strategy (i.e. daytime napping) but that this might do harm. Evidence also illustrates how hard FMS is to treat and that psychological therapies only have a moderate impact on health outcomes. This research reflects theories of illness cognitions and coping (see Chapter 8), theories of health behaviour and behaviour change (see Chapter 7) and research and evidence related to pain perception (see Chapter 11).

BOX 12.3
Critical Approaches to Health Psychology

Research and theories relating to HIV and cancer highlights some of the bigger issues in health psychology as follows:

Sex and gender: Much research into chronic conditions, particularly relating to HIV and cancer, assesses the role of individual differences and in particular the role of gender and sexuality. Until recently this described people as either male or female or heterosexual or gay (and sometimes bisexual). Over recent years the world has started to change and both gender and sexuality are seen as far more fluid than this and these dichotomies are considered limited and at times damaging. Health psychology research and theory therefore needs to move with the times and embrace the variability in both these constructs until at some point, eventually, they will become redundant and knowing what gender or what sexuality someone has (or is) will become a tiny or even irrelevant part of who they are.

The individual vs the social vs the political: Within research we explore the reasons why people develop chronic conditions (health beliefs, behaviours) and whether or not they adhere to treatment recommendations (medication, surgery, behaviour change). But these causes and solutions to illness exist very much in a social and political world. So whether someone adheres to their HIV medication or cancer treatment depends on whether they live in a community where it is available. It also depends on whether governments have invested in research to develop the treatments and whether, even if it is available, they can afford it. There are huge inequalities across the world both between and within communities which influence health outcomes and by addressing the role of individual factors these broader factors get ignored.

The role of agency and control: Different cultures place different emphasis on whether an individual has agency over their health and can influence their own mortality. Within the western world we tend to emphasize the individual and so research the role of individual beliefs and behaviours on health outcomes. This can be empowering for people but can also make them feel responsible when treatment stops working as they may feel they didn't try hard enough. Further, research into post-traumatic growth can also be positive but might also make people feel inadequate if they feel miserable about their illness and struggle to find any benefits. Therefore agency and control might be empowering for some but for others it can lead to guilt and blame when things go wrong.

7 | THINKING CRITICALLY ABOUT HIV AND CANCER RESEARCH

There are some problems with research in this area that need to be considered.

SOME CRITICAL QUESTIONS

When thinking about research relating to chronic conditions such as HIV and cancer ask yourself the following questions:

- Much research is carried out in the western world. What are the problems of this for understanding worldwide conditions such as HIV and cancer?
- How do we synthesize research when there have been many changes in the management of HIV and cancer?

- Chronic conditions illustrate the ways in which the mind influences the body. What does the mind–body link actually mean and how does it work?
- Are there ethical problems with emphasizing the psychological aspects in the cause of a chronic condition such as HIV or cancer?

SOME PROBLEMS WITH. . .

Here are some problems specific to research exploring chronic conditions such as HIV and cancer.

Generalizability across people: Much psychological research explores the predictors of becoming HIV-positive in terms of safer sex behaviour and needle-sharing. HIV, however, is a worldwide problem which affects people from all religions and cultural backgrounds. The reasons that people do or do not engage in risky behaviours are highly linked to their specific cultures. It is therefore very difficult to generalize from one study to populations outside the study group.

Research synthesis: The management of HIV and AIDS has changed enormously over the past 30 years, resulting in an increase in longevity due to combination therapies. HIV is now seen as a chronic illness rather than a terminal one. This means that combining research on longevity across the years is difficult as people at different times have been managed in very different ways.

Generalizability across conditions: Research on cancer shows some commonalities across different types of cancers. However, there are also vast differences in the ways in which different cancers impact upon people's lives and are and should be managed. Generalizations across cancers should therefore be limited to those areas where there is consistent cross-cancer variation.

Doing harm: Due to this variability between cancer types, while screening and early detection for some cancers can result in improved management and health outcomes, screening for other cancers may result in anxiety, a painful procedure and a recommendation of watchful waiting, which can make people regret knowing about their condition in the first place.

TO CONCLUDE

Psychology has a role to play in understanding chronic illness in terms of illness onset, adaptation, coping, illness progression and health outcomes. This chapter has focused on two examples, namely HIV/AIDS and cancer, although the theories and evidence presented are also relevant to any number of chronic illnesses.

QUESTIONS

1 Discuss the role of psychological factors in the progression to full-blown AIDS.
2 To what extent is the transmission of the HIV virus due to a lack of knowledge?
3 AIDS kills. Discuss.
4 Discuss the factors that may explain why patients do not take their medication for AIDS.
5 Describe the role of psychology in cancer onset.
6 Discuss the impact that cancer may have upon the individual.
7 To what extent do psychological factors relate to the recovery from cancer?
8 How does the breadth of psychology help to understand other chronic illness other than HIV or cancer?
9 Cancer is a very varied disease. What are the implications of this variability for research?

FOR DISCUSSION

Do you know anyone who has had either HIV or cancer? Think about how psychological factors such as behaviour, beliefs and coping have influenced their state of health.

FURTHER READING

Barraclough, J. (2007) *Cancer and Emotion: A Practical Guide to Psycho-oncology,* 3rd edn. Chichester: Wiley.

A thorough and accessible review of the research and theories exploring links between psychological factors and cancer in terms of onset, progression and recovery.

James, D. (2018) *F*** You Cancer: How to face the big C, live your life and still be yourself.* Ebury Digital.

This is an inspiring and very real account of what it is like to have cancer.

Scott, S., Walter, F., Webster, A. et al. (2013) The Model of Pathways to Treatment: Conceptualization and integration with existing theory, *British Journal of Health Psychology,* **18.** Doi: 10.1111/j.2044-8287.2012.02077.x.

This is an interesting theoretical paper that provides a framework for understanding pathways into and through the treatment process for cancer and other chronic conditions.

Vedhara, K. and Irwin, M. (eds) (2012) *Human Psychoneuroimmunology.* Oxford: Oxford University Press.

This book provides an excellent overview of the research on PNI and covers key concepts, research and methods.

Whitaker, K. (2019) Earlier diagnosis: the importance of cancer symptoms, *Lancet Oncology;* **21** (1): 6–8.

This is a well-argued editorial that makes a strong case for early diagnosis of cancer.

It's a Sin (2021). UK TV series. https://en.wikipedia.org/wiki/It%27s_a_Sin_(TV_series)

Please watch this! It is an amazing series about a group of gay men and their friends living in London between 1981 and 1991 during the AIDS epidemic. It is funny, enlightening and tragic. (And, speaking as someone who was at university in Brighton at this time, it felt very realistic.)

13

Chronic Illness: Obesity and Coronary Heart Disease

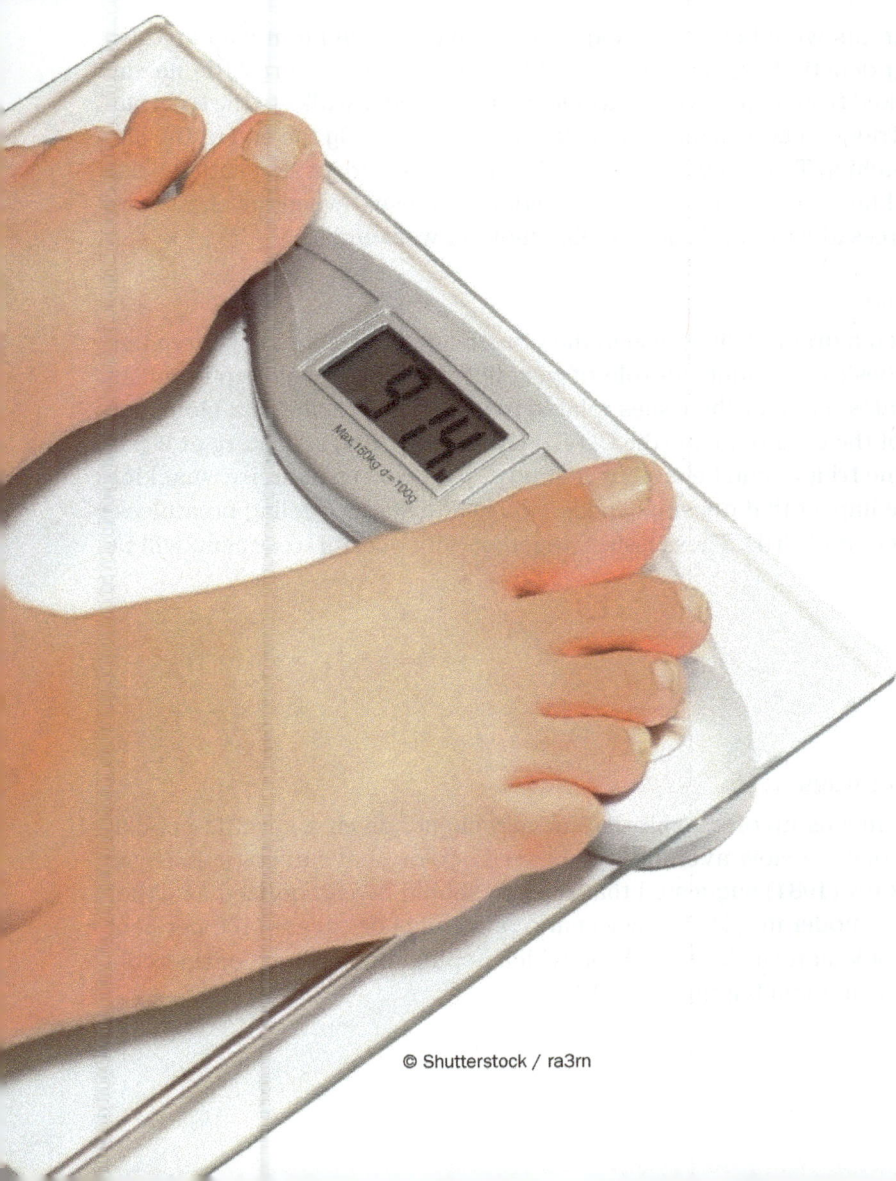

© Shutterstock / ra3rn

Learning Objectives

To understand:

1. Obesity
2. The Role of Psychology in the Study of Obesity
3. Obesity Treatment
4. Coronary Heart Disease
5. The Role of Psychology in the Study of CHD
6. Rehabilitation for Patients with CHD
7. Thinking Critically about Research into Obesity and CHD

CHAPTER OVERVIEW

This chapter focuses on obesity and coronary heart disease (CHD). First, it examines definitions of obesity, its prevalence and potential consequences. It then examines the role of genetics, the obesogenic environment and behaviour in causing obesity. The chapter then looks at obesity treatment with a focus on dietary management, medication and surgery and explores the factors associated with successful weight loss maintenance. In the second half, the chapter looks at CHD, describing what it is, how it is defined and the role of psychology in its aetiology. The psychological consequences of CHD are then explored, along with the role of psychology in patient rehabilitation. The chapter concludes with descriptions of the predictors of patient health outcomes, with a focus on quality of life and mortality. In line with the previous chapter, the many roles for psychology relevant to both obesity and CHD are also relevant to a wide range of both common and less common chronic conditions. These are illustrated throughout with case examples.

CASE STUDY

Saahil is 50 and overweight. His parents were both overweight and he has two children who are also overweight. He believes in a strong genetic basis to obesity and feels that there is very little he can do about it. Since COVID he has worked from home, which has meant he no longer walks to the train station and often grabs food from the fridge in between meetings to eat at his desk. By the end of the day he is exhausted and recovers by watching TV on the sofa with a beer and some crisps. Recently he has been feeling quite out of breath and he seems to get more indigestion than usual when his chest feels tight. He thinks that this is due to stress at work and tries to relax more at weekends.

Through the Eyes of Health Psychology. . .

Over the past 30 years there has been a dramatic increase in the prevalence of obesity in children and adults. The three key theories of obesity highlight the role of genetics, the obesogenic environment and behaviour. Saahil's story illustrates many of the issues related to obesity: the belief in a biological cause (runs in the family), the role of the environment (the COVID pandemic, being sedentary at work, working from home, working near the fridge) and behaviour (eating at the desk, no exercise, snacking in the evening). It also illustrates the impact that obesity can have on health status (feeling breathless) and the link to diseases such as cancer and CHD. These issues, together with obesity treatment, will be covered in this chapter.

1 OBESITY

WHAT IS OBESITY?

Obesity can be defined in a number of ways:

- *Population means.* Population means involve exploring mean weights, given a specific population, and deciding whether someone is below average weight, average or above average in terms of percentage overweight. Stunkard (1984) suggested that obesity should be categorized as either mild (20–40 per cent overweight), moderate (41–100 per cent overweight) or severe (100 per cent overweight). This approach is problematic as it depends on which population is being considered – someone could be defined as obese in India but not in the USA.

- *BMI.* Body mass index (BMI) is calculated using the equation weight (kg)/height (m²). This produces a figure that has been categorized as normal weight (20–24.9); overweight (25–29.9); clinical obesity (30–39.9); and severe obesity (40+). This is the most frequently used definition of obesity. However, it does not allow for differences in weight between muscle and fat – a bodybuilder could be considered obese.

- *Waist circumference.* BMI is the most frequently used measure of obesity but it does not allow for an analysis of the *location* of fat. This is important as some problems such as diabetes are predicted by abdominal fat rather than lower body fat. Researchers originally used waist:hip ratios to assess obesity but recently waist circumference on its own has become the preferred approach. For men, low waist circumference is < 94 cm; high is 94–102 cm and very high is > 102 cm. For women, low waist circumference is < 80 cm; high is 80–88 cm and very high is > 88 cm. Weight reduction is recommended when waist circumference is greater than 102 cm in men and 88 cm in women (Lean et al. 1995). A reduction in waist circumference is associated with a reduction in cardiovascular risk factors and abdominal obesity is associated with insulin resistance and the development of Type 2 diabetes (Chan et al. 1994; Han et al. 1997).

- *Percentage body fat.* As health is mostly associated with fat rather than weight per se, researchers and clinicians have also developed methods of measuring percentage body fat directly. At its most basic this involves assessing skinfold thickness using callipers, normally around the upper arm and upper and lower back. This is not suitable for those individuals who are severely obese and misses abdominal fat. At a more advanced level, body fat can be measured using bioelectrical impedence which involves passing an electrical current between a person's hand and foot. As water conducts electricity and fat is an insulator, the impedence of the current can be used to calculate the ratio between water and fat and therefore an overall estimate of percentage body fat can be made.

All measures of obesity have their problems but BMI is the one which is most commonly used as it is the easiest to measure for clinical and research purposes.

HOW COMMON IS OBESITY?

Since 1975, rates of obesity worldwide have nearly tripled. In 2016 it was estimated that 39 per cent of adults were overweight and 13 per cent were obese, while 41 million children under the age of 5 and 340 million children aged 5–19 years were overweight or obese. Worldwide, some of the highest rates of obesity of greater than 40 per cent are the Cook Islands, Samoa, Tonga and Qatar. Those at 30–40 per cent include Kuwait, Bahamas, Saudi Arabia, Libya and the USA and those at 20–39 per cent include New Zealand, Australia, UK, Mexico, Canada, Ireland and France. The lowest rates of 10–20 per cent include Finland, Sweden, Denmark, Germany and Portugal and those countries with less than 10 per cent rates of obesity include China, Nepal, Kenya, Sri Lanka and Japan. Figure 13.1 shows obesity rates across the world for men and Figure 13.2 shows rates for women for 2010.

In the UK the rates of obesity increased dramatically from 1993 to about 2007 but have been relatively stable for the past 10 years. Defined as a BMI greater than 30, reports show that in 1980, 6 per cent of men and 8 per cent of women were obese and that this had increased to 13 per cent and 16 per cent in 1994, to 18 per cent and 24 per cent respectively by 2005 and to 22 and 24 per cent respectively in 2009. In 2016 the obesity rate for adults was still about 26 per cent. The increase in obesity rates between 1994 to 2008 in the UK is shown in Figure 13.3.

For children in the UK, there was a similar dramatic increase in the rates of obesity from the 1970s but this has shown no real signs of slowing down and currently it is estimated that 16 per cent of children aged 2–15 years are obese and 12 per cent are overweight. Worldwide obesity rates for boys and girls in 2016 are shown in Figure 13.4.

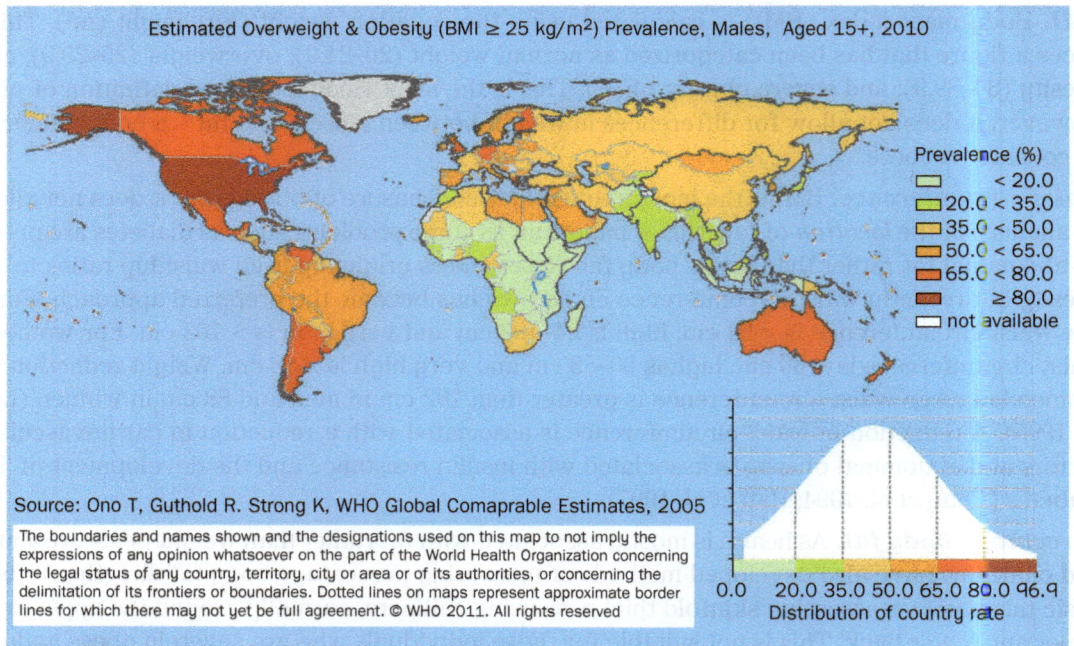

Figure 13.1 Worldwide obesity prevalence rates for men

SOURCE: WHO Global InfoBase (online)

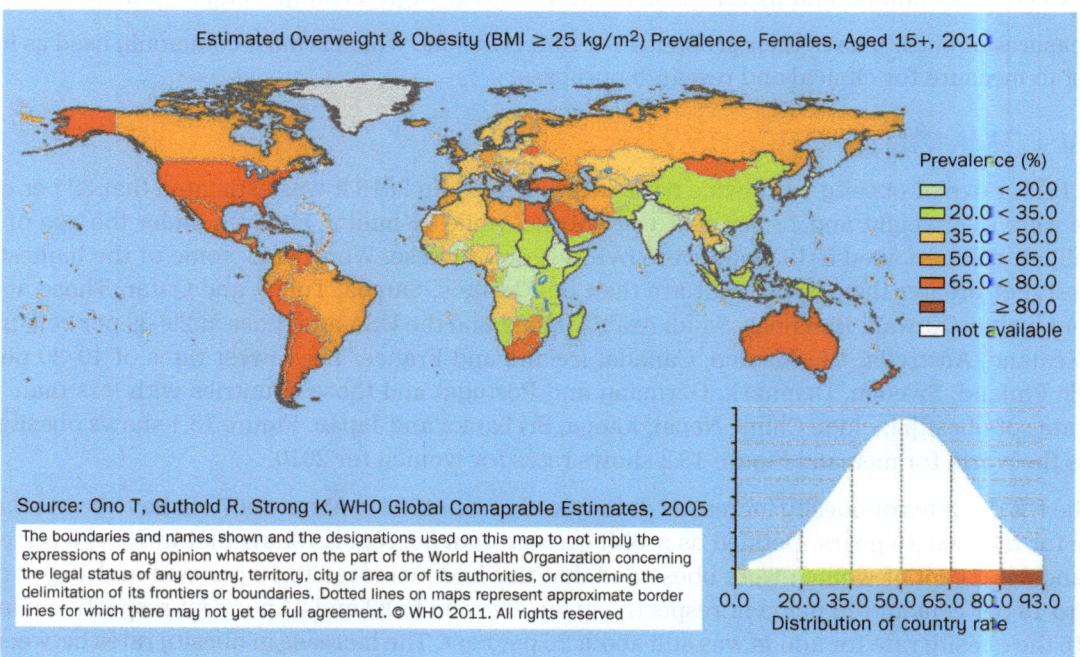

Figure 13.2 Worldwide obesity prevalence rates for women

SOURCE: WHO Global InfoBase(online)

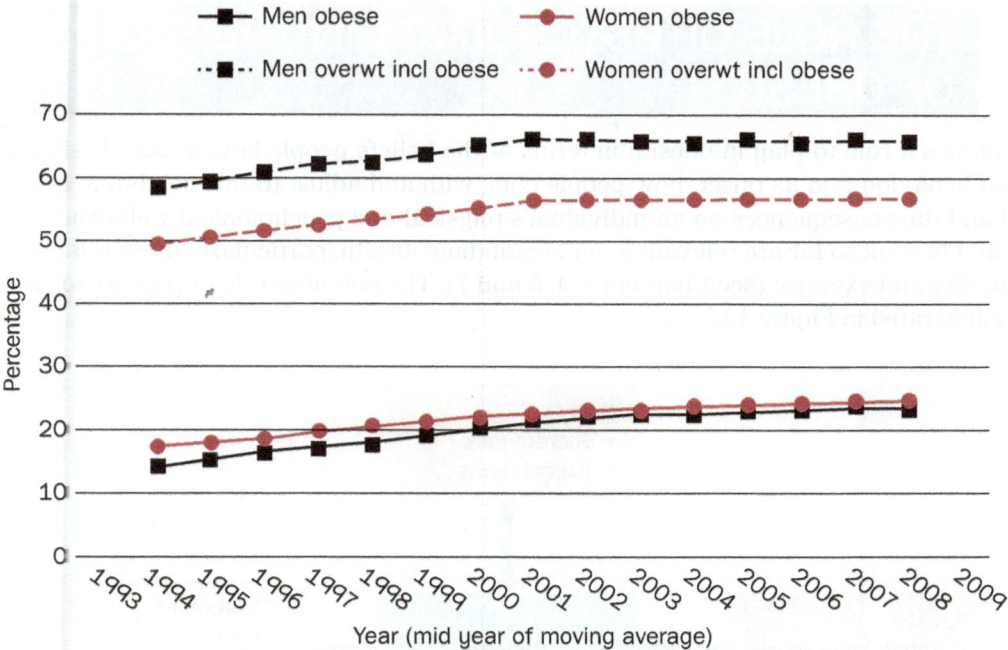

Figure 13.3 Obesity and overweight prevalence in the UK, 1993–2008

SOURCE: Copyright © 2011, Health and Social Care Information Centre annual report 2011 to 2012, Reproduced under the Open Government Licence v3.0.

https://www.nationalarchives.gov.uk/doc/open-government-licence/version/3/

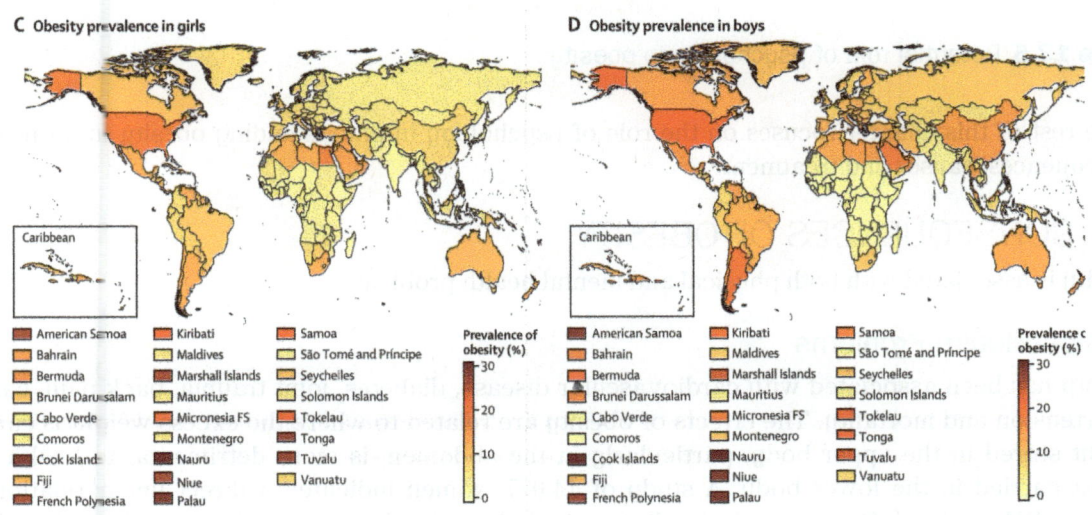

Figure 13.4 Worldwide obesity rates in boys and girls in 2016

NCD Risk Factor Collaboration (2017)

2   THE ROLE OF PSYCHOLOGY IN THE STUDY OF OBESITY

Psychology has a role to play in obesity in terms of the beliefs people hold about obesity, the role of beliefs and behaviours in its onset, how people cope with and adjust to this condition, how obesity is managed and the consequences on an individual's physical and psychological well-being. Most of the chapters in this book so far are relevant to understanding obesity, particularly those relating to beliefs, behaviour, diet and exercise (see Chapters 2, 4, 5 and 7). The potential role of psychological factors in obesity is illustrated in Figure 13.5.

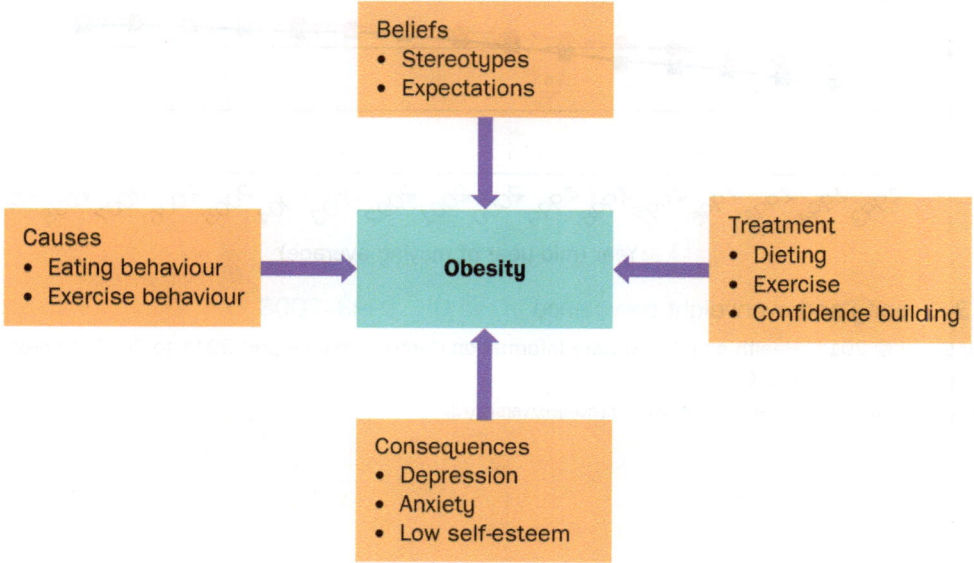

Figure 13.5 Potential role of psychology in obesity

The rest of this chapter focuses on the role of psychology in understanding obesity in terms of its consequences, causes and treatment.

THE CONSEQUENCES OF OBESITY

Obesity is associated with both physical and mental health problems.

Physical Health Problems

Obesity has been associated with cardiovascular disease, diabetes, joint trauma, back pain, cancer, hypertension and mortality. The effects of obesity are related to where the excess weight is carried; weight stored in the upper body, particularly in the abdomen, is more detrimental to health than weight carried in the lower body. A study of 14,077 women indicated a direct linear relationship between BMI and risk factors for heart disease including blood pressure, cholesterol and blood glucose (Ashton et al. 2001). Similar studies have also reported a relationship between BMI increases in the lower range of the spectrum and hypertension (National Institutes of Health 1998), diabetes (Ford et al. 1997) and heart attack (Willett et al. 1995). A recent review also showed an association between obesity and CHD and indicated that this association remained even when risk factors such as raised blood pressure and cholesterol were controlled for (Ortega et al. 2018). Moore et al. (2008) also explored the impact of BMI measured 10 years prior to death in a large cohort of 50,186 women.

The results showed a direct relationship between BMI and mortality (see Romero-Corral et al. 2006 for a systematic review of the literature). In 2014, a population-based cohort study in the UK of 5.24 million adults reported a link between obesity and 22 cancers and concluded that 41 per cent of uterine and 10 per cent or more of gallbladder, kidney, liver and colon cancers could be attributable to excess weight (Bhaskaran et al. 2014).

For children, the physical consequences of obesity mostly relate to being immobile and unfit and not being able to be as active as their friends and peer group. Some health problems do start early, however, and studies show a link between being obese as a child and having childhood asthma and Type 2 diabetes (Foresight 2007).

Psychological Problems

Research has examined the relationship between psychological problems and obesity. The contemporary cultural obsession with thinness, the aversion to fat found in both adults and children and the attribution of blame to people living with obesity may promote low self-esteem and poor self-image in those individuals who do not conform to the stereotypically attractive thin image. Further, those who are depressed or anxious may eat more as a means to manage their mood. Accordingly, psychological problems may be either a consequence or a cause of weight problems but much research shows that they are associated. For example, research indicates that adults who are obese also tend to show depression, anxiety, low self-esteem and high levels of body dissatisfaction (WHO 2016; Pereira-Miranda et al. 2017). Research also shows that patients attending for bariatric surgery often have complex psychological histories with issues including depression, anxiety, poor self-esteem and body image, eating disorder symptoms, self-harm, addiction or suicidality (see Busetto et al. 2018 for review). In line with this, Ogden and Clementi (2011) carried out a qualitative study of the experience of being obese and reported that people with obesity describe a multitude of negative ways in which their weight impacts upon their self-identity and that this is exacerbated by living in a society that stigmatizes their condition. There is also a large literature exploring weight bias which illustrates how people stigmatize those who are obese in terms of characterological blame (i.e. people with obesity are lazy, sloppy, incompetent and lack willpower) and behavioural blame (that they do not exercise enough and have excessive dietary consumption) and how this can lead to weight bias internalization and emotions such as shame, depression and poor self-esteem (see Pearl and Puhl 2018 for a review). Obesity in children has also been linked with psychological issues. For children, the most immediate consequences of being overweight or obese are psychological, with many showing body dissatisfaction, low self-esteem, anxiety, low mood and a general lack of confidence. Children who are overweight are also more likely to be bullied than thin children, which can lead to under-achievement or missing school (Foresight 2007).

WHAT CAUSES OBESITY?

The theories relating to the causes of obesity include a role for genetics, the impact of the obesogenic environment and behavioural theories.

Genetic Theories

Size appears to run in families and the probability that a child will be overweight is related to the parents' weight. For example, having one parent with obesity results in a 40 per cent chance of producing a child with obesity, and having two parents with obesity results in an 80 per cent chance. In contrast, the probability that thin parents will produce overweight children is very small, about 7 per cent (Garn et al. 1981). This observation has been repeated in studies exploring populations from different parts of the world living in different environments (Maes et al. 1997). However, parents and children share both environment and genetic constitution, so this likeness could be due to either factor. To address this problem, research has examined twins and adoptees and carried out detailed genetic analysis.

- *Twin studies.* Twin studies have examined the weight of identical twins reared apart, who have identical genes but different environments. Studies have also examined the weights of non-identical twins reared together, who have different genes but similar environments. The results show that the identical twins reared apart are more similar in weight than non-identical twins reared together. For example, Stunkard et al. (1990) examined the BMI in 93 pairs of identical twins reared apart and reported that genetic factors accounted for 66–70 per cent in the variance in their body weight, suggesting a strong genetic component in determining obesity. However, the role of genetics appears to be greater in lighter twin pairs than in heavier pairs.

- *Adoptee studies.* Research has also examined the role of genetics in obesity using adoptees. Such studies compare the adoptees' weight with both their adoptive parents and their biological parents. Stunkard et al. (1986) gathered information about 540 adult adoptees in Denmark, their adopted parents and their biological parents. The results showed a strong relationship between the weight class of the adoptee (thin, median weight, overweight, obese) and their biological parents' weight class but no relationship with their adoptee parents' weight class. This suggests a major role for genetics and was also found across the whole range of body weight. Interestingly, the relationship to the biological mother's weight was greater than the relationship with the biological father's weight.

- *Genetic analysis:* Obesity is found in some syndromes which are caused by individual genes such as Bardet-Biedl syndrome and Prader-Willi syndrome. These are known as *monogenic* types of obesity and are caused by genetic mutations. This form of obesity is very rare and only 78 cases worldwide have been attributed to mutations of seven distinct genes. The more common forms of obesity are probably caused by the interaction between different genes known as *polygenic* obesity. Sequence variations within a pool of 56 different genes have been reported as being related to obesity. Only ten of those genes, however, showed positive results in at least five different studies and within this, the role of each gene is very small (about 0.4 per cent) with gene interactions accounting for about 0.8 per cent of obesity rates (Willer et al. 2009). Some research has therefore turned to the interaction between genes and the environment known as *epigenetics*. This suggests that changes in the environment switch different genes on or off which then change body weight, possibly through behaviour (Foresight 2007; Rohde et al. 2019; Golden and Kessler 2020). There is good evidence for epigenetics *in utero* when the foetus is developing and even at preconception when it is influenced by the mother's own health status (e.g. Baird et al. 2017; Fleming et al. 2018). Evidence for epigenetics once fully developed is still in its early stages. From a more general perspective, research also suggests that some people have a *genetic predisposition* to obesity, possibly because they evolved with a 'thrifty gene' to enable them to survive famine, which makes them store food more efficiently and/or eat more when food is plentiful (Neel 1999). The search for this gene, however, has only managed to account for a very small percentage of the variance of the prevalence of obesity.

Research therefore suggests a role for genetics in predicting obesity. There are some problems with this approach, however, as follows:

Problems with twin/adoptee data: although the twin and adoptee data suggests a strong role for genetics in obesity there are problems with this data including assumptions of shared environments in both identical twins and non-identical twins (as siblings have different micro environments within families) and assumptions of different environments between biological and adoptee parents (children are often adopted by parents similar to their biological ones). Further, although this data indicates a major role for genetics, no subsequent genetic analysis has been able to match these high estimates of 66–70 per cent.

Predicting obesity rates: The variance predicted by genetics analysis is very small (ranging from approximately 0.4 per cent to 1.4 per cent) compared to the rates of obesity (up to 50 per cent). Something else other than genetics must be playing a role.

Changes over time: A genetic theory of obesity cannot explain why there has been such a huge increase in the prevalence of obesity over the past 30 years, as our genes have not changed during this time.

Migration data: When populations migrate from one country to another they quickly take on the body weight of their new environment (Misra and Ganda 2007). This cannot be explained by genetics as genetics do not change just because someone has moved. For example, for Nigerians living in Nigeria, the prevalence of obesity is 5 per cent, but for those Nigerians who move to the USA, the rate is 39 per cent. Similarly, for the Japanese living in Japan the rate of obesity is 4 per cent, but for the Japanese living in Brazil the rate is also 39 per cent.

Social contagion: A social network approach explores how BMI clusters within groups and shows that even though our body weight is similar to that of our parents, it is even more similar to that of our friends (Christakis and Fowler 2006). It also shows that over time our body weight becomes more similar to those around us even if they are not genetically related to us and that we either lose or gain weight depending upon the changes in weight of those we spend most time with. This has been called social contagion and cannot be explained by genetics as we do not share genes with our friends.

Therefore, although it would seem that obesity runs in families and that some people might have a genetic predisposition to gain weight, genetics cannot be the main cause of this problem. Researchers have therefore turned to both the environment and individual behaviour as more useful explanations.

The Obesogenic Environment

To address the dramatic increase in obesity since the 1970s, researchers have turned their attention to the role of the external world which has been labelled an *obesogenic environment* (Hill and Peters 1998). For example, they have highlighted the impact of the food industry with its food advertising, food labelling and the easy availability of energy-dense foods such as fast foods and takeaways. They have identified environmental factors which encourage us to live an increasingly sedentary lifestyle, such as a reduction in manual labour, the use of cars, computers and television and the design of towns whereby walking is prohibited through the absence of streetlights, pavements and large distances between residential areas and places of entertainment or shops, and they have focused on factors which make it more and more difficult to eat well and be active, such as the presence of lifts and escalators which detract from stair use and the cheapness of prepared foods which discourages food shopping and cooking. Accordingly, this obesogenic environment creates a world in which it is easy to gain weight. Furthermore, the changes in our environment coincide with the increased prevalence of obesity. From a public health perspective, therefore, environmental factors are key to understanding obesity and any attempts to prevent obesity onset should focus on changing the environment. In line with this, governments provide subsidies for leisure centres, trying to make them more accessible for everyone. There are local campaigns to encourage stair climbing by putting prompts near lifts and stairwells and there is legislation limiting food advertising. Furthermore, some companies encourage their staff to be active in their lunch breaks by organizing walking groups and offering

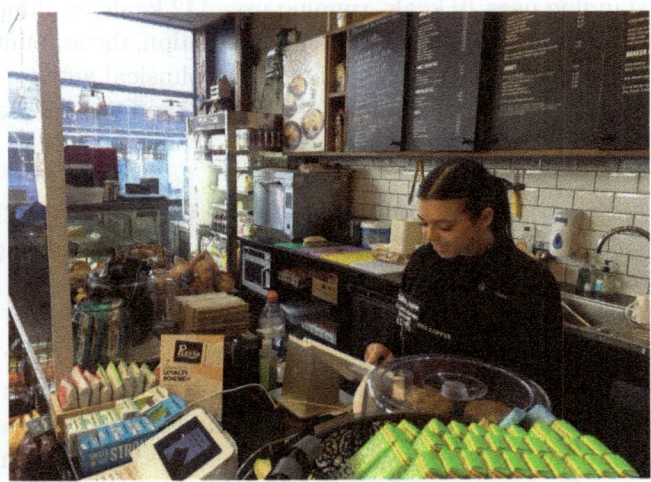

The obesogenic environment changes our behaviour

gym facilities, and school and work canteens are supported in their attempts to offer healthier meals. In the same way that many governments have now finally responded to the knowledge that smoking kills by banning it in public places, steps are being made to intervene at an environmental and policy level to control the obesity epidemic.

From a psychological perspective, understanding the environmental factors which promote obesity does not seem to be a sufficient explanatory model. Psychology focuses on beliefs and behaviour and as Prentice (1999: 38) argued, 'Obesity can only occur when energy intake remains higher than energy expenditure, for an extended period of time. This is an incontrovertible cornerstone on which all explanations must be based.' Research has therefore examined the role of behaviour in explaining obesity, and behavioural theories of obesity focus on physical activity and eating behaviour.

Behavioural Theories

Behavioural theories of obesity focus on physical activity and eating behaviour. Further details about physical activity and diet can be found in Chapters 4 and 5.

Physical Activity

Increases in the prevalence of obesity coincide with decreases in daily energy expenditure due to improvements in transport systems, and a shift from an agricultural society to an industrial and increasingly information-based one. As a simple example, in 1984 when everyone still had a landline, a telephone company in the USA suggested that having a phone extension upstairs as well as downstairs, saving the need to run downstairs to answer the phone, saved a person approximately one mile of walking per year – the equivalent of 2–3 lb of fat or up to 10,500 kcals (Stern 1984). Imagine how much energy a mobile phone saves! Further, at present only 20 per cent of men and 10 per cent of women are employed in active occupations and for many people leisure times are dominated by inactivity (see Figures 5.1–5.8 for descriptions of activity levels). Although data on changes in activity levels are problematic, there exists a useful database on TV viewing which shows that, whereas the average viewer in the 1960s watched 13 hours of TV per week, by 1994 in England this had doubled to 26 hours per week (OPCS 1994). Overall, data seem to indicate that the majority of people do not meet the recommended targets for activity, that generally people get more sedentary and less active as they get older and that men are more active than women particularly when young, but watch more TV than women as they get older. This is further exacerbated by the increased use of videos and computer games by both children and adults. It has therefore been suggested that obesity may be caused by inactivity. Further, exercise clearly burns up calories. For example, 10 minutes of sleeping uses up to 16 kcals, standing uses 19 kcals, running uses 142 kcals, walking downstairs uses 88 kcals and walking upstairs uses 229 kcals (Brownell 1989). In addition, the amount of calories used increases with the individual's body weight. To examine the role of physical activity in obesity, research has asked, 'Are changes in obesity related to changes in activity?' and 'Do people living with obesity exercise less?' These questions will now be examined.

Are Changes in Obesity Related to Changes in Activity?

This question can be answered in two ways: first, using epidemiological data on a population and second, using prospective data on individuals.

Epidemiological data: In 1995, Prentice and Jebb presented epidemiological data on changes in physical activity from 1950 to 1990, as measured by car ownership and TV viewing, and compared these with changes in the prevalence of obesity. The results from this study suggested a strong association between an increase in both car ownership and TV viewing and an increase in obesity. However, this data was only correlational so it remains unclear whether obesity and physical activity are related (the *third factor problem* – some other variable may be determining both obesity and activity), and whether decreases in activity cause increases in obesity or whether, in fact, increases in obesity actually cause decreases in activity (the problem of reverse causality). In addition, the data are at the population level and therefore could miss important individual differences (i.e. some people who become obese could be active and those who are thin could be inactive).

Prospective data: In an alternative approach to assessing the relationship between activity and obesity, a large Finnish study of 12,000 adults examined the association between levels of physical activity and excess weight gain over a five-year follow-up period (Rissanen et al. 1991). The results showed that lower levels of activity were a greater risk factor for weight gain than any other baseline measures. One study analysed data from 146 twin pairs as a means to assess the relative contribution of genetics and physical activity over a 30-year period (Waller et al. 2008). The results showed that persistent physical activity across the 30 years of the study was related to smaller waist circumference and a decreased weight gain as the active twin showed less weight gain than the inactive twin even though they shared the same genetic make-up and childhood environment. However, although these data were prospective, it is still possible that a third factor may explain the relationship (i.e. those with lower levels of activity at baseline were women, the women had children and therefore put on more weight). Unless experimental data are collected, conclusions about causality remain problematic.

Do People Living with Obesity Exercise Less?

Research has also examined the relationship between activity and obesity using a cross-sectional design to examine differences between those living with obesity and those not. In particular, several studies in the 1960s and 1970s examined whether people living with obesity obese exercised less than others. Using time lapse photography, Bullen et al. (1964) observed girls considered obese and those of healthier weight on a summer camp. They reported that during swimming the girls living with obesity spent less time swimming and more time floating, and while playing tennis those living with obesity were inactive for 77 per cent of the time compared with the girls of healthier weight, who were inactive for only 56 per cent of the time. In addition, research indicates that people living with obesity walk less on a daily basis and are less likely to use stairs or walk up escalators. For example, to assess the impact of stair climbing Shenassa et al. (2008) explored the relationship between BMI and floor of residence in nearly 3,000 healthier weight adults across eight European cities. The results showed that for men, higher floor was associated with lower BMI. This association was not, however, found for women. The authors concluded that daily stair climbing may reduce weight and therefore should be encouraged. Why the association was not there for women is unclear.

Cross-sectional data in 2008 from the UK also explored the relationship between body weight and being sedentary in the week and at the weekend. The results are shown in Figure 13.6 for men and women. The results from this data indicate that people living with obesity are more sedentary at both the weekend and in the week than either those who are overweight or those of healthier weight. These studies are cross-sectional and whether reduced exercise is a cause or a consequence of obesity is unclear. It is possible that those living with obesity take less exercise due to factors such as embarrassment and stigma and that exercise plays a part in the maintenance of obesity but not in its cause.

Heinonen et al. (2013) also explored the relationship between sedentary time (TV viewing, computer time, reading, music/radio listening and other relaxation) and waist circumference and BMI in 1084 women and 909 men aged 30–45 years in Finland. This study also controlled for a wide range of variables including age, occupational and leisure-time physical activity, sleep duration, SES and health behaviours such as smoking, alcohol intake, food intake and genetic variants associated with BMI and placed people into matched MET groups (metabolic equivalent index groups based on leisure time exercise and active commuting). The results showed that of the different types of sedentary activities, TV viewing was most consistently significantly related to higher BMI and waist circumference in both men and women. An additional hour of non-TV sedentary time was also significantly related to increased

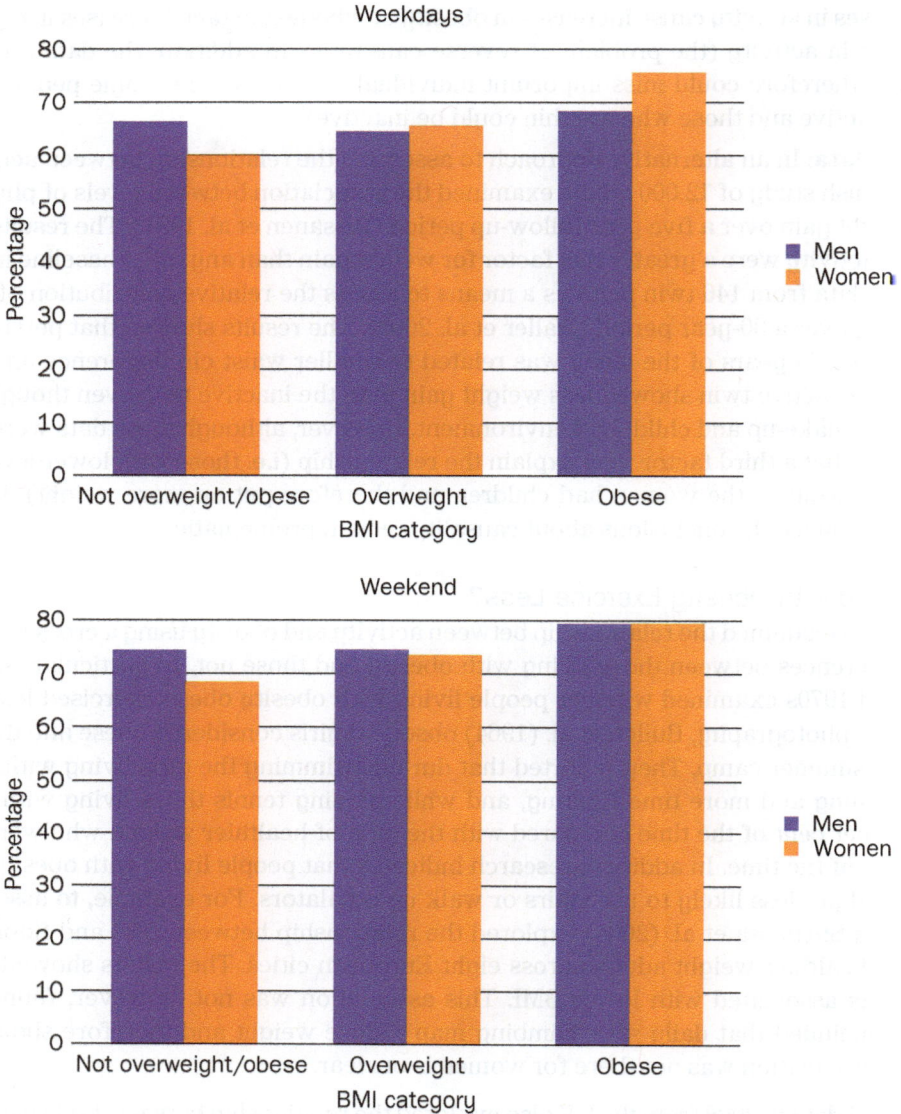

Figure 13.6 Body weight and being sedentary on a weekday and at the weekend

Adapted from Heinonen et al. (2013)

waist circumference in women but not in men. This data is illustrated in Figure 13.7. This study controlled for many possible third factors but is still correlational in design so still suffers with both the third factor problem and the possibility of reverse causality.

Eating Behaviour

To further understand the causes of obesity, research has also examined eating behaviour. Chapter 4 described a number of different approaches to understanding eating behaviour. These perspectives emphasize mechanisms such as exposure, modelling and associative learning, beliefs and emotions, body dissatisfaction and dieting, all of which can help explain obesity. For example, it is possible that those living with obesity have childhoods in which food is used to reward good behaviour, or have parents who overeat, or hold cognitions about food which drive eating behaviour. It is also possible that dieting when moderately overweight (or just feeling fat) triggers episodes of overeating

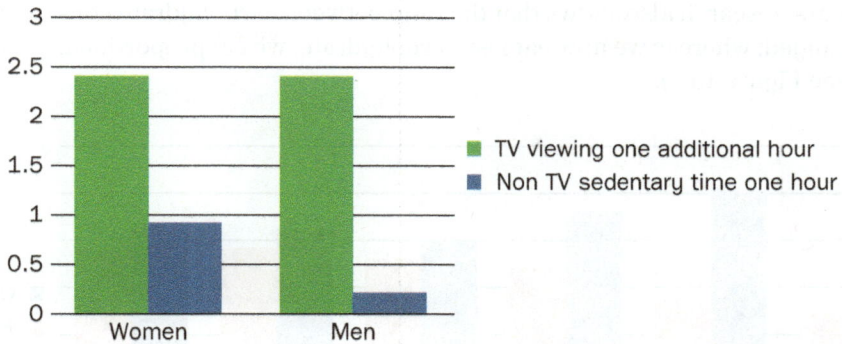

Figure 13.7 The impact of one additional hour of TV viewing and non-TV sedentary time on change in waist circumference (cm) in men and women (age adjusted) Adapted from Heinonen et al. (2013)

which cause increases in body fat. Research has therefore asked the following questions of the link between eating behaviour and obesity: 'Are changes in food intake associated with changes in obesity?', 'Do those who are living with obesity eat for different reasons than those of healthier weight?' and 'Do those who are living with obesity eat more than those of a healthier weight?'. These will now be described.

Are Population Changes in Food Intake Associated with Changes in Obesity?

The UK National Food Survey collects data on food intake in the home, which can be analysed to assess changes in food intake over the past 60 years. The results from this database illustrate that, although overall calorie consumption increased between 1940 and 1960, since 1970 there has been a distinct decrease in the amount of calories we eat (see Figure 13.8). However, this data relates *only* to food intake in the home and does not take into account meals and snacking in cafés and restaurants or on the move.

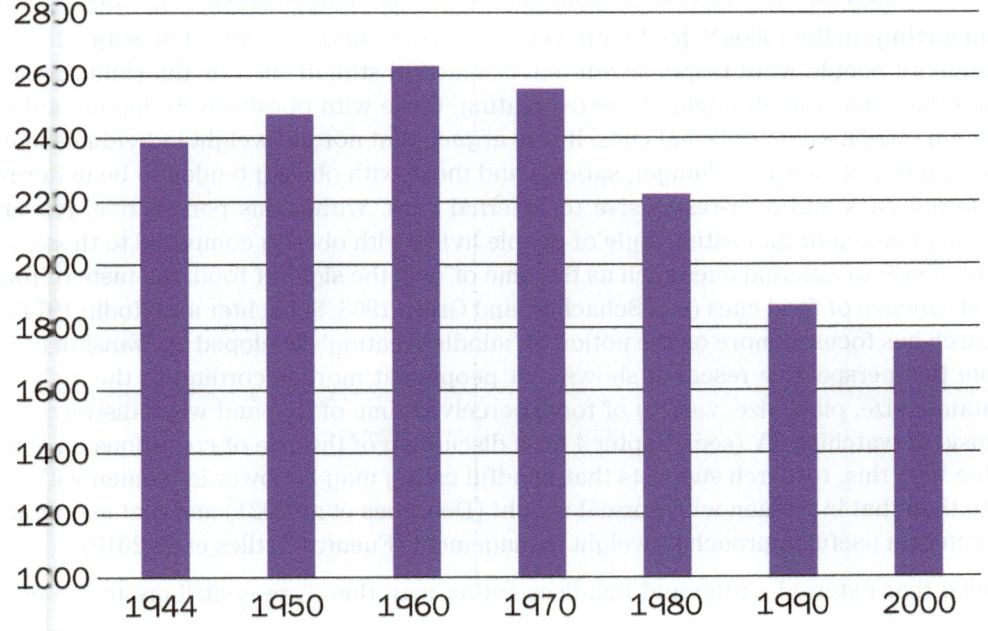

Figure 13.8 Changes in calorie intake per person per day, 1944–2000

SOURCE: Adapted from Department for Environment, Food and Rural Affairs (2011)

Over recent years, research also shows that the ratio between carbohydrate consumption and fat consumption has changed; whereas we now eat less carbohydrate, we eat proportionally more fat (Prentice and Jebb 1995; see Figure 13.9).

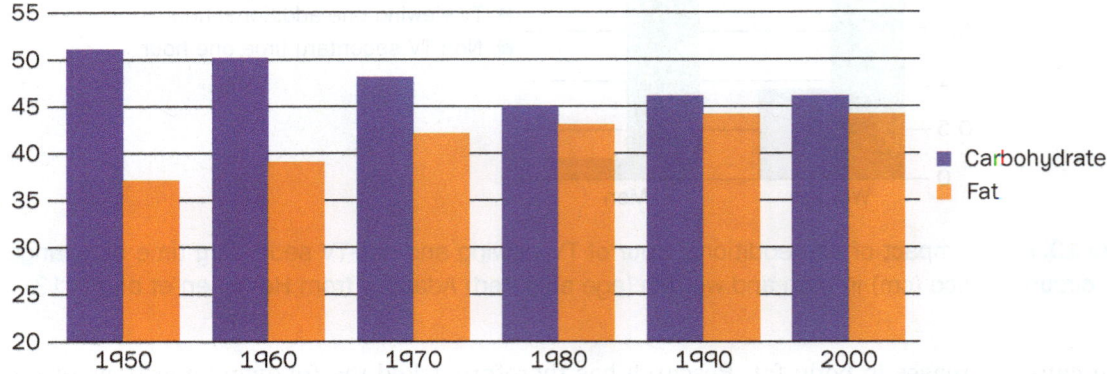

Figure 13.9 Changes in fat and carbohydrate consumption in the UK
SOURCE: Adapted from Prentice and Jebb (1995)

Prentice and Jebb (1995) examined the association between changes in food intake in terms of energy intake and fat intake and changes in obesity. Their results indicated no obvious association between the increase in obesity and the changes in food intake. Therefore, using population data, while we may eat fewer calories (at least in the home) and consume relatively more fat compared to carbohydrates, there appears to be no clear relationship between changes in food intake at a population level and changes in obesity.

Do those who are Living with Obesity Eat for Different Reasons than those of Healthier Weight?

Research has focused on external eating (sometimes now called mindless eating) and emotional eating.

External eating: In the 1960s Schachter developed his *externality theory* of obesity which suggested that, although all people were responsive to environmental stimuli such as the sight, taste and smell of food, and that such stimuli might cause overeating, those with obesity were highly and sometimes uncontrollably responsive to external cues. It was argued that normal-weight individuals mainly ate as a response to internal cues (e.g. hunger, satiety) and those with obesity tended to be under-responsive to their internal cues and over-responsive to external cues. Within this perspective, research examined the eating behaviour and eating style of people living with obesity compared to those of healthier weight in response to external cues such as the time of day, the sight of food, the taste of food and the number and salience of food cues (e.g. Schachter and Gross 1968; Schachter and Rodin 1974). Since the 1990s research has focused more on the notion of 'mindless eating' developed by Wansink (e.g. Wansink 2009). From this perspective research shows that people eat more according to the ambience of the room, container size, plate size, variety of food, perceived time of day and when distracted by factors such as music or watching TV (see Chapter 4 for a discussion of the role of cognitions on eating behaviour). In line with this, research suggests that mindful eating may be lower in women with overweight and obesity than that in women with normal weight (Demirbas et al. 2021) and that encouraging mindful eating can be a useful approach to weight management (Fuentes Artiles et al. 2019).

It is argued that external eating and mindless eating may therefore contribute to the development of obesity.

Emotional eating: Research has also addressed the *emotionality theory* of eating behaviour. For example, Bruch (e.g. 1974) developed a psychosomatic theory of eating behaviour and eating disorders which argued that some people interpret the sensations of such emotions as emptiness as similar to hunger and that food is used as a substitute for other forms of emotional comfort. Van Strien et al. (2009) explored the relationship between dietary restraint, emotional and external eating, overeating and BMI to assess how people resist (or not) the opportunity to become overweight offered by the obesogenic environment. The results showed that although overeating was associated with being overweight, this association was moderated by both restraint and emotional eating (not external eating). They drew two conclusions from their data. First, they argued that the impact of overeating is limited by dietary restraint; second, they argued that emotional eating is a better predictor of body weight than external eating.

Do those who are living with Obesity Eat more than those of Healthier Weight?

Research has also examined whether those who are obese eat more than the non-obese, focusing on the amount consumed per se, how they eat and the type of food consumed.

The Amount Eaten

Because it was believed that those who are obese ate for different reasons than the non-obese, it was also believed that they ate more. Early research in this area produced very inconsistent results and Spitzer and Rodin (1981) concluded from their analysis 'of twenty-nine studies examining the effects of body weight on amount eaten in laboratory studies. . . only nine reported that overweight subjects ate significantly more than their lean counterparts'. Over recent years, however, researchers have questioned this conclusion for the following reasons. First, much of the early research was based on self-report data, which are notoriously unreliable, with most people consistently under-reporting how much they eat (Prentice et al. 1986; Heitmann and Lissner 1995). Second, when those living with obesity and those of healthier weight are either over- or underfed in a controlled environment, these two groups gain or lose weight at the same rate, suggesting that those living with obesity must eat more in order to maintain their higher weight (Jebb et al. 1996). Finally, it has been argued that assessing food intake in terms of gross amount without analysing the *types* of food being eaten misses the complex nature of both eating behaviour and food metabolism (Prentice 1995). Bray and Bouchard (2020) recently carried out a systematic review of over 300 original papers dealing with the biology of overfeeding. They concluded that overfeeding resulted in weight gain in adolescents, adult men and women and in older men and that, in longer term studies, there was a highly significant relationship between energy ingested and weight gain and fat storage with only limited individual differences. Therefore increased body weight seems to be associated with increased food intake. Further, if overeating is defined as 'compared with what the body needs', it could be argued that those living with obesity overeat because they have excess body fat.

Eating Differently

One recent study asked whether those living with obesity eat at different times of day to those of healthier weight. Berg et al. (2009) used a sample of 3,610 women and men from Sweden and explored their BMI and meal patterns. The results showed that those who were living with obesity were more likely to skip breakfast, skip lunch and eat at night and reported larger portion sizes at meal times. Similarly, Aqeel et al. (2020) explored the association between temporal dietary patterns (TDPs) and obesity and concluded that those who had evenly spaced, energy balanced eating occasions had significantly lower mean BMI and some evidence indicates that a smaller feeding window (known as Time Restricted Feeding (TRF)) is associated with lower BMI (Chow et al. 2019). Similarly, Laessle et al. (2007) explored whether people with obesity ate differently in a laboratory study in Germany. The results showed that compared to healthier weight participants, those with obesity showed a faster initial rate of eating, took larger spoonfuls and had an overall greater intake of food. Likewise, Kolay et al. (2021) concluded from their systematic review that there was a consistent association between eating faster and higher body weight.

Type of Food

One theory that has been developed is that, although people with obesity may not eat more than people of healthier weight overall, they may eat proportionally more fat. Further, it has been argued that not all calories are equal (Prentice 1995) and that calories from fat may lead to greater weight gain than calories from carbohydrates. To support this theory, one study of 11,500 people in Scotland showed that men consuming the lowest proportion of carbohydrate in their diets were four times more likely to be obese than those consuming the highest proportion of carbohydrate. A similar relationship was also found for women, although the difference was only two- to threefold. Therefore it was concluded that relatively lower carbohydrate consumption is related to lower levels of obesity (Bolton-Smith and Woodward 1994). A similar study in Leeds also provided support for the fat proportion theory of obesity (Blundell and Macdiarmid 1997). This study reported that high fat eaters who derived more than 45 per cent of their energy from fat were 19 times more likely to be obese than those who derived less than 35 per cent of their energy from fat.

Some evidence also indicates that it may not just be fat per se but an intake of processed foods which causes weight gain. In line with this, Rauber et al. (2020) examined the association between the intake of ultra-processed foods and body weight in 6,143 participants aged 19 to 96 years sampled by the UK National Diet and Nutrition Survey (2008–16). Findings indicated that a higher consumption of ultra-processed food is associated with greater BMI and that a 10 per cent increase in the ultra-processed food consumptions was associated with an 18 per cent and 17 per cent increase in the prevalence of obesity in men and women, respectively.

WHAT DOES ALL THIS RESEARCH MEAN?

The evidence for the causes of obesity is therefore complex and can be summarized as follows:

- The twin and adoptee genetic evidence suggests a role for genetics but genetics analysis indicates that this role is small.
- Genetics theories cannot explain changes over time, migration data or social contagion data.
- The prevalence of obesity has increased at a similar rate to decreases in physical activity.
- There is some evidence that those who are living with obesity exercise less and are more sedentary than those of healthier weight.
- The prevalence of obesity has increased at a rate unrelated to the overall decrease in calorie consumption (but measured in the home).
- The relative increase in fat intake is parallel to the increase in obesity.
- There is inconsistent evidence as to whether those who are living with obesity eat more calories than those of healthier weight.
- Those who are living with obesity may eat differently and for different reasons than those of healthier weight.
- Those with obesity may eat proportionally more fat and more ultra-processed foods than those of healthier weight.

Therefore the following points would seem likely:

- Many people have a genetic predisposition to be obese.
- Whether they develop obesity depends upon the obesogenic environment, their level of activity and eating behaviour.

- Obesity is related to lack of exercise.
- Obesity is related to consuming more than the body needs. This might be driven by external eating and emotional eating and might involve eating relatively more fat and ultra-processed food and relatively fewer carbohydrates.

The causes of obesity remain complex and indicate that an integration of all theories is probably the most useful approach.

3 | OBESITY TREATMENT

The three main approaches to obesity treatment are dieting, medication and surgery. Psychology is key to all aspects of obesity treatment, even medication and surgery. These will now be considered.

DIETING

The traditional approach to obesity was a corrective one and early treatment encouraged people with obesity to eat 'normally' by putting them on a diet. Stuart and Davis (1972) developed a behavioural programme for obesity involving monitoring food intake, modifying cues for inappropriate eating and encouraging self-reward for appropriate behaviour, which was widely adopted by hospitals and clinics. In 1958, Stunkard concluded his review of the past 30 years' attempts to promote weight loss in those with obesity with the statement, 'Most obese persons will not stay in treatment for obesity. Of those who stay in treatment, most will not lose weight, and of those who do lose weight, most will regain it.'

The failure of traditional treatment packages for obesity resulted in psychologists, nutritionists, dieticians and endocrinologists taking a more multidimensional approach to obesity treatment. This involves a combination of the behaviour change strategies described in Chapter 7 together with theories of eating behaviour described in Chapter 4 alongside the nutritional and dietician skills and knowledge of those working with people who are trying to lose weight. For example, modern-day weight loss programmes often include self-monitoring, reinforcement, information, exercise, cognitive restructuring, motivational interviewing, attitude change and relapse prevention and encourage people with obesity to eat less than they do *usually* rather than encouraging them to eat less than those of a healthier weight. Many people also try to diet on their own without a formal programme. For example, studies indicate that about 42 per cent of the general population report trying to lose weight in the past year, that about 23 per cent report trying to maintain weight loss in the past year and about 70 per cent report having ever dieted to lose weight (Santos et al. 2017). This large-scale international study also explored the many different ways that people use to try to lose weight and identified 37 weight loss strategies, the most common being eating more fruit and vegetables, selecting food more consciously, eating soup and self weighing (Santos et al. 2017). Further, the researchers also identified 12 motivations, of which the most common were to improve well-being, to improve health and prevent disease and to improve fitness and appearance. At its essence, a diet is anything that suggests that you eat less than you usually would and impose some level of control over your eating in order to lose weight. Research has explored dieting in terms of its success and the possible psychological and physical consequences.

The Success of Dieting

The aim of dieting is to eat less and lose weight and evidence indicates that about 60 per cent of people who diet lose weight in the first six months. This is increased to about 70 per cent, with some form of sustained follow-up from a health professional. A review of the evidence by NICE indicated that by one year, those who had received best case behavioural management from either public sector or private sector weight management behaviour change services such as the NHS, Weight Watchers or Slimming World showed an average weight loss of 2.22 kg (Hartmann-Boyce et al. 2014). Similarly, a review of those interventions focusing on food intake and physical activity showed an average of 1.56 kg less weight regain by one year compared to controls (Dombrowski et al. 2014). In addition, a trial of those referred to a commercial weight loss company through the NHS indicated that while two-thirds lost less than 5 per cent of their body weight, one third lost more than 5 per cent after at least starting a 12-week course (Ahern et al. 2011). Even though weight losses can seem small following dieting attempts, evidence indicates that when people are overweight, even 10 per cent weight loss causes a dramatic reduction in the risk of heart disease and stroke, a reversal of Type 2 diabetes so that a person can start to regulate their own blood sugars again and a reduction in the risk of weight-related cancers such as breast cancer and endometrial cancer in women (Wing et al. 1987; Aucott 2008; Blackburn 1995). Weight loss can also improve a person's daily physical health through the reduction of symptoms such as breathlessness, back and knee pain and the susceptibility to minor infections. Losing weight can also lead to improved mood and a reduction in anxiety and depression and those who lose weight also report increases in self-confidence and body image, although this can sometimes take time as people need to internalize their new body size and sometimes report buying clothes that are too large while they learn to come to terms with their body shape (Ogden and Hills 2008; Epiphaniou and Ogden 2010).

There is always variation around these figures, however, with some people losing more weight and some losing less. In addition, research indicates that the majority of people show weight regain by 5 years follow-up. For example, a systematic review of 92 studies for the treatment of obesity concluded that the majority of the studies demonstrated weight regain either during treatment or post intervention (NHS Centre for Reviews and Dissemination 1997). Further, Fabricatore and Wadden (2006) argued that the weight losses achieved with non-surgical approaches 'have remained virtually unchanged over the past 20 years' and in real terms, between 90 percent and 95 per cent of those who lose weight, regain it within several years (Jeffrey et al. 2000).

Dieting can therefore result in weight loss and health benefits. But it can also do harm in terms of both physical and psychological consequences.

The Consequences of Dieting

Some research suggests that having periods of time in your life when you weigh less, even if this weight is regained, may be healthier in the same way that stopping smoking for the odd month or even year gives the lungs time to recover (Blackburn 1995). In contrast, other research indicates that yo-yo dieting or weight cycling (i.e. showing large fluctuations in weight) may be harmful – even more harmful than remaining at a more stable higher weight (Lissner et al. 1991). This is because when a person loses weight, they often lose muscle and fat, but when they put it back on, they regain proportionally more fat, making them not only heavier but fatter over time. In turn this has a negative impact on their cardiovascular health, can add to fatty liver disease and exacerbates their risk of diabetes (Hamm et al. 1989).

Dieting may also have negative psychological consequences. For example, Wadden et al. (1986) reported that dieting resulted in increased depression in a group of obese patients and Loro and Orleans (1981) indicated that obese dieters report episodes of bingeing precipitated by 'anxiety, frustration, depression and other unpleasant emotions'. This suggests that the obese respond to dieting in the same way as the non-obese, with lowered mood and episodes of overeating, both of which are detrimental to attempts at weight loss. The obese are encouraged to impose a cognitive limit on their food intake, which introduces a sense of denial, guilt and the inevitable response of overeating. Consequently any weight loss is precluded by episodes of overeating, which are a response to the many cognitive and emotional changes that occur during dieting (see Chapter 4 for a discussion of the consequences of dieting).

Restraint theory (see Chapter 4) suggests that dieting has negative consequences, and yet the treatment of obesity recommends dieting as a solution. This paradox can be summarized as follows:

- Obesity is a physical health risk, but dieting may promote yo-yo dieting which is also detrimental to health.
- Obesity treatment aims to reduce food intake, but dieting can promote overeating.

- The obese may suffer psychologically from the social pressures to be thin, but failed attempts to diet may leave them depressed, feeling a failure and out of control. For those few who do succeed in their attempts at weight loss, Wooley and Wooley (1984: 187) suggest that they 'are in fact condemned to a life of weight obsession, semi-starvation and all the symptoms produced by chronic hunger. . . and seem precariously close to developing a frank eating disorder'.

In Summary

The most common treatment of obesity involves some form of dieting and an attempt to eat less than usual. If successful, dieting can lead to physical and psychological benefits. Diets often fail, however, particularly in the longer term which can be detrimental to an individual's physical and psychological health.

MEDICATION

When dieting alone has failed, people who are overweight or living with obesity can turn to medication and as Hirsch said in 1998, 'Who would not rejoice to find a magic bullet that we could fire into obese people to make them permanently slim and healthy?' (Hirsch 1998). Doctors have been offering weight loss drugs for many years and often used to prescribe amphetamines, which was stopped due to the drug's addictive qualities. Nowadays, drug therapy is only legally available to patients in the UK with a BMI of 30 or more, and government bodies have become increasingly restrictive on the use of anti-obesity drugs. Current recommendations state that drugs should be used only when other approaches have failed, that they should not be prescribed for longer than three months in the first instance and should be stopped if a 10 per cent reduction in weight has not been achieved. Continued drug use beyond this time should be accompanied by review and close monitoring (Kopelman 1999).

There are currently three groups of anti-obesity drugs offered in conjunction with dietary and exercise programmes. Those in the first group work on the central nervous system and suppress appetite. Although there is some evidence for the effectiveness of these drugs, they can also be accompanied by side effects such as nausea, dry mouth and constipation. Recently all of these drugs (e.g. fenfluramine, dexfenfluramine, phentermine and lorcaserin) have been removed from the market due to the risk of heart attacks and lowered mood. The second group of drugs reduce fat absorption. Orlistat is one of these and can cause weight loss in obese subjects. It is, however, accompanied by a range of unpleasant side effects, including liquid stools, an urgent need to go to the toilet and anal leakage, which are particularly apparent following a high fat meal as the fat is blocked from entering the bloodstream. At present there is an over-the-counter version of orlistat which is a lower dose than that prescribed by the doctor but has a similar effect. The third group of drugs is new and show promise. These drugs were originally developed for treating diabetes and increase insulin secretion, thereby increasing sugar metabolism. There are currently two drugs being used and tested in the category called semaglutide and tirzepatide, which seem to reduce food intake and food craving by lowering appetite and slowing down digestion in the stomach. These drugs are also accompanied by unpleasant side effects including nausea, vomiting, diarrhea, abdominal pain and constipation, although so far these seem to be mild. Research has explored the effectiveness of orlistat, semaglutide and tirzepatide and some studies have examined the possible role of psychology in their use.

The Success of Medication

Orlistat has been shown to cause substantial weight loss in obese subjects (Sjostrom et al. 1998; Rossner et al. 2000). Phelps et al. (2021) further evaluated the impact of orlistat and concluded that it reduces BMI by about 2 kg/m^2 compared with placebo. Further, a review of evidence for weight loss and maintenance by non-surgical methods (prior to the development of semaglutide and tirzepatide) concluded that medication combined with behavioural modification, by one year follow-up, resulted in an average weight 1.8 kg greater than a placebo control group (Dombrowski et al. 2014). Over the past few years, evidence for the effectiveness of semaglutide and tirzepatide has been more impressive. For example, Wilding et al. (2021) carried out a double-blinded trial with adults (n = 1961) with a BMI of 30 or more who did not have diabetes, and randomly assigned them to 68 weeks of treatment with either once-weekly subcutaneous semaglutide or placebo, plus lifestyle intervention. The results showed that weekly semaglutide plus lifestyle intervention was associated with a mean reduction of −14.9 per cent body weight at 68 weeks compared to −2.4 per cent for the placebo. Likewise, Jastreboff et al. (2022) carried out a double-blind trial with non-diabetic adults (n = 2539) with a BMI or 30 or more who were randomized to receive once-weekly, subcutaneous tirzepatide at 3 different doses. The results showed that by week 72 the mean change in weight was −15.0 per cent with 5-mg dose, −19.5 per cent with 10-mg dose and −20.9 per cent with 15-mg dose compared to −3.1 per cent with placebo. A recent editorial by Rosen and Ingelfinger (2022) provides an excellent overview of the state of the art medications available for obesity management which concludes 'the "tides" are shifting, and there are now more options for people with obesity to lose weight'.

The Psychology of Medication

While orlistat, semaglitide and tirzepatide reflect a medical approach to the management of obesity, psychology still has a role to play in their effectiveness. Orlistat works by preventing the body from absorbing fat. It therefore causes unpleasant side effects as any fat eaten leaves the body in the form of anal leakage or oily stools. It probably therefore also has a deterrent effect as people start to avoid fatty foods once they experience the side effects. Ogden and Sidhu (2006) carried out a qualitative study exploring patients' experiences of taking orlistat. The results suggested that adherence to the drug was related to being motivated to lose weight by a life event rather than just the daily hassles of being obese. Further, if the unpleasant, highly visual side-effects were regarded as an education into the relationship between fat eaten and body fat, then they helped to change the patient's model of their problem by encouraging a model that emphasized behaviour. When orlistat works, it therefore does so by making people realize that their weight is caused by what they eat rather than just their biological makeup, as simply seeing the fat in their diet come out in such an unpleasant way helps them make the link between fat eaten and fat stored in the body. Such a behavioural model of obesity was then related to behaviour change (Hollywood and Ogden 2010). This is similar to the importance of coherent models described in Chapter 8 with beliefs about causes and solutions being matched. This medical approach to obesity treatment can therefore only work if people manage their food intake at the same time. Unfortunately, people sometimes eat a high fat diet, see the unpleasant consequences and stop taking the drugs rather than changing their diet. Or they use it as a lifestyle drug and choose when to take it according to what kinds of food they are going to eat. Hollywood and Ogden (2016) explored the experiences of those who took orlistat yet gained weight. They interviewed 10 patients and concluded that participants attributed their failed weight loss to mechanisms of the medication and emphasized a medical rather than behavioural model of obesity. They also considered their weight gain to be an inevitable part of their self-identity as a perpetual dieter which illustrated a self-fulfilling prophecy of expecting to fail and therefore failing.

To date, given the recentcy of their development, there is no research exploring the psychology behind the success of either semaglitide and tirzepatide. However, both require adherence to the medication regimen, both are self injected and both can result in some unpleasant side effects such as nausea, vomiting, diarrhea, abdominal pain, and constipation. This brings with it all the beliefs about illness and medication related to adherence discussed in Chapters 8 and 9 and may deter an individual from persisting with their medication. Both also, however, come with fairly substantial weight loss within a fairly short time frame which may well be reinforcing and, in line with theories of successful behaviour change discussed in Chapter 7, could promote weight maintenance in the longer term. Research is therefore needed to explore the longer term impact of these drugs and whether the patient's psychological response to taking them undermines or promotes their effectiveness.

In Summary

Some people living with obesity turn to medication to help them lose weight. There is some evidence for the effectiveness of medication although many obesity drugs are removed from the market due to dangerous side effects. At present there are two types of drugs available which can result in weight loss. Although a medical approach to obesity treatment, research indicates that it involves a strong role for psychology in terms of beliefs about medication, adherence and behaviour change.

SURGERY

Although there are a multitude of different surgical procedures for obesity (Kral 1995), the most popular are the vertical banded bypass, gastric bypass and gastric banding often known as bariatric surgery, metabolic surgery or weight loss surgery (WLS). The surgical management of obesity has been endorsed by expert committees in the USA (Institute of Medicine 1995) and the UK (Garrow 1997) and is recommended for those with a BMI over 40 (or > 35 with complications of obesity), who have not lost weight with dietary or pharmacological interventions, as long as they are made aware of the possible side-effects. Research has explored the success of surgery, the physical and psychological consequences of surgery, variability in outcomes after surgery and the role of psychological support in improving its effectiveness.

The Success of Surgery

Researchers in Sweden have carried out the large-scale Swedish Obese Subjects (SOS) study which explored nearly 1,000 matched pairs of patients who received either surgery or behavioural treatment for their obesity (Torgerson and Sjostrom 2001). The results showed an average weight loss of 28 kg in the surgical group after two years compared to only 0.5 kg in the behavioural group. After eight years the weight loss in the surgical group remained high (average of 20 kg) while the control group had gained an average of 0.7 kg. More recently, comprehensive reviews of the literature indicate that the majority of patients achieve clinically significant weight loss far exceeding that lost through lifestyle interventions alone (Picot et al. 2009; Gloy et al. 2013). In particular, a systematic review of weight loss surgery concluded that the mean percentage excess weight loss (EWL) for the Roux-en-Y gastric bypass was 67 per cent and for the gastric band was 42 per cent at one year. Standard behavioural interventions tend to show EWL of between 5 and 10 per cent by one year (O'Brien et al. 2006). Surgery is therefore currently the most effective method of treating obesity.

The Consequences of Surgery

Bariatric surgery clearly causes weight loss which in turn is associated with a reduction in diabetes and hypertension at two years and at eight years (Gloy et al. 2013; Ghiassi and Morton 2020; Wu et al. 2020). Obesity surgery, however, does not only affect weight. Some research has also explored post-operative changes in aspects of the individual's psychological state such as health status and psychological morbidity and a series of studies have shown significant improvements, particularly in those patients who show sustained weight loss. For example, cross-sectional research has illustrated improved quality of life in surgical patients compared to control subjects (De Zwann et al. 2002; Ogden et al. 2005) which has been supported by studies using either retrospective or longitudinal designs. In particular, in a large-scale follow-up of the SOS patients, Karlsson et al. (1998) reported an improvement in health-related quality of life operationalized in terms of mood disorders, mental well-being, health perceptions and social interaction. Bocchieri et al. (2002) carried out a comprehensive review of much of the literature examining the impact of obesity surgery on psychosocial outcomes and concluded that in general 'the empirical evidence. . . seems to be pointing in a positive direction'. In general, many patients show positive psychological outcomes after surgery such as improved self-identified health status, increased self-esteem, a decrease in the preoccupation with food and a decrease in depressive symptoms (Burgmer et al. 2014; Ogden et al., 2005, 2006a; Strain et al. 2014).

Variability in Outcomes after Surgery

Although the majority of patients show weight loss and maintenance after surgery and show many psychological benefits, this is not the case for all patients. For example, a minority show sub-optimal weight loss or weight regain and some show poorer psychological outcomes post surgery such as binge eating and difficulties with the transfer of addiction particularly to alcohol (King et al. 2017; Courcoulas et al. 2013; Karmali et al. 2013). Research has therefore explored the differences between those who do well after surgery versus those who do not. Some quantitative studies have explored the predictors or poor outcomes after a surgery and suggest a role for grazing, binge eating, lack of physical activity, cognitive function, personality, mental health and alcohol misuse as key contributors to weight regain (Wimmelmann et al. 2014a, 2014b). Qualitative research has also explored possible explanations for the success or failure of surgery. From the patients' perspective, studies indicate that whilst successful surgery was associated with a sense of being more in control of food intake, a reduction in hunger and preoccupation with food, less successful surgery was associated with feeling unprepared and unsupported for the changes required after surgery, a sense that psychological issues remain neglected and a belief that the surgery itself hadn't been effective (Ogden et al. 2006a, 2011). From the surgeon's perspective, Ward and Ogden (2019) concluded that surgeons considered less successful surgery to be related to challenges such as patient psychosocial issues, poor adherence and non-disclosure and limited resources. The surgeons also focused on the notion of 'responsibility' balanced between the patient, themselves and the health care system and all emphasized that they could only know what was disclosed by the patient, and felt that whether they had operated or not they were 'damned one way or the other'.

Psychological Support Pre- and Post-Surgery

Psychology is key to bariatric surgery in several ways. First many people presenting for bariatric surgery have complex psychological issues including depression, anxiety, poor self-esteem and body image, eating disorder symptoms, self-harm, addiction or suicidality (see Busetto et al. 2018 for review). Second, as described above, not all patients show optimal outcomes after surgery which may relate to psychological issues such as binge eating, depression or alcohol use. Third, some patients may develop new psychological problems in response to the surgery, such as grazing or alcohol addiction. As a result of this key role of psychology, several research teams have argued that bariatric patients should be managed by a multi-disciplinary team (MDT) and require psychological support pre- and post-surgery (Sogg et al. 2016). Research evaluating the effectiveness of psychological support is in its early stages but interventions have included lifestyle advice, education, CBT and health psychology input focusing on emotional eating, coping and behaviour change. This research has resulted in national and international guidelines for the provision of psychological support to patients before and after surgery (Ogden et al. 2019). Increasingly, therefore, psychologists are employed to support bariatric patients through the surgical journey.

In Summary

Surgery is the most effective treatment approach for managing obesity and promoting weight loss. Psychology plays a key role in bariatric surgery in terms of the problems faced by bariatric patients, the consequences of surgery and its success. Psychologists are therefore often involved as a core part of the clinical team.

THE SUCCESS STORIES

Losing weight and keeping it off is difficult but some people do show successful weight loss maintenance. Research has taken three different approaches to explore how some people manage to lose weight and keep it off, which is relevant to dieting, medication and surgery.

Approach 1: Qualitative Accounts of Success

Researchers have conducted a series of qualitative studies to explore the accounts of those who have lost weight and kept it off. These stories indicate the kinds of factors associated with success (Ogden and Sidhu 2006; Ogden and Hills 2008; Epiphaniou and Ogden 2010; Greaves et al. 2017).

Life events: Successful weight loss and weight loss maintenance often seem to happen after people have had a life event of some sort. People have called these events many things, such as 'seeing the light', 'an epiphany', 'reaching rock bottom' or 'a tipping point'. For some, this could be a relationship breakdown, a health condition such as a heart attack or the diagnosis of diabetes, a change of job, moving house, reaching a salient milestone such as having a significant birthday or simply going on holiday. These moments can help people to reset their thoughts and behaviours and start to re-establish new patterns.

Recognizing that behaviour is the problem: Many people who are overweight believe in a biological cause of their weight problem, saying, 'It runs in my family', 'I have a slow metabolism', 'It's my hormones' or 'My diabetes makes me overweight'. Although there is some evidence that weight is in part influenced by biology (see section on causes of obesity) this way of thinking does not help behaviour change. Those who show successful weight loss and maintenance tend to hold a more behavioural model of both the cause of their weight problem 'I overeat', and the solution, 'I need to eat less'; their model is coherent and emphasizes behaviour (see Chapter 8 on illness cognitions and coherence).

Disrupting the cost-benefit analysis: Most behaviours are governed by a simple cost-benefit analysis. Successful weight loss seems to occur when the benefits of the old unhealthy habits no longer outweigh the costs. For example, if an individual's marriage breaks up, food no longer needs to be their way to manage a problematic relationship.

Bringing the costs into the here and now: People are very good at future discounting and will ignore future costs in favour of focusing on any benefits in the here and now. For eating, this can be problematic as the benefits of eating are always immediate whereas the costs are always in the months and years to come. Successful dieting is also about changing the timing of these factors.

Investment in success: Weight loss can be extremely hard work as it involves changing habits that have been ingrained for a lifetime. Weight loss maintenance seems more likely to occur after initial weight loss if people recognize and can remember how difficult this initial stage was.

A new identity and the process of reinvention: Successful dieters seem to develop a new identity around being a thinner, healthier person, making it harder for them to regain their lost weight as this would no longer be in line with how they see themselves. For some, this new sense of self can be incorporated into their existing life, but for many it involves a process of reinvention and the establishment of a new way of being.

No more emotional eating: Being overweight can sometimes be the response to emotional eating as food is used for emotional regulation. Successful dieting is sometimes associated with finding alternative coping mechanisms.

A new eating routine: Part of losing weight for the longer term is the establishment of a new healthier routine which can persist onwards rather than just in the shorter term.

Hope: The final factor from the qualitative research that seems to relate to successful weight loss and maintenance is hope. For dieters, this sense of hope can come from hearing other people's success stories, taking full credit for times in their own lives when they have changed their behaviour or monitoring their behaviour to find small signs of change to offer hope that change is possible.

In-depth qualitative accounts of success stories are one approach to discovering the mechanisms behind successful dieting and indicate a number of processes.

Approach 2: Differences Between Those Who have Shown Successful Dieting and Those Who Haven't

The second approach to understanding successful weight loss maintenance has used quantitative methods to assess the characteristics of those who have managed to lose weight and kept it off versus those who have not. Some of this evidence comes from the National Weight Control Registry (NWCR) in the USA which is a database established in 1993 consisting of over 10,000 individuals who have shown more than 30 lbs (13.6 kg) weight loss which has been maintained for more than one year (Thomas et al. 2014; Wing et al. 2008; Wing and Phelan 2005). Research using the NWCR together with other research (e.g. Ogden 2000; Elfhag and Rossner 2005) has identified the following factors.

Profile factors: Successful dieters tend to be older, have dieted for longer and show greater initial weight loss. Some evidence also shows that men are more successful than women although the evidence is mixed.

Behaviour change: Success is also associated with increased physical activity, decreased intake of fat, increased dietary restraint (i.e. dieting efforts), maintaining a consistent diet regimen across the week rather than a more flexible approach to dieting, reaching a self-determined weight goal and eating regular meals throughout the day including breakfast.

Psychological factors: Those who show success often report a significant medical trigger, report a stronger behavioural and psychological model of their weight problem, show self-monitoring of their behaviour, good coping strategies and a sense of control, autonomy and responsibility.

Approach 3: Predicting Successful Dieting Over Time

The final approach to understanding successful dieting has explored the predictors of weight loss maintenance over time. One study used the NWCR data but with a 10-year follow-up period and found that 87 per cent were still maintaining a loss of at least 10 per cent of their initial body weight by this time (Thomas et al. 2014). The authors also found that larger weight losses and a longer duration of weight loss maintenance were related to increased physical activity in maintainers' leisure time, higher levels of dietary restraint, increased self-weighing, decreased intake of fat and a reduced number of episodes of overeating. Stubbs et al. (2011) pooled data across a number of reviews and individual studies and highlighted that successful dieting was associated with having a higher baseline weight, being male, showing early weight loss when part of an intervention, attendance at the weight loss intervention, increased length of treatment, increased social support, self monitoring of behaviours, goal setting, slowing rate of eating and increased physical activity. Similarly, Teixeira et al. (2015) identified factors associated with medium to longer weight control and highlighted the importance of autonomous motivation, self-regulation skills, self-efficacy, self-monitoring and positive body image. Finally, a comprehensive analysis by Hartmann-Boyce et al. (2014a) explored the predictors of weight loss by 12 months and reported key roles for calorie counting, greater contact with a dietician and the use of strategies which involved comparison with others.

Common Factors Associated with Successful Weight Loss and Maintenance

Using the three approaches described above, there are clearly a number of overlapping factors linked to successful dieting. These are shown in Table 13.1.

IN SUMMARY

Obesity is related to several health problems and a number of theories have been developed in an attempt to understand its aetiology. In particular, research has focused on the role of genetics, the obesogenic environment and behaviour. In terms of obesity treatment, the most common approaches are dieting, medication and surgery, all of which involve a key role for psychology. Overall, research indicates that promoting sustained weight loss and maintenance is hard but that the most effective

TABLE 13.1 Common factors explaining successful dieting

Success stories	Differences	Predictors of success
Life events	Life events, medical triggers	
Behavioural model	Reduced medical model	
Hope that things can change	Psychological consequences and motivations	
Disrupting costs and benefits of diet and physical activity	New benefits of being healthy	
Changing the timing of costs and benefits	Goal setting self determined goals	Self weighing, attendance at intervention, goal setting, length of treatment, contact with dietician
Investments made so far	More dieting attempts, initial weight loss	Early weight loss
New eating regiment	Breakfast, healthy eating, reduced fat, consistent routine, physical activity	Calorie counting decreased fat, physical activity
Less emotional eating	Good coping	Self regulation
New identity and reinvention		

SOURCE: Ogden (2018)

approach to date is obesity surgery. Further, research shows that in general successful dieting is linked to a number of profile, behavioural and psychological factors and can be understood using both qualitative and quantitative methods.

BOX 13.1
Less Common Chronic Conditions: Ménière's disease

Ménière's disease (MD) is a non-fatal disease of the inner ear associated with chronic vertigo, hearing loss, tinnitus and pressure or fullness in the ears and can cause severe dizziness and vomiting. The symptoms are intermittent and episodes generally last from 20 minutes to a few hours which means that it is very unpredictable and makes it hard to manage. To date there is no straightforward cure although possible interventions include medication to help with the nausea and anxiety, a low salt diet or diuretics or physical therapy to help with balance issues. From a health psychology perspective, research has addressed the impact of having MD and how people make sense of this condition.

Research indicates that MD has several negative consequences and is linked with anxiety and distress, leading to feelings of disorientation which can severely interrupt daily tasks (Yardley et al. 1992; Yardley 1994; Yardley et al. 2003). Some research, however, has also found evidence of positive change in areas such as interpersonal relationships, lifestyle and general health, and personal development (Stephens et al. 2007). Dibb (2009) used a longitudinal design to explore positive change in those with MD in more depth. Measures of disease severity, self-esteem, perceived control, optimism and social comparison variables were completed at baseline and at 10-month follow-up and a measure of Post-traumatic Growth was completed at follow up only. The results indicated that people with MD perceived positive change from their condition particularly in the domains of 'appreciation of life', 'relating to others', 'personal strength', 'new possibilities' and 'spiritual change'. The results also showed that social comparison was related to positive change and that both 'social comparison for information', whereby people compared themselves with others to gain information and 'downward positive comparison', whereby people make comparisons with those worse off than them, predicted a stronger sense of growth in 'personal strength.'

These findings illustrate the role of sense making in this less common chronic condition and find reflection in theories such as cognitive adaptation theory and the self regulatory model described in Chapter 8. They also illustrate how this condition can have a negative impact on aspects of health status as described in Chapter 14. Finally, this research also illustrates a role for the response shift also described in Chapter 14.

4 | CORONARY HEART DISEASE (CHD)

WHAT IS CORONARY HEART DISEASE? (CHD)

Cardiovascular diseases (CVDs) are a group of disorders of the heart and blood vessels. They include coronary heart disease (CHD; disease of the blood vessels supplying the heart muscle); cerebrovascular disease (disease of the blood vessels supplying the brain); peripheral arterial disease (disease of blood vessels supplying the arms and legs); deep vein thrombosis and pulmonary embolism (blood clots in the leg veins, which can dislodge and move to the heart and lungs).

Most research in health psychology has focused on CHD and cerebrovascular disease. CHD includes angina, acute myocardial infarction (AMI – heart attack) and sudden cardiac death. All these forms of CHD are caused by atherosclerosis which involves a narrowing of the arteries due to fatty deposits which obstruct the flow of blood. Angina is a powerful pain in the chest, which sometimes radiates down the left arm. It develops when blood flow to the coronary arteries is restricted to such an extent that the heart muscle is starved of oxygen. An AMI occurs when blood flow is restricted below a threshold level and some heart tissue is destroyed. It also seems to happen when a blood clot has further restricted blood flow to the heart. Sudden cardiac death typically occurs in patients who have already suffered damage to the heart through previous AMIs although it can occur in patients who previously seemed to have healthy arteries. In contrast, cerebrovascular disease causes stroke due to a blockage preventing blood from flowing to the brain.

THE PREVALENCE OF CVD

In 2017, CVD was the highest cause of death globally. In 2015, it was estimated that 31 per cent of all global deaths were due to CVD (about 17.7 million people) and, of these deaths, 7.4 million were due to coronary heart disease (CHD) and 6.7 million were due to stroke. CHD is responsible for 43 per cent of deaths in men across Europe and 54 per cent of deaths in women (Allender et al. 2008a, 2008b). In the UK, in 2008 CHD was responsible for 35 per cent of deaths in men and 34 per cent of deaths in women (Allender et al. 2008a). CHD is the main cause of premature death in the UK (i.e. under 75 years) and worldwide it is estimated that the highest death rates are in China, India and Russia. Deaths from CHD have declined in recent years in North America and across Europe mainly due to the decline in smoking and other lifestyle factors. The highest death rates from CHD are found in men and women in the manual classes, and men and women of Asian origin. In middle age, the death rate is up to five times higher for men than for women; this evens out, however, in old age when CHD is the leading cause of death for both men and women. In the UK about 150,000 people each year survive the acute stage of MI with women showing poorer recovery than men in terms of both mood and activity limitations. Deaths rates from CHD world wide in 2015 are shown in Figure 13.10.

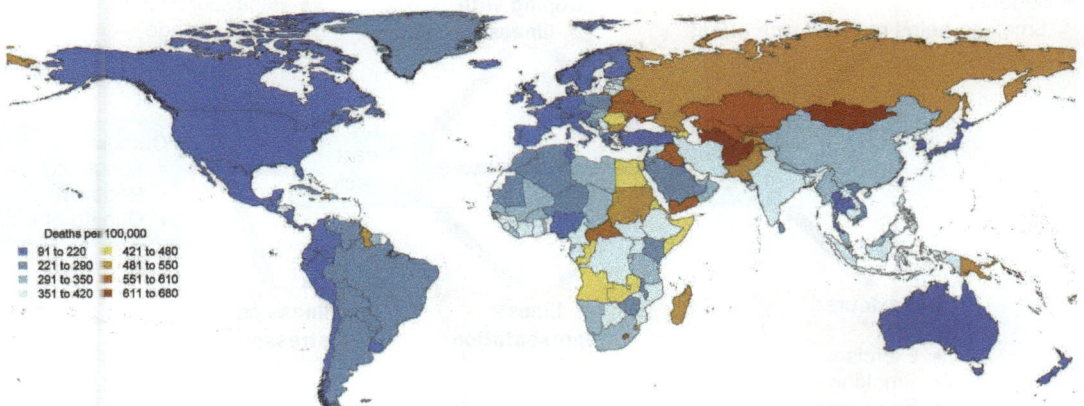

Figure 13.10 Worldwide deaths from CHD (2015)

WHO (2015); Roth et al. (2018)

For the purpose of this chapter, the term CHD will be used to cover CHD and cerebrovascular disease as this is the focus on most research in health psychology and addresses those health problems which show the strongest role for psychological factors (i.e. angina, heart attack, sudden cardiac death, stroke).

5 | THE ROLE OF PSYCHOLOGY IN THE STUDY OF CHD

CHD is another example of chronic illness which shows a strong role for a range of psychological factors. The potential role of psychology in CHD is shown in Figure 13.11.

The remainder of this chapter examines the risk factors for CHD, beliefs about CHD, the psychological impact of CHD, rehabilitation and the modification of risk factors, and the predictors of patient health outcomes.

RISK FACTORS FOR CHD

Many risk factors for CHD have been identified, such as educational status, social mobility, social class, age, gender, stress reactivity, family history, ethnicity, smoking, diet, obesity, sedentary lifestyle, perceived work stress and personality. Details of many of these factors can be found in Chapters 3, 4, 5, 10 and 13. Key modifiable risk factors are as follows:

1 *Smoking* One in four deaths from CHD is thought to be caused by smoking. Smoking more than 20 cigarettes a day increases the risk of CHD in middle age threefold. In addition, stopping smoking can halve the risk of another heart attack in those who have already had one. Smoking cessation is discussed in Chapter 3.

2 *Diet.* Diet, in particular cholesterol levels, has also been implicated in CHD. It has been suggested that the 20 per cent of a population with the highest cholesterol levels are three times more likely to die of heart disease than the 20 per cent with the lowest levels. Cholesterol levels may be determined by the amount of saturated fat consumed (derived mainly from animal fats). Cholesterol reduction

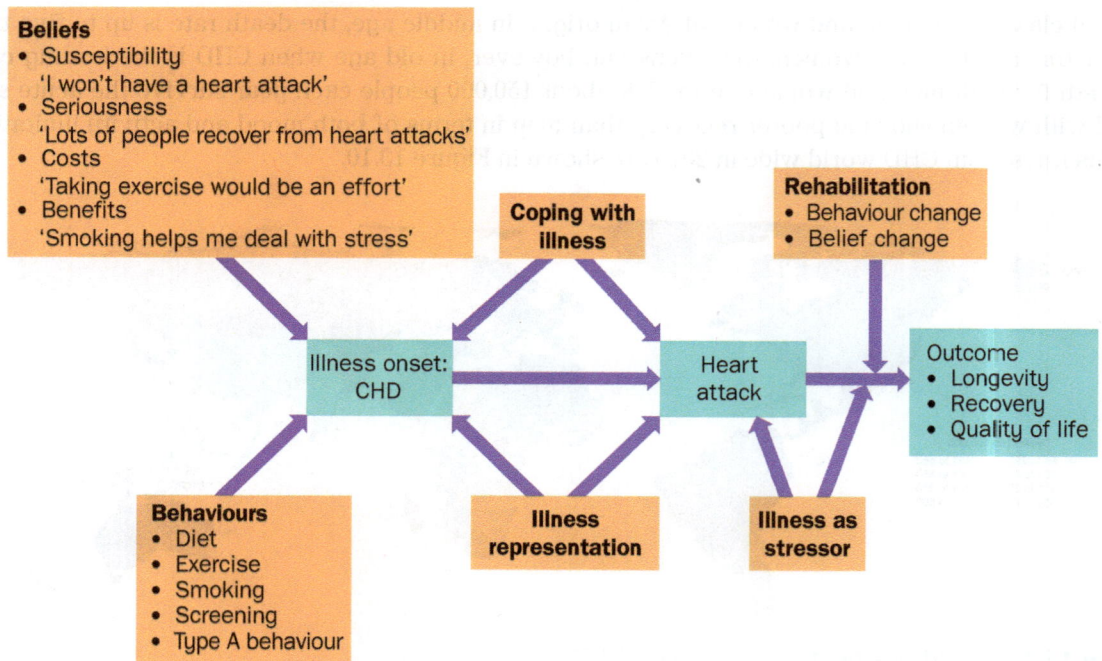

Figure 13.11 The potential role of psychology in CHD

can be achieved through a reduction in total fats and saturated fats, an increase in polyunsaturated fats and an increase in dietary fibre. Dietary change is discussed in Chapters 4, 7 and earlier in this chapter in the Obesity section.

3 *Obesity.* Obesity is a clear risk factor for CHD and stroke. This is in part through high blood pressure and cholesterol, which has generated a debate about whether healthy obesity exists if those who are obese take their medication to reduce these factors. The research indicates, however, that even if these factors are medically managed and levels normalized, obesity remains an independent risk factor for CHD and stroke (Hubert et al. 1983; Ortega et al. 2018). In particular, a large-scale review and meta analysis showed that metabolically healthy obese patients had higher risk of CHD and all-cause mortality than metabolically healthy normal weight patients (Ortega et al. 2018). This indicates that weight per se is a risk factor for CHD. This review also showed that metabolically healthy obese patients had a lower risk of CHD than metabolically unhealthy obese patients. This was mostly explained by their levels of fitness (see Chapter 5 for the benefits of exercise).

4 *High blood pressure.* High blood pressure is also a risk factor for CHD – the higher the blood pressure, the greater the risk. It has been suggested that a 10 mmHg decrease in a population's average blood pressure could reduce the mortality attributable to heart disease by 30 per cent. Blood pressure appears to be related to a multitude of factors such as genetics, obesity, alcohol intake and salt consumption. Some research also points to a role for caffeine intake (see Chapter 3).

5 *Type A behaviour and hostility.* Type A behaviour and its associated characteristic, hostility, are probably the most extensively studied risk factor for CHD (see Chapter 10 for details). Support for a relationship between type A behaviour and CHD is mixed (e.g. Johnston et al. 1987) with more recent research focusing on hostility, which has been shown to predict stress reactivity and to be linked to the development of CHD (e.g. Miller et al. 1996; Frederickson et al. 2000).

6 *Stress.* Stress has also been studied extensively as a predictor of CHD and research has shown links between stress reactivity and CHD, life events and CHD, and job stress and CHD (see Chapters 10 and 12). Stress management is used to reduce stress in people already diagnosed with CHD.

BELIEFS ABOUT CHD

Chapter 8 described the kinds of beliefs that people have about their illness and explored how these beliefs may influence the development and progression of the disease. Some research has specifically examined the beliefs that people have about CHD with a particular focus on beliefs about causes. For example, Stewart et al. (2016) explored beliefs about MI and stroke in older adults and found that many attributed their health problems to old age. They also found that a greater endorsement of old age as the cause predicted fewer lifestyle changes, more visits to the doctor and a greater risk of hospitalization over the next 3 years. Likewise, French et al. (2005a) explored people's beliefs about MI in 12 patients who had had an MI. The results showed that, while people were aware of many possible causes of MI, they tended to focus on a single cause for their MI which was often related to their symptoms. This was driven by a need to understand why they had had their MI 'now' which was further motivated by a desire not to blame themselves or others while at the same time trying to assert control over having another MI in the future. Gudmundsdottir et al. (2001) also explored people's beliefs about CHD but examined the beliefs of people who had had an MI in the past year. Using a longitudinal design they assessed the patients' beliefs within 72 hours of admission into hospital and interviewed the patients about the causes of their MI. Patients were then followed up three times over the next year. The results showed that the most common causes derived from all methods were 'smoking', 'stress', 'it's in the family', 'working' and 'eating fatty foods'. The results also showed some changes over time, with patients being less likely to blame their behaviour and/or personality as time went on. Beliefs about CHD can also impact upon others. Thomson et al. (2020) followed up 40 patient-caregiver dyads and reported that patient's perceptions of timeline and illness concerns at baseline predicted poorer mental health in their care giver at 6 months follow up.

People therefore have beliefs about CHD which might influence their subsequent risky behaviour and reflect a process of adjustment once they have become ill.

THE PSYCHOLOGICAL IMPACT OF CHD

Research has addressed the psychological impact of having an MI in terms of anxiety and depression, post-traumatic stress disorder (PTSD) and finding meaning.

Anxiety and Depression

Negative mood is very common in patients with CHD, particularly after a heart attack or stroke (Meijer et al. 2011). For example, Lane et al. (2002) used a longitudinal design to assess changes in depression and anxiety immediately post-MI, 2–15 days post-MI and after 4 and 12 months. The results showed that during hospitalization 30.9 per cent of patients reported elevated depression scores and 26.1 per cent reported elevated anxiety scores. The results also indicated that this increase in psychological morbidity persisted over the year of study. Holahan et al. (2006) explored gender and ethnic group differences in depressive symptoms in cardiac patients from the USA and reported that depressive symptoms were higher in women than men and in Hispanic patients compared to non-Hispanic white patients. The results also showed that higher levels of depression were predicted by greater physical and role limitations and less social support. Similarly, Gum et al. (2006) concluded that depressive symptoms 3 months after having a stroke were predicted by baseline levels of hopeful thinking about one's ability to fulfil one's own goals in the future. Further, Boersma et al. (2005) concluded from their study of patients post-MI that goal disturbance predicted both depression and health-related quality of life. Some research has also explored whether such changes in psychological morbidity can be modified. For example, Johnston et al. (1999b) evaluated the impact of nurse counsellor-led cardiac counselling compared to normal care. The study used a randomized design with a one-year follow-up and patients and their partners were recruited within 72 hours of the patients' first MI. The results showed that although patients did not show particularly raised levels of anxiety and depression while still in hospital, those who did not receive counselling showed an increase in these factors following discharge. Counselling seemed to minimize this increase. In contrast to the patients, the partners did show very high levels of anxiety and depression while the patients were still in hospital. This dropped to normal levels in those who received counselling.

PTSD

Research has also explored the prevalence and predictors of PTSD following either stroke or MI and indicates rates of about 17 per cent, with people experiencing intrusive thoughts, elevated levels of arousal, psychological numbing and avoidance of reminders of the trauma (e.g. Sheldrick et al. 2006; Bluvstein et al. 2013). Research also indicates that symptoms of PTSD vary over time and are strongly predicted and correlated with illness cognitions, particularly identity, time line, consequences and emotional representations (Sheldrick et al. 2006). In addition, such symptoms are associated with a history of psychological problems and dysfunctional coping strategies. Interestingly, Bluvstein et al. (2013) found that 71.2 per cent of their sample reported post-traumatic growth suggesting that although a heart attack or stroke may lead to negative mood states such as depression, anxiety or PTSD, some people find benefit in their condition.

Finding Meaning

Bury (1982) argued that illness can be seen as a form of biographical disruption which requires people to question 'what is going on here?' and results in a sense of uncertainty. Radley (1984, 1989) has drawn upon this perspective to explore how people adjust and respond to CHD. In particular, Radley argues that patients diagnosed with CHD try to resolve the dual demands of symptoms and society. He suggests that people with a chronic illness such as CHD need to establish a new identity as someone who has been ill but can be well again. This need occurs against a backdrop of family and friends who are worried about their health and often results in the ill person persistently acting in a 'healthy way' as a means to communicate that things are 'back to normal'. This approach finds reflection in theories of coping and the re-establishment of equilibrium described in Chapter 8. Research also indicates that finding meaning relates to health outcomes. For example, Vos (2021) carried out a systematic review and concluded that having concerns about meaning after CVD events (e.g. MI) was related to lower motivation to make lifestyle changes, more psychological stress, lower quality of life, worse physical well-being and increased risk of further CVD events.

6 | REHABILITATION FOR PATIENTS WITH CHD

Psychology also plays a role in the rehabilitation of individuals who have been diagnosed with CHD in terms of angina, stroke, atherosclerosis or heart attack. Rehabilitation programmes use a range of techniques including health education, relaxation training and counselling, and have been developed to encourage CHD sufferers to modify their risk factors (see Chapter 7 for a description of these techniques). Research has explored predictors of uptake of rehabilitation programmes and whether they can modify factors such as exercise, type A behaviour, general lifestyle factors, illness cognitions and stress.

PREDICTING UPTAKE OF REHABILITATION

Although MI is the primary cause of premature mortality in many western countries, over 60 per cent of patients will survive their MI. Furthermore, if risk factors can be modified then the likelihood of a further MI is greatly reduced. Rehabilitation programmes are therefore designed to reduce these risk factors. Despite the benefits of rehabilitation, however, many patients fail to attend either some or all of the classes. For example, in a systematic review of the literature, attendance rates across 15 studies varied from 13 to 74 per cent, although what constituted 'attendance' also varied from missing a few sessions to missing all sessions (Cooper et al. 2002). So why do people not turn up if rehabilitation can be effective? Cooper et al. (2002) explored the factors that predicted non-attendance in 15 studies of cardiac rehabilitation involving patients from Europe, the USA, Canada and New Zealand, and concluded that non-attenders were more likely to be older, to have lower income and greater deprivation, to deny the severity of their illness, to be less likely to believe that they can influence the outcome of their illness and to be less likely to perceive that their doctor recommends rehabilitation. Perceived lack of time is also considered a key barrier to attendance (Bennett et al. 2019) and women are less likely to be referred for rehabilitation than men, as are the elderly (Colella et al. 2015). Further, a qualitative study of South Asians post-MI indicated that their motivation to change comes from wanting to do it for others rather than for themselves (Dilla et al. 2020).

MODIFYING RISK FACTORS

Rehabilitation programmes encourage the modification of risk factors to improve the patient's quality of life and to reduce their risk of further cardiac events.

Exercise

Most rehabilitation programmes emphasize the restoration of physical functioning through exercise, with the assumption that physical recovery will in turn promote psychological and social recovery. Meta-analyses of these exercise-based programmes have suggested that they may have favourable effects on cardiovascular mortality and hospital admissions (e.g. Anderson et al. 2016). Whether these exercise-based programmes influence risk factors other than exercise, such as smoking, diet and type A behaviour, is questionable.

Type A Behaviour

The Recurrent Coronary Prevention project was developed by Friedman et al. (1986) in an attempt to modify type A behaviour. This programme was based on the following questions: can type A behaviour be modified? If so, can such modification reduce the chances of a recurrence of a heart attack? The study involved 1,000 subjects and a five-year intervention. Subjects had all suffered a heart attack and were allocated to one of three groups: cardiology counselling, type A behaviour modification or no treatment. Type A behaviour modification involved discussions of the beliefs and values of type A, discussing methods of reducing work demands, relaxation and education about changing the cognitive framework of the individuals. At 5 years, the results showed that the type A modification group had a reduced recurrence of heart attacks, suggesting that not only can type A behaviour be modified but that, when modified, there may be a reduction of reinfarction. However, the relationship between type A behaviour and CHD is still controversial, with recent discussions suggesting that type A may at times be protective against CHD.

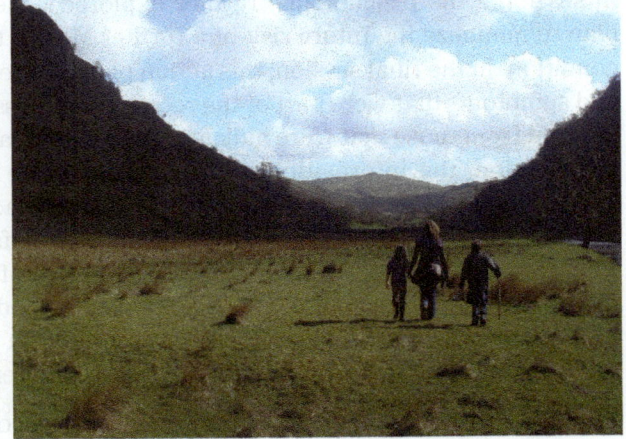

Exercise is a standard part of rehabilitation after a heart attack

General Lifestyle Factors

Rehabilitation programmes have been developed which focus on modifying other risk factors such as smoking and diet. For example, van Elderen et al. (1994) developed a health education and counselling programme for patients with cardiovascular disease after hospitalization, with weekly follow-ups by telephone. This was a small-scale study, but the results showed that after 2 months the patients who had received health education and counselling reported a greater increase in physical activity and a greater decrease in unhealthy eating habits. Further, this improvement was greater in those whose partners had also participated in the programme. Many of these improvements were maintained by 12 months.

More recently, however, van Elderen and Dusseldorp (2001) reported results from a similar study which produced more contradictory results. They explored the relative impact of providing health education, psychological input, standard medical care and physical training to patients with CHD and their partners after discharge from hospital. Overall, all patients improved their lifestyle during the first 3 months and showed extra improvement in their eating habits over the next 9 months. However, by one-year follow-up many patients had increased their smoking again and returned to their sedentary lifestyles. In terms of the relative effects of the different forms of intervention, the results were more complex than the authors' earlier work. Although health education and the psychological intervention had an improved impact on eating habits over standard medical care and physical training, some changes in lifestyle were more pronounced in the patients who had only received the latter. For example, receiving health education and psychological intervention seemed to make it more difficult to quit a sedentary lifestyle, and receiving health education seemed to make it more difficult to stop smoking. Therefore, although some work supports the addition of health education and counselling to rehabilitation programmes, at times this may have a cost. In 2010, Huttunen-Lenz et al. carried out a meta-analysis of psychoeducational interventions focusing on smoking cessation for CHD patients. Their analysis identified 14 studies and the results showed that although the interventions had no significant impact on mortality, they did significantly increase smoking cessation rates. Although research also indicates that depression may act as a barrier to smoking cessation post heart attack (Doyle et al. 2014).

Illness Cognitions

Research illustrates that patients' beliefs about their MI may relate to health outcomes in terms of attendance at rehabilitation, return to work and adjustment (see Chapter 8 for illness cognitions and outcomes). In line with this, Petrie et al. (2002) developed an intervention designed to change illness cognitions and explored the subsequent impact upon a range of patient outcomes. The intervention consisted of three sessions of about 40 minutes with a psychologist and was designed to address and change patients' beliefs about their MI. For session 1 the psychologist gave an explanation about the nature of an MI in terms of its symptoms and explored patients' beliefs about the causes of the MI. In session 2 the psychologist further explored beliefs about causes, helped the patient to develop a plan to minimize the future risk of a further MI and tried to increase patient control beliefs about their condition. In the final session, this action plan was reviewed, concerns about medication were explored and symptoms that were part of the recovery process such as breathlessness upon exercise were distinguished from those that were indicative of further pathology such as severe chest pain. Throughout the intervention, the information and discussion were targeted to the specific beliefs and concerns of the patient. The results showed that patients who had received the intervention reported more positive views about their MI at follow-up in terms of beliefs about consequences, time line, control/cure and symptom distress (see Chapter 8 for a description of these dimensions). In addition, they reported that they were better prepared to leave hospital, returned to work at a faster rate and reported a lower rate of angina symptoms. No differences were found in rehabilitation attendance. The intervention therefore seemed to change cognitions and improve patients' functional outcome after MI.

In a similar vein, Janssen et al. (2013) carried out a study with 158 cardiac patients to explore changes in illness cognitions during cardiac rehabilitation. The results showed that all illness cognitions (apart from timeline and personal control) changed over the course of rehabilitation and that patients generally viewed their illness as less threatening. In addition, the results showed that improved quality of life was related to a perception of fewer emotional consequences of the illness, a better understanding of the illness and attributing fewer symptoms to the illness.

Stress Management

Stress management involves teaching individuals about the theories of stress, encouraging them to be aware of the factors that can trigger stress, and teaching them a range of strategies to reduce stress, such as 'self-talk', relaxation techniques and general life management approaches, such as time management and problem-solving. Stress management has been used successfully to reduce some of the risk factors for CHD, including raised blood pressure (Johnston et al. 1993), blood cholesterol (Gill et al. 1985) and type A behaviour (Roskies et al. 1986). Further, some studies also indicate that it can reduce angina, which is highly predictive of heart attack and/or death (Gallacher et al. 1997; Bundy et al. 1998). Recently there has also been an interest in the use of other psychological interventions. For example, Parswani et al. (2013) delivered a mindfulness-based stress reduction programme to men with CHD and reported a reduction in anxiety, depression, perceived stress, blood pressure and BMI, which were maintained by 3 months follow-up. Further, Nourisaeed et al. (2021) compared Cognitive Behavioural Therapy (CBT) and Dialectical Behavioural Therapy (DBT) on perceived stress and coping skills in patients after MI and reported that DBT was more effective in improving emotion-focused coping than CBT.

Research has therefore explored ways to modify the risk factors for CHD and has specifically focused on behaviour, cognitions and stress.

PREDICTING PATIENT HEALTH OUTCOMES

Research has also explored the role of psychological factors in predicting patient health outcomes with a focus on quality of life and level of functioning, and mortality.

Predicting Quality of Life and Level of Functioning

Research exploring the predictors of quality of life and level of functioning in patients with CHD has focused on patient demographics, perceptions of control, goal disturbance, depression, social support and illness cognitions.

Patient Demographics

Research shows that a number of patient demographics are associated with quality of life post-MI. For example, Pocock et al. (2021) reported that poorer quality of life 1–3 years post-MI (n = 9000) was associated with having chronic comorbidities (e.g. angina, stroke), being female, older age, having obesity, smoking and having spent fewer years in education. Similarly, Kang et al. (2021) reported that poorer quality of life in the acute phase of MI was related to lower educational level, poorer financial status, diabetes, history of CVD and poorer mental health as measured by the DASS 21.

Perceptions of Control

Research shows a consistent link between baseline levels of perceived control and recovery from stroke in terms of level of functioning (e.g. Johnston et al. 2004; Bonetti and Johnston 2008). Johnston et al. (2006) developed a workbook-based intervention to change perceptions of control in patients who had just had a stroke and showed that at 6 months follow-up those receiving the intervention showed better disability recovery than those in the control group. In a similar vein, Chan et al. (2006) explored the role of resilience in predicting outcomes in CHD patients in Hong Kong. Resilience was defined as closely aligned to perceived control and was a composite measure including optimism, perceived control and self-esteem. The results showed that those high in resilience showed better outcomes after an 8-week rehabilitation programme in terms of lower cholesterol, higher physical and mental health status and a better performance on a 6 -minute walk test. In addition, personal resilience was also predictive of greater post-traumatic growth (see Chapter 8).

Goal Disturbance

MI and stroke often result in a reduction in physical functioning through impaired speech or movement. They can also trigger a sense of goal disturbance. According to goal theory (Carver and Scheier 1999) behaviour is driven by a hierarchy of goals that make life feel meaningful. Lower-order goals could involve eating, getting to work or getting enough sleep, while higher-order goals include 'supporting others' or 'ensuring my safety'. It has been argued that a major health event such as a stroke or MI can disturb an individual's usual means of attaining their goals, which in turn can challenge how an individual sees themselves or their future (e.g. Kuijer and De Ridder 2003). In terms of CHD, research indicates that goal disturbance at baseline predicts both depression and lowered health-related quality of life at follow-up (Boersma et al. 2005; Joekes et al. 2007).

Depression

Depression post-MI is quite common. Although for many patients levels of depressive symptoms reduce over time, research indicates a link between depression at baseline and health-related quality of life by 4 months follow-up (e.g. Lane et al. 2000).

Social Support

Research also shows a role for social support in predicting patient quality of life post-MI, although perceived rather than actual support is more important (e.g. Bosworth et al. 2001). Not all social support is positive, however, and although 'active engagement' by partners of those who have had an MI may predict better outcomes, 'over-protection' can result in decreased levels of physical functioning over time (Joekes et al. 2007).

Illness Cognitions

Research shows a role for beliefs in predicting recovery from MI and quality of life as measured by return to work and general social and occupational functioning. In particular, studies indicate that those with more negative beliefs about their work capacity (Maeland and Havik 1987), a greater perception of helplessness towards future MIs (called 'cardiac invalidism'; Riegel 1993) and beliefs that their MI has more serious consequences and will last a longer time at baseline (Petrie et al. 1996) show poorer outcomes. Further, beliefs that the illness can be controlled or cured at baseline predict attendance at rehabilitation classes which itself predicts better outcomes (Petrie et al. 1996) (see Chapter 8 for further details).

Predicting Mortality

Research has explored the predictors of survival or mortality in patients with CHD. There are many biological predictors including cholesterol levels, blood pressure, previous MIs, long-term health history and a number of biological markers. The results, however, also show a role for more psychological factors such as health-related behaviours, depression and anxiety and quality of life.

Health Behaviours

Research indicates that the behaviours which predict CHD onset also predict mortality. In addition, other health conditions, which are also related to health-related behaviours, also predict CHD mortality. For example, large-scale cohort studies and systematic reviews indicate that mortality post-MI or stroke is predicted by smoking, obesity and diabetes (Panagiotakos et al. 2003; Pearte et al. 2006; Prugger et al. 2008). Research also shows a similar pattern for predicting mortality after coronary artery bypass surgery (e.g. Ketonen et al. 2008). A recent meta-analysis showed a role for sleep duration with both low and long sleep duration being predictive of cardiovascular mortality (Cappuccio et al. 2011), although the mechanism of this association is less clear.

Depression and Anxiety

Research indicates that depression post-MI and stroke is common and can relate to an individual's subsequent quality of life (see p. 420). Research, however, also indicates that depression predicts mortality. Barth et al. (2004) carried out a meta-analysis of 20 studies and reported that although depression had no impact on mortality by 6 months, by 2 years those with clinical depression were twice as likely to have died. Similar results have been found when follow-up times were extended to 12 years, with depression being predictive of mortality in both men and women (Ahto et al. 2007). Likewise, anxiety is also common post MI and a meta-analysis by Wen et al. (2021) concluded that there was strong evidence that increased anxiety post-MI was associated with poorer prognosis in terms of both major adverse cardiac events and mortality. In particular, MI patients with anxiety had a 23 per cent increased risk of short-term complications and a 27 per cent increased risk of poorer long-term prognosis compared to those without anxiety.

Quality of Life

Quality of life can be considered an outcome post-MI and is predicted by a number of factors such as perceptions of control, depression, anxiety and social support as described above. Quality of life itself, however, can also be a predictor of health outcomes. Pocock et al. (2021) carried out a prospective study with almost 9000 patients from 25 countries across four continents 1–3 years post-MI. The results showed that, after adjustment for a wide range of patient factors, a lower health related quality of life score at enrolment was associated with a higher subsequent risk of all-cause death, of a major CV event and more hospitalizations over the next 2 years.

IN SUMMARY

CHD is a common cause of death across the Global South and North. It illustrates the role of psychology in illness in terms of the risk factors for its onset, beliefs people have about CHD, the psychological consequences of a diagnosis, rehabilitation, the modification of risk factors and the predictors of quality of life and mortality.

BOX 13.2
Less Common Chronic Conditions: Mild Traumatic Brain Injury (mTBI)

Mild traumatic brain injury (mTBI) lies at the lower end of the traumatic brain injury spectrum and is often used synonymously with the term 'concussion'. It accounts for about 70–90 per cent of all treated brain injuries and although most people show good recovery within 3 months about 5 per cent present with chronic symptoms. For this minority, symptoms can last for up to a year post-trauma and some still show symptoms up to 10 years and it has been questioned whether it should be called 'mild'. The range of physical, cognitive, emotional or behavioural changes reported following mTBI are known as post-concussive symptoms (PCS) and can include: headache, dizziness, anxiety, depression, fatigue, memory problems, irritability and noise sensitivity (Gouvier et al. 1992, King and Kirwilliam 2011). In addition, research indicates that people with mTBI also often suffer from sleep difficulties including insomnia and that this may prevent recovery over time (Theadom et al, 2015). From the perspective of health psychology, mTBI has been explored in terms of how people make sense and adjust to the mTBI and whether a health psychology-based intervention can improve their symptoms. One area of research has focused on mTBI in soldiers.

mTBI IN SOLDIERS

Over the past couple of decades there has been a dramatic increase in soldiers returning from combat with symptoms that cannot be accounted for by the more familiar physical injuries and/or mental health problems. Due to improved body armour and medical technology more soldiers are also surviving injuries and left to cope with debilitating consequences. Further, soldiers are exposed to an increase in the range of blasts. This has resulted in the increased prevalence of mTBI in front-line soldiers which has been labelled a 'signature injury' in the US (Tanielian and Jaycox 2008; Okie 2005) while the incidence in the UK is estimated at about 9.5 per cent of combat troops (Rona et al. 2012).

MAKING SENSE OF mTBI

Brunger et al. (2014) carried out a qualitative study to explore how soldiers, returning from combat experience, adjust after experiencing a mTBI. Participants (n = 16; male = 15; female = 1) were interviewed aged 19–53 years and came from the Royal Navy, the British Army and the Royal Air Force. Participants had sustained their mTBI in an IED blast (n = 8), from a fall (n = 4), from a sporting collision (n = 2) or from an assault (n = 1). Two also had a diagnosis of PTSD and three were amputees.

The first theme identified from the interviews related to **'Onset of the problem'**. Interestingly, those who received their mTBI through an IED seemed to see it as an occupational hazard, as if they had expected to be blown up while on duty. As one said:

'I went back to the area that we'd already cleared, following the safe route in, had a look at the device on the other side of the compound, came back out, briefed my team, grabbed my Team Commander and said 'I'll show you what we've found', and as we stepped through the opening on the other side of the compound, umm, which we'd all crossed, you know, 25–30 times, that's when a device that had been missed initiated because I'd stepped on it' (participant 15).'

In contrast, those who received their mTBI during their leisure time seemed to blame themselves more. One man who had a skiing accident described that he was *'getting a bit over-confident'* and

'I was skiing in the afternoon by myself, without a helmet, down a gentle slope. It was a blue slope so not a particularly hard slope. . . I can remember standing at the top of this long flat slope getting ready to ski down, and that was it' (participant 14)'.

The second theme described **'Symptom experience and impairment evaluation'** and participants described a wide a varied number of symptoms including 'intermittent headaches', 'nausea', 'tinnitus', 'dizziness' and 'poor concentration'. They also described how it impacted on their relationships and work life. One gave an insightful analogy for how he felt:

'It's a bit like a computer that's not been turned off properly. Instead of you know, going into proper shutdown, it's like when you pull the plug out and then when you reboot the computer; it takes a long time to get all the files organised. . . Sometimes it doesn't work quite right' (participant 3).

THE PSYCHOLOGICAL INTERVENTION

Brunger et al. (2014) also developed and evaluated a psychological intervention to support soldiers with mTBI. This involved a stepped care approach with soldiers only progressing through all four phases if deemed necessary:

Phase 1: All patients with mTBI received printed information about symptoms, patterns of recovery and strategies to prevent further injury.

Phase 2: Those with symptoms still present 3 weeks after the event received the following: a structured clinical interview and physical examination; tip cards relating to symptoms; a tailored and goal-driven treatment plan focusing on symptom-management, stress-reduction and relaxation training. Phase 2 was predominantly distance-based but patients received regular telephone counselling focusing on symptom management and how to resume work and social activities.

Phase 3: This involved an intensive 2-week group therapy programme with components of CBT, such as cognitive restructuring and behavioural activation.

Phase 4: This 'as-needed service' offered limited but ongoing support when needed to help with specific symptoms and maximize daily functioning.

EVALUATION

The intervention was run at DMRC Headley Court and given that all patients were required to have the intervention it was not possible to run a trial. Brunger et al.'s (2014) interviews with the soldiers, however, provided some insights into the success of the intervention.

The fourth theme from the interviews described '**Recovery**' and how this had been helped by the intervention. For some, this had been due to information giving and finding out about their condition:

'It's strange when you don't know anything about it, you don't know any better. Umm, so having come here and started to learn, it's just like opening a set of doors and realizing, well actually there is a world out there, beyond the mTBI and that' (participant 16).

For some, the benefits came from goal setting and some of the strategies they had learned from CBT:

'Right, you need to go and try this and try that', you know, 'if you can keep a diary of it, do, if you don't, just let me know how you feel about it' (participant 6).

Finally, soldiers then described a level of '**Acceptance**'. As one soldier said:

'I know I've got problems, and I understand that I've got some problems, but I don't want it to get in the way of my life' (participant 8).

Some had also managed to incorporate their symptoms into identity:

'I now don't consider them symptoms; I consider them [me]. If that makes sense, this is now who I am' (participant 13).

And at times this was attributed to the intervention:

'It proved to be a catalyst and a very good excuse to, err, sit down and work out work patterns, work life balance. . .so that's been something positive that's come out of this, through not being able to work' (participant 14)

Overall, research on mTBI illustrates how health psychology can support patients with this less common chronic condition and finds reflection in research exploring illness cognitions and coping (see Chapter 8), stress and stress management (Chapter 10), symptom perception and pain (see Chapter 8 and 11) and relates to the management of other chronic conditions as described in this chapter and Chapter 12.

BOX 13.3
Critical Approaches to Health Psychology

Research and theories relating to obesity and CHD highlights some of the bigger issues in health psychology as follows:

The individual vs social vs political: Health psychology tends to focus on the role of individual variables such as beliefs, behaviours, personality and coping in the experience of chronic conditions such as obesity and CHD. Yet these conditions exist within a broader social and political context. Obesity may well be the result of eating more than the body needs but this is influenced by government policies around food production, marketing and availability. Fat intake might be reduced if people ate less fat but if governments encourage fat intake by making it cheap to buy it is much harder for people to eat less. Likewise rehabilitation might be effective after a heart attack but this involves exercise which in turn involves councils to invest in parks, cycle lanes and gyms and this requires government support.

The mind vs body: Chronic conditions illustrate the interaction between the mind and the body as what we think changes what we do which in turn changes our health status. But while this emphasizes an interaction between the mind and body at the same time it defines them as discrete.

Individual differences: Research into chronic conditions such as obesity and CHD often emphasizes individual differences by variables such as gender, age, social class, or even between people with or without a health condition. But most of these variables are actually on a continuum and analysing data in this way oversimplifies who we are and can create false dichotomies.

7 | THINKING CRITICALLY ABOUT RESEARCH INTO OBESITY AND CHD

There are some problems with research and theory relating to chronic conditions such as obesity and CHD.

SOME CRITICAL QUESTIONS

When thinking about research in this area ask yourself the following questions.

- Obesity is a highly stigmatized condition. How should we research obesity without exacerbating this stigma?
- Some theories of obesity onset are too simple. What do they miss and what are the problems with this approach?
- Some theories of obesity are extremely complex. What are the problems with this approach?
- Can treatment for chronic conditions do harm?
- What does research data about the causes or treatment of a chronic condition such as obesity or CHD actually tell us about any individual with a chronic condition?

SOME PROBLEMS WITH. . .

Below are some problems with research in this area that you may wish to consider.

Measurement: Measuring and defining obesity are problematic as they rely upon assessments of body weight and body size, whereas the factor that is most linked to health status is probably body fat. Therefore research can show contradictory evidence for the consequences of obesity which probably illustrates the drawbacks of using proxy measures (i.e. BMI and waist circumference) for what the real measurement should be (i.e. body fat).

Simple or complex models: Obesity is a product of biological factors (e.g. genetics), the obesogenic environment (e.g. the food industry, town planning) and psychological factors (e.g. diet, exercise, beliefs). Research tends to focus on the contribution of one set of these factors. How they all interact remains unclear. This means that most research misses the complexity of the obesity problem. However, if research were to try to address all these factors, the studies would become unwieldy and the conclusions would be too complex to put into practice.

Tailored research: There are different stages of obesity: weight gain, weight maintenance and weight loss. Different factors might be involved at each of these stages (i.e. genetics, obesogenic environment, behaviour). Research tends to treat all stages the same.

Doing harm: We tend to assume that treatment is always beneficial. Obesity illustrates how treatment can also sometimes do harm. Any health care professional or researcher therefore always needs to weigh up the costs and benefits of any treatment approach.

Blame vs control: Obesity is a stigmatized condition with much research indicating that the negative attitudes to obesity can cause emotional problems and exacerbate overeating and weight. Such stigma often relates to blame. Taking away blame, however, can also take away responsibility and a perception of control. This can lead people to feel powerless and out of control. Somehow a middle ground is needed where people with weight problems can be encouraged to feel in control and responsible for their behaviour without feeling blamed or judged.

The ecological fallacy: Much data on obesity and CHD is at the population level (i.e. changing dietary patterns, levels of smoking, physical activity). There is always a problem when population data is used to draw conclusions about an individual. Therefore just because population data shows an increase in eating fat which corresponds to an increase in obesity, or a decrease in smoking which corresponds to a decrease in CHD, it does not tell us how individual people with either obesity or CHD behave. This is called the ecological fallacy.

TO CONCLUDE

Illnesses such as obesity and CHD illustrate the role of psychology throughout the course of an illness. For example, psychological factors play a role in illness onset (e.g. health beliefs, health behaviours, personality, coping mechanisms), illness progression (e.g. psychological consequences, adaptation, health behaviours) and longevity (e.g. health behaviours, coping mechanisms, quality of life). These psychological factors are also relevant to a multitude of other chronic and acute illnesses, such as diabetes, asthma, chronic fatigue syndrome and multiple sclerosis. This suggests that illness is best conceptualized not as a biomedical problem but as a complex interplay of physiological and psychological factors.

QUESTIONS

1 To what extent can obesity be explained by genetics?
2 Discuss the role of behaviour in the recent increase in the prevalence of obesity.
3 To what extent is obesity a social problem?
4 Treating obesity causes more problems than it solves. Discuss.
5 How can obesity be treated effectively?
6 What role does psychology play in the medical and surgical management of obesity?
7 CHD is a product of lifestyle. Discuss.
8 How might beliefs about CHD influence its onset and progression?
9 What are the psychological consequences of CHD?
10 To what extent can a heart attack be prevented?
11 Is death from a heart attack inevitable?

FOR DISCUSSION

In the light of the literature on obesity and CHD, discuss the possible role of psychological factors throughout the course of an alternative chronic illness (e.g. diabetes, rheumatoid arthritis, multiple sclerosis).

FURTHER READING

Brownell, K.D., Kersh, R., Ludwig, D.S., et al. (2010) Personal responsibility and obesity: a constructive approach to a controversial issue, *Health affairs (Project Hope),* **29**(3): 379–87. Doi.org/10.1377/hlthaff.2009.0739

This paper discusses the emphasis on patient responsibility for health and suggests that encouraging the obese to diet may be an example of attempting to control the uncontrollable. It is an interesting paper as it challenges the core of much health psychology thinking by suggesting that some illnesses are beyond the control of the individual. It is a good paper to generate debate.

Harris, R. (2019) *ACT Made Simple: An easy-to-read primer on acceptance and commitment therapy.* Oakland, CA: New Harbinger Publications.
This is a great book showing you how to do ACT, which is of relevance to all chronic conditions including obesity and CHD but also less common conditions, such as Ménière's disease, brain trauma, spinal cord injury and fibromyalgia, as covered in these two chapters.

Ogden, J. (2010) *The Psychology of Eating: From Health to Disordered Behaviour,* 2nd edn. Oxford: Blackwell.
This book provides an account of the continuum of eating behaviour from healthy eating, through dieting and body dissatisfaction, to obesity and eating disorders. In particular, it provides a detailed analysis of obesity and its treatment.

Ogden, J. (2018) *The Psychology of Dieting.* London: Routledge.
This book provides a clearer overview of the causes, consequences and treatments for obesity and how it can be managed well. It was written for those who want to lose weight or those who want to help others do the same.

Ortega, F.B., Cadenas-Sanchez, C., Migueles, J.H. et al. (2018) Role of physical activity and fitness in the characterization and prognosis of the metabolically healthy obesity phenotype: a systematic review and meta-analysis, *Progress in Cardiovascular Diseases,* **61**(2): 190–205.
Over the past decade there has been a debate about the notion of healthy obesity. This paper presents a thorough review of the literature and explores the role of body weight per se together with behaviour and metabolic risk factors on CHD and mortality.

Pearl, R.L. and Puhl, R.M. (2018) Weight bias internalization and health: a systematic review, *Obesity Reviews,* **19**(8): 1141–63.
Over recent years there has been a proliferation of papers exploring weight stigma and weight bias. This paper provides an excellent review of this literature.

Vyas, M.V. Chaturvedi, N., Hughes, A.D. et al. (2021) Cardiovascular disease recurrence and long-term mortality in a tri-ethnic British cohort, *Heart,* **107**: 996–1002.
This is a really interesting study exploring ethnic differences in cardiac events and mortality over time in the UK.

14

Health Status and Quality of Life

CHAPTER OVERVIEW

Health varies across many dimensions including geographical location, social economic status (SES), gender and time. Health is also the focus of much research from disciplines such as medicine, all the professionals allied to medicine including nursing and physiotherapy and the social sciences that study health including health psychology. All these research areas require health to be measured. This chapter examines health inequalities and how health varies by geographical location and SES. It also explores variation for the COVID pandemic. It then describes the different ways in which health status has been measured from mortality rates to quality of life. In addition, it describes the ways in which quality of life has been used in research both in terms of the factors that predict quality of life (quality of life as an outcome variable) and the association between quality of life and longevity (quality of life as a predictor). Finally, it describes the notion of a response shift and the ways in which a person's evaluation of their quality of life changes over the course of an illness.

CASE STUDY

Frances has recently had her first baby. Due to complications during labour she had an emergency Caesarian section which was quite traumatic as she had to be rushed to the operating theatre in order to get the baby out safely. She is now recovering at home two days later. The midwife visits her to check on her stitches, which are doing fine, and to help her with breastfeeding. The midwife asks her how she is feeling. She describes the following: massive relief that the baby is healthy and safe; upset that she failed to have a vaginal delivery which she feels is a failure; shock from what she went through; gratitude to the hospital staff for looking after her; frustration at her husband for not understanding how upset she feels about having to have a Caesarian; pain from the operation; tired from being up all night; totally in love with the baby; anxious about breastfeeding properly; pain from breastfeeding; irritated with her family for all visiting at the same time and expecting cups of tea; happy that she is now home. All of these make up the notion of health!

Through the Eyes of Health Psychology. . .

Health is a very broad construct and can be conceptualized and measured in many different ways. Frances's case illustrates that health can mean many different things such as positive mood (relief, love), negative mood (upset, anxiety), pain (of the operation), physical symptoms (tired), outcomes (the healthy baby, stitches are OK). This chapter will explain the ways in which health is measured and how these measures are used in research. It illustrates the complexity of health and how difficult it is to capture this complexity in a meaningful way.

1 HEALTH INEQUALITIES

Due to the internet and the publication of online reports there is now a huge volume of data available from respected bodies such as the World Health Organization (WHO) and the Office for National Statistics (ONS), health charities such as British Heart Foundation (BHF), Cancer Research UK (CRUK), the British Diabetes Association (BDA) and the American Cancer Society (ACS) as well as academic groups such as the European Heart Network. These data provide insights into health inequalities across the world and within individual countries, and evidence generally indicates that the diseases people are diagnosed with and whether or not they die from them vary according to four key dimensions: geographical location; time; socioeconomic status (SES) and gender. Time (i.e. changes throughout history) will not be explored independently as most available data includes this dimension in its analyses. Variation by gender is explored in Chapter 15. The following provides a preliminary insight into the notion of variation and health inequalities and how health varies by geographical location and SES. It also explores variation for the COVID pandemic. Please do not expect it to be an exhaustive or systematic analysis of this vast database.

GEOGRAPHICAL LOCATION

It is clear that the prevalence of a range of diseases and their mortality rates vary both between and within countries. For example, worldwide death rates in 2009 are shown in Figure 14.1 per 1,000 population. The figure illustrates huge variations across the world, with the highest death rates being in sub-Saharan Africa, Afghanistan, Russia and Eastern Europe.

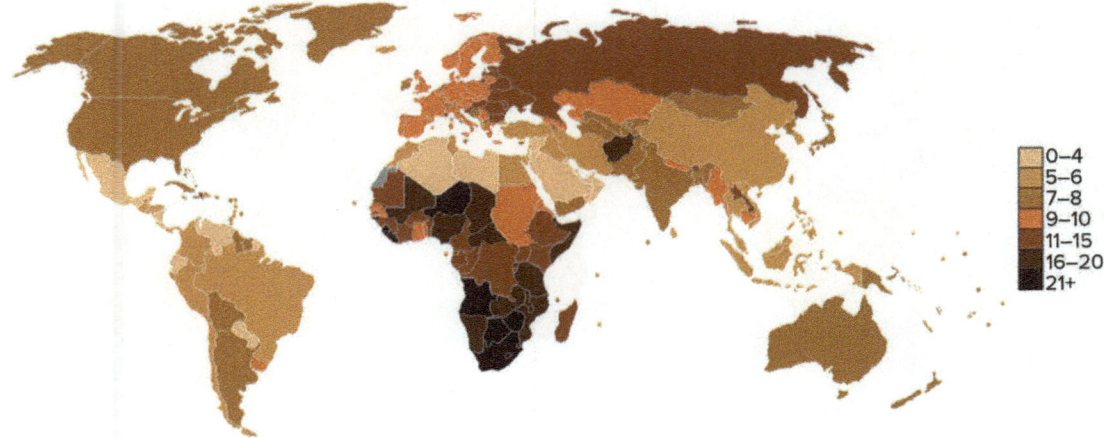

Figure 14.1 Death rates by geographical area worldwide in 2009 per 1,000 population

SOURCE: CIA Factbook (2009)

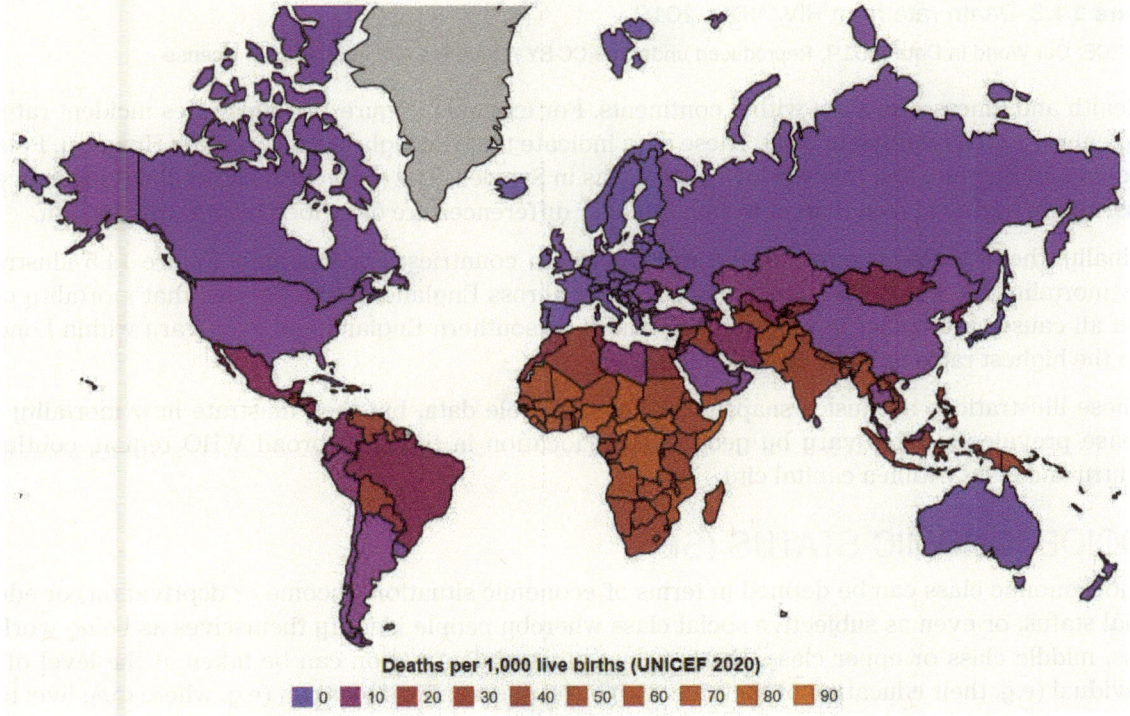

Figure 14.2 Infant mortality rates by country (2020)

SOURCE: World population review (2020); Unicef (2020)

Infant mortality rates also vary by geographical area. For example, data from the WHO (2020) shown in Figure 14.2 illustrate that the highest infant mortality rates in 2020 were in Africa and the South-East Asian region with the lowest rates being in Europe and North and Central America.

There are also geographical differences in specific diseases. For example, the global prevalence of people living with HIV infection in 2017 is shown in Figure 14.3, which shows that the highest rates were in sub-Saharan Africa, Brazil, the US and India.

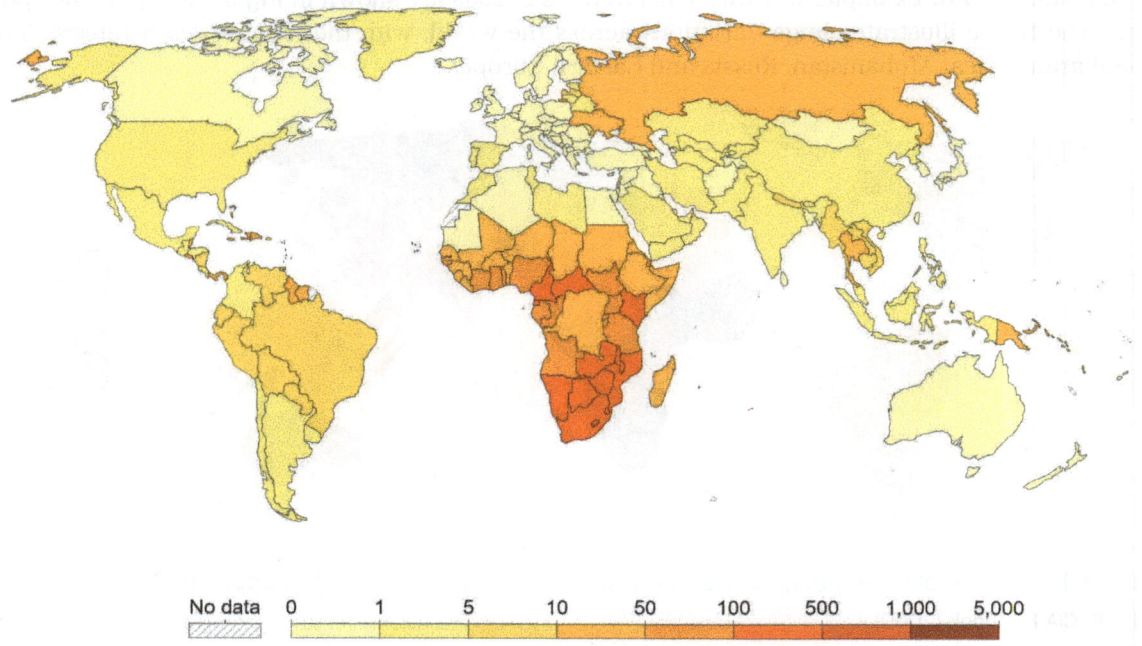

Figure 14.3 Death rate from HIV/AIDS, 2019

SOURCE: Our World in Data (2019, Reproduced under the CC-BY Attribution 4.0 International License

Health and illness also vary within continents. For example, Figure 14.4 illustrates incident rates of lung cancer across Europe in 2008. These data indicate that the highest rates were in Hungary, Poland, Estonia and Belgium and that the lowest rate was in Sweden. The graph also shows that lung cancer is consistently higher in men than in women. Gender differences are described later in this section.

Finally, there is also geographical variation within countries. For example, Figure 14.5 illustrates how mortality rates in people aged under 75 vary across England. It can be seen that mortality rates from all causes are higher in northern England than southern England and even vary within London, with the highest rates being in East London.

These illustrations are just a snapshot of the available data, but they illustrate how mortality and disease prevalence rates vary by geographical location in terms of broad WHO region, continent, country and even within a capital city.

SOCIOECONOMIC STATUS (SES)

Socioeconomic class can be defined in terms of economic situation (income or deprivation) or educational status, or even as subjective social class whereby people identify themselves as being working class, middle class or upper class. Further, measures of deprivation can be taken at the level of the individual (e.g. their education or their income) or by geographical location (e.g. where they live: town

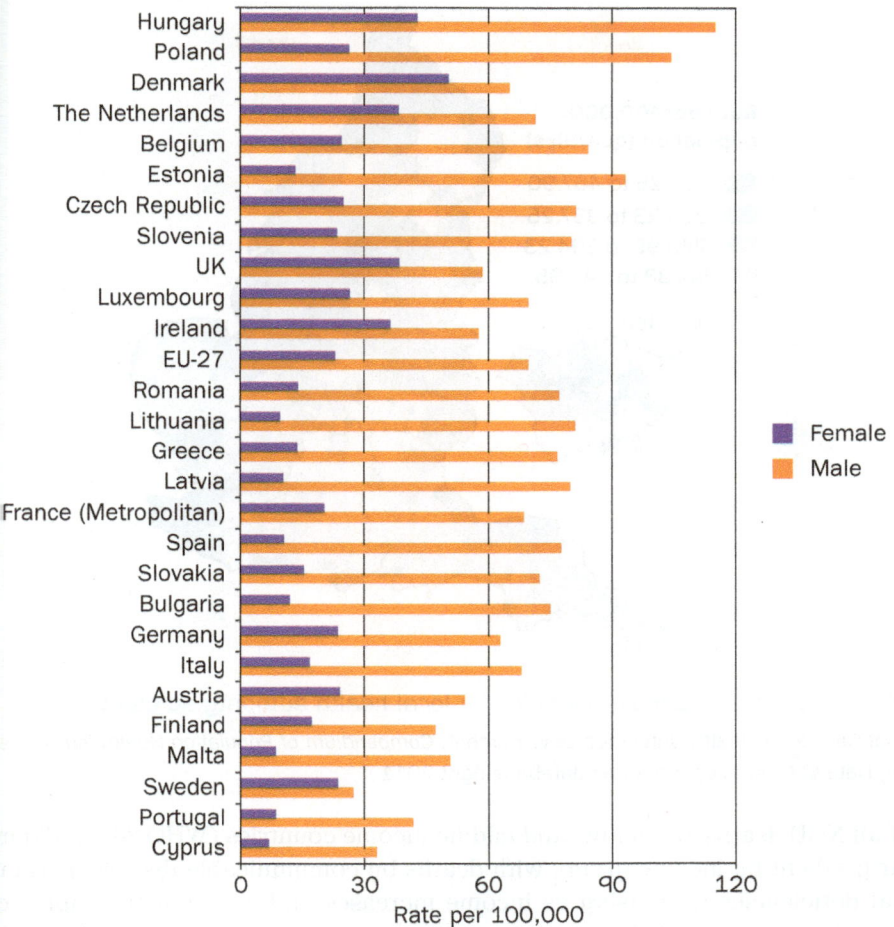

Figure 14.4 Lung cancer incident rates across Europe, 2008
SOURCE: Cancer Research UK (2011)

or city, region, country etc.). For the purposes of this chapter the term socioeconomic status (SES) will be used. Whatever definition is used, a consistent relationship emerges between SES, health, illness and mortality. Chronic conditions are also classified as non-communicable diseases (NCDs) which kill 41 million people each year, equivalent to 71 per cent of all deaths globally (WHO 2020). The WHO has classified the countries of the world into three income groups: low income, middle income and high income, and has explored the relationship with premature mortality (i.e. < 75). Each year, 85 per cent of these 'premature' deaths from NCDs occur in low- and middle-income countries and

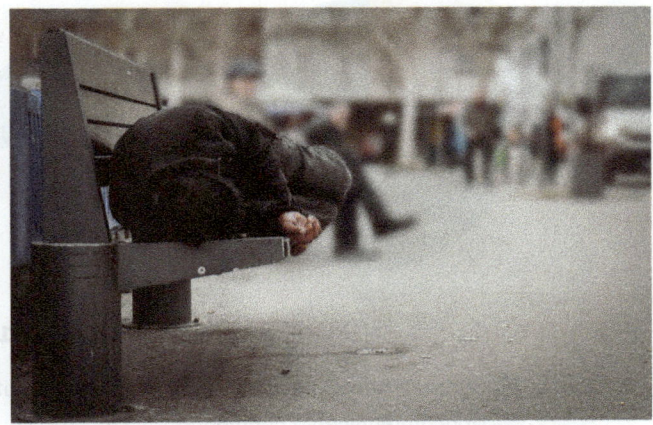

What difference does homelessness or low income make to people's health situation?

SOURCE: © Shutterstock / Srdjan Randjelovic

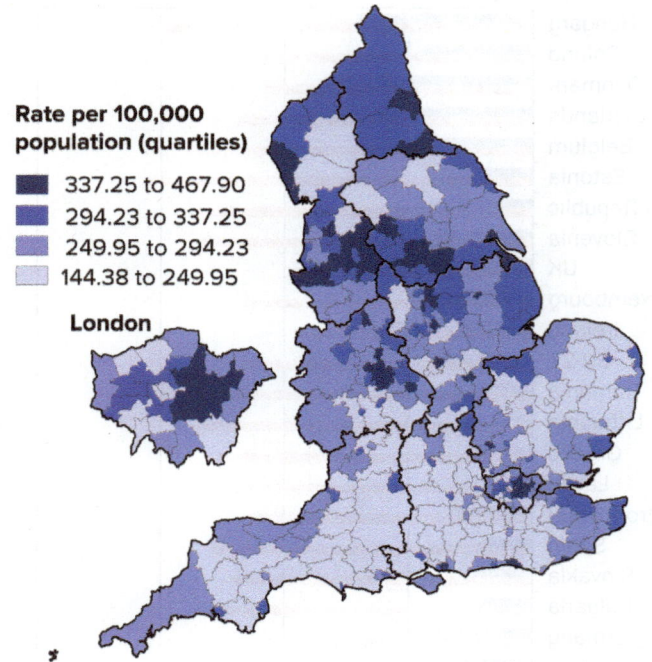

Figure 14.5 Mortality rates in people under 75 by local health authority across England

SOURCE: National Centre for Health Outcomes Development, *Compendium of Population Health Indicators,* Contains Ordnance Survey Data © Crown copyright and database right 2011

77 per cent of all NCD deaths are in low- and middle-income countries (WHO 2020). Figure 14.6 demonstrates a clear gradient by income group, with deaths by communicable disease, perinatal conditions and nutritional deficiencies decreasing as income increases and non-communicable conditions (e.g. cancer, coronary heart disease, diabetes) increasing as income increases. Interestingly, death by injury is highest in the middle income group.

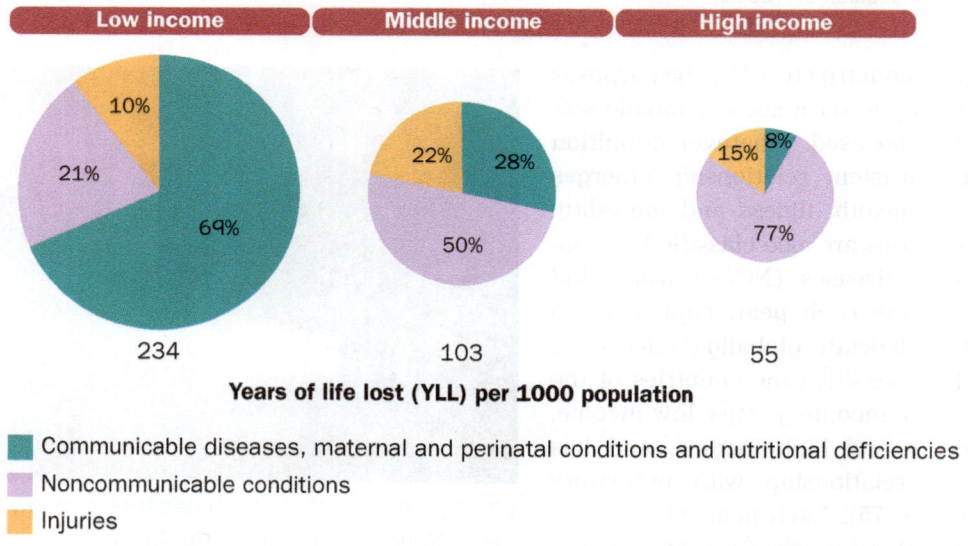

Figure 14.6 Premature mortality (i.e. < 75 years) worldwide by country income group, 2004

SOURCE: WHO (2010)

Data from England up to 2018 shows a similar pattern and illustrates the impact of deprivation on mortality rates measured in terms of deaths per se and premature deaths (before 75 years), (see Figure 14.7).

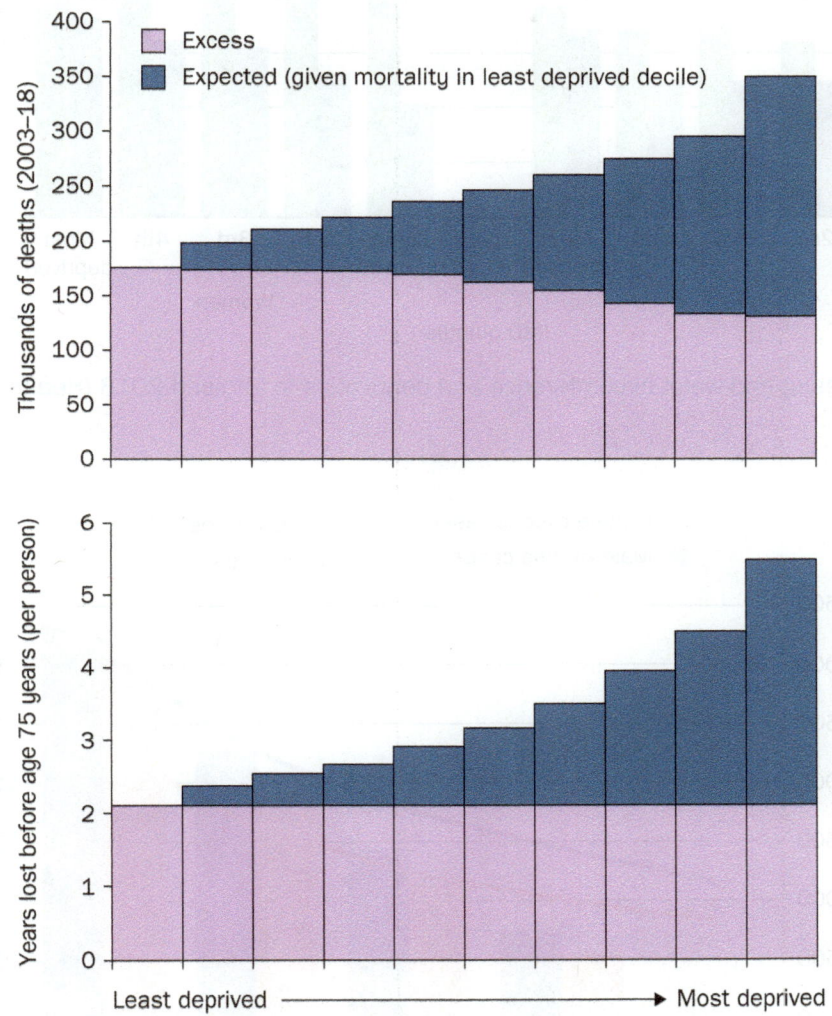

Figure 14.7 Mortality attributable to socioeconomic inequality and years lost to inequality in England, 2003–18 by index of deprivation (Lewer et al. 2020)

The prevalence of individual health conditions also varies by SES. For example, variation of obesity by deprivation levels in England is shown in Figure 14.8. These data indicate that for women there is a clear relationship between deprivation and both obesity and waist circumference, with body weight increasing as deprivation increases. The pattern for men is similar but less pronounced.

Lung cancer rates can also be seen to vary by SES as measured by deprivation category (see Figure 14.9). These data indicate a clear relationship between an increase in deprivation and an increase in lung cancer in England. This gradient can be seen for both men and women, although rates in men are much higher.

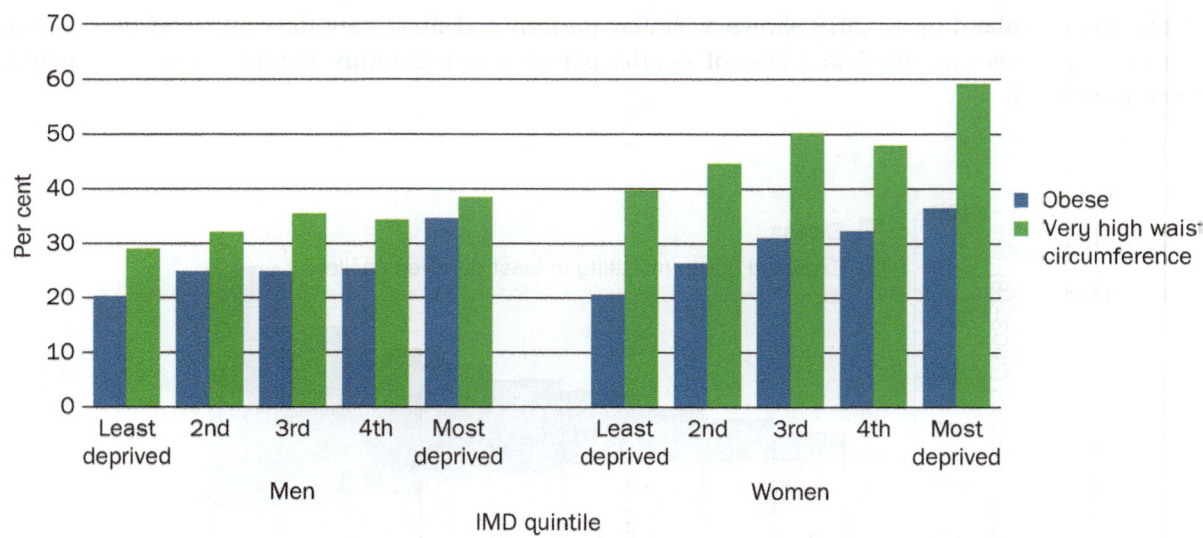

Figure 14.8 Obesity and waist circumference and deprivation in England 2018 (Health Survey for England 2018)

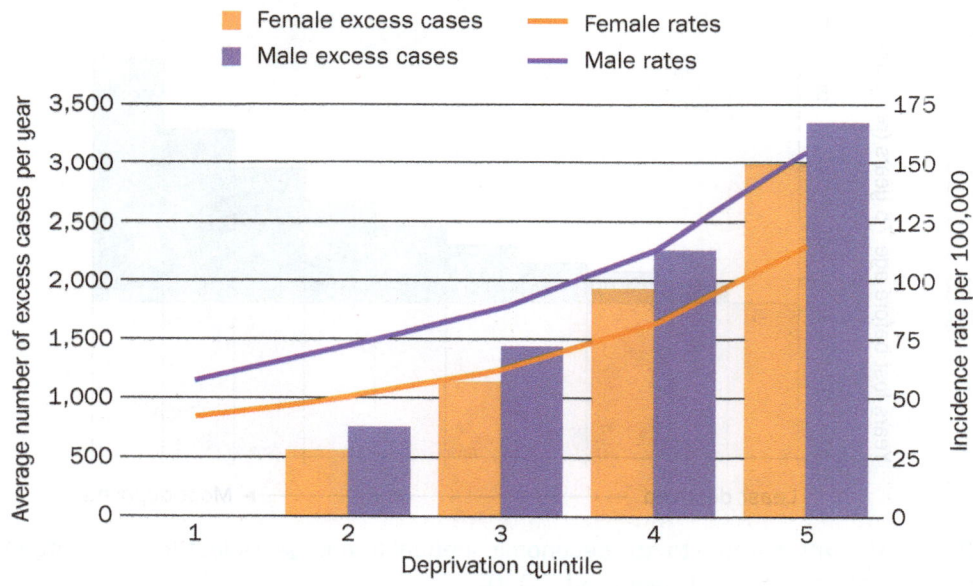

Figure 14.9 Estimated Average Number of Excess Cases of lung cancer per Year and European Age-Standardized Incidence Rates per 100,000 Population, by Deprivation in England, 2013–2017 (Cancer Research UK 2022)

Furthermore, it is not only the prevalence of individual conditions that vary by SES but also death from these conditions. For example, Figures 14.10 and 14.11 illustrate how mortality from Type 1 diabetes is higher in those with lower SES than those with higher SES from 2006 to 2015.

The data therefore show variation in mortality rates, causes of mortality, specific conditions and death rates from these conditions by SES, with those in the lower SES groups (measured by a range of approaches) having consistently poorer health than those in the higher SES groups. Overall, there are

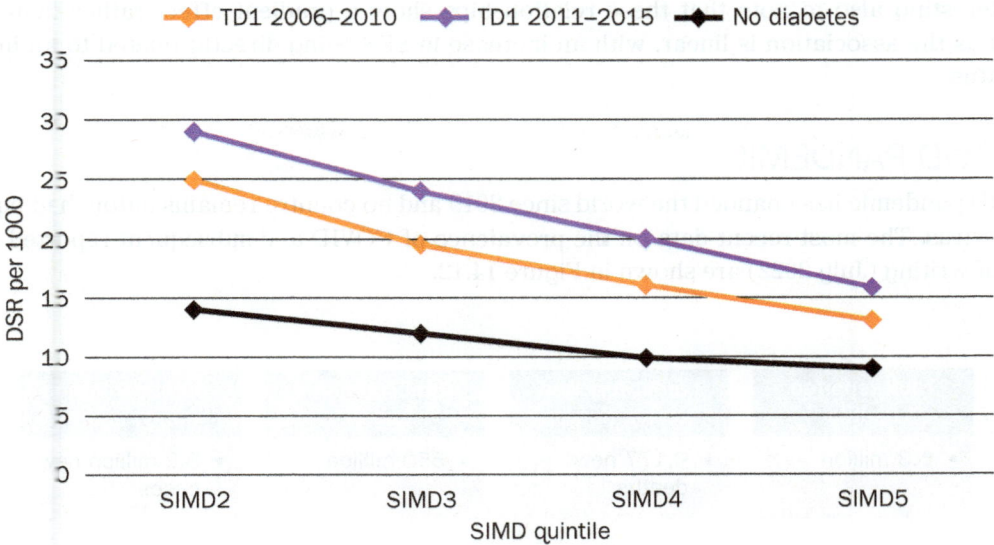

Figure 14.10 Mortality for men with type 1 diabetes by deprivation gradient in scotland 2006–2011 and 2011–2015 (Campbell et al. 2020)

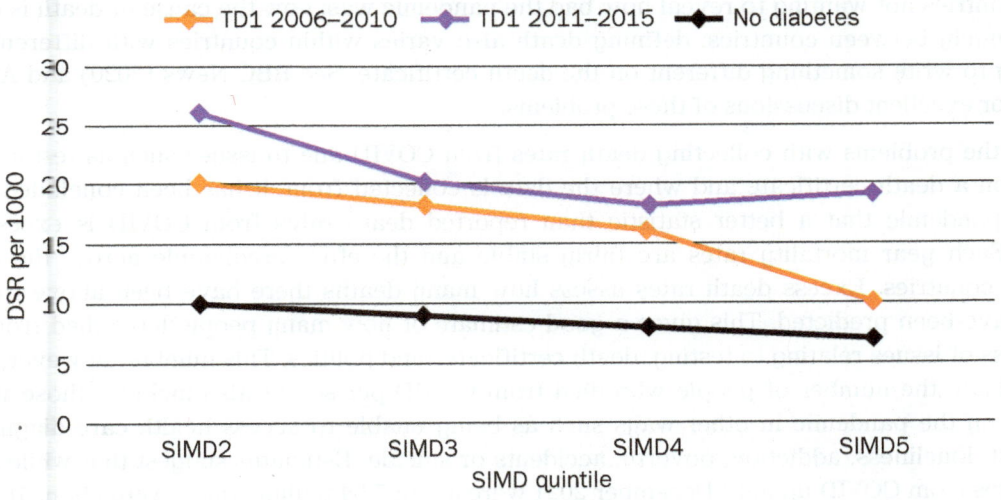

Figure 14.11 Mortality for women with type 1 diabetes by deprivation gradient in scotland 2006–2011 and 2011–2015 (Campbell et al. 2020)

three consistent findings concerning the relationship between SES and health as follows (see Marmot and Wilkinson 2005). As SES increases (however measured) there is:

- an improvement in mortality rates, disease progression and life expectancy
- a reduction in infant mortality, chronic disease and psychiatric morbidity
- an increase in self-reported mental and physical health.

It is interesting also to note that these relationships show a gradient effect rather than a thresh-old effect as the association is linear, with an increase in SES being directly related to an increase in health status.

THE COVID PANDEMIC

The COVID pandemic has changed the world since 2019 and no country remains untouched by this new strand of virus. The most recent data on the prevalence of COVID and subsequent reported deaths at the time of writing (July 2022) are shown in Figure 14.12.

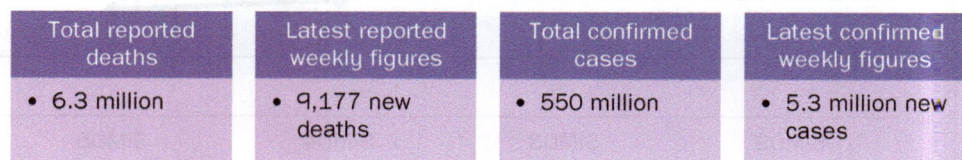

Total reported deaths	Latest reported weekly figures	Total confirmed cases	Latest confirmed weekly figures
• 6.3 million	• 9,177 new deaths	• 550 million	• 5.3 million new cases

Figure 14.12 COVID numbers around the world (After BBC News, 17/7/2022)

Counting COVID cases and deaths is problematic for many reasons: cases from early in the pandemic were often not confirmed due to the absence of testing; different countries use different ways of collecting their data for both cases and deaths; COVID became very politicized very quickly, with some countries not wanting to reveal how bad the pandemic was; how the cause of death is classified varies hugely between countries; defining death also varies within countries with different doctors choosing to write something different on the death certificate. See BBC News (2020) and Armstrong (2021), for excellent discussions of these problems.

Given the problems with collecting death rates from COVID due to issues such as testing, what is written on a death certificate and where the data is collected from, it has been concluded through-out the pandemic that a better statistic than reported death rates from COVID is excess deaths per se. Each year mortality rates are fairly stable and therefore predictable across the year and between countries. Excess death rates assess how many deaths there have been above that which would have been predicted. This gives a good estimate of how many people have died from COVID regardless of issues relating to testing, death certificates and politics. This number, however, does not only indicate the number of people who died from COVID per se but also includes those who were affected by the pandemic in other ways such as being unable to access health care diagnoses and treatment, loneliness, addiction, poverty, accidents or suicide. Estimates suggest that while recorded death rates from COVID up until December 2021 were about 5.94 million, there were about 18.2 million excess deaths worldwide (COVID Excess Mortality Collaborators 2022), indicating that the pandemic may have caused 3 times more deaths than has been reported previously.

COVID shows a very strong case for health inequalities and varies by demographics such as geographical location, gender, SES and co-morbidities.

COVID and Geographical Location

While COVID has spread all round the world, the highest number of confirmed cases are in the US, India and Brazil followed by France, Germany and the UK. The worldwide spread of COVID can be seen in Figure 14.13.

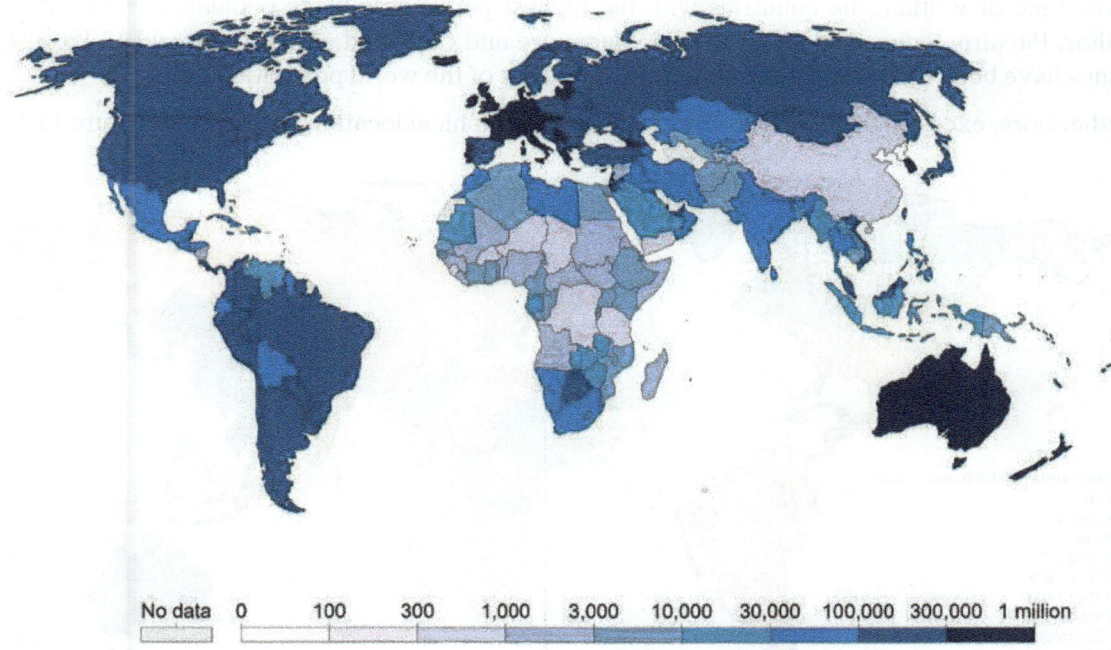

Figure 14.13 confirmed cases of COVID worldwide (Our World in Data 2022)

It is not only COVID cases that vary by geographical location but also vaccination rollout, as shown in Figure 14.14.

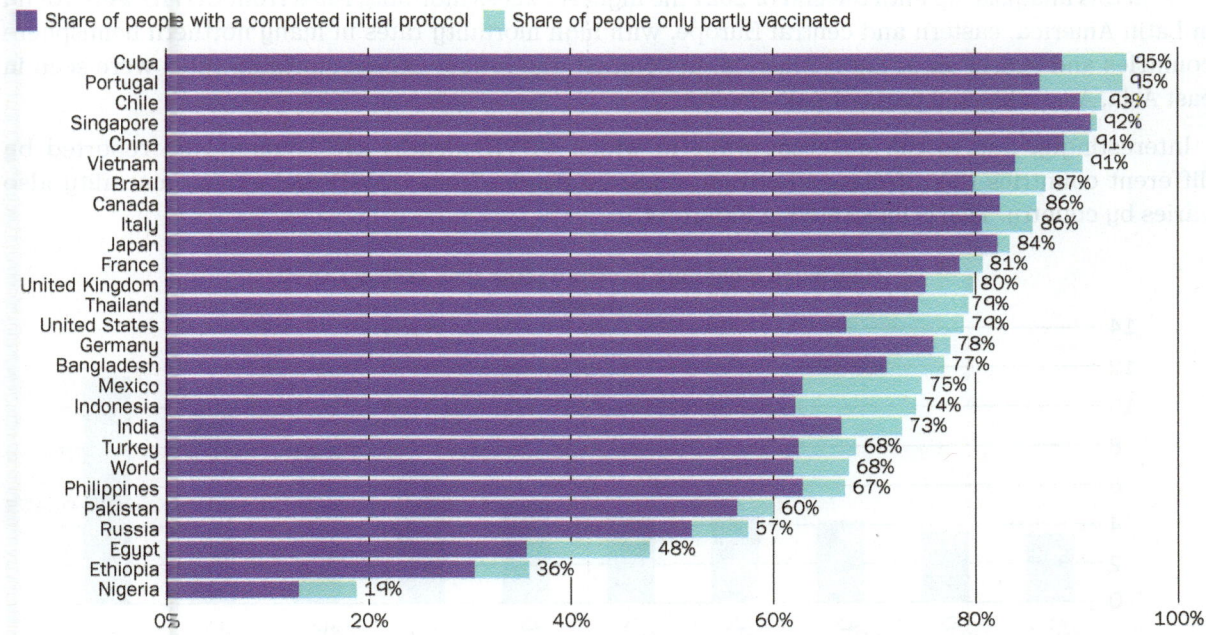

Note: Alternative definitions of a full vaccination, e.g. having been infected with SARS-CoV-2 and having 1 dose of a 2-dose protocol, are ignored to maximize comparability between countries.

Figure 14.14 COVID vaccination rollout (Our World in Data 2022)

At the time of writing, the countries with the highest percentage of its population vaccinated are Gibraltar, Pitcairn, Samoa, UAE and Brunei, Singapore and Chile and across the world 12,120,524,547 vaccines have been delivered, accounting for 61 per cent of the world population.

Furthermore, excess mortality rates also vary by geographical location, as shown in Figure 14.15.

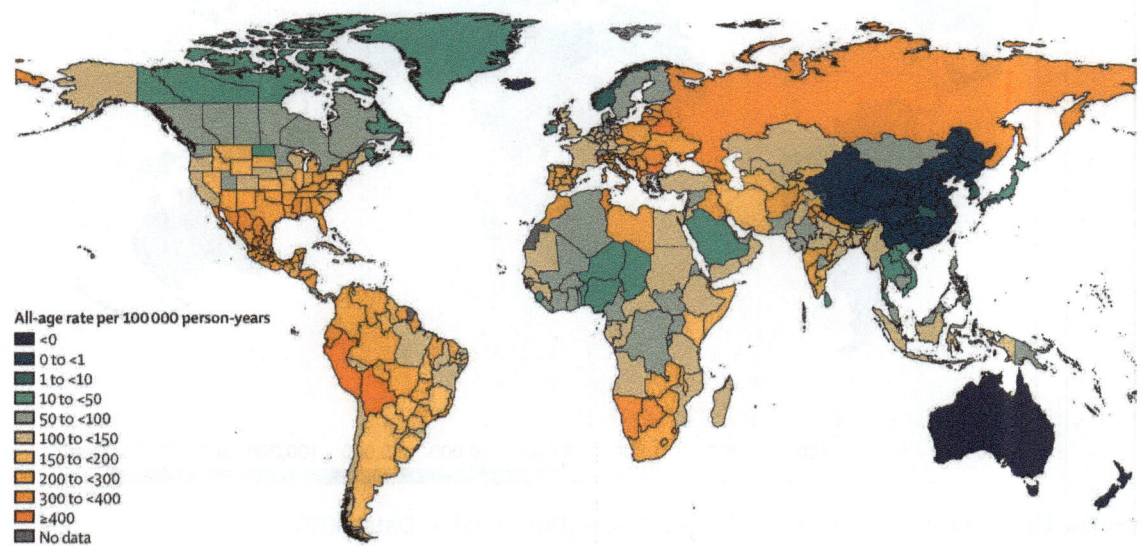

All-age rate per 100000 person-years
- <0
- 0 to <1
- 1 to <10
- 10 to <50
- 50 to <100
- 100 to <150
- 150 to <200
- 200 to <300
- 300 to <400
- ≥400
- No data

Figure 14.15 Global distribution of estimated excess mortality rate due to the COVID-19 pandemic, for the cumulative period 2020–21 (COVID excess mortality collaborators 2022)

From this analysis, up until the end of 2021 the highest excess mortality rates from COVID were found in Latin America, eastern and central Europe, with high mortality rates in many northern hemisphere countries and nearly all of Latin America. In contrast, the lowest excess mortality rates were seen in east Asia, Australia, and parts of Asia Pacific.

Interestingly, due to the different ways in which COVID deaths are counted and reported by different countries the difference between reported deaths from COVID and excess mortality also varies by country. This is illustrated in Figure 14.16.

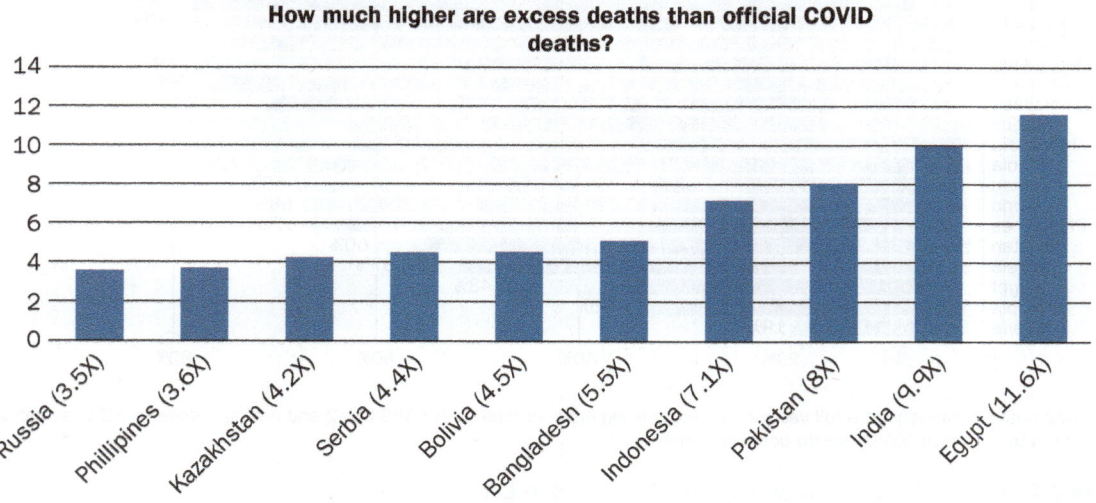

How much higher are excess deaths than official COVID deaths?

Figure 14.16 Ratio between reported COVID deaths and excess deaths (After WHO 2020; BBC News 2020)

This data illustrates the degree of under-reporting of COVID deaths and how this varies by country and suggests that Egypt's and India's actual numbers were about 10 times higher than those reported and that Russia deaths are 3 and half times higher than reported.

COVID and Gender

COVID did not affect men and women equally around the world. This is shown in Figure 14.17.

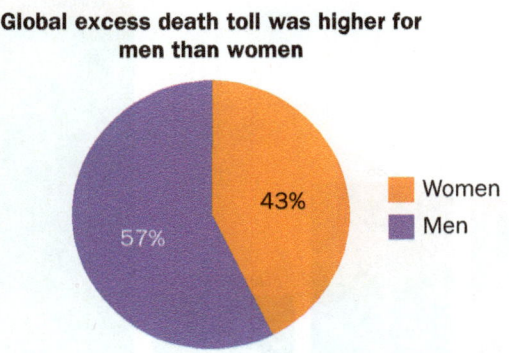

Global excess death toll was higher for men than women

43% Women
57% Men

Figure 14.17 COVID varies by gender (After WHO 2020; BBC News 2020)

COVID and Socioeconomic Status

COVID rates of cases and death rates have also been examined by measures of SES measured at both an individual and population level. The data from these analyses seem more complex than those for geography or gender. For example, some data indicates a clear association between country level income and death rates as shown in Figure 14.18.

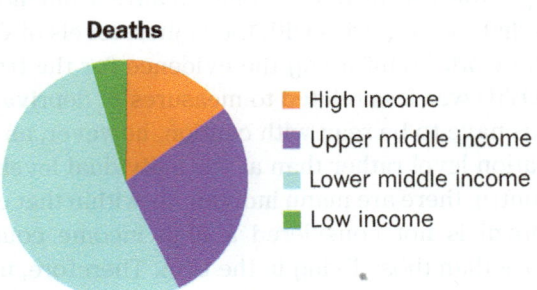

Deaths

High income
Upper middle income
Lower middle income
Low income

Figure 14.18 Excess deaths by level of income of country (After WHO 2020; BBC News 2020)

From this analysis by the WHO (2020) the highest rates of deaths are in lower-middle income countries. This could indicate that being a population of people who earn less than those in higher income countries increases the chances that COVID will kill you. It could also, however, simply indicate that there are more people in these lower-middle income countries and therefore more people died.

Using a different metric for analysis, researchers have explored the relationship between COVID excess death rates and GBD regions of the world (COVID Excess Mortality Collaborators 2022). The Global Burden of Disease (GBD) regional classification system defined seven super regions of the world as: South-East Asia, East Asia and Oceania; South Asia; North Africa and Middle East; Sub-saharan Africa; Latin America and Caribbean; Central Europe, Eastern Europe and Central Asia; high income countries (which includes 34 countries from Western Europe, Southern Latin America,

North America, Australasia and Asia Pacific). This classification is based upon epidemiological similarity and geographic closeness. The COVID Excess Mortality Collaborators (2022) explored the relationship between excess deaths during the COVID pandemic and these seven regions. The results are shown in Figure 14.19.

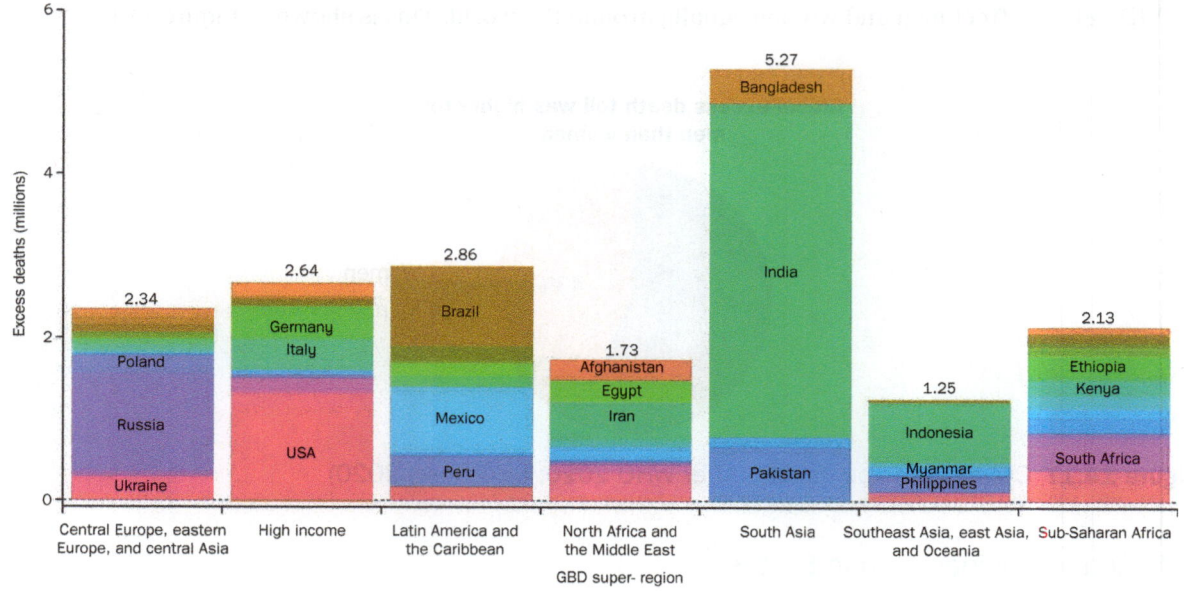

Figure 14.19 COVID excess death rates by the 7 GBD super regions (COVID excess mortality collaborators 2022)

The results from this analysis indicate that while South Asia clearly has the highest excess death rates, the pattern seems comparable for the high income countries and most other regions. The authors conclude from their analysis that the countries with the highest levels of COVID deaths 'are distributed across all GBD regions of the world, reinforcing the evidence for the truly global nature of the pandemic'. This suggests that COVID was less related to measures of deprivation such as income and SES than predicted. These findings have to be read with caution, however, as GBD regions measure epidemiological data at the population level rather than at the individual level. Therefore, while the USA is considered a high income country, there are many individuals within that country who do not have high incomes. Similarly, while Brazil is not considered a high income country, some people living in Brazil will have higher incomes than those living in the USA. Therefore, until we have data at the individual level relating to both cause of death and individual SES, the link between COVID and SES will remain unclear.

COVID and Co-morbidities

COVID also varies by co-morbidities and research increasingly indicates that those with other health conditions are more likely to develop a severe illness after contracting COVID, defined as being hospitalized, needing intensive care, requiring a ventilator to help them breathe or dying. These conditions include asthma, cancer, cerebrovascular disease, chronic kidney disease, chronic liver disease, COPD, diabetes, heart conditions, HIV and obesity (CDC 2022). For example, Földi et al. (2020) concluded from their systematic review and meta-analysis that obesity was a significant risk factor for both admission to an ICU with COVID (OR = 1.21, CI: 1.002–1.46; I2 = 0.0 per cent) as well as for requiring ventilation (OR = 2.05, CI: 1.16–3.64; I2 = 34.86 per cent) in COVID-19. Likewise, de Almeida-Pititto et al. (2020) concluded that pre-existing diabetes and hypertension were moderately associated with both the severity and mortality for COVID-19 (diabetes [OR 2.35 95 per cent, CI 1.80–3.06 and OR 2.50 95 per cent, CI 1.74–3.59]; hypertension: [OR 2.98 95 per cent, CI 2.37–3.75 and OR 2.88 (2.22–3.74)] and that pre-existing cardiovascular disease was strongly associated with both severity and mortality [OR 4.02 (2.76–5.86) and OR 6.34 (3.71–10.84)].

IN SUMMARY

Health varies by a number of dimensions including geographical location, gender, time and SES. Given that health varies so dramatically, and that it is the focus of much research in both medicine and disciplines such as health psychology, nursing, medical psychology and medical anthropology, researchers and clinicians require measures of health. The rest of this chapter focuses on the constructs of health status and quality of life and how these have been measured and used in research.

2   OBJECTIVE HEALTH STATUS

Objective health status refers to those approaches to health which are considered uncontaminated by bias and subjectivity.

MORTALITY RATES

At its most basic, a measure of health status takes the form of a very crude mortality rate, which is calculated by simply counting the number of deaths in one year compared with either previous or subsequent years. The question asked is, 'Has the number of people who have died this year gone up, gone down or stayed the same?' An increase in mortality rate can be seen as a decrease in health status and a decrease as an increase in health status. This approach, however, requires a denominator: a measure of who is at risk. The next most basic form of mortality rate therefore includes a denominator reflecting the size of the population being studied. Such a measure allows for comparisons to be made between different populations: more people may die in a given year in London when compared with Bournemouth, but London is simply bigger. In order to provide any meaningful measure of health status, mortality rates are corrected for age (Bournemouth has an older population and therefore we would predict that more people would die each year) and sex (men generally die younger than women and this needs to be taken into account). Furthermore, mortality rates can be produced to be either age specific, such as infant mortality rates, or illness specific, such as sudden death rates. As long as the population being studied is accurately specified, corrected and specific, mortality rates provide an easily available and simple measure: death is a good reliable outcome.

MORBIDITY RATES

Laboratory and clinical researchers and epidemiologists may accept mortality rates as the perfect measure of health status. However, the juxtaposition of social scientists to the medical world has challenged this position to raise the now seemingly obvious question, 'Is health really only the absence of death?' In response to this, there has been an increasing focus upon morbidity. However, in line with the emphasis upon simplicity inherent within the focus on mortality rates, many morbidity measures still use methods of counting and recording. For example, the expensive and time-consuming production of morbidity prevalence rates involves large surveys of 'caseness' to simply count how many people within a given population suffer from a particular problem. Likewise, sickness absence rates simply count days lost due to illness and caseload assessments count the number of people who visit their general practitioner (GP) or hospital within a given time frame. Such morbidity rates provide details at the level of the population in general. However, morbidity is also measured for each individual using measures of functioning.

MEASURES OF FUNCTIONING

Measures of functioning ask the question, 'To what extent can you do the following tasks?' and are generally called activity of daily living scales (ADLs). For example, Katz et al. (1970) designed the Index of Activities of Daily Living to assess levels of functioning in the elderly. This was developed for the therapist and/or carer to complete and asked the rater to evaluate the individual on a range of dimensions including bathing, dressing, continence and feeding. ADLs have also been developed for individuals themselves to complete and include questions such as, 'Do you or would you have any difficulty: washing down/cutting toenails/running to catch a bus/going up/down stairs?' Measures of functioning can either be administered on their own or as part of a more complex assessment involving measures of subjective health status.

3 | SUBJECTIVE HEALTH STATUS

Over recent years, measures of health status have increasingly opted for measures of subjective health status, which all have one thing in common: they ask the individual to rate their own health. Some of these are referred to as subjective health measures, while others are referred to as either quality of life scales or health-related quality of life scales. Research has also addressed other related outcome variables such as benefit-finding, post-traumatic growth, adjustment and meaning-making which all reflect the ways in which an illness impacts upon an individual's life (see Chapter 8). The literature in the area of subjective health status and quality of life is plagued by two main questions: 'What is quality of life?' and 'How should it be measured?'

WHAT IS QUALITY OF LIFE?

Reports of a Medline search on the term 'quality of life' indicate a surge in its use from 40 citations (1966–74), to 1,907 citations (1981–85), to 5,078 citations (1986–90) (Albrecht 1994). Quality of life is obviously in vogue. However, to date there exists no consensus as to what it actually *is*. For example, it has been defined as 'the value assigned to duration of life as modified by the impairments, functional states, perceptions and social opportunities that are influenced by disease, injury, treatment or policy' (Patrick and Ericson 1993), 'a personal statement of the positivity or negativity of attributes that characterise one's life' (Grant et al. 1990) and by the World Health Organization (WHO) as 'a broad ranging concept affected in a complex way by the person's physical health, psychological state, level of independence, social relationships and their relationship to the salient features in their environment' (WHOQoL Group 1993). Further, while some researchers treat the concepts of quality of life as interchangeable, others argue that they are separate (Bradley 2001).

Such problems with definition have resulted in a range of ways of operationalizing quality of life. For example, following the discussions about an acceptable definition of quality of life, the European Organization for Research on Treatment of Cancer operationalized quality of life in terms of 'functional status, cancer and treatment specific symptoms, psychological distress, social interaction, financial/economic impact, perceived health status and overall quality of life' (Aaronson et al. 1993). In line with this, their measure consisted of items that reflected these different dimensions. Likewise, the researchers who worked on the Rand Corporation health batteries operationalized quality of life in terms of 'physical functioning, social functioning, role limitations due to physical problems, role limitations due to emotional problems, mental health, energy/vitality, pain and general health perception', which formed the basic dimensions of their scale (e.g. Stewart and Ware 1992). Furthermore, Fallowfield (1990) defined the four main dimensions of quality of life as psychological (mood, emotional distress, adjustment to illness), social (relationships, social and leisure activities), occupational (paid and unpaid work) and physical (mobility, pain, sleep and appetite).

Creating a Conceptual Framework

In response to the problems of defining quality of life, researchers have recently attempted to create a clearer conceptual framework for this construct. In particular, they have divided quality of life measures either according to who devises the measure or in terms of whether the measure is considered objective or subjective.

Who Devises the Measure?

Browne et al. (1997) differentiated between the standard needs approach and the psychological processes perspective. The first of these is described as being based on the assumption that 'a consensus about what constitutes a good or poor quality of life exists or at least can be discovered through investigation' (Browne et al. 1997: 738). In addition, the standard needs approach assumes that needs rather than wants are central to quality of life and that these needs are common to all, including the researchers. In contrast, the psychological processes approach considers quality of life to be 'constructed from individual evaluations of personally salient aspects of life' (Browne et al. 1997: 737). Therefore Browne et al. conceptualized measures of quality of life as being devised either by researchers or by the individuals themselves.

Is the Measure Objective or Subjective?

Muldoon et al. (1998) provided an alternative conceptual framework for quality of life based on the degree to which the domains being rated can be objectively validated. They argued that quality of life measures should be divided into those that assess objective functioning and those that assess subjective well-being. The first of these reflects those measures that describe an individual's level of functioning, which they argue must be validated against directly observed behavioural performance, and the second describes the individual's own appraisal of their well-being.

Therefore some progress has been made to clarify the problems surrounding measures of quality of life. However, until a consensus among researchers and clinicians exists, it remains unclear what quality of life is, and whether quality of life is different to subjective health status and health-related quality of life. In fact, Annas (1990) argued that we should stop using the term altogether. However, 'quality of life', 'subjective health status' and 'health-related quality of life' continue to be used and their measurement continues to be taken. The range of measures developed will now be considered in terms of: (1) unidimensional measures and (2) multidimensional measures.

HOW SHOULD IT BE MEASURED?
Unidimensional Measures

Many measures focus on one particular aspect of health. For example, Goldberg (1978) developed the General Health Questionnaire (GHQ), which assesses mood by asking questions such as, 'Have you recently: been able to concentrate on whatever you're doing/spent much time chatting to people/been feeling happy or depressed?' The GHQ is available as long forms, consisting of 30, 28 or 20 items, and as a short form, which consists of 12 items. While the short form is mainly used to explore mood in general and provides results as to an individual's relative mood (i.e. is the person better or worse than usual?), the longer forms have been used to detect 'caseness' (i.e. is the person depressed or not?). Other unidimensional measures include the following: the Hospital Anxiety and Depression Scale (HADS) (Zigmond and Snaith 1983) and the Beck Depression Inventory (BDI) (Beck et al. 1961), both of which focus on mood; the McGill Pain Questionnaire, which assesses pain levels (Melzack 1975); measures of self-esteem, such as the Self-esteem Scale (Rosenberg 1965) and the Self-esteem Inventory (Coopersmith 1967); measures of social support (e.g. Sarason et al. 1983, 1987); measures of satisfaction with life (e.g. Diner et al. 1985); and measures of symptoms (e.g. deHaes et al. 1990).

These unidimensional measures assess health in terms of one specific aspect of health and can be used on their own or in conjunction with other measures.

Multidimensional Measures

Multidimensional measures assess health in the broadest sense. However, this does not mean that such measures are always long and complicated. For example, researchers often use a single item such as, 'Would you say your health is: excellent/good/fair/poor?' or 'Rate your current state of health on a scale ranging from "poor" to "perfect"'. Further, some researchers simply ask respondents to make a relative judgement about their health on a scale from 'best possible' to 'worst possible'. In addition to these measures of self-reported health, researchers have also assessed self-reported fitness (Phillips et al. 2010). Although these simple measures do not provide as much detail as longer measures, they have been shown to correlate highly with other more complex measures and to be useful as outcome measures (Idler and Kasl 1995). Furthermore, they have also been shown to be good predictors of mortality at follow-ups ranging from 2 to 28 years even when a wide range of factors including demographics, smoking and medical diagnoses are taken into account (Idler and Benyamini 1997; Phillips et al. 2010). This indicates that how healthy people think they are predicts when they die!

Composite Scales

In the main, researchers have tended to use *composite scales*. Because of the many ways of defining quality of life, many different measures have been developed. Some focus on particular populations, such as the elderly (McKee et al. 2002), children (Jirojanakul and Skevington 2000), or those in the last year of life (Lawton et al. 1990). Others focus on specific illnesses, such as diabetes (Bradley et al. 1999), arthritis (Meenan et al. 1980), heart disease (Rector et al. 1993), HIV (Skevington and O'Connell 2003) and renal disease (Bradley 1997). In addition, generic measures of quality of life have also been developed, which can be applied to all individuals. These include the Nottingham Health Profile (NHP) (Hunt et al. 1986), the Short Form 36 (SF36) (Ware and Sherbourne 1992), the Sickness Impact Profile (SIP) (Bergner et al. 1981) and the WHOQoL-100 (Skevington et al. 2004a, 2004b). Research using these generic measures has explored quality of life in people from different cultures, with different levels of health and different levels of economic security (e.g. (Skevington et al. 2004a, 2004b). All of these measures have been criticized for being too broad and therefore resulting in a definition of quality of life that is all-encompassing, vague and unfocused. In contrast, they have also been criticized for being too focused and for potentially missing out aspects of quality of life that may be of specific importance to the individual concerned. In particular, it has been suggested that by asking individuals to answer a predefined set of questions and to rate statements that have been developed by researchers, the individuals' own concerns may be missed. This has led to the development of individual quality of life measures.

Individual Quality of Life Measures

Measures of subjective health status ask the individual to rate their own health. This is in contrast to measures of mortality, morbidity and most measures of functioning, which are completed by carers, researchers or an observer. However, although such measures enable individuals to rate their own health, they do not allow them to select the dimensions along which to rate it. For example, a measure that asks about an individual's work life assumes that work is important to this person, but they might not want to work. A measure that asks about family life might be addressing the question to someone who is glad not to see their family. How can one set of individuals who happen to be researchers know what is important to the quality of life of another set of individuals? In line with this perspective, researchers have developed individual quality of life measures, which not only ask the subjects to rate their own health status but also to define the dimensions along which it should be rated. One such measure, the Schedule for Evaluating Individual Quality of Life (SEIQoL) (McGee et al. 1991; O'Boyle et al. 1992) asks subjects to select five areas of their lives that are important to them, to weight them in terms of their importance and then to rate how satisfied they currently are with each dimension.

Patient Reported Outcome Measures (PROMS)

Over the past few years there has been an increased interest in the use of Patient Reported Outcome Measures (PROMS; see Black 2013 for a review). These ask patients to rate aspects of their health, usually before and after a clinical procedure such as a hip replacement or varicose vein surgery, but they may also be used throughout the course of a chronic condition such as cancer or dementia. PROMS can be either disease-specific (i.e. specific to the hip) or generic (i.e. self-care, mood, ADLs). PROMS clearly overlap with the measures of quality of life described above as they can be unidimensional (i.e. hip only), multidimensional (i.e. self-care and mood), designed by the researcher but completed by the patient. PROMS were initially used in research, but were then adopted by health professionals to improve the management of individual patients. Over recent years some PROMS have been standardized so that patient outcomes can be compared between different healthcare providers. If made public, this data could enable patients to choose where they go for any specific clinical intervention.

4   A SHIFT IN PERSPECTIVE

Health status can be assessed in terms of objective measures such as mortality rates, morbidity and levels of functioning or subjective health measures which focus on the perspective of the individual and overlap with measures of quality of life and health-related quality of life. These different measures illustrate a shift among a number of perspectives (see Figure 14.20).

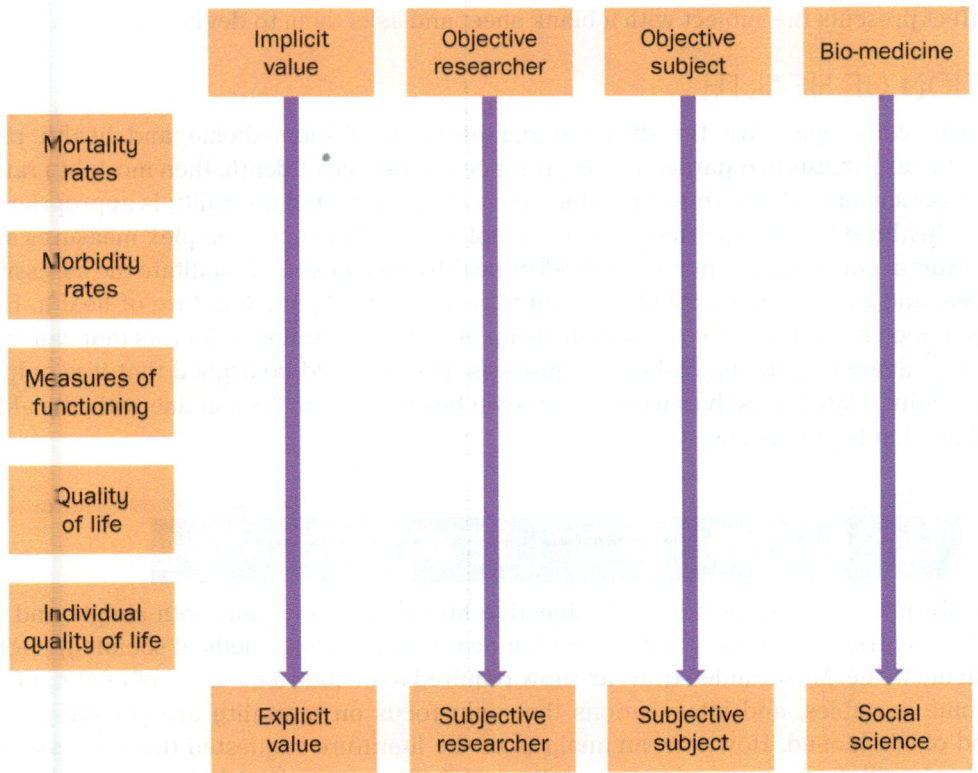

Figure 14.20 A shift in perspective in measuring health

VALUE

The shift from mortality rates to subjective health measures represents a move from implicit value to attempts to make this value explicit. For example, mortality and morbidity measures assume that what they are measuring is an absolute index of health. The subjects being studied are not asked, 'Is it a bad thing that you cannot walk upstairs?' or the relatives asked, 'Did they want to die?' Subjective health measures attempt to make the value within the constructs being studied explicit by asking, 'To what extent are you prevented from doing the things you would like to do?'

SUBJECTIVITY OF THE SUBJECT

Mortality and morbidity measures are assumed to be objective scientific measures that access a reality that is uncontaminated by bias. In contrast, subjective measures make this bias the essence of what they are interested in. For example, mortality data are taken from hospital records or death certificates, and morbidity ratings are often made by the health professionals rather than the individuals being studied. However, subjective health measures ask the individual for their own experiences and beliefs in terms of 'How do you rate your health?' or 'How do you feel?' They make no pretence to be objective and, rather than attempting to exclude the individuals' beliefs, they make them their focus.

SUBJECTIVITY OF THE RESEARCHER

In addition, there is also a shift in the ways in which measures of health status conceptualize the researcher. For example, mortality and morbidity rates are assumed to be consistent regardless of who collected them; the researcher is assumed to be an objective person. Subjective measures, however, attempt to address the issue of researcher subjectivity. For example, self-report questionnaires and the use of closed questions aim to minimize researcher input. However, the questions being asked and the response frames given are still chosen by the researcher. In contrast, the SEIQoL (O'Boyle et al. 1992) in effect presents the subject with a blank sheet and asks them to devise their own scale.

DEFINITION OF HEALTH

Finally, such shifts epitomize the different perspectives of biomedicine and health psychology. Therefore, if health status is regarded as the presence or absence of death, then mortality rates provide a suitable assessment tool. Death is a reliable outcome variable and mortality is appropriately simple. If, however, health status is regarded as more complex than this, more complex measures are needed. Morbidity rates account for a continuum model of health and illness and facilitate the assessment of the greyer areas, and even some morbidity measures accept the subjective nature of health. However, if health psychology regards health status as made up of a complex range of factors that can only be both chosen and evaluated by the individuals themselves, then it could be argued that it is only measures that ask the individuals themselves to rate their own health that are fully in line with a health psychology model of what health means.

5   USING QUALITY OF LIFE IN RESEARCH

Quality of life measures, in the form of subjective health measures and both simple and composite scales, play a central role in many debates within health psychology, medical sociology, primary care and clinical medicine. Most funded trials are now required to include a measure of quality of life among their outcome variables, and interventions that only focus on mortality are generally regarded as narrow and old-fashioned. However, an analysis of the literature suggested that the vast majority of published trials still do not report data on quality of life. For example, following an assessment of the Cochrane Controlled Trials Register from 1980 to 1997, Sanders et al. (1998) reported that, although the frequency of reporting quality of life data had increased from 0.63 to 4.2 per cent for trials from all disciplines, from 1.5 to 8.2 per cent for cancer trials and from 0.34 to 3.6 per cent for cardiovascular trials, less than 5 per cent of all trials reported data on quality of life. Furthermore, they showed that this proportion was below 10 per cent even for cancer trials. In addition, they indicated that, while 72 per cent of the trials used established measures of quality of life, 22 per cent used measures developed by the authors themselves. Therefore it would seem that, although quality of life is in vogue and is a required part of outcome research, it still remains underused. For those trials that do include a measure of quality of life, it is used mainly as an outcome variable and the data are analysed to assess whether the intervention had an impact on the individual's health status, including their quality of life. Sometimes, quality of life is used a predictor variable and has shown to be associated with mortality. The use of quality of life as an outcome variable and as a predictor of mortality will now be discussed.

QUALITY OF LIFE AS AN OUTCOME MEASURE

At its simplest, research using cross-sectional and longitudinal designs has explored the impact of an illness on an individual's quality of life. For example, Wiczinski et al. (2009) explored the association between obesity and quality of life in 2,732 participants from Germany. The results indicated that obesity was associated with reduced physical but not mental quality of life as measured by the SF-12 in men and women and that this link was mediated by strong social support, but only in men. Research has examined how a range of interventions influence an individual's quality of life using a repeated-measures design. For example, a trial of breast reduction surgery compared women's quality of life before and after the operation (Klassen et al. 1996). The study involved 166 women who were referred for plastic surgery, mainly for physical reasons, and their health status was assessed using the SF36 to assess general quality of life, the 28-item GHQ to assess mood and Rosenberg's self-esteem scale. The results showed that the women reported significantly better quality of life both before and after the operation than a control group of women in the general population and, further, that the operation resulted in an improvement in the women's physical, social and psychological functioning, including their levels of 'caseness' for psychiatric morbidity. Accordingly, the authors concluded that breast reduction surgery is beneficial for quality of life and should be included in NHS purchasing contracts.

Quality of life has also been included as an outcome variable for disease-specific randomized controlled trials to illustrate how one form of intervention may be more effective than another. For example, Koevska et al. (2019) concluded from their randomized control trial that exercise can improve quality of life in post-menopausal women with osteoporosis; the DAFNE study group (2002) concluded that teaching diabetic patients flexible intensive treatment which combines dietary freedom and insulin adjustment (dose adjustment for normal eating – DAFNE) improved both the patients' glycaemic control and their quality of life at follow-up and Bond et al. (2015) concluded that a physical activity intervention pre-bariatric surgery not only increased physical activity but also improved mental HRQoL compared with those receiving standard care. Likewise, Fayazi et al. (2020) concluded from their trial that self-care education can increase the quality of life among patients with coronary artery disease and Mardani et al. (2021) reported that exercise can improve the quality of life of prostate cancer survivors.

At times, Quality of Life has also been used as an outcome variable showing that interventions are equivalent. For example, Grunfeld et al. (1996) examined the relative impact of providing either hospital (routine care) or primary care follow-ups for women with breast cancer. The study included 296 women with breast cancer who were in remission and randomly allocated them to receive follow-up care either in hospital or by their GP. Quality of life was assessed using some of the dimensions from the SF36 and the HADS. The results showed that general practice care was not associated with any deterioration in quality of life. In addition, it was not related to an increased time to diagnose any recurrence of the cancer Therefore the authors concluded that general practice care of women in remission from breast cancer is as good as hospital care. Similarly, Armstrong et al. (2019) carried out a pragmatic, randomized controlled equivalency trial which concluded that an online, collaborative connected-health model resulted in equivalent improvements in quality of life compared with in-person care for psoriasis. Likewise, Shepperd et al. (1998) examined the relative effectiveness of home versus hospital care for patients with a range of problems, including hip replacement, knee replacement and hysterectomy. Quality of life was assessed using tools such as the SF36 and disease-specific measures, and the results showed no differences between the two groups at a three-month follow-up. The authors concluded that if there are no significant differences between home and hospital care in terms of quality of life, then the cost of these different forms of care becomes an important factor.

PROBLEMS WITH USING QUALITY OF LIFE AS AN OUTCOME MEASURE

Research uses quality of life as an outcome measure for trials that have different designs and are either focused on specific illnesses or involve a range of problems. However, there are the following difficulties with such studies:

- Different studies use different ways of measuring quality of life: generalizing across studies is difficult.
- Some studies use the term 'quality of life' while others use the term 'subjective health status': generalizing across studies is difficult.
- Some studies report results from the different measures of quality of life, which are in the opposite direction to each other: drawing conclusions is difficult.
- Some studies report the results from quality of life measures, which are in the opposite direction to mortality or morbidity data: deciding whether an intervention is good or bad is difficult.

QUALITY OF LIFE AS A PREDICTOR OF MORTALITY

Most research using quality of life explores its predictors and therefore places this variable as the end-point. However, it is possible that quality of life may also be a predictor of future events, particularly mortality. This is illustrated indirectly by several studies that indicate that mortality is higher in the first six months after the death of a spouse, particularly from heart disease or suicide (e.g. Schaefer et al. 1995; Martikainen and Valkonen 1996). It is also illustrated directly by studies measuring quality of life at baseline and then collecting follow up measures of mortality. For example, Terrin et al. (2015) found that emotional, physical and role functioning together with global HRQL all predicted transplant-related mortality in a paediatric sample and Höfer et al. (2014) found that a deterioration of ≥ 0.5 points in MacNew HRQL global scores predicted mortality by 4 years in patients with coronary artery disease. Similarly, Pocock et al. (2021) carried out a prospective study with almost 9000 patients 1–3 years post-MI and reported that a lower health-related quality of life score at enrolment was associated with a higher subsequent risk of all-cause death, of a major CV event and more hospitalizations over the next 2 years.

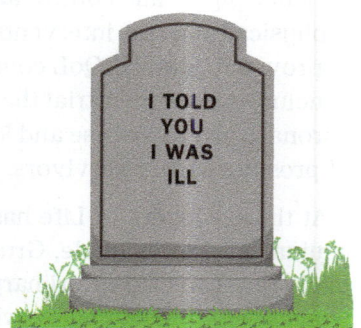

Not all measures of quality of life need to be this complex, however, and research indicates that simple self-report measures of health status that ask an individual to rate their own health using single item scales are predictive of mortality at follow-ups ranging from 2 to 28 years (Idler and Benyamini 1997; Phillips et al. 2010). In fact, the comedian Spike Milligan was reported to have joked that he wanted the words 'I told you I was ill' on his tombstone. Milligan recognized that subjective health status was a good predictor of mortality! Therefore quality of life may not only be an outcome variable in itself but a predictor of further outcomes in the future.

Subjective health status can predict mortality: Spike Milligan's joke about his tombstone

To test the impact of quality of life on mortality, Phillips et al. (2010) analysed data from a large cohort study called the West of Scotland Twenty-07 study which involved participants from the Glasgow region. For this study, wave 2 data were selected as the baseline (data collected in 1991/92) as this database included measures of both self-reported health and self-reported fitness. At baseline the sample (n = 858) were almost all white, 46 per cent were male, 38 per cent were current smokers, 71 per cent had a long-standing illness and participants had a mean age of 59. Participants completed two very simple single items measures of health status: **Self-reported health:** 'would you say that for someone your own age your own health is. . .' with the response options being excellent/good/fair/poor and **Self-reported fitness:** 'would you say that for someone your own age your fitness is. . .' with the response options being very good/good/moderate/poor/very poor. Mortality data was then collected after 16.5 years when 247 of the original sample had died. The mean age of death was 69 and the most common causes were cardiovascular disease (39 per cent), cancer (34 per cent), respiratory disease (13 per cent) and other (14 per cent). The data was then analysed to explore the role of both these measures of health status in predicting death 16.5 years later while controlling for potential confounding variables (sex, occupational group, smoking status, body mass index (BMI), blood pressure, longstanding illness). Overall, the results showed that those with either poor ratings of health or poor ratings of fitness at baseline were 2 times more likely to have died by 16.5 years follow-up. Further, in the individual models both self-reported health and self-reported fitness were individually significant predictors of mortality. In addition, when both measures of health status were entered into the equation, both remained significant with those participants with both poor health and poor fitness at baseline being 2.7 times more likely to have died by follow-up. This indicates that self-reported health and self-reported fitness predicted mortality independently of each even when other possible risk factors had been controlled for. Furthermore, the existence of both poor self-reported health and poor self-reported fitness appeared to be a particularly lethal combination. These simple single item measures of health status were powerful predictors of death.

6 | THE RESPONSE SHIFT

Quality of life research is often inconsistent, presenting challenges to those involved in its measurement. For example, people often rate their quality of life differently at different time points even though there are no observable changes to their lives and often there seems to be no relationship between any objective assessment of quality of life and the person's own ratings of their health status. Some of this variation has been attributed to measurement error. Increasingly, however, it is seen as an illustration of the appraisal processes involved in making quality of life assessments and has been addressed within the context of the *response shift* (Rapkin and Schwartz 2004). Rapkin and Schwartz argued that each time a person judges their quality of life they must establish a 'frame of reference' which determines how they comprehend the questions being asked (what do the words 'health', 'mood', 'family', 'work' mean to them?). Next they decide upon 'standards of comparison', which include both between- and within-subject comparisons, to decide whether to judge their quality of life in terms of their own past history, their expectations

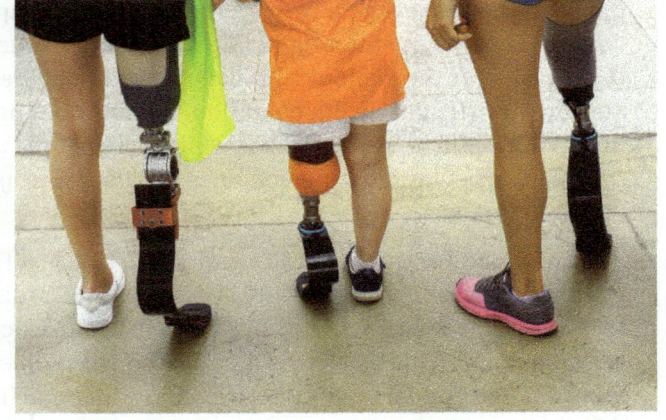

People can show an improvement in their quality of life even after a serious illness or injury – the response shift

SOURCE: © Shutterstock / Dmitry Markov152

of themselves or other people they know ('Am I better off or worse off than I have been or than other people?'). Then they decide upon a 'sampling strategy' to determine which parts of their life they should assess ('Should I think of right now or how far back should I go?'). People then combine these three sets of appraisals to formulate a response. From this perspective, inconsistencies in the quality of life literature are no longer seen as a product of measurement error but as illustrations of the complex ways in which people make judgements about their health. In line with this, Ogden and Lo (2012) compared aspects of health status between people who were homeless, students and those living in the town. The results indicated some strange findings, such as those who were homeless rating themselves as less tired, more healthy and less lonely. Using the qualitative data as a comparison it was argued that this reflected a form of the response shift with ratings on the Likert scales being influenced by three factors: i) frame of reference (current salient issues influence how questions are interpreted); ii) within subject comparisons (ratings are based on past experiences); iii) time frame (people can habituate to difficult circumstances). Therefore people who are homeless may rate aspects of their quality of life as better due to immediate benefits (finding a hostel bed), having been in an even worse situation in the past and having got used to being homeless.

In the context of physical health, studies show that although immediately after diagnosis of an illness or the occurrence of a serious injury people's rated quality of life might be poor, several months later it may well be high again even though their physical condition has remained constant. For example, Dempster et al. (2010) concluded from their study of cardiac patients that the response shift occurred over the course of a cardiac rehabilitation programme and that it was related to changes in an individual's internal standards and correlated with active coping strategies. Similarly, the response shift has been reported in parents of children diagnosed with epilepsy (Sajobi et al. 2017) and in patients with Parkinson's disease (Yang et al. 2017).

BOX 14.1
Critical Approaches to Health Psychology

Research and theories relating to health status and quality of life highlight some of the bigger issues in health psychology as follows:

Individual differences: There are clear health inequalities across a range of dimensions such as age, gender, geographical location and sexuality. These inequalities need to be mapped and recognized so that we can understand the factors behind them and develop strategies to reduce them. At the same time however, the process of mapping can create false dichotomies and even contribute towards stereotyping by different demographic variables. This process also illustrates the problem of the ecological fallacy – there may be a link between gender and health status, or age and a particular health condition, but this does not mean that at the level of the individual this observation still holds. Therefore while older people may have poorer health than younger people, this one particular older person does not necessarily have poorer health than this one particular younger person.

Mind vs body: Quality of life and subjective health status reflect how a person perceives their health, whereas illness status or a diagnosis of a disease reflect an objective version of health. Likewise, how someone feels about their health is considered different from what their body is actually doing. This illustrates a divide between objective and subjective health and between the mind and the body. In reality, however, there is much more interaction between these factors than this suggests. So an objective version of health probably still has an element of subjectivity and a biological marker of the body will influence and be influenced by the mind. We often create separation between variables when they are much more blurred than we acknowledge.

The individual vs the social vs the political: While we may focus on health as an individual variable, how an individual perceives their health will very much depend on the social norms of their society. For example, a culture that expects people to live a long time will rate an illness in an individual at the age of 75 as more serious than a culture which sees that illness as nature taking its course. Likewise, a culture that has access to medical treatment will rate illness as more problematic than one which is more fatalistic or one which has never known treatments to work. Health very much exists within a social and political world and often this gets lost from a psychological viewpoint.

7 | THINKING CRITICALLY ABOUT HEALTH STATUS AND QUALITY OF LIFE

There are many problems with research exploring health status and quality of life.

SOME CRITICAL QUESTIONS

When thinking about research in this area ask yourself the following questions.

- What are the problems with measuring health status?
- What are the implications of the different approaches to measurement for research and clinical practice?
- How might the chosen measure of health status influence the rationing of health services?
- What do you think is the most important patient health outcome?
- How might politics get in the way of understanding the impact of COVID?
- How might psychological factors influence what is considered the cause of death from COVID?

SOME PROBLEMS WITH. . .

Below are some specific problems with research in this area that you may wish to consider.

Measurement: Health status can be measured using either tools that include predefined domains or those that rely on the individual themselves to generate the domains. Both are problematic. Even the definition and recording of cause of death can be influenced by subjective factors.

Simple vs complex: Quality of life measures are sometimes criticized for missing important domains and for being too simple. Sometimes they are criticized for being over-inclusive, unwieldy and difficult to use. The choice of measure therefore has to be pragmatic and based upon what a particular person is deemed able to complete at any particular time rather than perfect theoretical principles.

Research synthesis: Research measuring health outcomes often includes a range of health status, quality of life and physiological measures. Often these measures contradict each other. For example, while an intervention may improve longevity, it may be detrimental to quality of life. How these different outcomes are combined is unclear and can cause conflict or confusion for health professionals.

From research into practice: Policy makers use outcome measures to decide where funding should be spent. For example, should the health service fund drug A, drug B, counselling or surgery? This decision is based upon a calculation of both the clinical effectiveness and the cost effectiveness of any given intervention. If a drug improves longevity but reduces quality of life, while counselling improves quality of life but reduces longevity, it will mean these decisions are complex and often hotly debated.

TO CONCLUDE

Health varies hugely by a number of factors including geographical location, time, gender and SES. This is particularly apparent with the impact of the COVID pandemic and how this has varied around the world. Health is also the focus of much research not only in medicine and allied health professions, such as nursing and physiotherapy, but also in health psychology. Researchers therefore need to measure health status. This chapter has explored the different ways of measuring health status. In particular, it has examined the use of objective measures such as mortality rates, morbidity rates, measures of functioning and measures of subjective health status and quality of life. It then described how the change from mortality rates to quality of life reflects a shift from implicit to explicit value, an increasing subjectivity on behalf of both the subject being studied and the researcher, and a change in the definition of health from a biomedical dichotomous model to a more complex psychological one. Further, it explored definitions of quality of life and the vast range of scales that have been developed to assess this complex construct, and their use in research. Finally, it described the use of quality of life in research as an outcome variable, as a predictor of mortality and within the context of the response shift.

QUESTIONS

1 Health varies by geography, SES, time and gender. What are the problems with making comparisons across these variables?
2 COVID clearly varies around the world. What factors could influence our understanding of the impact of the pandemic in terms of cases and deaths?
3 Mortality rates are the most accurate measure of health status. Discuss.
4 The views of the subject get in the way of measuring health. Discuss.
5 The views of the researcher get in the way of measuring health. Discuss.
6 To what extent is quality of life a useful construct?
7 Should all outcome research include an assessment of quality of life?
8 To what extent can quality of life predict mortality?
9 Describe the mechanisms of the response shift and how this could help our understanding of how people respond to illness or trauma.

FOR DISCUSSION

Consider the last time you felt that your quality of life was reduced. What did this mean to you and would this be addressed by the available measures?

FURTHER READING

Armstrong, D. (2021) The COVID-19 pandemic and cause of death. *Sociology of Health & Illness*, **43**(7): 1614–26. Doi.org/10.1111/1467-9566.13347.

This is an interesting paper which explores problems with death rates from COVID and addresses issues such as what influences what goes on a death certificate

Black, N. (2013) Patient reported outcome measures could help transform healthcare, *BMJ (Clinical research ed.)*, **346**: f167. Doi.org/10.1136/bmj.f167.
Patient reported outcomes (PROMS) are increasingly used in clinical care and emphasize the patient perspective alongside that of the clinician. This paper provides a useful overview of what they are and the challenges involved in bringing them into routine care.

Bowling, A. (2017) *Measuring Health: A Review of Subjective Health, Well-being and Quality of Life Measurement Scales*, 4th edn. Maidenhead: Open University Press.
This is an extremely comprehensive overview of the different scales that have been developed to assess quality of life. It also includes two interesting chapters on what quality of life is and theories of measurement.

Joyce, C.R.B., O'Boyle, C.A. and McGee, H.M. (eds) (1999) *Individual Quality of Life*. London: Harwood.
This edited book provides details on the conceptual and methodological principles of quality of life and focuses on individual measures. It then provides some examples of using these measures, together with some ideas for future directions.

Marmot M. (2007) *Status Syndrome: How your social standing directly affects your health and life expectancy*. London: Bloomsbury Publishing Plc.
This book by Michael Marmot pulls together many of his ideas and the data exploring health inequalities. It is easier to read than some of the reports in this area!

Marmot M and Allen J. (2020) COVID-19: exposing and amplifying inequalities, *Journal of Epidemiology and Community Health*, **74**:681–682.
Much has been written about the impact of the COVID pandemic on health inequalities. This is a really interesting commentary which locates COVID within previous 'plagues' and discusses whether it is a leveller or an exacerbator of differences across society.

Marmot M., Allen J., Boyce T., et al. (2020) *Health Equity in England: the Marmot review 10 years on*. London, UK: Institute of Health Equity, UCL.
Michael Marmot is a world-leading epidemiologist who writes extensively about health inequalities and the impact of social deprivation on health outcomes. I would read anything from his web page! But this is a good start as it takes the initial report from 2010 and explores what has changed in the past 10 years.

Rapkin, B.D. and Schwartz, C.E. (2004) Towards a theoretical model of quality of life appraisal: implications of findings from studies of response shift, *The Social Causes of Illness Health and Quality of Life Outcomes*, **2**: 14.
This is an excellent paper that describes the notion of the response shift and outlines the mechanisms that might be involved in this process of change and adaptation.

15
Gender and Health

© Shutterstock / Dmytro Gilitukha

CHAPTER OVERVIEW

Health status varies by geographical location, social class, ethnic group and time. It also varies by gender. This chapter first explores the impact of gender on health and illness. The chapter then addresses health conditions specific to women with a focus on miscarriage, termination of pregnancy and menopause. These have been chosen as they can generate strong emotional reactions, all involve some interaction with the health system and illustrate how the choice of intervention can change a woman's experience. Next, the chapter focuses on men's health and describes men's health behaviour and recent theories which have analysed why men behave differently to women. The chapter addresses three case examples which highlight many of the key issues for men's health: prostate cancer, suicide and coronary heart disease (CHD). The chapter then addresses health issues specific to the LGBTQ+ community with a focus on stigma, prejudice and the impact upon help seeking behaviour. Finally, the chapter considers problems with research in this area including the impact of ideology and methodological issues.

CASE STUDY

Isaac and Yasmin are twins in their mid-thirties. They have always been very close and still live near each other. But they are very different. Yasmin likes to look after herself and so she eats well, walks as much as she can, doesn't smoke and drinks only occasionally. Isaac, however, has always been a bit wild and thinks he is immortal. He likes to drive his car at top speed on the motorway and still has big nights out with his friends where they take drugs and drink too much even though they all have jobs to get up for in the morning. He also lives on his own and often doesn't cook and so misses meals or eats takeaways. Yasmin loves her brother but thinks that it is time he grew up. She also worries about his health as he is very thin and often looks quite pale. Recently, he has started to seem quite low and depressed although he says everything is fine when she asks him about it.

Through the Eyes of Health Psychology. . .

Health is clearly gendered and, although much has changed over the past one hundred years in terms of gender equality, men and women still show different patterns of health behaviours and illness. Isaac and Yasmin's stories illustrate some of the reasons why men and women have different health patterns in terms of beliefs (feeling immortal vs wanting to look after herself), behaviours (smoking, drug use, risk taking, drinking vs eating well, walking) and beliefs about masculinity (being wild, not growing up vs liking to look after herself). This chapter explores these differences and outlines theories of why these differences still exist.

A NOTE ON GENDER

Research commonly explores differences between men and women and, in the case of health psychology, highlights differences in terms of beliefs, behaviour and health outcomes. There are several problems with this approach. First, it may promote a stereotypical approach to men and women emphasizing the differences *between* these groups rather than similarities. Second, in emphasizing these differences between men and women it also minimizes any differences *within* men and *within* women. It therefore promotes the notion that men are more similar to men and women are more similar to women than they are to each other. We therefore start to ignore variability within all men and within all women and treat each gender as a simple homogenous group. Third, it assumes that gender is a binary construct consisting of only men and women. Over recent years this notion has been hotly debated and the idea of gender fluidity is increasingly accepted in academic circles. Accordingly, whereas some people may identify themselves as male or female, others may find this dichotomy too simplistic for their sense of identity.

This chapter therefore explores gender differences in health and describes conditions of most relevance to women and those of most relevance to men as this is the format of the existing literature. In addition, it explores some of the health issues pertinent to the LGBTQ+ community. So when reading this chapter please keep your critical hat on and engage in some of the wider debates covered at the end of the chapter in the 'Thinking Critically...' section.

1 GENDER DIFFERENCES IN HEALTH

In the twenty-first century there are still gender differences in health and illness in terms of life expectancy, physical symptoms and illness.

LIFE EXPECTANCY

In 2015, the average life expectancy worldwide was 70.5 years; for men it was 68.4 and for women it was 72.8 (WHO 2018) In general, women tend to live longer than men although this varies country by country. For example, the countries with the longest life expectancies for men are Switzerland (81.3), Iceland (81.2), South Korea (78.8), Sweden (80.7) and Israel (80.6) whereas for women the countries are Japan (86.8), Singapore (86.1), Spain (85.5), South Korea (85.5) and France (85.4). The lowest life expectancy is in Sierra Leone which is 49.5 for men and 50.8 for women (WHO 2018). In the UK, life expectancy has gradually increased over the past 40 years driven mostly by improved health care, living and working conditions which has increased

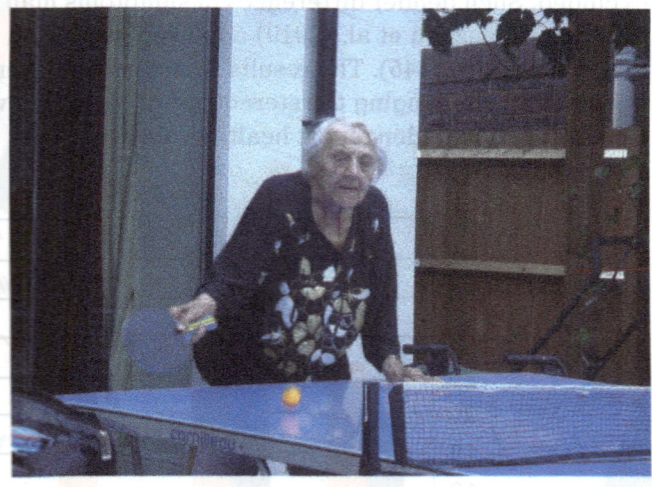

Going strong at 98: women generally live longer than men (This is my Gran who died at 100 after a very long, active and happy life!)

longevity in those of older age. The most recent data for between 2018 and 2020 indicates that life expectancy at birth in the UK was 79.0 years for males and 82.9 years for females. Figure 15.1 shows

Figure 15.1 Life expectancy in men and women, 1982–2020

SOURCE: Office for National Statistics (2020)

an increase for both men and women between 1982 and 2020, with wo...
although this gap is gradually closing (Office for National Statistic...

PHYSICAL SYMPTOMS

In 1996, MacIntyre et al. carried out an ...
der differences in physical sympt...
were no differences for su...
were more likely to ...
having kidney ...
commu...

---

or bisexual men and women reporting poor self-rated health were about 1.2 times higher than for heterosexual people. To date, it seems clear that the health of the LGBTQ+ community is poorer than that of heterosexuals. This is considered further, later on in this chapter.

WHY ARE THERE DIFFERENCES BY GENDER AND SEXUALITY?

There are therefore consistent differences between men and women, with men dying younger than women worldwide and being more likely to develop and die from the leading causes of death such as CHD and cancer. Such gender differences have been understood in terms of the role of biological factors such as oestrogen, which improves lipid profiles and can protect against cardiovascular disease, and the general robustness of females illustrated by the higher neonatal death rate of male babies compared to females. Furthermore, in evolutionary terms women may need to be stronger than men in order to survive childbirth and, whereas maternal mortality reduced women's life expectancy in the past, women have now overtaken men because the risk of dying during labour is much reduced. However, these biological differences cannot be the complete picture as the gap between men and women's life expectancy is not only changing over time but also shows great variation across geographical location, suggesting a strong role for psychological and social factors. Further, biology cannot explain differences in health status for the LBGTQ+ community.

These differences by gender and sexuality can also be understood in terms of all the factors described throughout this book such as health beliefs and behaviour, symptom perception, help-seeking, coping, adherence to medication and behaviour change. There are, however, a few health problems which are gender-specific. For example, while women get breast cancer, endometriosis and uterine cancer, men suffer from baldness, impotence and prostate cancer. Women also suffer miscarriages, receiv... terminations of pregnancy and experience the menopause and men are more likely to get prosta... cancer, die by suicide or have a heart attack. In addition, members of the LGBTQ+ community ... also have a different experience of health, illness and health care due to issues such as stigma, la... of understanding by health care professionals and a reluctance to seek help. This chapter will ... explore some of the gender-specific issues and conditions that women, men and members of ... LGBTQ+ community have to deal with.

Figure 15.:
SOURCE: Adap

ILLNESS

In this analysis ...
They reported tha...
respiratory disorde...
piles, digestive disor...
(see Figure 15.3.)

In addition, women ...
men. Therefore, in gene...
and yet live longer. Intere...
services, are less likely to...
fewer hospital admissions ...
(DH 2001; Bayram et al. 20...
diagnosed with depression, m...
(see later in this chapter).

2 WOMEN'S HEALTH: MISCARRIAGE AND TERMINATION OF PREGNANCY

Regardless of gender, people can become ill with many common health conditions such as ... obesity, cancer and CHD as well as less common health conditions such as MS and fibr... Yet women also have gender-specific conditions to deal with, such as breast cancer (althoug... ity of cases are male), endometrial cancer, endometriosis and cervical cancer. The next two... this chapter will focus on three problems which are more specific to women: miscarriage, ... of pregnancy and the menopause. These problems have been chosen as they generate stro... in those experiencing them, they illustrate the ways in which the mode of intervention ... vs non surgical) can change these experiences and also closely reflect the interests ... psychology community.

MISCARRIAGE

Miscarriage is a relatively common phenomenon occurring in 15–20 per cent of ... cies, with 80 per cent of these occurring within the first trimester (Broquet 1999... 'spontaneous abortion' has been defined as the unintended end of a pregnancy be... survive outside the mother, which is recognized as being before the twentieth...

This chapter therefore explores gender differences in health and describes conditions of most relevance to women and those of most relevance to men as this is the format of the existing literature. In addition, it explores some of the health issues pertinent to the LGBTQ+ community. So when reading this chapter please keep your critical hat on and engage in some of the wider debates covered at the end of the chapter in the 'Thinking Critically. . .' section.

1 GENDER DIFFERENCES IN HEALTH

In the twenty-first century there are still gender differences in health and illness in terms of life expectancy, physical symptoms and illness.

LIFE EXPECTANCY

In 2015, the average life expectancy world-wide was 70.5 years; for men it was 68.4 and for women it was 72.8 (WHO 2018) In general, women tend to live longer than men although this varies country by country. For example, the countries with the longest life expectancies for men are Switzerland (81.3), Iceland (81.2), South Korea (78.8), Sweden (80.7) and Israel (80.6) whereas for women the countries are Japan (86.8), Singapore (86.1), Spain (85.5), South Korea (85.5) and France (85.4). The lowest life expectancy is in Sierra Leone which is 49.5 for men and 50.8 for women (WHO 2018). In the UK, life expectancy has gradually increased over the past 40 years driven mostly by improved health care, living and working conditions which has increased

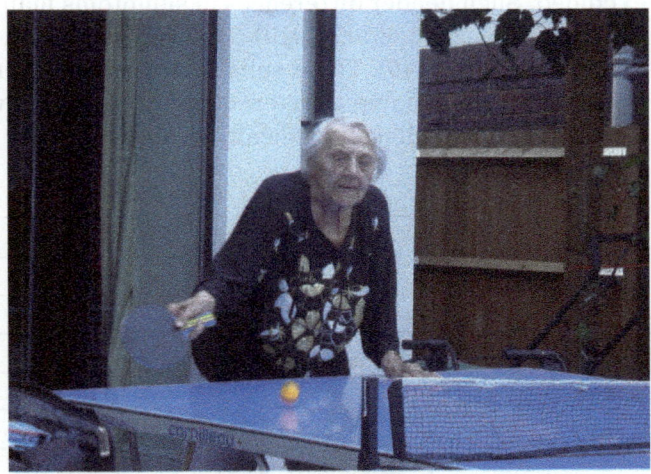

Going strong at 98: women generally live longer than men (This is my Gran who died at 100 after a very long, active and happy life!)

longevity in those of older age. The most recent data for between 2018 and 2020 indicates that life expectancy at birth in the UK was 79.0 years for males and 82.9 years for females. Figure 15.1 shows

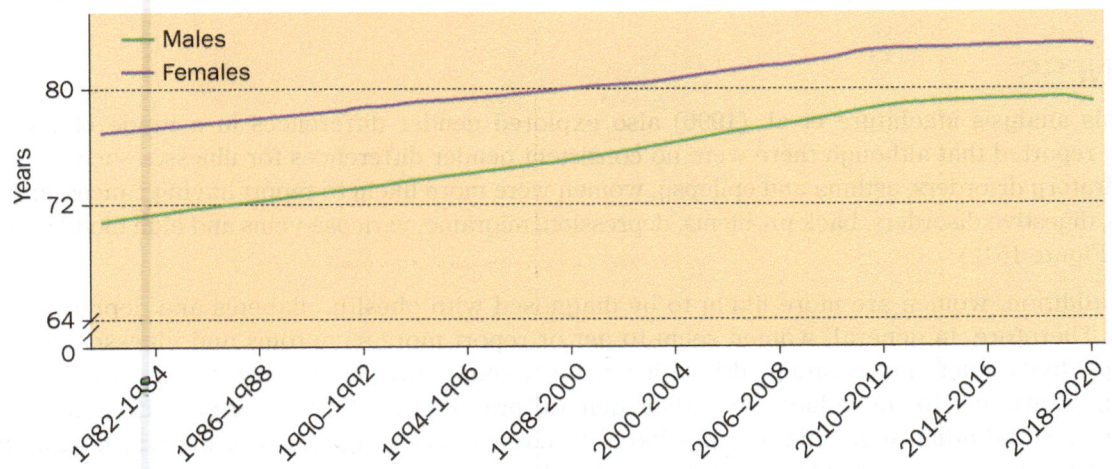

Figure 15.1 Life expectancy in men and women, 1982–2020

SOURCE: Office for National Statistics (2020)

an increase for both men and women between 1982 and 2020, with women living longer than men, although this gap is gradually closing (Office for National Statistics 2020).

PHYSICAL SYMPTOMS

In 1996, MacIntyre et al. carried out an analysis of two large British data sets and explored gender differences in physical symptoms (see Figure 15.2.) The results indicate that although there were no differences for symptoms relating to eyes, ears, colds, flu, palpitations or coughs, women were more likely to report feeling tired, having headaches, constipation, feeling faint or dizzy and having kidney or bladder problems. These findings were replicated in 2001 in both medical and community samples (Barsky et al. 2001) which showed that women report more frequent, intense and numerous physical symptoms even when reproductive and gynaecological symptoms are excluded. Such gender differences in symptoms may not be as clear cut as sometimes believed. For example, Oksuzyan et al. (2019) analysed data from the Survey of Health, Ageing and Retirement in Europe (n = 27345). The results found no clear gendered patterns in reporting for either poor or good health challenging the stereotype of 'sensitive women and stoical men' and that women over-report and men under-report health problems.

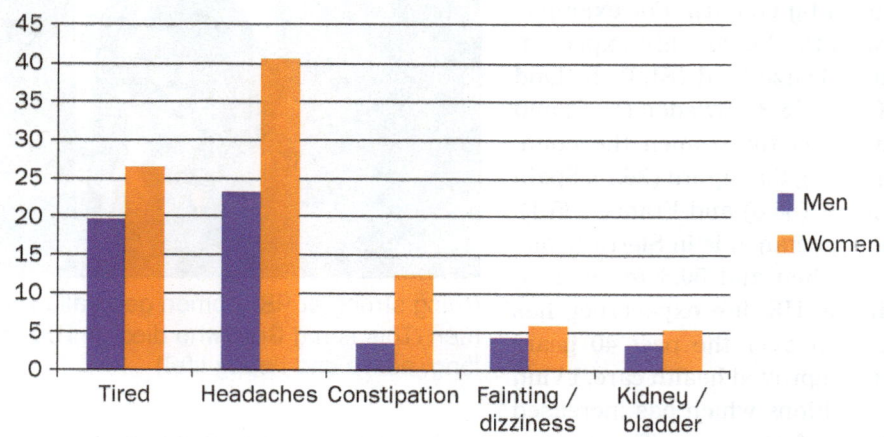

Figure 15.2 Gender differences in physical symptoms

SOURCE: Adapted from MacIntyre et al. (1996)

ILLNESS

In this analysis MacIntyre et al. (1996) also explored gender differences in a range of illnesses. They reported that although there were no consistent gender differences for illnesses such as hernia, respiratory disorders, asthma and epilepsy, women were more likely to report having cancer, arthritis, piles, digestive disorders, back problems, depression, migraine, varicose veins and high blood pressure (see Figure 15.3.)

In addition, women are more likely to be diagnosed with obesity, diabetes and depression than men. Therefore, in general, women seem to get or report more symptoms and illnesses than men and yet live longer. Interestingly, although men die younger, they have less contact with health care services, are less likely to have seen their general practitioner (GP) in the past 12 months, have fewer hospital admissions and are less likely to have a screening test or a general health check (DH 2001; Bayram et al. 2003; Eurostat 2007). Further, although women are more likely to be diagnosed with depression, men are about four times more likely to die from suicide than women (see later in this chapter).

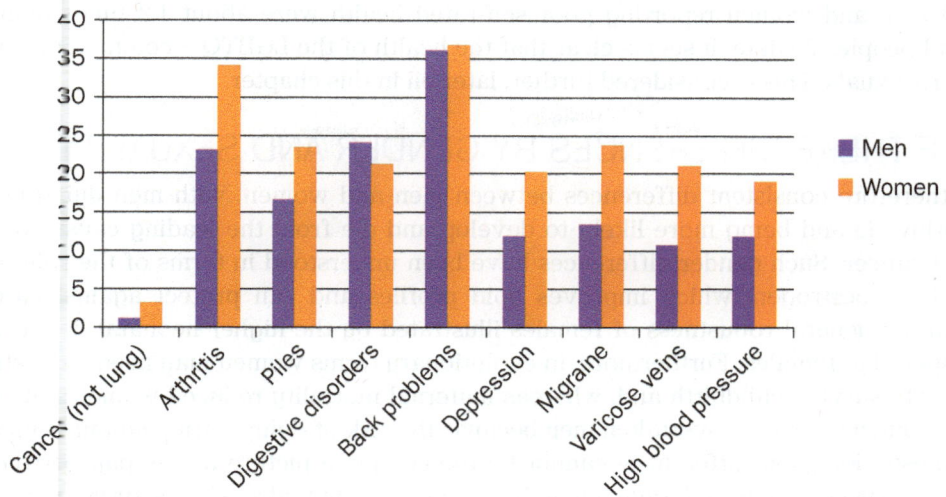

Figure 15.3 Gender differences in a range of illnesses reported

SOURCE: Adapted from MacIntyre et al. (1996)

Worldwide, we also know the following about gender differences in health (see Lee and Glynn Owens 2002 for a comprehensive review):

- Worldwide, men live three years less than women.
- This varies across regions.
- In Eastern Europe men live on average 11 years less than women.
- In the UK men live on average 4 years less than women; 6 years less in the USA.
- In Australia indigenous men live on average 23 years less than non-indigenous women and 19 years less than non-indigenous men.
- In Afghanistan men live on average 1 year longer than women.
- Men are twice as likely to develop and die from the 10 most common cancers which affect both men and women.
- Although CHD is a leading cause of death for both men and women, men die younger from this illness than women.
- Of those who die from a heart attack in the USA under the age of 65, nearly 75 per cent are men.

HEALTH OF THE LGBTQ+ COMMUNITY

Over recent years, as well as focusing on differences between men and women, research has also increasingly explored the health status of members of the LGBTQ+ community. For example, Bränström et al. (2016) analysed data from 60,922 individuals (16–84 years of age) from nationwide population-based health surveys in Sweden collected between 2008 and 2013. In the sample, 0.7 per cent (n = 430) self-identified as gay/lesbian and 1.3 per cent (n = 757) self-identified as bisexual. The results showed that LGB individuals reported poorer self-rated health, more physical health symptoms (e.g. pain, insomnia, dermatitis, tinnitus, intestinal problems) and more health conditions (e.g., diabetes, asthma, high blood pressure) than heterosexuals. In addition, these differences were greater in adolescents and young adults and were related to health behaviours and experiences of perceived discrimination, victimization, and threats of violence. Likewise, in a recent analysis of data by the International Longevity Centre UK (2019) from 24 different surveys, the odds of lesbian, gay, or bisexual men and women reporting poor self-rated health were about 1.2 times higher than for heterosexual people. To date, it seems clear that the health of the LGBTQ+ community is poorer than that of heterosexuals. This is considered further, later on in this chapter.

WHY ARE THERE DIFFERENCES BY GENDER AND SEXUALITY?

There are therefore consistent differences between men and women, with men dying younger than women worldwide and being more likely to develop and die from the leading causes of death such as CHD and cancer. Such gender differences have been understood in terms of the role of biological factors such as oestrogen, which improves lipid profiles and can protect against cardiovascular disease, and the general robustness of females illustrated by the higher neonatal death rate of male babies compared to females. Furthermore, in evolutionary terms women may need to be stronger than men in order to survive childbirth and, whereas maternal mortality reduced women's life expectancy in the past, women have now overtaken men because the risk of dying during labour is much reduced. However, these biological differences cannot be the complete picture as the gap between men and women's life expectancy is not only changing over time but also shows great variation across geographical location, suggesting a strong role for psychological and social factors. Further, biology cannot explain differences in health status for the LBGTQ+ community.

These differences by gender and sexuality can also be understood in terms of all the factors described throughout this book such as health beliefs and behaviour, symptom perception, help-seeking, coping, adherence to medication and behaviour change. There are, however, a few health problems which are gender-specific. For example, while women get breast cancer, endometriosis and uterine cancer, men suffer from baldness, impotence and prostate cancer. Women also suffer miscarriages, receive terminations of pregnancy and experience the menopause and men are more likely to get prostate cancer, die by suicide or have a heart attack. In addition, members of the LGBTQ+ community can also have a different experience of health, illness and health care due to issues such as stigma, lack of understanding by health care professionals and a reluctance to seek help. This chapter will now explore some of the gender-specific issues and conditions that women, men and members of the LGBTQ+ community have to deal with.

| 2 | WOMEN'S HEALTH: MISCARRIAGE AND TERMINATION OF PREGNANCY |

Regardless of gender, people can become ill with many common health conditions such as diabetes, obesity, cancer and CHD as well as less common health conditions such as MS and fibromyalgia. Yet women also have gender-specific conditions to deal with, such as breast cancer (although a minority of cases are male), endometrial cancer, endometriosis and cervical cancer. The next two sections of this chapter will focus on three problems which are more specific to women: miscarriage, termination of pregnancy and the menopause. These problems have been chosen as they generate strong emotions in those experiencing them, they illustrate the ways in which the mode of intervention (e.g. surgical vs non surgical) can change these experiences and also closely reflect the interests of the health psychology community.

MISCARRIAGE

Miscarriage is a relatively common phenomenon occurring in 15–20 per cent of known pregnancies, with 80 per cent of these occurring within the first trimester (Broquet 1999). Miscarriage or 'spontaneous abortion' has been defined as the unintended end of a pregnancy before a foetus can survive outside the mother, which is recognized as being before the twentieth week of gestation

(Borg and Lasker 1982). Despite the frequency with which miscarriage occurs, it has only been in the last 30 years that research has begun to identify and explore the consequences of early pregnancy loss. This section explores the psychological consequences of miscarriage in terms of the quantitative and qualitative research, the impact on couples and then examines the impact of how miscarriage is managed on women's experiences of this event.

QUANTITATIVE RESEARCH

Quantitative research has tended to conceptualize women's reactions to miscarriage in terms of grief, depression and anxiety, or coping.

- *Grief.* One main area of research has conceptualized miscarriage as a loss event, assuming that after miscarriage women experience stages of grief parallel to that of the death of a loved one (Herz 1984). The main symptoms identified are sadness, yearning for the lost child, a desire to talk to others about the loss and a search for meaningful explanations (Herz 1984; Athey and Spielvogel 2000). In addition, research has highlighted grief reactions that are unique to the miscarriage experience. For example, women often perceive themselves as failures for not being able to have a healthy pregnancy and this loss is often not acknowledged by the community because there are no rituals that can be performed (Herz 1984). In 2018, Volgsten et al. published a longitudinal study which followed women up one week and four months after miscarriage. The results showed that while grief was high immediately after the miscarriage this reduced with time. The results also showed that the experience of grief was higher in those who had suffered a previous miscarriage or undergone fertility treatment while having previous children helped the women adjust.

- *Depression and anxiety.* Other research has focused on depression and anxiety following miscarriage. Friedman and Gath (1989) used the Present State Examination (PSE) to assess psychiatric 'caseness' in women four weeks post-miscarriage. They found that 48 per cent of the sample had sufficiently high scores on the scale to qualify as 'case' patients, which is over four times higher than that in women in the general population. When analysed, these women were all classified as having depressive disorders. Klier et al. (2000) similarly found that women who had miscarried had a significantly increased risk of developing a minor depressive disorder in the six months following their loss, compared to a cohort drawn from the community. Thapar and Thapar (1992) also found that women who had miscarried experienced a significant degree of anxiety and depression at both the initial interview and at the six-week follow-up compared to the control group. In contrast, Prettyman et al. (1993) used the Hospital Anxiety and Depression Scale (HADS) and found that anxiety rather than depression was the predominant response at 1, 6 and 12 weeks after miscarriage. Further, Beutel et al. (1995) reported that immediately after the miscarriage the majority of the sample experienced elevated levels of psychological morbidity compared to a community cohort and a pregnant control group, much of which persisted up until the 12-month follow-up. The authors concluded that depression and grief should be considered as two distinct reactions to pregnancy loss, with grief being the normal reaction and depression only developing when certain circumstances are met. This study also showed that a large minority reported no negative emotional reaction post-miscarriage, suggesting that a focus on anxiety, depression and grief may only tap into a part of the miscarriage experience. In 2018, Farren et al. carried out a systematic review of 28 studies to evaluate the evidence for depression, anxiety and post-traumatic stress disorder (PTSD) following a miscarriage or an ectopic pregnancy. Their analysis found evidence of significant depression and anxiety in the first month following early pregnancy loss in women. There was also evidence of post-traumatic stress symptoms in three studies.

- *Coping.* Some studies have considered the experience of miscarriage from a coping viewpoint. For example, Madden (1988) completed 65 structured interviews with women two weeks post-miscarriage and concluded that, rather than self-blame, external blame for the miscarriage and the ability to be able to control the outcome of future pregnancies were predictive of depressive symptoms post-miscarriage. Tunaley et al. (1993) drew upon the theory of cognitive adaptation (Taylor 1983) which focuses on meaning, self-enhancement and mastery, to explore the miscarriage experience (see Chapter 8). They found that 86 per cent of the sample had established their own set of reasons as to why the miscarriage had occurred, ranging from medical explanations to feelings of punishment and judgement, which finds reflection in work on attributions for heart disease (e.g. French et al. 2001) and breast cancer (Taylor 1983). In terms of self-enhancement, 50 per cent of the sample made downward social comparisons with women who had reproductive problems. By comparing themselves with women who were worse off than themselves, they were able to increase their own self-esteem. The search for mastery was less visible. There was little evidence that the women in the sample tried to gain control over their lives in general. Although 81 per cent of the sample believed that they could make changes to prevent future miscarriage, they had little or no confidence in the difference these changes would make to future outcomes (Tunaley et al. 1993).

The quantitative research has therefore explored the reaction to miscarriage in terms of grief, anxiety and depression and coping. Other research has used a qualitative method to assess women's broader experience of having a miscarriage.

QUALITATIVE RESEARCH

In an early study, Hutti (1986) conducted in-depth interviews at two time points with two women. The results showed that although both women referred to a similar inventory of events, the significance that they attached to these events was different and dependent upon their previous experience. For example, one woman had had a previous miscarriage and was described as taking more control over her medical treatment; she found her grief to be less severe than with her first miscarriage. In contrast, the woman who had experienced her first miscarriage represented the miscarriage as a 'severe threat to her perception of herself as a childbearing woman' (p. 383). On a larger scale, Bansen and Stevens (1992) focused on 10 women who had experienced their first pregnancy loss of a wanted pregnancy. The authors concluded that miscarriage was a 'silent event' which was not discussed within the wider community. The women were described as being unable to share their experiences and felt isolated as a result. When they did get the opportunity to talk about their loss, they realized how common miscarriage is and that was a source of comfort to them. The authors concluded that miscarriage constituted a major life event that changed the way in which women viewed their lives in the present and affected the way in which they planned for the future.

Maker and Ogden (2003) carried out in-depth interviews with a heterogeneous sample of 13 women in the UK who had experienced a miscarriage up to five weeks previously. The women described their experiences using a range of themes which were conceptualized into three stages: turmoil, adjustment and resolution. For the majority, the turmoil stage was characterized by feelings of being unprepared and negative emotions. Some women who had had an unwanted pregnancy described their shock at the physical trauma of miscarriage but described the experience as a relief. The women then described a period of adjustment involving social comparisons, sharing and a search for meaning. The latter included a focus on causality which left a minority, particularly those who had had previous miscarriages, feeling frustrated with the absence of a satisfactory medical explanation. The final resolution stage was characterized by a decline in negative emotions, a belief by some that the miscarriage was a learning experience and the integration of the experience into their lives. This resolution seemed more positive for those with children and more negative if the miscarriage was not their first. The authors argued that, rather than being a trigger to psychological morbidity, a miscarriage should be conceptualized as a *process* involving the stages of turmoil, adjustment and resolution. Likewise, Carolan and Wright (2016) conducted interviews with 10 older women (aged 35 years plus) and reported themes relating to physical, emotional, temporal and social context that included intense loss and grief, having a sense of otherness, a continuous search for meaning, and feelings of regret and self-blame.

Some research has also explored how women cope with having a miscarriage. For example, Fernández-Basanta et al. (2021) interviewed 16 Spanish women about their experiences of miscarriages and stillbirths and concluded that they use two opposing strategies. First, the results showed that the women talk with their family, friends, others with similar experiences and with co-workers as it provides relief, helps them normalize their feelings, because others can empathize with them and because they do not want to pretend. In contrast, however, they also use avoidant behaviours as they often anticipate negative responses and want to avoid the discomfort of retelling the story which reflects the complexity of making sense of having a miscarriage. Bailey et al. (2019) carried out a qualitative study to explore how having a miscarriage influences future pregnancies and interviewed 14 women in the early stages of a new pregnancy after a miscarriage. The results showed that the women adopt a range of coping strategies designed to maintain hope while bracing themselves for a further miscarriage such as keeping distracted and being busy, not allowing themselves to think about the pregnancy, blocking it out and preferring support from others who were in a similar situation. In addition, many women also reported changing their lifestyles to reduce the risk of miscarriage, such as reducing strenuous exercise or improving their diets, but at times these became quite extreme such as never opening the window on a car journey to avoid pollution or avoiding taking baths or showers.

RESEARCH IN COUPLES

One neglected area of research is the impact of a miscarriage on couples. To address this, Volgsten et al. (2018) used a longitudinal design to explore changes in the responses of men and women. The results showed that women reported stronger emotional experiences of miscarriage in general, greater depressive symptoms and grief than their male partners. Over time whereas their depressive symptoms and grief decreased, no changes were found for their emotional experience of miscarriage. Similarly, Huffman et al. (2015) conducted secondary analysis on data from 341 couples as part of the couple's miscarriage healing project. They found that women's scores were higher than men's on all psychological outcome measures. They also found that feelings of isolation and grief were higher in younger couples when either partner had previously been treated for anxiety or depression and that younger couples were also more likely to feel more devastated than older couples. Likewise the results from Farren et al.'s (2018) systematic review showed that while male partners reported anxiety, depression and grief after miscarriage these were generally lower than for the women.

IMPACT OF MODE OF TREATMENT

Miscarriages can occur throughout a pregnancy but most occur during the first trimester (Steer et al. 1999). Until recently, the standard management of first trimester miscarriages involved the evacuation of the retained products of conception (ERPC), also sometimes known as a D&C (dilatation and curettage). This uses either a general or local anaesthetic and surgically removes the lining of the womb and the foetus if it is still there. This occasionally causes infection, uterine perforation and bowel damage and brings with it all the associated risks of an anaesthetic. Expectant management is a possible alternative and has been increasingly adopted by clinics across the UK. This involves letting the miscarriage take its natural course and enables the woman to be at home as the miscarriage occurs. Trials suggest that expectant management might produce less infection (Neilson and Hahlin 1995) and observational studies show that it usually results in complete evacuation of the products of conception (Sairam et al. 2001; Luise et al. 2002). It would seem to be feasible, effective and safe and may be the preferred treatment by many women (Luise et al. 2002). Rates of surgical management of miscarriage vary by age and are shown in Figure 15.4.

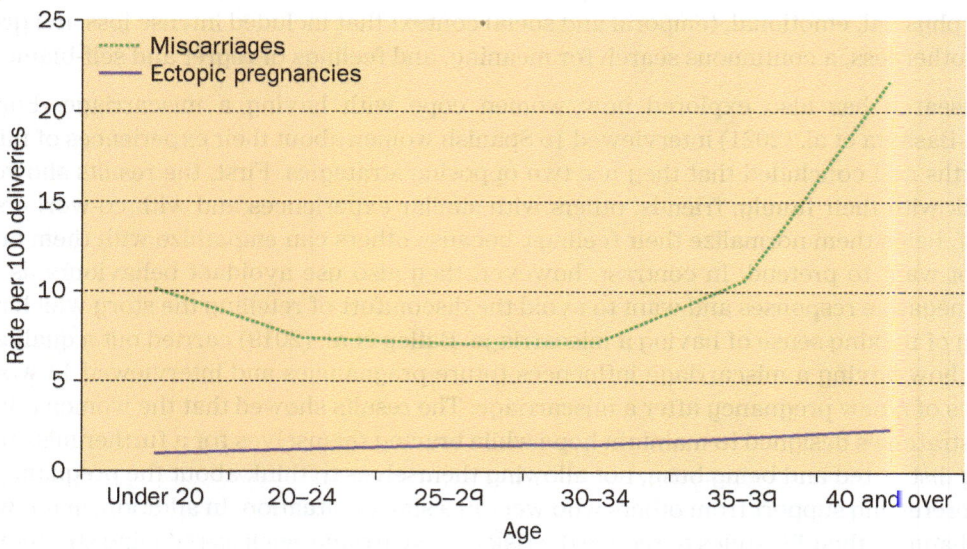

Figure 15.4 Rates of miscarriage that require a hospital stay vary by age of mother

SOURCE: Adapted from Department of Health (2005)

Little is known about what women expect, or about their subsequent experiences of each management approach. Ogden and Maker (2004) assessed women's reasons for deciding upon a given treatment and the impact of treatment type upon their subsequent experiences. The choice of expectant management was motivated by a desire for a natural solution and a fear of surgery. Women described how pain and bleeding had made them anxious that something was wrong and how they felt unprepared for how gruelling the experience would be. Some also described how their support had dwindled as the miscarriage progressed. In contrast, women who chose surgery valued a quick resolution and focused on the support from hospital staff, although some commented that their emotional needs had not always been met. The mode of treatment therefore seemed to influence how the miscarriage was experienced. Furthermore, even though expectant management is becoming increasingly common, women feel unprepared for how this will make them feel. Some research has also addressed the impact of place on the miscarriage experience. For example, MacWilliams et al. (2016) interviewed eight women who had been managed in the emergency department of a hospital. They found that participants felt that their loss was dismissed and that they perceived a lack of discharge education on follow-up care, which created a sense of marginalization. In 2022, Galeotti et al. synthesized the findings from 30 studies exploring the experiences of women and men experiencing miscarriage in hospital settings. Their analysis indicated that both women and men's emotional wellbeing was influenced by the hospital environment and they described a lack of understanding among healthcare professionals of the significance of their loss and need for emotional support. They also reported feeling that their distress was exacerbated by a lack of information, support, and feelings of isolation and expressed concerns about the lack of privacy.

IN SUMMARY

Research exploring the psychological impact of having a miscarriage has used both quantitative and qualitative research methods. The results indicate that miscarriage can result in feelings of grief, anxiety and depression. Women also experience their miscarriage as a *process*, involving a series of stages which can result in women reassessing both their past and future experiences. Furthermore, even though a miscarriage affects both partners, women's experiences seem to be more intense than men's. Further, research indicates that a woman's experience is clearly influenced by how it is managed, and that, although the medical management of miscarriage brings with it the risks associated with surgery and the lack emotional support and privacy that can come from being in hospital, a more 'natural' approach can leave women feeling misinformed and unprepared.

TERMINATION OF PREGNANCY

In 1967 the Abortion Act was passed in the UK and abortions (also known as termination of pregnancy – TOP) were made legal. Although this did not mean that abortions were available simply 'on demand', the Act was welcomed by many women who could subsequently gain access to a legal abortion on the grounds that it was considered to be less physically and mentally harmful than childbirth. Nowadays, abortions can be obtained through the National Health Service (NHS), through private for-profit services or alternatively through the specialist non-profit services set up by charitable organizations shortly after the introduction of the Act. The latter of these continue to lead the way in developing and implementing improved provision both within their own organizations and within the NHS, including such practices as day care, the use of local anaesthetics and, more recently, the introduction of medical abortions. Further, with the introduction of agency contracts such specialist services have enabled health authorities and general practitioners (GPs) to deal with inadequate abortion provision within the NHS. Although the law places the abortion decision in the hands of doctors (Greenwood 2001), in practice women make this decision and their choice is respected (Lee 2003). Abortion is also legal in the USA (although still hotly contested and some cities have no abortion clinics) and most European countries. In England and Wales one in three women is likely to have an abortion in their lifetime. Debate continues over the moral status of a human foetus and consequently also over that of abortions (Gillon 2001). The changes in the abortion rates per 1,000 women in the UK between 2007 and 2017 by age is shown in Figure 15.5. (DHSC 2017).

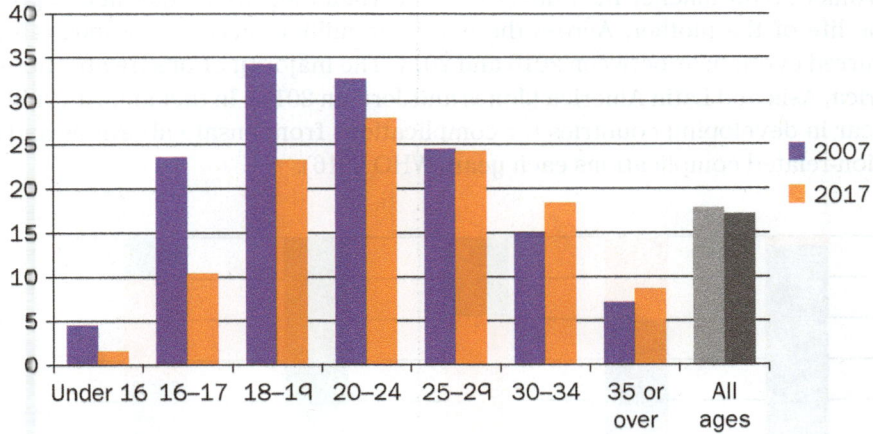

Figure 15.5 Abortion rate per 1,000 women in England and Wales by age, 2007 and 2017

SOURCE: Adapted from DHSC (2017)

Until recently, all abortions involved the surgical removal of the foetus using a D&C and a general anaesthetic. Nowadays, however, women can choose to have their abortion using either the D&C with a general or local anaesthetic, a suction technique which can involve general or local anaesthetic or no anaesthetic, or the abortion pill which induces a miscarriage (later abortions may be managed through inducing labour). The type of abortion procedure depends upon the gestation of the pregnancy, the preference of the woman and the methods preferred by the clinic involved. In the UK an abortion is legal up until the 24th week of gestation although the large majority of abortions occur within the first trimester. While legal in the UK, the laws were different in Northern Ireland and until recently abortion remained illegal with many women and girls travelling to England. After much debate, however, abortion is now legal in Northern Ireland although access to services remains very limited and contentious. In the Republic of Ireland, in 2018 a large majority of Irish citizens voted in a referendum to repeal the constitutional amendment and replace it with the wording: 'Provision may be made by law for the regulation of termination of pregnancy.' As a result, abortions became legal in Ireland in December 2018 and the first abortion clinics became operational on 1 January 2019. Abortion is still illegal in a number of countries in all circumstances except to save a woman's life. These include Brazil, Mexico, Venezuela, Angola, Congo, Mali, Niger, Nigeria, Uganda, Malta, Afghanistan, Iran, Egypt, Libya, Syria, Bangladesh and Malta. In addition, many countries only allow abortion to protect a woman's health. These include Argentina, Chile, Peru, Cameroon, Ethiopia, Malawi, Zimbabwe, Kuwait, Saudi Arabia, Pakistan, Thailand and Poland. At the time of writing (2022) the Supreme Court in the US has just changed the abortion laws throughout the country by voting to overturn the Roe vs Wade and Doe vs Bolton cases that enabled the legalization of abortion in 1973. As a result of this vote, each state can have it own local abortion law. According to the Centre for Reproductive Rights, it is predicted that at least 25 states will now ban abortion and that others will limit abortion access. It is also predicted that this will result in a drop in safe abortions but an increase in unsafe abortions together with an increase in medical abortions with women buying medication from the internet and an increase in travel abortions.

During 2010–2014, an estimated 56 million safe and unsafe abortions occurred each year worldwide (Guttmacher Institute 2018). The percentages of safe versus unsafe abortions worldwide are shown in Figure 15.6. Rates of unsafe abortions are shown in Figure 15.7. This data shows that abortions continue at about the same rate regardless of whether they are legal (34 per 1,000 women) or restricted (37 per 1,000 women) (Guttmacher Institute 2018). But when they are illegal they happen in an unsafe way risking the life of the mother. Across the world, 25 million unsafe abortions (45 per cent of all abortions) occurred every year between 2010 and 2014. The majority of unsafe abortions (97 per cent), occurred in Africa, Asia and Latin America (Jones and Jerman 2017). In fact almost 7 million women are treated each year in developing countries for complications from unsafe abortions and at least 22,000 die from abortion-related complications each year (WHO 2016).

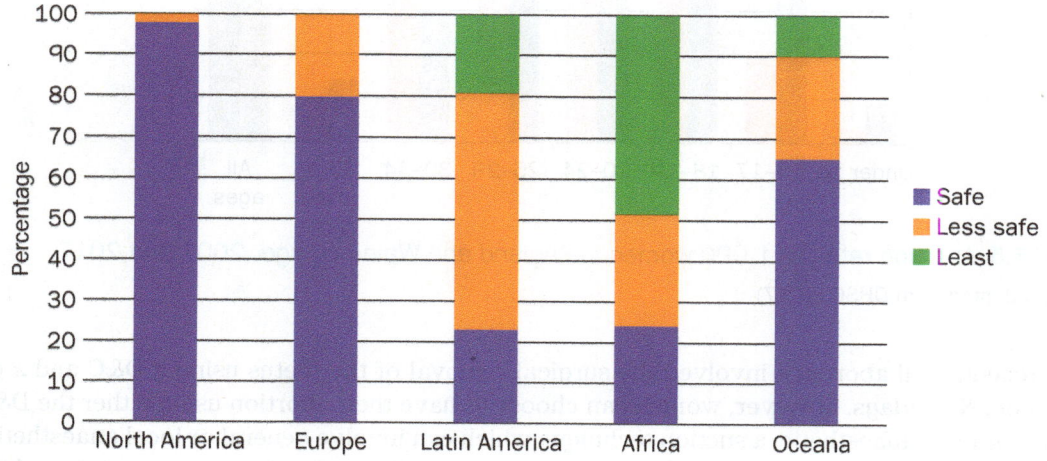

Figure 15.6 Safe vs less safe vs least safe abortions worldwide

SOURCE: Adapted from WHO (2018)

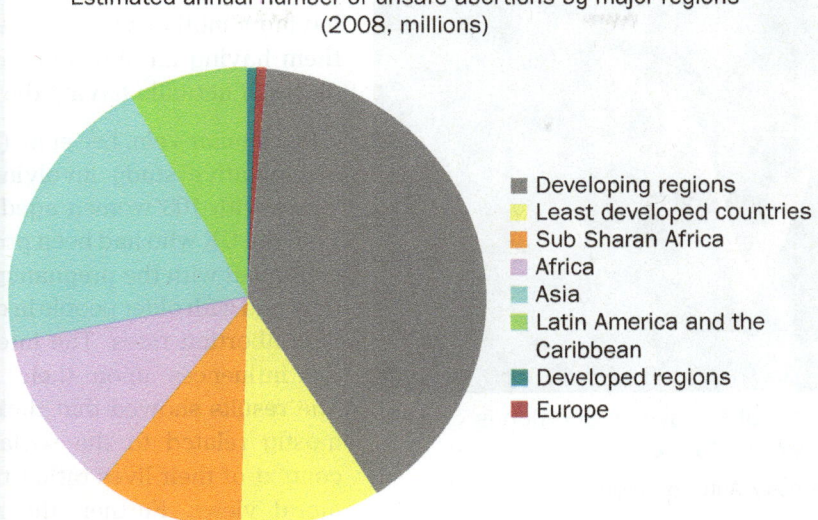

Estimated annual number of unsafe abortions by major regions (2008, millions)

- Developing regions
- Least developed countries
- Sub Sharan Africa
- Africa
- Asia
- Latin America and the Caribbean
- Developed regions
- Europe

Figure 15.7 Worldwide rates of unsafe abortions

SOURCE: Adapted from WHO (2008)

Research focusing on abortions has addressed a range of issues including deciding to have an abortion, women's experiences of having an abortion, the longer term consequences of having an abortion and the impact of the mode of intervention used.

DECIDING TO HAVE AN ABORTION

Some research has explored the experience of deciding to have an abortion. For example, Kjelsvik et al. (2018) conducted a qualitative study on 13 pregnant Norwegian women who were struggling to finalize their decision over whether to have an abortion or not. They were interviewed before and after their decision and described the experience as a lonely journey which challenged their values. In addition, research has also explored how women decide whether or not to have an abortion and what factors influence this decision. Freeman and Rickels (1993) reported the results from the Penn State study in the USA which followed over 300 black teenagers aged 13–17 for two years who were either pregnant and intending to keep the baby (n = 137), had terminated their first pregnancy (n = 94) or who had never been pregnant (n = 110). The results were analysed to explore what factors related to whether or not the teenager decided to continue with their pregnancy. Using quantitative data, the results illustrated that those who opted for an abortion had more employment in their households, were more likely to still be in school, showed better course grades at school and reported having friends and family who did not approve of early childbearing. The results also indicated that believing that their mother did not approve

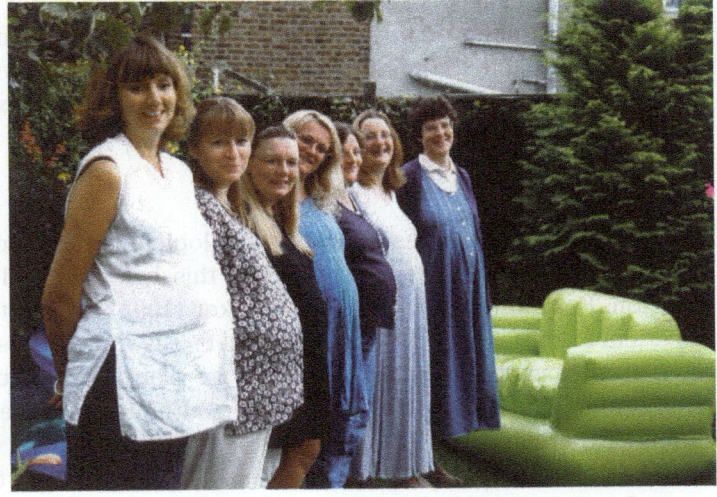

Social support can be important for new mothers

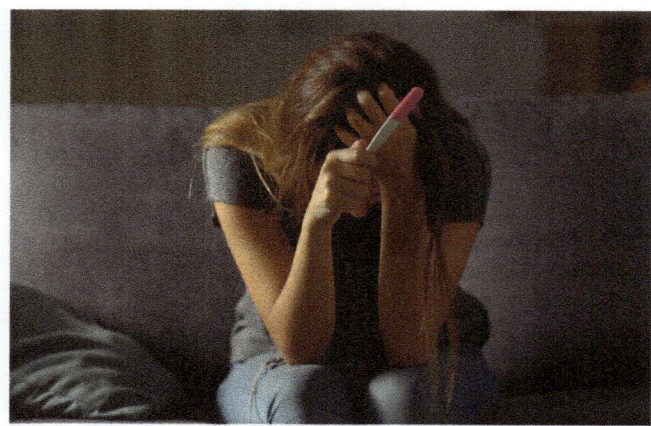

Deciding whether or not to have an abortion is influenced by the views of others

SOURCE: © Shutterstock / Antonio Guillem

of having a child while still a teenager and having a mother who was very supportive of them having an abortion were the best predictor of actually having the procedure.

In a similar vein, Lee et al. (2004) carried out a qualitative study involving in-depth interviews with 103 women aged between 15 and 17 in the UK who had been pregnant and either continued with the pregnancy or had an abortion, and with older people in communities with high abortion rates. The interviews explored the influences upon their decision-making. The results showed that their decisions were mostly related to the social and economic context of their lives rather than any abstract moral views. Further, the results indicated that similar factors influenced the decision-making processes for women regardless of their age. For example, the decision to have an abortion was related to social deprivation. In particular, the results indicated that although there are higher numbers of conceptions in young women in deprived areas, these women are less likely to terminate their pregnancy than those in less deprived areas. In addition, those who believed that their future life would include higher education and a career, who had higher expectations of their life in the present, who had a lack of financial independence and who felt that they lacked the stable relationships to support them if they became a mother were more likely to have an abortion. In contrast, keeping the baby was related to a positive view of motherhood that was not associated with lack or loss, and those who viewed motherhood as rewarding, associating it with responsibility and seeing it as an achievement, were more likely to carry on with the pregnancy. Further, the decision-making process seemed to be highly related to the views of the women's family and community.

For example, some women described how having children early was considered by their world to be acceptable and normal, and these tended to have the baby. In contrast, those who went on to have an abortion described how their parents saw abortion in a pragmatic way, regarding young motherhood as a more negative event. Finally, although most women had made up their minds whether or not to have an abortion before they had any contact with a health professional, the results showed an association between the abortion rate and provision of local family planning provision, higher proportions of female GPs and a greater independent sector providing abortion services. This suggests that, although much of the decision-making process is influenced by social and economic factors prior to professional contact, structural factors such as service provision also have a role to play. Deciding to have an abortion seems to relate to the context of the woman's life and the beliefs and support offered by those important to her.

PSYCHOLOGICAL IMPACT

Much research has addressed the psychological consequences of abortion (see Coleman et al. 2005 for a comprehensive review). Some of this has explored the extent of emotional reactions post-abortion. For example, Zolese and Blacker (1992) argued that approximately 10 per cent of women experience depression or anxiety that is severe or persistent after an abortion. Other authors have used case studies of women who are distressed to suggest that this may be more widespread (Butler and Llanedeyrn 1996). In contrast, although Major et al. (2000) found that 20 per cent of their sample experienced clinical depression within two years of an abortion, they argued that this is equivalent to population rates. Adler et al. (1990) reviewed the most methodologically sound US studies and concluded that incidence of severe negative responses was low, that distress was greatest before an abortion and reactions were often positive. They argued that abortion can be considered within a stress and coping framework and that the small numbers of women who experience distress are insignificant from a public health perspective.

Some research has also considered what type of psychological reactions occur after an abortion. Söderberg et al. (1998) conducted interviews with a large sample of Swedish women (n = 845) a year after their abortion and found that 55 per cent experienced some form of emotional distress. In contrast, however, Kero et al. (2004) interviewed 58 women in Sweden a year after their abortion and concluded that most reported no distress and that more than half reported only positive experiences. Other researchers have found that relief is commonly expressed after an abortion (Rosenfeld 1992) and Major et al. (2000) found that 72 per cent of their sample were satisfied with their decision two years after. Similarly, Alex and Hammarström (2004) conducted a study in Sweden of five women's experiences and concluded that the women reported gaining a sense of maturity and experience.

Harden and Ogden (1999a) interviewed 54 women aged between 16 and 24 up to three hours after their abortion about their experiences. They reported that, overall, having an unwanted pregnancy was experienced as a rare event which was accompanied by feelings of lack of control and loss of status. Further, the process of arranging and having an abortion led to a reinstatement of status, control and normality. However, this process was sometimes hindered by inaccessible information, judgemental health professionals and the wider social context of abortion in which it is seen as a generally negative experience. In the main, however, most of these negative experiences were associated with accessing the abortion service and the professionals who act as gatekeepers to the service rather than those who work within the service itself. Therefore, although young women's experiences were wide-ranging and varied, most were positive and at times even negative expectations were compensated by supportive staff.

LONGER-TERM IMPACT

It would therefore seem that, although some women experience emotional distress post-abortion, others experience more positive reactions such as relief, a return to normality and satisfaction. But do these emotional states persist over time? Russo and Zierk (1992) followed up women eight years after their abortion and compared them to those who had kept the child. They found that having an abortion was related to higher global self-esteem than having an unwanted birth, suggesting that any initial negative reactions decay over time. In a similar vein, Major et al. (2000) explored the variation in emotional reactions over time and reported that negative emotions increased between the time of the abortion and two years, and satisfaction with the decision decreased. These results also suggest a linear pattern of change but one towards worse rather than better adaptation. In contrast, however, some researchers have argued that emotional responses do not always alter in a linear way. For example, Kumar and Robson (1987) found that neurotic disturbances during pregnancy were significantly higher in those who had had a previous termination than those who had not, and suggested that this is due to unresolved feelings about the abortion that had been reawakened by the pregnancy. In contrast, however, Adler et al. (1990) argued that research from other life stressors has found that if no severe negative responses are present from a few months to a year after the event, it is unlikely that they will develop later.

The research therefore illustrates variability both in terms of the initial emotional reactions to an abortion and how these reactions change over time. Some research has addressed which factors may explain variability in the initial response. For example, immediate distress has been reported as being higher in those women who belong to a society that is antagonistic towards abortion (Major and Gramzow 1999), in those who experienced difficulty making the decision (Lyndon et al. 1996), and in those who are younger, unmarried, have the abortion later in pregnancy (which may be due to the features of women who delay), show low self-esteem or an external locus of control, have had multiple abortions, and self-blame for the pregnancy or abortion (Harris 2004). Further, believing in the human qualities of the foetus has also been associated with higher levels of distress (Conklin and O'Connor 1995). Goodwin and Ogden (2006) explored women's reactions to their abortion up to nine years later and examined how they believed their feelings about the abortion had changed over time. The results showed that, although a few women reported a linear pattern of change in their emotions, some also described different patterns including persistent upset that remained ongoing many years after the event, negative reappraisal some time after the event and a positive appraisal at the time of the event with no subsequent negative emotions. The results also provide some insights into this variability. Those who described how they had never been upset or experienced a linear recovery also tended to conceptualize the foetus as less human, reported having had more social support and described either a belief that abortions are supported by society or an ability to defend against a belief that society is judgemental. In contrast, patterns of emotional change involving persistent upset or negative appraisal were entwined with a more human view of the foetus, a lack of social support and a belief that society is either overly judgemental or negates the impact that an abortion can have on a woman.

The key problem with research exploring the impact of having an abortion is that it mostly explores the experiences of those who have had an abortion per se, without comparing these experiences to having an unwanted baby. To address this problem, Biggs et al. (2017) conducted a cohort study observing 956 women over the course of 5 years and compared those who had an abortion to those who were denied having an abortion. The results showed that those who were denied an abortion were more anxious, had lower self-esteem and lower life satisfaction. Therefore, compared with having an abortion, being denied an abortion was associated with poorer psychological outcomes although over time these outcomes did improve.

IMPACT OF MODE OF INTERVENTION

An abortion can be carried out using a D&C (surgical), vacuum aspiration (suction) or the abortion pill (medical) and may or may not involve a general or local anaesthetic. Some research has explored the relative impact of type of procedure on women's experiences. For example, Slade et al. (1998) examined the impact of having either a medical or surgical abortion. The results showed that those opting for surgical procedure had to wait longer and were more advanced by the time of the abortion but that the two groups showed similar emotional responses prior to having the abortion. After the abortion, however, the medical procedure was seen as more stressful and was associated with more post-termination problems. It was also seen as more disruptive to life. Further, seeing the foetus was associated with more intrusive events such as nightmares, flashbacks and unwanted thoughts. Fifty-three per cent of the medical group said they would have the same procedure again whereas 77 per cent of the surgical group felt this. Similarly, Goodwin and Ogden (2007) suggest from their study that the abortion pill technique may result in a more negative experience for several women than other methods, as some women described seeing the foetus as it was expelled from their bodies. In contrast, Lowenstein et al. (2006) compared surgical and medical management of abortion and reported no differences in anxiety by two weeks following the abortion. In line with this, Howie et al. (1997) reported no differences in emotional change two years after having either a medical abortion or vacuum aspiration. In a large-scale study on 1,832 pregnant women, Di Carlo et al. (2016) compared patient satisfaction between medical (mifepristone taken orally followed after 3 days by sublingual misoprostol) and surgical (vacuum aspiration) abortion. Participants chose either surgical (n = 885) or medical (n = 947) abortions. The results showed higher satisfaction for the surgical approach compared to medical management. The results also showed that surgical abortion was preferred by those who had had a previous abortion and that those who already had a child showed greater satisfaction following the medical abortion. Mode of intervention may therefore have an impact on women's experience of having an abortion, but this may differ according to whether immediate or longer-term impacts are explored.

IN SUMMARY

Research exploring abortions has focused on women's decision to have an abortion, the short- and longer-term impact of having an abortion and the impact of the mode of treatment on women's experiences. In general, the research indicates that although some women report negative mood changes following an abortion, many describe a return to normality and relief, although this varies according to a range of individual and social factors as well as the type of intervention used.

3 | THE MENOPAUSE

The word 'menopause' means the end of monthly menstruation and for the average woman in the UK and across most of Europe and the US this occurs at the age of 51 years, with 80 per cent of women reaching the menopause by age 54 (NHS 2018). In general, the menopause is considered to be a transition which has been classified according to three stages (WHO 1996). The *pre-menopause* refers to the whole of the woman's reproductive life up until the end of the last menstrual period. The *peri-menopause* is the time prior to the final menstrual period when hormonal changes are taking place and continues until a year after the last menstrual period. The *post-menopause* stage refers to any time after the last menstrual period but has to be defined retrospectively after 12 months of no menstruation. Therefore the menopause reflects the end point of a gradual change in biological function which is finally lost as the woman stops releasing eggs and the level of oestrogen produced is reduced as it is no longer required to stimulate the lining of the womb in preparation for fertilization. The cessation of menstruation for 12 consecutive months is the required period of time for a doctor to define a woman as menopausal, with research showing that around 75 per cent of women present to their doctor about the menopause (Hope et al. 1998). Although there is a strong genetic determinant of the time of the menopause, with mothers and daughters tending to become menopausal at a similar age, smoking can result in an earlier menopause and being heavier can result in a later menopause (Ballard, 2003). In addition to the cessation of periods, the menopause brings with it other symptoms while it is happening and results in longer-term physical changes due to the reduction in female hormones.

SYMPTOMS

During the menopause women report a range of symptoms, some of which are clearly linked to a reduction in oestrogen while others have unclear origins. These illustrate the complex nature of symptoms and the role of social and psychological factors in influencing symptom perception. The most common symptoms are the following:

- change in pattern and heaviness of periods
- hot flushes
- night sweats
- tiredness
- poor concentration
- aches and pains in joints
- vaginal dryness
- changes in the frequency of passing urine.

As part of a large-scale survey, 413 women completed a questionnaire about their experiences of menopausal symptoms and their perceptions of severity, and the results showed that the most common symptoms were hot flushes, night sweats and tiredness, and of these, night sweats seemed to cause the most distress with over a third describing their night sweats as severe (Ballard 2003). The results from this study are illustrated in Figure 15.8.

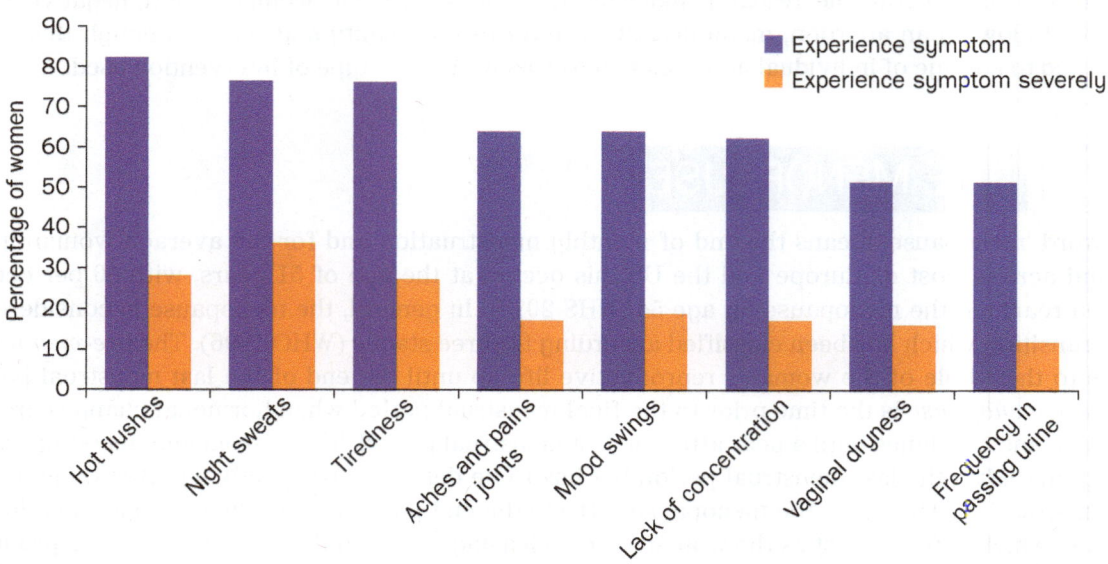

Figure 15.8 The frequency and severity of menopausal symptoms

SOURCE: Adapted from Ballard (2003)

PHYSICAL CHANGES

Women also experience a range of physical changes which persist after the menopause has passed. In particular they show changes in their breasts and it is suggested that older women should have regular mammograms to check for breast cancer. There is a post-menopausal increase in cholesterol in the blood which places women more at risk of heart disease; bone loss becomes more rapid, increasing the chance of osteoporosis; the urinary organs can become less elastic and pliable, resulting in many women suffering from incontinence; and finally women experience vaginal dryness, making sexual intercourse uncomfortable.

The menopause therefore signifies the end of a woman's reproductive capacity and brings with it a wide range of symptoms and physical changes. Ballard (2003) describes how the menopause experience is influenced by a range of social, cultural and biological factors which in turn have a psychological impact upon the individual. This reflects why the menopause is also referred to as 'the change of life'. This is illustrated in Figure 15.9.

Research exploring the impact of the menopause has highlighted the experience as a life transition and the social and psychological factors that affect this transition.

THE MENOPAUSE AS A TRANSITION

As part of a larger-scale cohort study which has collected data regularly from people born during the first week of March 1946 (see Wadsworth 1991; Wadsworth and Kuh 1997; Ballard et al. 2001), 1,572 women described their menopausal years. The women completed questions about their symptoms and health in general and then 65 per cent also completed a 'free comments' section.

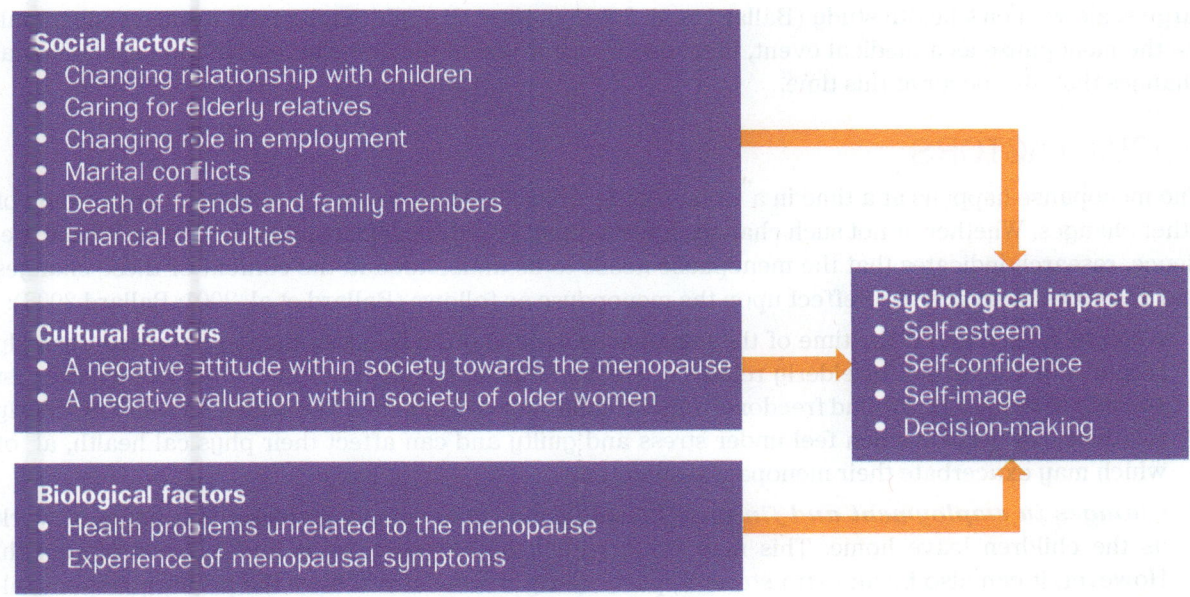

Figure 15.9 The menopause as a biopsychosocial event

These data were then analysed using both quantitative and qualitative methods. From this study the authors conclude that women experience the menopause as a 'status passage' which involves five stages. These are as follows:

1 *Expectations of symptoms.* The results illustrate that, prior to the menopause onset, women are searching for symptoms and looking for signs of any biological changes. At this point some women seek help from the doctor and start to find further information.

2 *Experience of symptoms and loss of control.* Women then start to experience symptoms such as night sweats, hot flushes and mood swings, which for some interfere with their sense of well-being and can make them feel out of control.

3 *Confirmation of the menopause.* Once women sense a loss of control, they then try to confirm the onset of the menopause by visiting their doctor as a means to regain control. The doctor can use blood tests to measure hormone levels to confirm the onset of the menopause and at this stage many women are offered hormone replacement therapy (HRT).

4 *Regaining control.* Women try to regain control in several ways. Some try to minimize the impact of their symptoms by taking HRT while others try a range of methods, such as wearing different clothes to cope with hot flushes or taking alternative medicines.

5 *Freedom from menstruation.* The end of menstruation is often welcomed by women who can feel relieved that they do not have to experience the pain and bleeding from periods any more and the inconvenience that this can cause.

The menopause is therefore seen as a process through which women go, which starts with a sense of expectation and loss of control and finishes with a sense of freedom and regained control. For many women and doctors this transition is managed through the use of HRT as the symptoms and changes associated with the menopause are attributed to changes in hormone levels. For some researchers, however, this perspective has been seen as over-medicalizing the menopause which provides a platform for medicine to take control of women's bodies (Oakley 1984; Doyal 1994). The results from the large-scale women's health study (Ballard et al. 2001) suggest that, although many women conceptualize the menopause as a medical event, they also locate it within the complex social and psychological changes that also occur at this time.

SOCIAL FACTORS

The menopause happens at a time in a woman's life when she is probably also experiencing a range of other changes. Whether or not such changes have a direct or indirect effect upon the menopausal experience, research indicates that the menopause needs to be understood in the context of these changes and describes them and their effect upon the menopause as follows (Ballard et al. 2001; Ballard 2003):

1 *Elderly relatives.* At the time of the menopause women often find that they are also increasingly responsible for caring for elderly relatives. Further, this may come at a time when women are just starting to enjoy a newfound freedom from the children leaving home. The added pressure of elderly relatives can make women feel under stress and guilty and can affect their physical health, all of which may exacerbate their menopausal symptoms.

2 *Changes in employment and finance.* In middle life many women increase their hours of work as the children leave home. This may bring with it new opportunities and a sense of rebirth. However, it can also be an extra stressor, particularly if women still have the primary responsibility for the home. In contrast, some women retire in middle life which brings with it its own sets of stresses in terms of readjustment and a need to develop a new self-image. Both these types of changes in employment can influence the menopause and its associated symptoms.

3 *Changing relationships.* At the time of the menopause women often experience changes in their role as a mother as this is the time when children leave home, and a change in their relationship with their partner as they renegotiate a new life without children. Such changes can make the menopause seem more pertinent as it reflects the end of an era.

4 *Death of family or friends.* As women reach their fifties they may experience the death of similar-age family or friends. The menopause may represent a sense of mortality which can be exacerbated by a sense of loss.

According to Ballard et al. (2001) these social factors coexist alongside the time of the menopause and can influence the ways in which the menopause is experienced. In turn they result in subsequent changes in the individual's psychological state.

PSYCHOLOGICAL EFFECTS

Psychological factors influence the menopause in terms of symptom perception because symptoms such as hot flushes, night sweats, lack of concentration and tiredness are all influenced by processes such as distraction, focus, mood, meaning and the environment (see Chapter 8). In addition, the menopause has more direct effects upon the individual's psychological state. Ballard (2003) describes these as the following:

1 *Changes in body image.* The menopause brings with it physical changes such as drier skin, changing fat distribution and softer breasts, which can all impact upon a woman's body image. In addition, becoming 50 is also seen as a milestone, particularly within a society that associates getting older with being less attractive. Ballard provides interesting descriptions of how women can suddenly catch themselves in a mirror and think 'it's my mum' or 'you are getting old'. Such changes in body image and body dissatisfaction are in line with those described in Chapter 4.

2 *Mood changes.* Some women report experiencing moods such as anxiety and depression and some report having panic attacks. Given the many life changes that co-occur with the menopause, it is

not surprising that women experience changes in their mood. However, many women view their emotional shifts as directly linked to their changing hormone levels. This therefore raises the problem of attribution as there is a danger of all menopausal women's emotional shifts being attributed to their biological state, which makes them seem 'unstable'. However, there is also the converse problem that 'real' biological mechanisms are ignored and that emotions are inappropriately attributed to more social reasons.

3 *Self-esteem and self-confidence.* Some women also report decreases in their self-esteem and self-confidence. They describe not feeling confident in everyday tasks such as cooking or work, and feeling less able to manage relationships.

4 *Lack of concentration.* Several surveys report that women describe how the menopause disrupts their cognitive function in terms of concentration and memory (Rubin and Quine 1995; Ballard et al. 2001). Experimental studies in controlled conditions, however, show no evidence for any cognitive decline that could be attributed to the menopause above and beyond standard age effects (Herlitz et al. 1997).

About 1 in 100 women experience premature menopause which is defined as occurring before the age of 40. A review of the research indicates that this might be particularly upsetting and is associated with longer-term increased anxiety and depression, adverse effects on cognition and sexual health and an increased risk of early mortality (Faubion et al. 2015).

MODE OF MANAGEMENT

The menopause can be managed in a range of ways. Some women simply carry on with their lives and wait for the symptoms to pass. They may manage these symptoms using 'tricks of the trade' – such as wearing layered clothes rather than thick jumpers to make removing clothes easier should they have a hot flush, sleeping with the window open to cope with night sweats and buying lubricants to manage vaginal dryness – but they do not necessarily present their symptoms to the doctor. Others may try alternative medicines for symptom relief including herbal remedies, homeopathy and acupuncture, preferring a more natural approach. Many, however, do visit their doctor and are prescribed HRT and the numbers of women taking HRT increased threefold between 1981 and 1990, up to 19 per cent, and increased to a rate of 60 per cent by 2000 (Moorhead et al. 1997; Kuh et al. 2000; Ballard 2002). These numbers then dropped, however, following the publication of the WHI report (2002) which raised concerns about the risks to health. Recently, however, reviews of the evidence argue that these risks were overstated and currently it is generally concluded that while HRT results in a very small increase in the risk of breast and endometrial cancer and thrombosis it is also protective against all-cause mortality and risks of coronary disease, osteoporosis and dementia, particularly if taken within 10 years since the onset of menopause or by symptomatic women under 60 years of age (see Beral et al. 2005; Cagnacci and Venier 2019 Fait 2019; Langer et al. 2021 for comprehensive reviews). Recently, uptake of HRT has started to increase and, in 2018, Kuh et al. analysed data from a British birth cohort study of women going through the menopause and reported that in a sample of 1,315 women, 63.5 per cent of women had taken HRT and of these 17.5 per cent had used it for less than 3 years, 18.7 per cent had used it for 3–6 years, 16.4 per cent had used it for 7–10 years and 10.2 per cent had used it for more than 10 years.

IN SUMMARY

The menopause reflects the end of a woman's reproductive life and brings with it a range of symptoms and longer-term physical changes. Research has explored how women experience the menopause and suggests that it is considered a life transition which results in a range of psychological shifts and changes. However, the research also suggests that, although some of these changes may be directly related to the biological nature of the menopause, they are also created or exacerbated by the multitude of social changes that occur in a woman's life at the same time. The menopause is therefore best understood as a time where biological, social and psychological factors come together.

4   UNDERSTANDING MEN'S HEALTH

So why do men die earlier than women? And why are they more likely to die once they become ill? Research points to a key role for behaviour in terms of health behaviours, risky behaviours and help-seeking behaviours. It also points to the impact of social norms of masculinity and emotional expression as explanations as to why men behave the way they do. These factors are illustrated below in Figure 15.10.

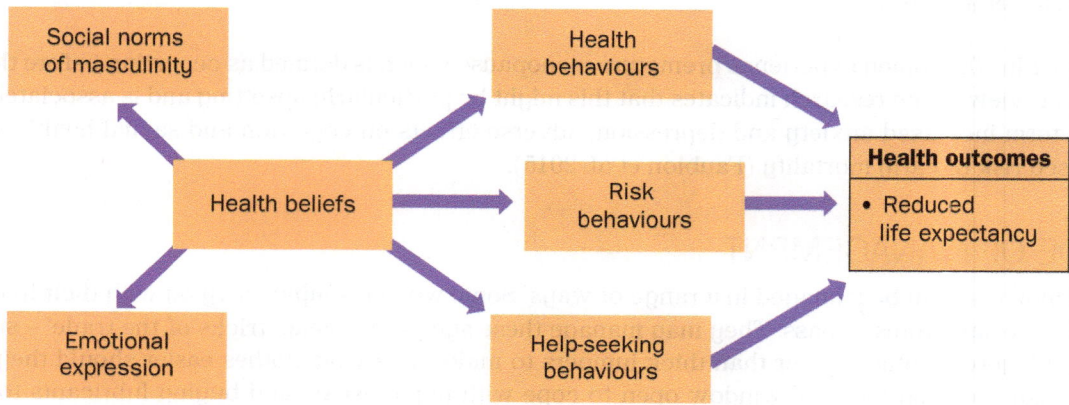

Figure 15.10 Explaining men's health

HEALTH BEHAVIOURS

This book has extensively described the role of health behaviours in health and illness. For example, Chapters 2–7 described behaviours such as smoking, alcohol use, diet, exercise and safe sex and how these can be predicted by beliefs and changed using a number of different interventions. Furthermore, Chapter 10 illustrated how stress may trigger unhealthy behaviours which in turn cause disease and Chapters 12 and 13 illustrated the role of behaviour in chronic illness. Much research indicates that men are often more likely to engage in unhealthy behaviours than women. For example, Courtenay et al. (2002) carried out a survey of 1,816 students from the USA and concluded that men showed more risky unhealthy behaviours than women in terms of their diet and substance use. In particular, men eat more meat, fat and salt and less fibre and fruit and vegetables than women and are more likely to smoke and show higher levels of alcohol and drug use. Similar results have also been found from surveys in Germany, Austria Scotland, China, the US and Korea across a range of age groups (Uitenbroek et al. 1996; Stronegger et al. 1997; Reime et al. 2000; Chang et al. 2019; Zhang et al. 2019; Al-Rousan et al. 2022). Men also show less motivation to engage in lifestyle changes than women and whereas older men believe it is 'too late' to change, younger men believe that they don't need to change 'yet' (Gabhainn et al. 1999). In addition, following divorce or widowhood, men show a greater deterioration in their diet, use of alcohol and drugs than women (Byrne et al. 1999). In fact, the only health-related behaviour that men consistently perform more than women is physical activity (e.g. Guthold et al. 2018). Interestingly, however, while men still seem to drink more than women, the gap between men and women is closing with women increasingly showing binge drinking, particularly those aged 30 to 40 and over 60, and in particular, drinking more following lockdown orders due to the COVID pandemic (Barbosa et al. 2021; White 2020; Keyes et al. 2019).

Therefore men show fewer health-promoting behaviours than women, which may explain gender differences in life expectancy and causes of mortality.

RISK-TAKING BEHAVIOURS

In addition to general health-related behaviours, men also show more risky behaviours. For example, not only are they more likely to smoke, drink alcohol and take drugs than women but they are also more likely to do these behaviours to excess (Courtenay et al. 2002). Men also have more sexual partners than women, are more likely to take part in high-risk sports and leisure activities such as rugby, snowboarding, sky-diving, bungee-jumping and rally driving (Courtenay et al. 2002). These risky behaviours are reflected in higher rates of accidental injury and death among men. For example, research shows the following:

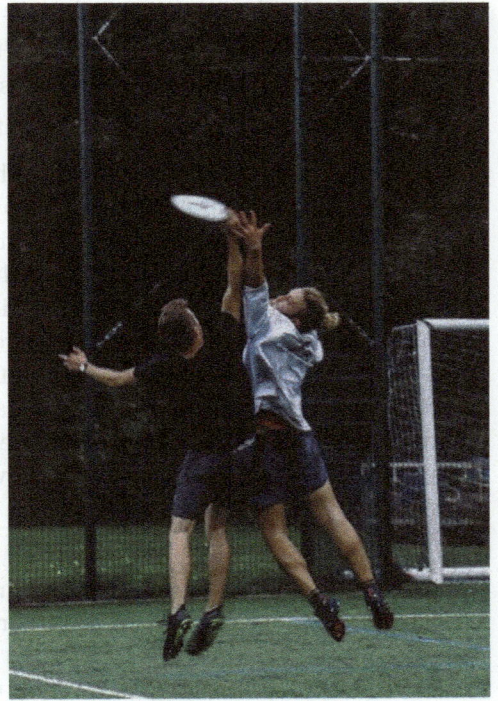

Physical exercise – a positive part of men's health behaviour

- An Australian study showed that boys are twice as likely to die in play-related accidents (Lam et al. 1999) and a study from Denmark showed that men are more likely to die or suffer serious injury from accidents at work (Arbeidstilsynet 2012).

- A study of 201 Australian adults indicated that men had significantly higher intentions to drive through floodwater than women together with significantly lower barrier self-efficacy, risk perception, anticipated regret, perceived susceptibility, and perceived severity with respect (Hamilton et al. 2018).

- A US study showed boys are twice as likely to die or be injured from falling out of a window (Stone et al. 2000).

- Using data from the Nationwide Emergency Department Sample, White et al. (2018) report that men account for the majority of alcohol-related medical emergencies and deaths in the US.

- In Argentina boys are more likely to suffer from head injuries (Murgio et al. 1999).

- The death rate for men is higher than women for motor vehicle accidents and drowning (Courtenay et al. 2002).

- The large majority of all fatal and non-fatal injuries recorded in hospitals are for men (Watson and Ozanne-Smith 2000).

- Men are four times more likely than women to fracture their clavicle (e.g. from sporting accidents) and sustain spinal cord injuries (e.g. from diving) than women (Van Asbeck et al. 2000).

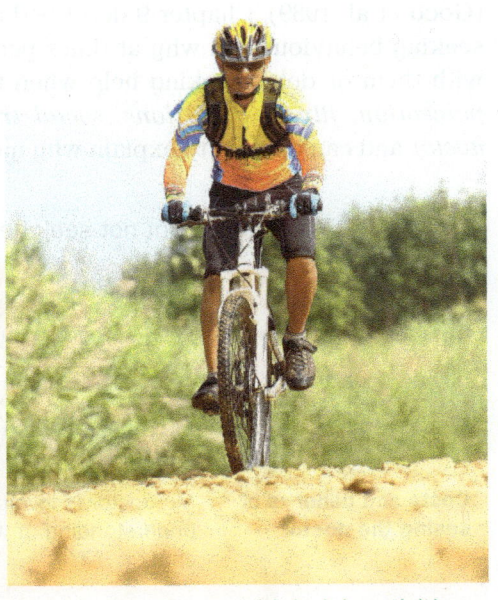

Men engage in more high-risk activities than women

SOURCE: © Shutterstock / wandee007

- In New Zealand, men recorded more moderate-to-serious and serious injury claims than females across most sports (cricket, rugby league, rugby union and football) (King et al. 2019).
- Men are more likely to have accidents of any kind when snowboarding in Austria (Rugg et al. 2021)
- Many of these injuries are sustained after heavy drinking (Kolakowsky-Hayner et al. 1999).

Men therefore engage in more risky behaviours than women and are also more likely to be injured or die as a result. Interestingly, the data also indicate that, in the main, accidental injury or death is directly related to the level of exposure to the high-risk activity. This means that more men die from injuries because they engage in more activities that expose them to risk. There are two good examples of this. First, research shows that men are more likely to die from accidental injury while employed in the armed forces. However, although the armed forces are overwhelmingly men, when this is accounted for, men in the army are more likely to be injured than women (Snedecor et al. 2000). Likewise, although overall men have more motor vehicle accidents, accidents are best predicted by being younger, heavy drinking and not wearing a seatbelt than by gender per se (Bell et al. 2000). Accordingly, men are more likely to be injured or die from their injuries than women because they are more likely to behave in risky ways.

HELP-SEEKING BEHAVIOURS

One core component of being healthy and staying well is the appropriate use of health care services. Chapter 9 described a number of factors involved in the use of health care including help-seeking behaviour and screening which bring individuals into contact with health care professionals. Research indicates that in general men use health care services less than women and show greater delay in seeking help and identifying symptoms (e.g. Gijsbers van Wijk et al. 1999; Schappert 1999). Further, they are less likely to have seen their general practitioner (GP) in the past 12 months, have fewer hospital admissions and are less likely to have a screening test or a general health check (DH 2001; Bayram et al. 2003; National Statistics Online 2006; Eurostat 2007). Importantly, these differences persist even when reproductive and sex-specific conditions are accounted for but start to diminish when a health problem is serious (Courtenay 2000a, 2000b). A similar pattern can also be seen for mental health problems with only one-third of all clients seeking psychological support being men and with men delaying help-seeking until their problems are more serious and entrenched (Good et al. 1989). Chapter 9 described a series of psychological processes that help to explain help-seeking behaviour and why at times people either go to their doctor when they have nothing wrong with them or delay seeking help when they have a serious problem. These processes are *symptom perception, illness cognitions, social triggers* and the *perceived costs and benefits of going to the doctor* and can be used to explain why men use health care less than women (see Table 15.1).

TABLE 15.1 Why men might not seek help: the role of psychological processes

	Help-seeking	Delay
Symptom perception	I have a pain in my stomach	I am too busy to think about myself
Illness cognitions	This pain could be serious	I will try to ignore it until it goes away
Social triggers	My friends tell me that this pain isn't normal	My colleagues tell me to stop making a fuss
Costs and benefits of seeing the doctor	My doctor is lovely. She will be really understanding. It will be nice to have a chat	I feel embarrassed about seeing a doctor/I should be able to manage this on my own/I don't want someone I don't know interfering
Help-seeking	I will see the doctor after I have dropped the kids at school	I don't have a doctor/I am too busy at work/I work a long way from my doctor

EXPLAINING MEN'S HEALTH-RELATED BEHAVIOURS AND ILLNESS PROFILES

So why do men behave in ways that are damaging to their health? Yousaf et al. (2015) conducted a systematic review of 41 papers investigating the factors associated with delays in medical and psychological help-seeking among men. They found that the most common barriers to help-seeking were reluctance to express emotions/concerns about health, embarrassment, anxiety and fear and poor communication with health-care professionals. Some of the key factors are described below:

Health Beliefs

Chapter 2 described the ways in which health beliefs predict health behaviours such as smoking, diet, exercise and alcohol use. Similarly, Chapter 9 explored the factors involved in help-seeking, screening and adherence to medication. Research indicates that men may have different beliefs about their health which in turn influence their behaviours.

Risk Perception

In general, men appear to underestimate their risk for illness or injury compared to women. For example, research indicates the following:

- Men of all ages perceive that they are less at risk from smoking cigarettes or e-cigarettes, drug or alcohol use or smoking related cancers (e.g. Kauffman et al. 1997; Gustafson 1998; Pepper et al. 2015).
- Men perceive that they are less at risk of skin cancer and rate the risks of sun exposure as less than women (e.g. Flynn et al. 1994).
- Even though men are more likely to have HIV/AIDs than women, they perceive that they are less at risk of contracting the HIV virus than women rate their own risk (Flynn et al. 1994).
- Men also rate the risks of dangerous driving as less than women (Savage 1993).
- Men also perceive lower risks from driving through floodwater (Hamilton et al. 2018).

Perceived Control

The research into perceptions of control is less clear-cut although some studies indicate that men believe that they have less control over their health than women (Furnham and Kirkcaldy 1997). However, Magoc et al. (2016) investigated beliefs in 298 college students and found that men reported having greater self-efficacy for physical activity, greater perceived ability to set goals and make plans for physical activity and greater expectancies that physical activity would produce psychological effects (e.g. reduced stress), improve their body image and enhance their competitive ability.

Perceived Health Status

Ironically, although men die younger than women and tend to seek help at a later stage of disease, research indicates that men rate their subjective health status as higher than women rate theirs (Ross and Bird 1994). In addition, men also rate their behaviours as healthier than their peers whereas women tend to see their own behaviour as worse or comparable to those around them (Rakowski 1986). This suggests a mismatch between 'objective' and 'subjective' assessments of health which may relate to symptom perception and illness cognitions, as discussed above.

Readiness to Change Behaviour

Chapter 2 described the stages of change (SOC) model which emphasizes behaviour change as progressing through a series of discrete stages. At times research using this approach has explored gender differences and illustrates that men are less likely to be contemplating changing their behaviour,

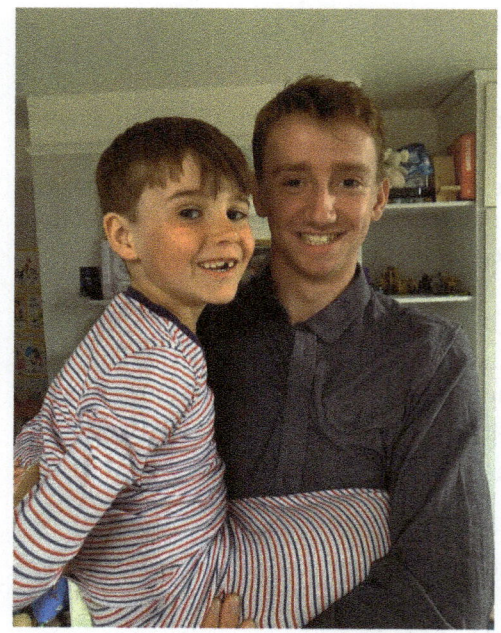

What is your idea of masculinity?

less likely to be maintaining any healthy behaviour changes and more likely to deny that their behaviours are problematic (e.g. Leforge et al. 1999; Weinstock et al. 2000).

Men therefore show a profile of health beliefs which may contribute to behaving in less healthy ways and in turn having shorter life expectancy than women.

Social Norms of Masculinity

Within men's health research there has been an increasing interest in the impact of social norms of masculinity on the ways in which men behave and how this might impact upon their health (see Courtenay 2000a; Lee and Glynn Owens 2002; Robertson 2007; Gough and Robertson 2010 for comprehensive debates).

Central to this literature is the notion of 'hegemonic masculinity' which reflects dominant ideals of masculinity within any given context (Carrigan et al. 1985). From this perspective hegemonic masculinity represents that version of masculinity which has become a 'male script', illustrating and describing the most acceptable way for men to think, feel and behave (Lohan 2010). In contemporary society concern for health is considered a feminine characteristic while 'men are positioned as naturally "strong", resistant to disease, unresponsive to pain and physical distress and unconcerned with minor symptoms' (Lee and Glynn Owens 2002). Furthermore, society encourages men to engage in stereotypically male behaviour to define themselves as 'not female' and the ways in which they do this often involve unhealthy behaviours. From this perspective hegemonic masculinity promotes a version of being male which encourages beliefs and behaviours which are ultimately damaging to health and longevity. Research indicates that more traditional beliefs about masculinity in men have been shown to be associated with:

- Health behaviours including smoking, diet, alcohol and drug use, and sexual behaviour (e.g. Eisler et al. 1988).
- Higher stress reactivity following stressors (see Chapter 10 for discussion).
- Slower help-seeking when ill (O'Neil et al. 1995).
- Poorer adherence to medication and recommended lifestyle changes following a diagnosis of heart disease (Helgeson 1994).

Thus, hegemonic masculinity encourages men to engage in unhealthy behaviours and they are also slower to seek help when ill. In line with this, some behaviour change interventions have been based upon the assumed relationship between hegemonic masculinity and health behaviours. For example, interventions have targeted men at their place of work, have been offered during work-friendly hours and have been made available at places occupied by men (e.g. Watson 2000; McKinlay 2005). In addition, health-related messages have been framed in 'male friendly' language with unhealthy bodies being described as cars which need tuning (Doyal 2001). To date, such initiatives have not been overly effective which has raised three questions about the link between hegemonic masculinity and men's health. First, it has been argued that it is not only men themselves that limit their help-seeking behaviour; health professionals' gendered beliefs may also be a barrier to men who want to seek help (Robertson and Williamson 2005; Hale et al. 2010). Second, it has been argued that although social norms of masculinity may well impact upon men's health, men are not a homogenous group and not all men adhere to the same male script of how they should be (Robertson 2007). This has led to a call for understanding the plurality of masculinity and a recognition that the stereotype of maleness is not a case of 'one size fits all'. Finally, it has been argued that masculinity is not all bad and that there are some benefits to being male. In particular, the masculine traits of being independent, decisive and assertive may help men cope with cancer and chronic illness (Charmaz 1995; Gordon 1995).

Emotional Expression

One central component to current social norms of masculinity is the focus on men not sharing their emotions or asking for help when upset (Petersen 1998). Lupton (1998) has also argued that men who express their emotions are considered weak, effeminate and possibly gay, and that they are expected to show mastery and control over their feelings. To reflect this, research indicates that men are less likely to cry than women and overall report less fear and emotional distress (Courtenay et al. 2002). Furthermore, men express fewer negative internally focused emotions such as grief and fewer positive externally focused emotions such as tenderness, than do women (Brody 1999; Lee and Glynn Owens 2002). Such lowered levels of emotional expression have implications for health and behaviour. For example, Chapter 12 described how emotional expression through writing or talk relates to a wide range of health outcomes including mood, immune functioning and return to work (see Chapter 12 for discussion). Similarly, research also describes how repressive coping and denial may be detrimental to one's health status (Myers 2000; Solano et al. 2001). The one exception in terms of emotional expression is anger, and research indicates that men express more anger and hostility than women (Brody 1999). In line with research on type behaviour described in Chapter 12 the expression of negative emotions may be linked to cardiovascular disease which is the leading cause of death in men (Rosenman 1978). Men also report higher thresholds for and greater tolerance of pain (Unruh et al. 1999). This may reflect biological factors such as hormones which may influence pain perception. It may, however, also reflect a determination not to acknowledge pain in order to present a more masculine image to the world. In line with this, men have been shown to express less pain in front of female compared to male health professionals (Puntillo and Weiss 1994). Accordingly the perception of pain may be influenced by issues relating to identity ('I am not the kind of person to feel pain'). It may also relate to the processes of symptom perception ('I am too busy to think about my pain') and illness cognitions ('This pain is nothing and will go away'), which were discussed earlier (see Chapter 13 for a discussion of pain perception).

Men in general are therefore less emotionally expressive than women which may relate to their health behaviours, help-seeking and experience of illness. The data in this area, however, are not always consistent and research indicates that not all men conform to this stereotypical presentation of their ways of coping with their lives. For example, Lucas and Gohm (2000) collated data from several large-scale surveys from different countries and concluded that although there was a tendency for men to be less expressive of some negative emotions, this certainly wasn't consistent for all men and for all emotions. Accordingly, in line with the call to consider the plurality of masculinity, it would seem that patterns of emotional inexpression are more varied than they are sometimes presented as being.

IN SUMMARY

In summary, research indicates consistent gender differences for life expectancy and illness that can be attributed to men's behaviour, with men being more likely to engage in unhealthy and risky behaviours and less likely to perform health-protective or help-seeking behaviours. From this perspective, differences in health and illness can be seen as 'gendered' as they reflect the ways in which men and women behave within the confines of what is expected. This will now be explored in the context of three case examples: prostate cancer, suicide and CHD.

5	HOW BEING MALE CAN IMPACT UPON HEALTH: CASE EXAMPLES

CASE 1: PROSTATE CANCER

Prostate cancer is now the most common form of male cancer and accounts for 23 per cent of all new male cancer diagnoses (Cancer Research UK 2006). There has been a significant increase in the prevalence of prostate cancer since the 1980s and whereas it used to be said that 'men die with it not of it' as many elderly men have prostate cancer but die from another cause, this is now changing, with more younger men both being diagnosed with and dying from this disease (Broom 2004). In 2015, there were 47,151 new cases of prostate cancer in the UK; 11,631 deaths from prostate cancer in 2016, with an 84 per cent survival rate of prostate cancer for 10 or more years (Cancer Research UK 2016). Prostate cancer illustrates many of the issues relating to men's health in the following ways.

Help-Seeking

The most common symptoms of prostate cancer are dribbling after urination, a frequent need to urinate, urination during the night and a feeling that the bladder is never empty. Although these symptoms are intrusive and upsetting, they are not always qualitatively different from normal urination behaviour which means that they can be normalized or ignored. Research indicates that many men choose to manage their symptoms on their own and delay seeking help. Hale et al. (2007) carried out a qualitative study of men's help-seeking behaviour for prostate symptoms and concluded that the men tended to ignore their symptoms or put them down to age or general 'wear and tear'. They also described how the men didn't want to inconvenience the doctor and as one participant said: 'I'm not the sort of person who would necessarily bother a GP or run to a GP, you know, sort of straight away.' This lack of help-seeking resulted from embarrassment and a desire not to trouble anyone else with their problems due to a need to live up to traditional images of masculinity. This in turn led to an absence of any social messages from others about their condition.

Broom (2010) similarly carried out a study on men in Australia and illustrated how men wanted to manage their health. Participants' responses included, 'I think it's part of the male image thing' and 'I'm not going to let anyone else know I've got the problem and I'm going to figure it out myself.' Eventual help-seeking was often triggered by the appearance of blood in the urine or pain which was seen as a more legitimate symptom that required formal help. Similarly, Ezenwankwo et al. (2021) identified several factors that could deter help-seeking in 27 men with symptoms of prostate cancer in Nigeria. These were classified as: intrapersonal (knowledge of prostate cancer, risk factors, perceived risk and symptom awareness); interpersonal (lack of family history of prostate cancer, non-disclosure of symptoms, perception of symptoms by family/friends and socioeconomic status); and institutional/community level factors (past medical experiences and dysfunctional societal beliefs). Some of these findings are also reflected in the review of eight qualitative studies carried out by Kannan et al. (2019) which focused on men who had not been diagnosed with prostate cancer about their perspectives on prostate care and prostate cancer. The authors concluded that men did not always understand screening, prostate anatomy or their prostate cancer risk. They also concluded that concerns about masculinity could deter men from having health checks and that doctor–patient communication should be improved to enable doctors to identify early warning signs. Together these findings help explain why many men present late with their symptoms when the disease has already progressed.

Uptake of Tests

Once deciding to seek help, a man with prostate symptoms will need to undergo tests to determine whether the problem is cancer, prostate disease or simply a normal variation of urination. These tests are painful, intrusive and embarrassing and involve inserting a probe either into the man's anus and/or into the end of the penis. Broom (2010) concluded from his qualitative study of men at varying stages of prostate diagnosis and treatment that these intrusive procedures impacted 'upon the participants' perceptions of being men' (p. 189) and were associated with feelings of 'shame', 'humiliation' and 'embarrassment'. The anticipation of the feelings such as these could therefore be a barrier to seeking help, exacerbating problems of delayed help-seeking. As one man said, 'My brother said he is not going to let anyone stick anything up his backside. That's an issue for a lot of people' (Broom 2010: 186–7).

Treatment

The most common treatments for prostate cancer are radical prostatectomy and radiation treatments which are painful and can result in serious and unpleasant side-effects such as incontinence and impotence. Although studies indicate that most men are prepared to trade potency for survival (Kunkel et al. 2000), Broom (2010) argued that concerns about masculinity were central both to a patient's decision about choice of treatment and their adaptation after treatment. For some men in Broom's study these concerns resulted in their choosing to have alternative treatments as a means to maintain their sense of masculinity. As one man said: 'My sexual performance is very important even to an older bloke like me . . . if you take that away from the male, you change the male . . . you change him entirely' (2010: 194). Others had the treatment but found it hard to adjust to their diminished sex lives. One man said: 'Masculinity is an incredibly important thing . . . my wife and I had reached a stage in our lives where sex had become really important . . . I was 55, my boys were off at uni and we had some time to ourselves . . . we've never got that back' (2010: 193).

Prostate cancer is increasingly common and illustrates many of the issues relating to men's health. In particular, many men delay seeking help by normalizing their symptoms and not talking to others about their problem. Furthermore, the tests and treatments are embarrassing, impacting directly on aspects of masculinity which may further exacerbate problems with delay and also influence men's choice of intervention.

CASE 2: SUICIDE

There are two common sayings about gender and health. The first is 'women get ill but men die younger' and the second is 'women get depressed but men die by suicide'. Research shows that the rates of suicide are higher in men than women across all age groups with child, adolescent and adult males being four times more likely to take their own lives than females of comparable age in most western societies (Taylor et al. 1998; Lee et al. 1999). In the UK, of the 5,965 suicides registered, 4,508 were male and 1,457 were female (Office for National Statistics 2016b). In contrast, rates of suicide are equal in Hong Kong for men and women and in China the rates are slightly lower for men (Yip et al. 2000). Suicide in men illustrates some of the factors described earlier in this chapter in terms of health, risky and help-seeking behaviours, emotional expression and social norms of masculinity. For example, the evidence shows the following:

- Men who are marginalized from mainstream society are more at risk of suicide (e.g. gay, migrant or indigenous populations, Lee et al. 1999). Such marginalization seems to affect men more than women, perhaps because they have fewer social resources to draw upon.

- Suicide attempts and actual suicide are strongly associated with other unhealthy and risky behaviours such as alcohol and drug use, smoking and fighting (Woods et al. 1997). Men show more of all these behaviours.

- Men tend to use more immediate forms of suicide such as shooting (rather than poisoning) which are less likely to be discovered and prevented. It has been argued that failed suicide is seen as weak and effeminate (Canetto 1997).
- Men respond more negatively to divorce or bereavement than women and are more likely to die by suicide (Kposowa 2000). This may reflect their lower levels of emotional expression and help-seeking.
- Although more women are diagnosed with depression, many men are depressed but delay seeking help. This may result in suicide as their emotional needs are not acknowledged or met (Lee and Glynn Owens 2002).

Men are therefore more likely to die by suicide than women. This seems to reflect the factors discussed in this chapter in terms of their health and risky behaviours, levels of emotional expression and social norms of masculinity.

CASE 3: CHD

About half of all male deaths are caused by CHD across Europe and in 2008 in the UK CHD was responsible for 35 per cent of deaths in men and 34 per cent of deaths in women (Allender et al. 2008a). Worldwide it is estimated that 17 million people die from CHD each year with the highest death rates being in China, India and Russia. In middle age, the death rate is up to five times higher for men than for women but this evens out in old age (see Chapter 13 for a detailed discussion of CHD in terms of prevalence, causes and consequences). CHD takes the form of angina, heart attack or sudden death and highlights many of the issues central to understanding men's health as follows:

- Unhealthy behaviours such as poor diet and smoking are key causes of CHD. Men are more likely to show these behaviours than women (see Chapters 3 and 4).
- Heart attack can be treated more effectively the earlier it is diagnosed. Men are more likely to delay help-seeking for symptoms of heart attack such as chest pain (see Chapters 8, 9 and 13).
- Following a heart attack, patients will be offered cardiac rehabilitation which encourages behaviour changes and often offers cognitive behavioural therapy (CBT) to change health-related cognitions. Men are less likely to attend rehabilitation than women (see Chapter 13).
- CHD is linked to stress, including chronic stressors such as work. Men are more likely to work full time, have a poorer work–life balance and are more likely to ruminate after work than women. This may be linked to the onset of their CHD (see Chapter 10).
- Men, however, are more physically active than women which is protective of CHD (see Chapter 5).

CHD is therefore a common cause of death in men and is linked to an unhealthy lifestyle, particularly poor diet and smoking. Men often have poorer lifestyles. Furthermore, recovery can be facilitated through early help-seeking, attending a rehabilitation programme and subsequent behaviour change. Men, however, may be less likely to seek help either before or after they have had a heart attack. All these aspects of CHD can be seen to be gendered, which may help to explain gender differences in life expectancy and causes of mortality.

IN SUMMARY

Health is clearly gendered and while women still tend to live longer than men, women also report and are diagnosed with more symptoms and more health conditions. This section has explored how 'being male' may result in different health beliefs, health behaviours, risk taking, help seeking and emotional expression, all of which relate to social norms of masculinity that in turn influence what men do and how healthy (or ill) they become. It has also addressed the impact of being male with a focus on prostate cancer, suicide and CHD.

6   LGBTQ+ HEALTH ISSUES

Over the past decade an increasing number of research studies have addressed the health issues of the LGBTQ+ community and have explored the impact of both gender and sexuality on health outcomes. This section will explore differences in health in terms of the prevalence of health conditions and the possible mechanisms underlying these differences.

THE PREVALENCE OF HEALTH CONDITIONS

Much research indicates that members of the LGBTQ+ community have poorer physical and mental health.

Physical Health

A comprehensive review of the health of young people in the US indicates that those identifying as LGBTQ+ are at higher risk for a number of physical health conditions such as sexually transmitted diseases (STDs), cancers, cardiovascular diseases and obesity (Hafeez et al. 2017). For adults, the evidence shows a similar pattern with young gay and bisexual men in the US accounting for 83 per cent (6,385) of all new HIV diagnoses in people aged 13 to 24 in 2019 (Centers for Disease Control and Protection 2021) and men who have sex with men are about 20 times as likely as heterosexual men to develop anal cancer which has been linked to the human papilloma virus (HPV) (Patel et al. 2018). Further, data from Behavioral Risk Factor Surveillance System surveys 2014–2017 (Azagba et al. 2019) reported that bisexual and lesbian women were more likely to be overweight or obese than women identifying as heterosexual, whereas gay men were less likely to be obese than straight men. There is also some evidence for higher rates of breast cancer and cervical cancer in lesbian and bisexual women than straight women (Valanis et al. 2000) although the evidence for this is problematic in terms of sampling as sexual orientation is not routinely collected as part of cancer registry data or large cohort studies (Meads and Moore 2013). Finally, evidence also suggests that LGBTQ adults (particularly lesbian, bisexual and transgender women) have poorer cardiovascular health metrics (Caceres et al. 2020).

Mental Health

Research shows a similarly negative picture for mental health. For example, in their comprehensive review of the literature in the US, Hafeez et al. (2017) concluded that young people who identify as LGBTQ+ are more likely to experience bullying, isolation, rejection, anxiety, depression and suicide. In line with this, Becerra-Culqui et al. (2018) carried out a large cohort study (n = 2164) and found that transgender and/or gender nonconforming (TGNC) youth were more likely to have attention deficit disorders and depressive disorders than non-TGNC youth. In adults, the pattern is similar. For example, following their survey of 5000 adults in the UK, Stonewall (2018) concluded that half of LGBTQ+ people (52 per cent) had experienced depression in the last year. Further, while some of the findings are conflicting, evidence seems to indicate that substance use and abuse is more prevalent in the LGBTQ+ community than in non-LGBTQ+ groups for smoking, drug use and alcohol use (Centers for Disease Control and Protection 2018; Boyd et al. 2019). Further, a meta-analysis of 12 surveys in the UK found higher rates of poor mental health and lower well-being in LGB adults, particularly younger and older adults (Semlyen et al. 2016) and a review by Parker and Harriger (2020) found that gay, bisexual and transgender adults and adolescents show a higher incidence of eating disorders than their heterosexual and cisgender counterparts, although the results were mixed for lesbian adults and adolescents.

MECHANISMS OF POORER HEALTH STATUS

Research therefore shows a fairly consistent pattern for poorer physical and mental health status for members of the LGBTQ+ community. There are several possible explanations for this including enacted stigma in general and from health care professionals, perceptions of stigma by the LBBTQ+ community, delayed help-seeking and health-related behaviours. These will now be considered and are illustrated in a spiral model of health in Figure 15.11.

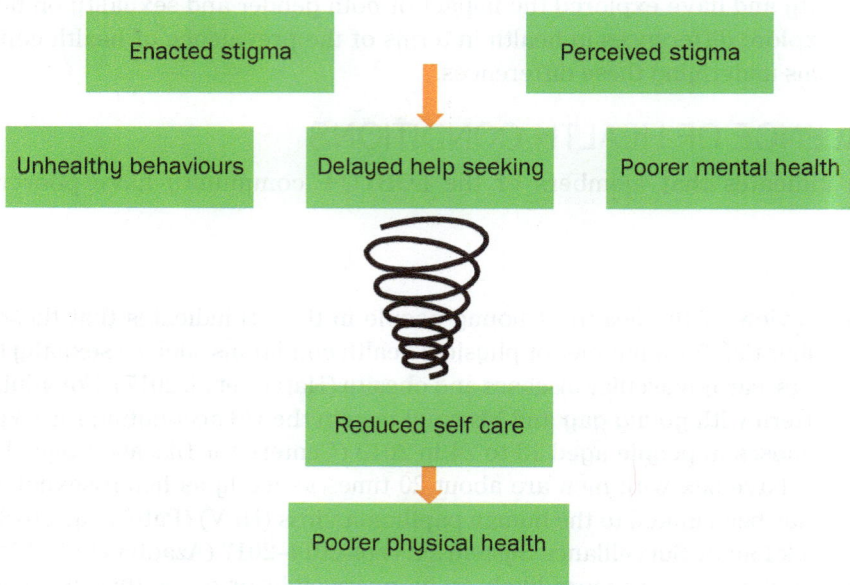

Figure 15.11 A spiral model of physical health for the LGBTQ+ community

Stigma

There is a wealth of evidence that members of the LGBTQ+ community experience stigma both in their day-to-day lives and when accessing health care. This research can be understood in terms of the enacted stigma (coming from others) and perceived stigma (experienced by the individual).

Enacted stigma: Many members of the LGBTQ+ community experience enacted stigma from others in their personal and working lives which may well impact their health. For example, a large survey in the US in 2020 (Center for American Progress 2020) reported that in the previous year more than 36 per cent of LGBTQ Americans had faced discrimination in their public, work and personal lives, and this increased to 62 per cent for those identifying as transgender. Respondents also described how this had impacted to a moderate or significant degree in the past year upon their psychological well-being (56 per cent), spiritual well-being (36 per cent) and physical well-being (32 per cent). In addition, research also indicates a degree of enacted stigma from health care professions. For example, this same survey (Center for American Progress 2020) concluded that more than 1 in 10 LGBTQ Americans faced mistreatment by a doctor or health care provider, and that transgender Americans face specific issues such as doctors being visibly uncomfortable, doctors intentionally misgendering or using the wrong name and doctors refusing to give health-care related to gender transition. Similarly, a review by Hafeez et al. (2017) concluded that healthcare providers lack awareness of gender and sexuality issues and that they are often insensitive to the unique needs of this community. They also concluded that health care providers may lack adequate training on the specific needs and challenges faced by this community which can perpetuate prejudice and discrimination, in turn leading to poorer medical care and an increase in disease and associated risk factors. In line with this, Parameshwaran et al. (2017) carried out an anonymous survey (n = 166) of UK medical students. The results showed that 84.9 per cent of participants reported a lack of LGBTQ+ health care education. In particular, they described a lack of confidence for a range of activities including clarifying unfamiliar sexual and gender terms, deciding the ward in which to nurse transgender patients, finding support resources and discussing domestic abuse with LGBTQ+ patients. The majority also stated that they would not clarify gender pronouns or ask about gender or sexual identity in mental health or reproductive health settings. Many participants, however, did hold positive attitudes towards LGBTQ+ patients and findings indicated that more positive attitudes positively correlated with greater knowledge about LGBTQ terminology. Reflecting these findings, the Stonewall report in the UK (Stonewall 2018) concluded that LGBT people face widespread discrimination in health care settings.

Perceived stigma: Reflecting the enacted stigma from health care professionals and their lack of knowledge and training, members of the LGBTQ+ community also report perceived stigma when considering or actually interacting with the health care system. For example, the large National LGBT survey in the UK (GOV.UK 2017) had over 108,000 responses and described how LGBT communities face discrimination, felt that their specific needs were not being met, had a poorer health care experience and expressed major concerns about accessing healthcare. For example, the findings reported that 16 per cent of respondents reported that their sexual orientation had negatively impacted on their access to public health services and 38 per cent said that their experiences had been negatively impacted by their gender identity. Likewise, 51 per cent of survey respondents said they had to wait too long for mental health services, 27 per cent were worried, anxious or embarrassed about going to seek mental health support and 16 per cent said their GP was not supportive.

Delayed Help-Seeking

The poorer physical and mental health experienced by those identifying as LGBTQ+ may also be related to delayed help seeking (also see Chapter 9 and the section on men's health in this chapter). There are several possible reasons for this. Primarily, delayed help seeking may be the result of both enacted and perceived stigma which can make people concerned about interacting with health care professionals. For example, the large survey in the UK by GOV.UK (2017) concluded that many members of the LGBTQ+ community avoid help seeking through feeling anxious or embarrassed about going to the doctor. Likewise, the Stonewall report in the UK (2018) concluded from their survey of 5000 people that one in seven LGBT people (14 per cent) avoid seeking healthcare for fear of discrimination from staff. Similarly, the Center for American Progress (2020) report concluded that 15 per cent of respondents (including 28 per cent of transgender respondents), reported postponing or avoiding help-seeking when they were sick or injured due to fear of disrespect or discrimination. In line with this, the LGBTQ+ community has been identified as a 'health disparity population' by the National Institute on Minority Health and Health Disparities (2016) due to their reduced access to health care. It may also, however, not only be due to enacted or perceived stigma but the actual availability of care itself. For example, in the US where there is a reliance upon health care insurance it has been argued that 43 per cent of those identifying as transgender face health care insurance discrimination which limits their ability to seek help (National Institute on Minority Health and Health Disparities 2016). Furthermore, a study by Buchmueller and Carpenter (2010) of over 800,000 men and women found that women in same-sex relationships were less likely to have had a recent mammogram or Pap test than heterosexual women which was linked to the availability of health insurance.

Health Behaviours

Individuals who identify as LGBTQ+ are therefore likely to have poorer mental and physical health which may be linked to enacted and perceived stigma which in turn may result in delayed help seeking. It is possible, however, that poorer health outcomes are also linked to health-related behaviours and that all these factors are interlinked. For example, if members of the LGBTQ+ community are more likely to smoke use drugs or over consume alcohol (e.g. Centers for Disease Control and Protection 2018; Boyd et al. 2019) then this in turn would be linked to higher rates of chronic conditions such as cancer and heart disease (Caceres et al. 2020; Valanis et al. 2000). Likewise, increased rates of anal cancer (Patel et al. 2018) could be linked to higher rates of STIs (Hafeez et al. 2017) and higher rates of obesity (Azagba et al. 2019) could be linked to higher rates of alcohol use (Centers for Disease Control and Protection 2018; Boyd et al. 2019) and to higher rates of cancer and heart disease

(Caceres et al. 2020; Valanis et al. 2000). Further, given the clear crossover between mental and physical health (Seligman and Nemeroff 2015), the higher rates of anxiety and depression may well be linked to higher rates of cancer and heart disease.

IN SUMMARY

Members of the LGBTQ+ community clearly have poorer health outcomes in terms of both physical and mental health issues. This section has explored how this relates to both enacted and perceived stigma which in turn can lead to delayed help seeking. Furthermore, there is also a role for health-related behaviours. From this perspective, the poorer health found in the LGBTQ+ community can be conceptualized as resulting from enacted and perceived stigma which in turn leads to delayed help-seeking and unhealthier behaviours. Further, this can create an ongoing downward spiral with poorer mental health then resulting in less self care, unhealthier behaviours and poorer physical health (see Figure 15.11).

BOX 15.1
Critical Approaches to Health Psychology

Research and theories relating to gender and health highlight some of the bigger issues in health psychology as follows:

Gender differences: For centuries research has explored differences between men and women and gender has been treated as a dichotomous variable. Increasingly, gender is seen as more fluid than this and research in health psychology needs to embrace this fluidity. This will initially result in gender differences between the spectrum of genders. Eventually, it may well mean that gender loses its significance as a way of understanding who we are.

Sexuality: Similarly research has focused on differences between people who are heterosexual or gay and treated sexuality as a dichotomous variable. In line with gender, sexuality is also becoming more fluid as we recognize how limited this classification system has been.

Biology vs experience: Research into the gendered nature of health also highlights the relationship between the biology behind an experience and the person's actual experience. For example, we may have hormones, but is how we experience them what really contributes to our health? Likewise, we may have different bodily parts or biological processes but what is more important to our health: the biological component or the way we live and experience this biology? This is a debate which will run and run but needs to happen if we are to understand the best ways to maximize someone's health status.

---

7 | THINKING CRITICALLY ABOUT GENDER AND HEALTH

There are several issues with research exploring gender and health that need to be considered.

SOME CRITICAL QUESTIONS

When thinking about research into gender and health ask yourself the following questions.

- Much research treats gender as a binary construct and explores differences between men and women. Is this approach useful or could it do harm?
- Can research ever be unbiased by the researcher's own values?
- To what extent can we generalize from research participants to people in general?

- How can we synthesize between research using qualitative and quantitative methods? Should we?
- This chapter has mostly focused on gender. How might sexuality also impact upon health? How are gender and sexuality interlinked?

SOME PROBLEMS WITH . . .

Below are some problems with research and theory exploring gender and health.

Stereotypes: Research often makes very clear distinctions between men and women, emphasizing how different they are. This can result in a highly stereotypical version of gender differences and emphasizes differences rather than similarities. It is important to remember that not all men behave like 'men' and not all women behave like 'women', and that there is much variability in the ways in which both men and women think and act.

Classification: Research not only differentiates between men and women but also between members of the LGBTQ+ community and 'others'. Is it fair to group together all members of the LGBTQ+ community and suggest that they have something in common? Is it fair to group together those who are *not* in the LGBTQ+ community and suggest they have something in common? Is it fair to suggest that people within the LGBTQ+ community have more in common with each other than with those not in the LGBTQ+ community? How do we decide which label most suits us? Am I mostly a woman? Straight? A mother? White? A psychologist? And is my colleague mostly a man? Gay? Italian? All these classification processes help research by giving us a way to organize data and look for differences. But they don't tell us much about individuals as we all belong to more than one classification and the very process of classification can help generate the stereotypes they are sometimes trying to break down.

Gender as binary: Over the past few years there has been a debate about the notion of *cisgenderism* – the prejudicial belief that there are only two genders (i.e. men and women). In line with this, some researchers have called for an understanding of a multitude of different genders and have highlighted many different cultures in which a binary version of gender doesn't exist. The focus on men's and women's health as presented in this book falls into the camp of cisgenderism as it reinforces the belief that the world can be broken down into only two genders.

The gender gap is changing: At the beginning of the twentieth century men generally lived longer than women as many women died in childbirth. Then this turned around and women started to live longer as childbirth became less risky. Nowadays, however, the gap between men's and women's life expectancy is getting smaller year on year. Soon we may all be equal in terms of life expectancy or men may start living longer than women again. Any analysis of gender and health needs to take this historical perspective into account.

Biased by ideology: Much women's health research generates political and ideological perspectives. For example, miscarriage, termination and menopause management can create a strong sense of what is right or wrong. Research in these areas may therefore be biased in terms of what questions are asked, how data are collected and how the results are interpreted and presented. For example, someone who is more anti-medicalization may favour the natural management of miscarriages and the menopause, while someone in favour of medicine may take the opposite view. Likewise, a pro-life/anti-abortion researcher may focus on the harms of termination while a pro-choice researcher may focus on the benefits.

The problem of stigma: Some issues addressed by psychology are stigmatized conditions which can influence the research process. For example, mental health problems such as anxiety and depression which may accompany physical health problems; issues relating to sexuality such as sexual health; reproduction issues such as termination of pregnancy and childlessness; and issues relating to gender identity may all be stigmatized by society or perceived as stigmatized by those having these experiences. Such stigma may influence research in several ways including limiting those willing to come forward and share their experiences; the degree of openness and honesty people are prepared to show when involved in research; the willingness of researchers to carry out research in these areas; the response of reviewers to research papers in these areas.

Research is changing: Many areas of women's health are constantly changing. For example, the use of hormone replacement therapy (HRT) for the menopause, the management of miscarriages and that of terminations change from year to year. Summarizing results within these areas across time is therefore difficult.

The problem of case mix: Research can only be done on those participants who identify that they have a problem and/or come into contact with health care professionals. Miscarriage is very common and the menopause happens to every woman. Yet some miscarriages are considered to be late periods or miscarriages that will resolve themselves without medical intervention. Likewise, many women consider the menopause to be just part of life and wait on their own for it to end. To date, most research focuses on those who seek help and requires the participants to identify that they are having the problem. This offers an unrepresentative sample and means that very little is known about those women who experience miscarriage and menopause but never seek help.

The problem of comparison: Research often explores experiences of difference conditions (i.e. prostate cancer, CHD, abortion, miscarriage, menopause). In doing, so it assumes that these experiences are worse (or better) than the experiences of those without the condition. For some conditions this can be actually tested with a comparison group (i.e. no prostate cancer, no CHD, no miscarriage). But for abortion this is more difficult. Therefore, we might find that an abortion is upsetting but this can only be compared to those who don't have an abortion. It is hard to compare this to those who wanted an abortion but ended up with an unwanted baby. The results are therefore biased. Further, all women go through the menopause. So it is again hard to find an appropriate comparison group. As a result, we cannot work out whether the effects we see are actually due to the menopause or the stage of life when a menopause happens.

The problem of culture: Miscarriages and the menopause happen to all women regardless of class, culture or time. Most research to date, however, has explored the experiences of western women for whom these are often seen as an event that needs to be managed medically. It is likely that other cultures have very different beliefs about both miscarriages and the menopause and that this influences their management strategies and women's subsequent experiences. We know very little about these cross-cultural differences.

Triangulation: Research exploring miscarriage and termination tends to use either quantitative or qualitative methods. To date, there has been no use of mixed methods or any real integration of the two literatures.

TO CONCLUDE

Research indicates that women have more symptoms and illnesses than men but live longer and that when men get ill they are more likely to die sooner. It also indicates that those from the LGBTQ+ community have poorer health in terms of both mental and physical health issues. Health is therefore clearly gendered. This chapter has first focused on three aspects of women's health that most closely reflect the interests of the health psychology community. Miscarriage, termination of pregnancy and the menopause are generally regarded as negative events that women have to endure. The results from the studies described in this chapter indicate that, although these are difficult and often unpleasant times for women, many women report how they can also see the benefit in these experiences. In particular, miscarriage is sometimes seen as a pivotal point in a woman's life, enabling her to re-evaluate her past and future self; termination is often accompanied by feelings of relief and a return to normality; and the menopause introduces a new period of life and a sense of liberation. Furthermore, the research illustrates how women's experiences of these events are influenced by the mode of management as all can be managed medically, surgically or by letting them happen in their own time without medical intervention. This chapter then explored how being male can impact health in terms of risk and help-seeking behaviours, health beliefs, social norms of masculinity and emotional expression. It has then illustrated these processes with a focus on prostate cancer, suicide and CHD. Next the chapter explored health issues pertinent to the LGBTQ+ community in terms of the prevalence of physical and mental health problems and how these might relate to enacted and perceived stigma, delayed help seeking and health-related behaviours. Gender therefore impacts health in a number of ways and highlights the inter-relationship between behaviour, individual beliefs and those held by society as a whole.

QUESTIONS

1 In what ways is women's health worse than men's?
2 Why do women live longer than men but have more illnesses and/or symptoms?
3 To what extent are women's responses to miscarriage similar to those following bereavement?
4 What factors influence the decision to have an abortion?
5 To what extent are women's experiences of the menopause a response to the biological changes that occur at this time?
6 How are women's experiences of their health problems influenced by whether they are managed medically, surgically or left to happen in their own time?
7 What are some of the problems with carrying out research into controversial areas of health such as termination of pregnancy?
8 How might behaviour influence men's health status?
9 Consider the evidence that men are less emotionally expressive than women.
10 Where might men's beliefs about their health come from?
11 Why are health issues specific to the LGBTQ+ community?
12 How does stigma influence help seeking?
13 How does delayed help seeking impact health and illness?
14 Considering the issues faced by the LGBTQ+ community, how might mental and physical health interrelate?

FOR DISCUSSION

Consider how someone you know (your mother, friend, etc.) experienced the menopause. Reflect upon how this experience may have been affected by other factors that were changing at the same time.

Talk to a male friend about their health beliefs and behaviour. Consider to what extent they are (or are not) conforming to social norms of masculinity.

Talk to someone from the LGBTQ+ community and ask them how they feel their gender or sexuality has influenced their health.

FURTHER READING

Courtenay, W.H. (2000) Constructions of masculinity and their influence on men's well being: a theory of gender and health, *Social Science and Medicine,* **50**(10): 1385–1401.
Will Courtenay has written extensively on male health issues. This is one of his more theoretical papers which provides an interesting discussion on masculinity and health. Other papers by him are also useful and can be found in the reference list at the end of this book.

Frostrup, M. and Smellie, A. (2021) *Cracking the Menopause. While Keeping Yourself Together.* London: Bluebird: Pan Macmillan.
This book was written for a lay audience but draws upon lots of research evidence and expert accounts (including from me!) and provides a great overview of the experiences of those going through the menopause.

Gough, B. and Robertson, S. (eds) (2010) *Men, Masculinities and Health: Critical Perspectives.* Basingstoke: Palgrave Macmillan.
This is an edited collection of an interesting series of studies which explore men's health issues such as fatherhood, body image and chest pain. The book takes a critical perspective and has an excellent introductory chapter outlining the theoretical stance being used.

Lee, C. (1998) *Women's Health: Psychological and Social Perspectives.* London: Sage.
This book covers a wide range of issues relating to women's health not covered by the present chapter, including pre-menstrual syndrome, post-partum depression and fertility control. It therefore offers a useful background into the areas not addressed by this book.

Lee, C. and Glynn Owens, R. (2002) *The Psychology of Men's Health.* Maidenhead: Open University Press.
This is an excellent text which clearly describes a range of aspects of men's health and locates them within a sense of gender and notions of masculinity.

Moulder, C. (1998) *Understanding Pregnancy Loss: Perspectives and Issues in Care.* London: Macmillan.
This is an excellent book that draws upon the experiences of women who have had a miscarriage, termination or stillbirth and locates their experiences within the existing literature. It explores a range of factors including health care prior to admission, experiences of being in hospital, health professionals' views and care after discharge.

Spiers, M.V., Geller, P.A. and Kloss, J.D. (eds) (2013) *Women's Health Psychology.* Hoboken, NJ: Wiley.
This edited collection covers a breadth of issues relating to health psychology ranging from the more traditional domains such as obesity, smoking, alcohol and pregnancy to the more specific such as infertility, body adornment and the impact of employment.

Wood, G.W. (2018) *The psychology of gender.* Routledge: London.
This little book explores the complexities of sex and gender in a thorough yet accessible way.

Methodology glossary

B

Between-subjects design: this involves making comparisons between different groups of subjects; for example, males versus females, those who have been offered a health-related intervention versus those who have not.

C

Case-control design: this involves taking a group of subjects who show a particular characteristic (e.g. lung cancer – the dependent variable), selecting a control group without the characteristic (e.g. no lung cancer) and retrospectively examining these two groups for the factors that may have caused this characteristic (e.g. did those with lung cancer smoke more than those without?).

Condition: experimental studies often involve allocating subjects to different conditions; for example, information versus no information, relaxation versus no relaxation, active drug versus placebo versus control condition.

Cross-sectional design: a study is described as being cross-sectional if the different variables are measured at the same time as each other.

D

Dependent variable: the characteristic that appears to change as a result of the independent variable; for example, changing behavioural intentions (the independent variable) causes a change in behaviour (the dependent variable).

E

Experimental design: this involves a controlled study in which variables are manipulated in order to specifically examine the relationship between the independent variable (the cause) and the dependent variable (the effect); for example, does experimentally induced anxiety change pain perception?

I

Independent variable: the characteristic that appears to cause a change in the dependent variable; for example, smoking (the independent variable) causes lung cancer (the dependent variable).

L

Likert scale: variables can be measured on a scale marked by numbers (e.g. 1 to 5) or terms (e.g. never/seldom/sometimes/often/very often). The subject is asked to mark the appropriate point.

Longitudinal design

Longitudinal design: this involves measuring variables at a baseline and then following up the subjects at a later point in time (sometimes called prospective or cohort design).

P

Prospective design: this involves following up subjects over a period of time (sometimes called longitudinal or cohort design).

Q

Qualitative study: this involves methodologies such as interviews in order to collect data from subjects. Qualitative data is a way of describing the variety of beliefs, interpretations and behaviours from a heterogenous subject group without making generalizations to the population as a whole. It is believed that qualitative studies are more able to access the subjects' beliefs without contaminating the data with the researcher's own expectations. Qualitative data are described in terms of themes and categories.

Quantitative study: this involves collecting data in the form of numbers using methodologies such as questionnaires and experiments. Quantitative data are a way of describing the beliefs, interpretations and behaviours of a large population and generalizations are made about the population as a whole. Quantitative data are described in terms of frequencies, means and statistically significant differences and correlations.

R

Randomly allocated: subjects are randomly allocated to different conditions in order to minimize the effects of any individual differences; for example, to ensure that subjects who receive the drug versus the placebo versus nothing are equivalent in age and sex. If all the subjects who received the placebo happened to be female, this would obviously influence the results.

Repeated-measures design: this involves asking subjects to complete the same set of measures more than once; for example, before and after reading a health information leaflet.

S

Subjects: these are the individuals who are involved in the study. They may also be referred to as participants, clients, respondents or cases.

V

Variable: a characteristic that can be measured (e.g. age, beliefs, fitness).

Visual analogue scale: variables such as beliefs are sometimes measured using a 100 mm line with anchor points at each end (such as not at all confident/extremely confident). The subject is asked to place a cross on the line at the appropriate point.

W

Within-subjects design: this involves making comparisons within the same group of subjects. How do subjects respond to receiving an invitation to attend a screening programme? How does a belief about smoking relate to the subjects' smoking behaviour?

References

Aaronson, N.K., Ahmedzai, S. and Bergman, B. et al. (1993) The European Organisation for Research and Treatment of Cancer, QLQ-C30: a quality of life instrument for use in international clinical trials in oncology, *Journal for the National Cancer Institute*, **85**: 365–76.

Aarts, H., Verplanken, B. and van Knippenberg, A. (1998) Predicting behaviour from actions in the past: repeated decision making or matter of habit? *Journal of Applied Social Psychology*, **28**: 1355–74.

Abbey, J.G., Rosenfeld, B., Pessin, H. and Breitbart, W. (2006) Hopelessness at the end of life: the utility of the hopelessness scale with terminally ill cancer patients, *British Journal of Health Psychology*, **11**: 173–83.

Abbott, S. and Freeth, D. (2008) Social capital and health: starting to make sense of the role of generalized trust and reciprocity, *Journal of Health Psychology*, **13**(7): 874–83.

Abraham, C. and Michie, S. (2008) A taxonomy of behaviour change techniques used in interventions, *Health Psychology*, **27**: 379–87.

Abraham, C. and Sheeran, P. (1993) In search of a psychology of safer-sex promotion: beyond beliefs and text, *Health Education Research: Theory and Practice*, **8**: 245–54.

Abraham, C. and Sheeran, P. (2005) The health belief model, in M. Conner and P. Norman (eds) *Predicting Health Behaviour*, 2nd edn. Maidenhead: Open University Press.

Abraham, S., Sheeran, P., Abrams, D. and Spears, R. (1996) Health beliefs and teenage condom use: a prospective study, *Psychology and Health*, **11**: 641–55.

Abrams, D., Abraham, C., Spears, R. and Marks, D. (1990) AIDS invulnerability: relationships, sexual behaviour and attitudes among 16–19-year-olds, in P. Aggleton, P. Davies and G. Hart (eds) *AIDS: Individual, Cultural and Policy Dimensions*. London: Falmer Press.

Achstetter, L.I., Schultz, K., Faller, H. and Schuler, M. (2019) Leventhal's common-sense model and asthma control: Do illness representations predict success of an asthma rehabilitation? *Journal of Health Psychology*, **24**(3): 327–36.

Acuff, S.F., Strickland, J.C., Tucker, J.A. and Murphy, J.G. (2022) Changes in alcohol use during COVID-19 and associations with contextual and individual difference variables: a systematic review and meta-analysis, *Psychology of Addictive Behaviors*, **36**(1): 1–19.

Adam, B.D., Husbands, W., Murray, J. and Maxwell, J. (2005) AIDS optimism, condom fatigue, or self-esteem? Explaining unsafe sex among gay and bisexual men, *Journal of Sex Research*, **42**(3): 238–48.

Adamczyk, W.M., Buglewicz, E., Szikszay, T.M. et al. (2019) Reward for pain: hyperalgesia and allodynia induced by operant conditioning: systematic review and meta-analysis, *The Journal of Pain*, **20**(8): 861–75.

Ader, R. and Cohen, N. (1975) Behaviourally conditioned immuno suppression, *Psychosomatic Medicine*, **37**: 333–40.

Ader, R. and Cohen, N. (1981) Conditioned immunopharmacologic responses, in R. Ader (ed.) *Psychoneuroimmunology*. New York: Academic Press.

Alder, N., David, H., Major, B.N. et al. (1990) Psychological responses after abortion, Science, 248: 41–4.

Afrisham, R., Paknejad, M., Soliemanifar, O. et al. (2019) The influence of psychological stress on the initiation and progression of diabetes and cancer, *International Journal of Endocrinology and Metabolism*, **17**(2): e67400.

Afriyie, J. and Essilfie, M.E. (2019) Association between risky sexual behaviour and HIV risk perception among in-school adolescents in a municipality in Ghana, *Ghana Medical Journal*, **53**(1): 29–36.

Aggio, D., Papachristou, E., Papacosta, O. et al. (2018) Trajectories of self-reported physical activity and predictors during the transition to old age: a 20-year cohort study of British men. *International Journal of Behavioral Nutrition and Physical Activity*, **15**(1): 14.

Aggleton, P. and Homans, H. (1988) *Social Aspects of AIDS*. London: Falmer Press.

Aggleton, P. (1989) HIV/AIDS education in schools: constraints and possibilities, *Health Education Journal*, **48**: 167–71.

Ahern, A.L., Olson, A.D., Aston, L.M. and Jebb, S.A. (2011) Weight Watchers on prescription: an observational study of weight change among adults referred to Weight Watchers by the NHS, *BMC Public Health*, **11**: 434.

Ahmed, A.K., Weatherburn, P., Reid, D. et al. (2016) Social norms related to combining drugs and sex ('chemsex') among gay men in South London, *International Journal of Drug Policy*, **38**: 29–35.

Ahto, M., Isoaho, R., Puolijoki, H. et al. (2007) Stronger symptoms of depression predict high coronary heart disease mortality in older men and women, *International Journal of Geriatric Psychiatry*, **22**(8): 757–63.

Ainsworth, M.D.S., Blehar, M.C., Waters, E. and Wall, S. (1978) *Patterns of Attachment: A Study of the Strange Situation*. Hillsdale, NJ: Erlbaum.

Ajayi, A.I., Ismail, K.O. and Akpan, W. (2019) Factors associated with consistent condom use: a cross-sectional survey of two Nigerian universities, *BMC Public Health*, **19**(1): 1–11.

Ajzen, I. and Madden, T.J. (1986) Prediction of goal-directed behavior: attitudes, intentions, and perceived behavioral control, *Journal of Experimental Social Psychology*, **22**: 453–74.

Ajzen, I. (1988) *Attitudes, Personality and Behavior*. Chicago, IL: Dorsey Press.

Alamnia, T.T., Tesfaye, W. and Kelly, M. (2022) The effectiveness of text message delivered interventions for weight loss in developing countries: a systematic review and meta-analysis, *Obesity Reviews*, **23**(1): e13339.

Albarracín D., Johnson, B.T., Fishbein, M. and Muellerleile, P.A. (2001) Theories of reasoned action and planned behaviour as models of condom use: a meta-analysis. *Psychological Bulletin*, **127**: 142–61.

Albrecht, G.L. (1994) Subjective health status, in C. Jenkinson (ed.) *Measuring Health and Medical Outcomes*. London: UCL Press.

Alder, N., David, H., Major, B.N. et al. (1990) Psychological responses after abortion, *Science*, **248**: 41–4.

Alderson, T. and Ogden, J. (1999) What mothers feed their children and why, *Health Education Research: Theory and Practice*, **14**: 717–27.

Alex, L. and Hammarström, A. (2004) Women's experiences in connection with induced abortion: a feminist perspective, *Scandinavian Journal of Caring Sciences*, **18**: 160–8.

Ali, N., Lifford, K.J., Carter, B. et al. (2015) Barriers to uptake among high-risk individuals declining participation in lung cancer screening: a mixed methods analysis of the UK Lung Cancer Screening (UKLS) trial. *BMJ Open*, **5**(7): e008254.

Allen, I. (1991) *Family Planning and Pregnancy Counseling Projects for Young People*. London: Policy Studies Institute.

Allender, S., Peto, V., Scarborough, P. et al. (2008a) *Coronary Heart Disease Statistics*. London: British Heart Foundation.

Allender, S., Scarborough, P., Peto, V. et al. (2008b) *European Cardiovascular Disease Statistics*. Brussels: European Heart Network.

Almedon, A.M. (2005) Social capital and mental health: an interdisciplinary review of primary evidence, *Social Science and Medicine*, **61**: 943–64.

Almqvist, E.W., Brinkman, R.R., Wiggins, S. et al. (2003) Psychological consequences and predictors of adverse events in the first 5 years after predictive testing for Huntington disease, *Clinical Genetics*, **64**: 300–9.

Alonso, J., Black, C., Norregaard, J.C. et al. (1998) Cross-cultural differences in the reporting of global functional capacity: an example in cataract patients, *Medical Care*, **36**: 868–78.

Al-Rousan, T., Moore, A.A., Han, B.H. et al. (2022) Trends in binge drinking prevalence among older US men and women, 2015 to 2019, *Journal of the American Geriatrics Society*, **70**(3): 812–19.

American Lung Association. (2002b) *Trends in Tobacco Use*, www.lungusa.orgdata/smoke/smoke1.pdf.

American Lung Association (2002a) *Adolescent Smoking Statistics*, www.lungusa.org/press/tobacco/not_stats.html.

Amialchuk, A. and Gerhardinger, L. (2015) Contraceptive use and pregnancies in adolescents' romantic relationships: Role of relationship activities and parental attitudes and communication, *Journal of Developmental and Behavioral Pediatrics*, **36**(2): 86–97.

An, K.Y., Kang, D.W., Morielli, A.R., Friedenreich, C.M., Reid, R.D., McKenzie, D.C., Courneya, K.S. et al. (2020) Patterns and predictors of exercise behavior during 24 months of follow-up after a supervised exercise program during breast cancer chemotherapy, *International Journal of Behavioral Nutrition and Physical Activity*, **17**(1): 1–11.

Analogbei, T., Dear, N., Reed, D. et al. (2020) Predictors and barriers to condom use in the African cohort study, *AIDS Patient Care and STDs*, **34**(5): 228–36.

Anderson, H.R., Freeling, P. and Patel, S.P. (1983) Decision making in acute asthma, *Journal of the Royal College of General Practitioners*, **33**: 105–8.

Anderson, K.G. (2017) Adverse childhood environment: relationship with sexual risk behaviours and marital status in a large American sample, *Evolutionary Psychology*, **15**(2), doi: 1474704917710115.

Anderson, L., Oldridge, N., Thompson, D.R. et al. (2016) Exercise-based cardiac rehabilitation for coronary heart disease: Cochrane systematic review and meta-analysis, *Journal of the American College of Cardiology*, **67**(1): 1–12.

Annas, G.J. (1990) Quality of life in the courts: early spring in fantasyland, in J.J. Walter and T.A. Shannon (eds) *Quality of Life: The New Medical Dilemma*. New York: Paulist Press.

Antoni, M.H. and Dhabhar, F.S. (2019) The impact of psychosocial stress and stress management on immune responses in patients with cancer. *Cancer*, **125**(9): 1417–31.

Antoni, M.H., Carrico, A.W., Durán, R.E. et al. (2006) Randomized clinical trial of cognitive behavioral stress management on human immunodeficiency virus viral load in gay men treated with highly active anti retroviral therapy, *Psychosomatic Medicine*, **68**: 143–51.

Antoni, M.H., Cruess, D.G., Cruess, S. et al. (2000) Cognitive–behavioral stress management intervention effects on anxiety, 24-hr urinary norepinephrine output and T-cytotoxic/suppressor cells over time among symptomatic HIV-infected gay men, *Journal of Consulting and Clinical Psychology*, **68**(1): 31–45.

Antoni, M.H., Cruess, D.G., Klimas, N. et al. (2002) Stress management and immune system reconstitution in symptomatic HIV-infected gay men over time: effects on transitional naive T cells (CD4+CD45RA−CD29+), *American Journal of Psychiatry*, **159**(1): 143–5.

Antoni, M.H., Cruess, D.G., Klimas, N. et al. (2005) Increases in marker of immune system reconstitution are predated by decreases in 24-hr urinary cortisol output depressed mood during a 10-week stress management intervention in symptomatic HIV-infected men, *Journal of Psychosomatic Research*, **58**(1): 3–13.

Antoni, M.H., Lehman, J.M., Klibourn, K.M. et al. (2001) Cognitive-behavioral stress management intervention decreases the prevalence of depression and enhances benefit finding among women under treatment for early-stage breast cancer, *Health Psychology*, **20**(1): 20–32.

Anzman, S.L., Rollins, B.Y. and Birch, L.L. (2010) Parental influence on children's early eating environments and obesity risk: implications for prevention, *International Journal of Obesity*, **34**: 1116–24.

Appels, A., Golombeck, B., Gorgels, A. et al. (2002) Psychological risk factors of sudden cardiac arrest, *Psychology and Health*, **17**: 773–81.

Aqeel, M.M., Guo, J., Lin, L. et al. (2020) Temporal dietary patterns are associated with obesity in US adults, *The Journal of Nutrition*, **150**(12): 3259–68.

Aranguren, M. (2022) Face mask use conditionally decreases compliance with physical distancing rules against COVID-19: gender differences in risk compensation pattern, *Annals of Behavioral Medicine*, **56**(4): 332–46.

Arbejdstilsynet (2012) Anmeldte arbejdsulykker 2006-11-Arbejdstilsynets a°rsopgørelse 2011. Arbejdstilsynet, August: 87-7534-603-6.

Arcò, D., Raggi, A. and Ferri, R. (2016) Cognitive behavioral therapy for insomnia in breast cancer survivors: a review of the literature. *Frontiers in Psychology*, **7**: 1162.

Armitage, C.J. (2007b) Efficacy of a brief worksite intervention to reduce smoking: the roles of behavioural and implementation intentions, *Journal of Occupational Health Psychology*, **12**: 376–90.

Armitage, C.J. (2007a) Effects of an implementation intention-based intervention on fruit consumption, *Psychology and Health*, **22**(8): 917–28.

Armitage, C.J. and Conner, M. (2000) Social cognition models and health behaviour: a structured review, *Psychology and Health*, **15**: 173–89.

Armitage, C.J. and Conner, M. (2001) Efficacy of the theory of planned behaviour: a meta-analytic review, *British Journal of Social Psychology*, **40**: 471–99.

Armitage, C.J. and Harris, P.R. (2006) The influence of adult attachment on symptom reporting: testing a meditational model in a sample of the general population, *Psychology and Health*, **21**(3): 351–66.

Armitage, C.J. (2004) Evidence that implementation intentions reduce dietary fat intake: a randomized trial, *Health Psychology*, **23**(3): 319–23.

Armitage, C.J. (2005) Can the theory of planned behaviour predict the maintenance of physical activity? *Health Psychology*, **24**(3): 235–45.

Armitage, C.J. (2008) A volitional help sheet to encourage smoking cessation: a randomized exploratory trial, *Health Psychology*, **27**(5): 557–66.

Armitage, C.J. (2009a) Effectiveness of experimenter-provided and self-generated implementation intentions to reduce alcohol consumption in a sample of the general population: a randomized exploratory trial, *Health Psychology*, **28**(5): 543–53.

Armstrong D. (2021) The COVID-19 pandemic and cause of death, *Sociology of Health & Illness*, **43**(7): 1614–26. Doi.org/10.1111/1467-9566.13347.

Armstrong, A.W., Ford, A.R., Chambers, C.J. et al. (2019) Online care versus in-person care for improving quality of life in psoriasis: a randomized controlled equivalency trial, *Journal of Investigative Dermatology*, **139**(5): 1037–44.

Arvola, A., Vassallo, M., Dean, M. et al. (2008) Predicting intentions to purchase organic food: the role of affective and moral attitudes in the theory of planned behaviour, *Appetite*, **50**: 443–54.

Ashton, W., Nanchahal, K. and Wood, D. (2001) Body mass index and metabolic risk factors for coronary heart disease in women, *European Heart Journal*, **22**: 46–55.

Asimakopoulou, K. and Newton, J.T. (2015) The contributions of behaviour change science towards dental public health practice: a new paradigm. *Community Dentistry and Oral Epidemiology*, **43**(1): 2–8.

Athey, J. and Spielvogel, A. (2000) Risk factors and interventions for psychological sequelae in women after miscarriage, *Primary Care Update for Obstetrics and Gynaecology*, **7**: 64–9.

Atkins, L., Francis, J., Islam, R., et al. (2017) A guide to using the Theoretical Domains Framework of behaviour change to investigate implementation problems, *Implementation Science*, **12**(1): 77.

Atkins, L., Wood, C. and Michie, S. (2015) How to design and describe behaviour change interventions, *Health Psychology Update*, **24**: 36–42.

Attie, I. and Brooks-Gunn, J. (1989) Development of eating problems in adolescent girls: a longitudinal study, *Developmental Psychology*, **25**: 70–9.

Aucott, L.S. (2008) Influences of weight loss on long-term diabetes outcomes, *Proceedings of the Nutrition Society*, **67**(1): 54–9.

Aujla, N., Walker, M., Sprigg, N. et al. (2016) Can illness beliefs, from the common-sense model, prospectively predict adherence to self-management behaviours? A systematic review and meta-analysis, *Psychology and Health*, **31**(8): 931–58.

Avery, A.R., Tsang, S., Seto, E.Y. and Duncan, G.E. (2020) Stress, anxiety, and change in alcohol use during the COVID-19 pandemic: findings among adult twin pairs, *Frontiers in Psychiatry*, 1030. https://doi.org/10.3389/fpsyt.2020.571084

Aveyard, P., Lawrence, T., Cheng, K.K. et al. (2006) A randomized controlled trial of smoking cessation for pregnant women to test the effect of a transtheoretical model-based intervention on movement in stage and interaction with baseline stage, *British Journal of Health Psychology*, **11**: 263–78.

Axelson, M.L., Brinberg, D. and Durand, J.H. (1983) Eating at a fast-food restaurant: a social psychological analysis, *Journal of Nutrition Education*, **15**: 94–8.

Ayerdi Aguirrebengoa, O., Vera García, M., Arias Ramírez, D. et al. (2021) Low use of condom and high STI incidence among men who have sex with men in PrEP programs, *PloS one*, **16**(2): e0245925.

Ayling, K., Jia, R., Coupland, C. et al. (2022) Psychological predictors of self-reported COVID-19 outcomes: results From a prospective cohort study, *Annals of Behavioral Medicine: a Publication of the Society of Behavioral Medicine*, **56**(5): 484–97. Doi.org/10.1093/abm/kaab106.

Azagba, S., Shan, L. and Latham, K. (2019) Overweight and obesity among sexual minority adults in the United States, *International Journal of Environmental Research and Public Health*, **16**(10): 1828.

Bélanger-Gravel, A., Godin, G. and Amireault, S. (2013) A meta-analytic review of the effect of implementation intentions on physical activity, *Health Psychology Review*, **7**(1): 23–54.

Bagozzi, R.P. (1993) On the neglect of volition in consumer research: a critique and proposal, *Psychology and Marketing*, **10**: 215–37.

Bahri, N., Fathi Najafi, T., Homaei Shandiz, F. et al. (2019) The relation between stressful life events and breast cancer: a systematic review and meta-analysis of cohort studies, *Breast Cancer Research and Treatment*, **176**(1): 53–61.

Bailey, J.V., Webster, R., Hunter, R. et al. (2016) The Men's Safer Sex project: intervention development and feasibility randomised controlled trial of an interactive digital intervention to increase condom use in men, *Health Technology Assessment*, **20**(91): 1–124.

Bailey, S.L., Boivin, J., Cheong, et al. (2019) Hope for the best. . . but expect the worst: a qualitative study to explore how women with recurrent miscarriage experience the early waiting period of a new pregnancy, *BMJ Open*, **9**(5): e029354.

Baillie, C., Smith, J., Hewison, J. and Mason, G. (2000) Ultrasound screening for chromosomal abnormality: women's reactions to false positive results, *British Journal of Health Psychology*, **5**: 377–94.

Bain, D.J.G. (1977) Patient knowledge and the content of the consultation in general practice, *Medical Education*, **11**: 347–50.

Baird, J., Jacob, C.M., Barker, M. et al. (2017) Developmental origins of health and disease: a lifecourse approach to the prevention of noncommunicable diseases, *Healthcare (Basel)*, **5**(1). Doi: 10.3390/healthcare5010014

Ballard, K., Kuh, D.J. and Wadsworth, M.E.J. (2001) The role of the menopause in women's experiences of the 'changes of life', *Sociology of Health and Illness*, **23**(4): 397–424.

Ballard, K. (2002) Understanding risk: women's perceived risk of menopause-related disease and the value they place on preventive hormone replacement therapy, *Family Practice*, **19**(6): 591–5.

Ballard, K. (2003) *Understanding Menopause*. Chichester: John Wiley.

Ballenger, J.C., Davidson, J.R., Lecrubier, Y. et al. (2001) Consensus statement on transcultural issues in depression and anxiety from the International Consensus Group on Depression and Anxiety, *Journal of Clinical Psychiatry*, **62**(Suppl. 13): 47–55.

Bandura, A. (1986) *Social Foundations of Thought and Action*. Englewood Cliffs, NJ: Prentice Hall.

Bandura, A. (1977) Self efficacy: toward a unifying theory of behavior change, *Psychological Review*, **84**: 191–215.

Bansen, S. and Stevens, H.A. (1992) Women's experiences of miscarriage in early pregnancy, *Journal of Nurse-Midwifery*, **37**: 84–90.

Barbosa, C., Cowell, A. J. and Dowd, W. N. (2021) Alcohol consumption in response to the COVID-19 pandemic in the United States, *Journal of Addiction Medicine*, **15**(4): 341–44.

Barkhordari, A., Malmir, B. and Malakoutikhah, M. (2019) An analysis of individual and social factors affecting occupational accidents, *Safety and Health at Work*, **10**(2): 205–12.

Barraclough, J., Pinder, P., Cruddas, M. et al. (1992) Life events and breast cancer prognosis, *British Medical Journal*, **304**: 1078–81.

Barsky, A.J., Peekna, H.M. and Borus, J.F. (2001) Somatic symptom reporting in women and men. *Journal of General Internal Medicine*, **16**(4): 266–75.

Barth, J., Schumacher, M. and Herrmann-Lingen, C. (2004) Depression as a risk factor for mortality in patients with coronary heart disease: a meta-analysis, *Psychosomatic Medicine*, **66**(6): 802–13.

Barthomeuf, L., Rousset, S., and Droit-Volet, S. (2007) Emotion and food: do the emotions expressed on other people's faces affect the desire to eat liked and disliked food products? *Appetite*, **48**: 211–17.

Bascour-Sandoval, C., Salgado-Salgado, S., Gómez-Milán et al. (2019) Pain and distraction according to sensory modalities: current findings and future directions, *Pain Practice*, **19**(7): 686–702.

Basu, S., Goswami, A.G., David, L.E. and Mudge, E. (2022) Psychological stress on wound healing: A silent player in a complex background, *The International Journal of Lower Extremity Wounds*, 1:1534346221077571, 1–7.

Battle, R.S., Cunradi, C.B., Moore, R.S. and Yerger, V.B. (2015). Smoking cessation among transit workers: beliefs and perceptions among an at-risk occupational group. *Substance Abuse Treatment, Prevention, and Policy*, **10**(1): 19.

Baucom, D.H. and Aiken, P.A. (1981) Effect of depressed mood on eating among obese and non-obese dieting and nondieting persons, *Journal of Personality and Social Psychology*, **41**: 577–85.

Baum, A., Fisher, J.D. and Solomon, S. (1981) Type of information, familiarity and the reduction of crowding stress, *Journal of Personality and Social Psychology*, **40**: 11–23.

Bavik, Y.L., Shaw, J.D. and Wang, X.H. (2020) Social support: multidisciplinary review, synthesis, and future agenda, *Academy of Management Annals*, **14**(2): 726–58.

Bayram, C., Britt, H., Kelly, Z. and Valenti, L. (2003) *Male Consultations in General Practice in Australia 1999–00: General Practice Series No. 11*. Canberra: Australian Institute of Health and Welfare.

BBC News (2020) https://www.bbc.co.uk/news/52311014

BBC News (2020) https://www.bbc.co.uk/news/health-61327778

BBC News (2022) https://www.bbc.co.uk/news/world-61235105

Becerra-Culqui, T.A., Liu, Y., Nash, R. et al. (2018) Mental health of transgender and gender nonconforming youth compared with their peers, *Pediatrics*, **141**(5): e20173845.

Beck, A.T., Mendelson, M., Mock, J. et al. (1961) Inventory for measuring depression, *Archives of General Psychiatry*, **4**: 561–71.

Beck, F., Gillison, F. and Standage, M. (2010) A theoretical investigation of the development of physical activity habits in retirement, *British Journal of Health Psychology*, **15**(3): 663–79.

Beck, K.H. and Lund, A.K. (1981) The effects of health threat seriousness and personal efficacy upon intentions and behaviour, *Journal of Applied Social Psychology*, **11**: 401–15.

Becker, M.H. (ed.) (1974) The health belief model and personal health behavior, *Health Education Monographs*, **2**:324–508.

Becker, M.H. and Rosenstock, I.M. (1984) Compliance with medical advice, in A. Steptoe and A. Mathews (eds) *Health Care and Human Behaviour*. London: Academic Press.

Becker, M.H. and Rosenstock, I.M. (1987) Comparing social learning theory and the health belief model, in W.B. Ward (ed.) *Advances in Health Education and Promotion*. Greenwich, CT: JAI Press.

Beecher, H.K. (1955) The powerful placebo, *Journal of the American Medical Association*, **159**: 1602–6.

Beecher, H.K. (1956) Relationship of significance of wound to the pain experienced, *Journal of the American Medical Association*, **161**: 1609–13.

Belar, C.D. and Deardorff, W.W. (1995) *Clinical Health Psychology in Medical Settings: A Practitioner's Guidebook*. Hyattsville, MD: APA.

Bell, N.S., Amoroso, P.J., Yore, M.M. et al. (2000) Self-reported risk-taking behaviors and hospitalization for motor vehicle injury among active duty army personnel, *American Journal of Preventive Medicine*, **18**(Suppl. 3): 85–95.

Bellack, A.S. and DiClemente, C.C. (1999) Treating substance abuse among patients with schizophrenia. *Psychiatric Services*, **50**(1): 75–80.

Bellisle, F. and Dalix, A. (2001) Cognitive restraint can be offset by distraction, leading to meal intake in women. *American Journal of Clinical Nutrition*, **74**: 197–200.

Bellissimo, N., Pencharz, P.B., Thomas, S.G. and Anderson, G.H. (2007) Effect of television viewing at mealtime on food intake after a glucose preload in boys. *Pediatric Research*, **61**(6): 745–9.

Belloc, N.B. and Breslow, L. (1972) Relationship of physical health status and health practices, *Preventative Medicine*, **1**: 409–21.

Beltz, A.M., Loviska, A.M. and Kelly, D. (2019) No personality differences between oral contraceptive users and naturally cycling women: implications for research on sex hormones, *Psychoneuroendocrinology*, **100**: 127–30.

Bendtsen, M., McCambridge, J., Åsberg, K. and Bendtsen, P. (2021) Text messaging interventions for reducing alcohol consumption among risky drinkers: systematic review and meta-analysis, *Addiction*, **116**(5): 1021–33.

Bennebroek Evertsz, F., Sprangers, M.A., Sitnikova, K. et al. (2017) Effectiveness of cognitive–behavioral therapy on quality of life, anxiety, and depressive symptoms among patients with inflammatory bowel disease: a multicenter randomized controlled trial, *Journal of Consulting and Clinical Psychology*, **85**(9): 918–25.

Bennett, G., Young, E., Butler, I. and Coe, S. (2021) The impact of lockdown during the COVID-19 outbreak on dietary habits in various population groups: a scoping review, *Frontiers in Nutrition*, **8**: 1–10.

Bennett, K.K., Smith, A.J., Harry, K.M. et al. (2019) Multilevel factors predicting cardiac rehabilitation attendance and adherence in underserved patients at a safety-net hospital, *Journal of Cardiopulmonary Rehabilitation and Prevention*, **39**(2): 97–04.

Bentley, M.R., Mitchell, N., Sutton, L. and Backhouse, S.H. (2019) Sports nutritionists' perspectives on enablers and barriers to nutritional adherence in high performance sport: A qualitative analysis informed by the COM-B model and theoretical domains framework, *Journal of Sports Sciences*, **37**(18): 2075–85.

Bentley, R, Kavanagh, A. and Smith, A. (2009) Area disadvantage, socioeconomic position and women's contraception use: a multilevel study in the UK, *The Journal of Family Planning and Reproductive Health Care*, **35**(4): 221–6.

Beral, V., Reeves, G. and Banks, E. (2005) Current evidence about the effect of hormone replacement therapy on the incidence of major conditions in postmenopausal women, *BJOG: An International Journal of Obstetrics and Gynaecology*, **112**(6): 692–5.

Berg, C., Lappas, G., Wolk, A. et al. (2009) Eating patterns and portion size associated with obesity in a Swedish population, *Appetite*, **52**(1): 21–6.

Bergner, M., Bobbitt, R.A., Carter, W.B. and Gilson, D. (1981) The sickness impact profile: development and final revision of a health status measure, *Medical Care*, **19**: 787–805.

Berkman, L.F. and Syme, S.L. (1979) Social networks, lost resistance and mortality: a nine year follow up study of Alameda County residents, *American Journal of Epidemiology*, **109**: 186–204.

Berry, D.C., Michas, I.C. and Bersellini, E. (2003) Communicating information about medication: the benefits of making it personal, *Psychology and Health*, **18**(1): 127–39.

Berry, D.C., Michas, I.C., Gillie, T. and Forster, M. (1997) What do patients want to know about their medicines, and what do doctors want to tell them? A comparative study, *Psychology and Health*, **12**: 467–80.

Berry, D.C. (2004) *Risk Communication and Health Psychology*. New York: Open University Press.

Best, E., Lokuge, B., Dunlop, A. and Dunford, A. (2021) Unmet need for postpartum long-acting reversible contraception in women with substance use disorders and/or socioeconomic disadvantage, *Australian and New Zealand Journal of Obstetrics and Gynaecology*, **61**(2): 304–09.

Beta-blocker Heart Attack Trial Research Group (BHAT) (1982) A randomized trial of propranolol in patients with acute myocardial infarction: I–mortality results, *Journal of the American Medical Association*, **247**: 1707–14.

Beutel, M., Deckhardt, R., von Rad, M. and Weiner, H. (1995) Grief and depression after miscarriage: their separation, antecedents and course, *Psychosomatic Medicine*, **57**: 517–26.

Bhaskaran, K., Douglas, I., Forbes, H. et al. (2014) Body-mass index and risk of 22 specific cancers: a population-based cohort study of 5·24 million UK adults, *Lancet*, **384**(9945): 755–65.

Bieliauskas, L.A. (1980) Life stress and aid seeking, *Journal of Human Stress*, **6**: 28–36.

Biello, K.B., Edeza, A., Montgomery, M.C. et al. (2019) Risk perception and interest in HIV pre-exposure prophylaxis among men who have sex with men with rectal gonorrhea and chlamydia infection, *Archives of Sexual Behavior*, **48**(4): 1185–90.

Biesecker, B.B. (2019) The psychological well-being of pregnant women undergoing prenatal testing and screening: a narrative literature review, *Hastings Center Report*, **49**: S53–S60.

Biggs, M.A., Upadhyay, U.D., McCulloch, C.E. and Foster, D.G. (2017) Women's mental health and well-being 5 years after receiving or being denied an abortion: a prospective, longitudinal cohort study, *JAMA Psychiatry*, **74**(2): 169–78.

Binse, Z. (2021) The representation of women who have sex with women (WSW) in sexual health promotion in England: a frame analysis, *The British Student Doctor Journal*, **5**(2): 4–20.

Birch, L.L. and Anzman, S.L. (2010) Learning to eat in an obesogenic environment: a developmental systems perspective on childhood obesity, *Child Development Perspectives*, **4**: 138–43.

Birch, L.L. and Deysher, M. (1986) Caloric compensation and sensory specific satiety: evidence for self-regulation of food intake by young children, *Appetite*, **7**: 323–31.

Birch, L.L. and Fisher, J.O. (2000) Mothers' child-feeding practices influence daughters' eating and weight, *American Journal of Clinical Nutrition*, **71**: 1054–61.

Birch, L.L. and Marlin, D.W. (1982) I don't like it; I never tried it: effects of exposure on two-year-old children's food preferences, *Appetite*, **23**: 353–60.

Birch, L.L., Birch, D., Marlin, D. and Kramer, L. (1982) Effects of instrumental eating on children's food preferences, *Appetite*, **3**: 125–34.

Birch, L.L., Gunder, L., Grimm-Thomas, K. and Laing, D.G. (1998) Infant's consumption of a new food enhances acceptance of similar foods, *Appetite*, **30**: 283–95.

Birch, L.L., McPhee, L., Shoba, B.C. et al. (1987) What kind of exposure reduces children's food neophobia? Looking vs tasting, *Appetite*, **9**: 171–8.

Birch, L.L., Zimmerman, S. and Hind, H. (1980) The influence of social affective context on preschool children's food preferences, *Child Development*, **51**: 856–61.

Birch, L.L. (1980) Effects of peer models' food choices and eating behaviors on preschoolers' food preferences, *Child Development*, **51**: 489–96.

Birch, L.L. (1989) Developmental aspects of eating, in R. Shepherd (ed.) *Handbook of the Psychophysiology of Human Eating*, pp. 179–203. Chichester: Wiley.

Birch, L.L. (1999) Development of food preferences, *Annual Review of Nutrition*, **19**: 41–62.

Bish, A., Sutton, S. and Golombok, S. (2000) Predicting uptake of a routine cervical smear test: a comparison of the health belief model and the theory of planned behaviour, *Psychology and Health*, **15**: 35–50.

Bishop, G.D. and Converse, S.A. (1986) Illness representations: a prototype approach, *Health Psychology*, **5**: 95–114.

Black, N. (2013) Patient reported outcome measures could help transform healthcare, *BMJ (Clinical research ed.)*, **346**: f167. Doi.org/10.1136/bmj.f167.

Black, R.B. (1989) A 1 and 16 month follow up of prenatal diagnosis patients who lost pregnancies, *Prenatal Diagnosis*, **9**: 795–804.

Blackburn, G. (1995). Effect of degree of weight loss on health benefits. *Obesity Reviews*, 3(Supplement 2): 211s–216s.

Blair, S.N., Kampert, J.B., Kohl, H.W. et al. (1996) Influences of cardiorespiratory fitness and other precursors on cardiovascular disease and all-cause mortality in men and women, *Journal of the American Medical Association*, **276**: 205–10.

Blair, S.N., Kohl, H.W., Gordon, N.F. and Paffenbarger, R.S. (1992) How much physical activity is good for health? *Annual Review of Public Health*, **13**: 99–126.

Blair, S.N., Kohl, H.W., Paffenbarger, R.S. et al. (1989) Physical fitness and all-cause mortality: a prospective study of healthy men and women, *Journal of the American Medical Association*, **262**: 2395–401.

Blair, S.N. (1993) Evidence for success of exercise in weight loss and control, *Annals of Internal Medicine*, **199**: 702–6.

Blass, E.M., Anderson, D.R., Kirkorian, H.L. et al. (2006) On the road to obesity: television viewing increases intake of high-density foods. *Physiology and Behaviour*, **88**(4): 597–604.

Blaxter, M. (1990) *Health and Lifestyles*. London: Routledge.

Blok, D.J., de Vlas, S.J., van Empelen, P. and van Lenthe, F.J. (2017) The role of smoking in social networks on smoking cessation and relapse among adults: a longitudinal study. *Preventive Medicine*, **99**: 105–10.

Bloom, J.R. (1983) Social support, accommodation to stress and adjustment to breast cancer, *Social Science and Medicine*, **16**: 1329–38.

Blundell, J. and Macdiarmid, J. (1997) Fat as a risk factor for over-consumption: satiation, satiety and patterns of eating, *Journal of the American Dietetic Association*, **97**: S63–9.

Bluvstein, I., Moravchick, L., Sheps, D. et al. (2013) Posttraumatic growth, posttraumatic stress symptoms and mental health among coronary heart disease survivors, *Journal of Clinical Psychology in Medical Settings*, **20**(2): 164–72.

Bocchieri, L.E., Meana, M. and Fisher, B.L. (2002) A review of psychosocial outcomes of surgery for morbid obesity, *Journal of Psychosomatic Research*, **52**: 155–65.

Boersma, S.N., Maes, S. and Elderen, T. (2005) Goal disturbance predicts health-related quality of life and depression 4 months after myocardial infarction, *British Journal of Health Psychology*, **10**(4): 615–30.

Bolderdijk, J., Steg, L., Geller, E. et al. Comparing the effectiveness of monetary versus moral motives in environmental campaigning. *Nature Clim Change* **3**, 413–416 (2013). https://doi.org/10.1038/nclimate1767

Boldero, J., Moore, S. and Rosenthal, D. (1992) Intention, context, and safe sex: Australian adolescents' responses to AIDS, *Journal of Applied Social Psychology*, **22**: 1374–98.

Bolton-Smith, C. and Woodward, M. (1994) Dietary composition and fat to sugar ratios in relation to obesity, *International Journal of Obesity*, **18**: 820–8.

Bommelé, J., Hopman, P., Walters, B.H. et al. (2020) The double-edged relationship between COVID-19 stress and smoking: implications for smoking cessation, *Tobacco Induced Diseases*, **18**: 63.

Bond, D.S., Thomas, J.G., King, W.C. et al. (2015) Exercise improves quality of life in bariatric surgery candidates: results from the Bari-Active trial, *Obesity*, **23**(3): 536–42.

Bonetti, D. and Johnston, M. (2008) Perceived control predicting the recovery of individual-specific walking behaviours following stroke: testing psychological models and constructs, *British Journal of Health Psychology*, **13**(3): 463–78.

Boon, B., Stroebe, W., Schut, H. and Ijntema, R. (2002) Ironic processes in eating behaviour of restrained eaters, *British Journal of Health Psychology*, **7**: 1–10.

Boon, B., Stroebe, W., Schut, H. and Ijntema, R. (2002) Ironic processes in the eating behaviour of restrained eaters. *British Journal of Health Psychology*, **7**(1): 1–10.

Boreham, C.A., Wallace, W.F. and Nevill, A. (2000) Training effects of accumulated daily stairclimbing exercise in previously sedentary young women, *Preventive Medicine*, **30**: 277–81.

Borg, S. and Lasker, J. (1982) *When Pregnancy Fails: Coping with Miscarriage, Stillbirth and Infant Death*. London: Routledge & Kegan Paul.

Borland, R., Owens, N., Hill, D. and Chapman, S. (1990) Changes in acceptance of workplace smoking bans following their implementation: a prospective study, *Preventative Medicine*, **19**: 314–22.

Borrayo, E. and Jenkins, S. (2001) Feeling indecent: breast cancer-screening resistance of Mexican descent women, *Journal of Health Psychology*, **6**(5): 537–49.

Bortner, R.W. (1969) A short rating scale as a potential measure of pattern A behaviour, *Journal of Chronic Disease*, **22**: 87–91.

Bosgraaf, R.P., Ketelaars, P.W., Verhoef, V.J. et al. (2014) Reasons for non-attendance to cervical screening and preferences for HPV self-sampling in Dutch women, *Preventive Medicine: An International Journal Devoted to Practice and Theory*, **64**: 108–13.

Bosworth, H.B., Siegler, I.C., Olsen, M.K. et al. (2001) Social support and quality of life in patients with coronary heart disease, *Quality of Life Research*, **9**: 829–39.

Boulton, M., Schramm Evans, Z., Fitzpatrick, R. and Hart, G. (1991) Bisexual men: women, safer sex, and HIV infection, in P. Aggleton, P.M. Davies and G. Hart (eds) *AIDS: Responses, Policy and Care*. London: Falmer Press.

Bowen, S., Witkiewitz, K., Clifasefi, S.L. et al. (2014) Relative efficacy of mindfulness-based relapse prevention, standard relapse prevention, and treatment as usual for substance use disorders: a randomized clinical trial. *JAMA Psychiatry*, 71(5): 547–56.

Bower, J.E., Kemeny, M.E., Taylor, S.E. et al. (1998) Cognitive processing, discovery of meaning, CD 4 decline, and AIDS-related mortality among bereaved HIV seropositive men, *Journal of Consulting and Clinical Psychology*, **66**: 979–86.

Bowlby, J. (1973) *Attachment and Loss: Vol. II. Separation: Anxiety and Anger*. New York: Basic Books.

Boyce, W.T., Alkon, A., Tschann, J.M. et al. (1995) Dimensions of psychobiologic reactivity: cardiovascular responses to laboratory stressors in preschool children, *Annals of Behavioural Medicine*, **17**: 315–23.

Boyd, C.J., Veliz, P.T., Stephenson, R. et al. (2019) Severity of alcohol, tobacco, and drug use disorders among sexual minority individuals and their "not sure" counterparts, *LGBT Health*, **6**(1): 15–22.

Boyle, C.M. (1970) Differences between patients' and doctors' interpretations of common medical terms, *British Medical Journal*, **2**: 286–9.

Bränström, R., Hatzenbuehler, M. L. and Pachankis, J. E. (2016) Sexual orientation disparities in physical health: age and gender effects in a population-based study, *Social Psychiatry and Psychiatric Epidemiology*, **51**(2), 289–301.

Bradley, C., Todd, C., Symonds, E. et al. (1999) The development of an individualized questionnaire measure of perceived impact of diabetes on quality of life: the ADDQoL, *Quality of Life Research*, **8:** 79–91.

Bradley, C. (1997) Design of renal-dependent individualized quality of life questionnaire, *Advances in Peritoneal Dialysis*, **13**: 116–20.

Bradley, C. (2001) Importance of differentiating health status from quality of life, *Lancet*, **357**(9249): 7–8.

Bradt, J., Dileo, C. and Shim, M. (2013) Music interventions for pre-operative anxiety, *Cochrane Database of Systematic Reviews*, **6.**

Bray, G.A. and Bouchard, C. (2020) The biology of human overfeeding: a systematic review, *Obesity Reviews*, **21**(9): e13040.

Brechbiel, J.K. and Keeley, J.W. (2019) Pathways linking clinician demographics to mental health diagnostic accuracy: an international perspective, *Journal of Clinical Psychology*, **75**(9): 1715–29.

Breslow, L. and Enstrom, J. (1980) Persistence of health habits and their relationship to mortality, *Preventive Medicine*, **9**: 469–83.

Breuer, J. and Freud, S. (1890) *Studies in Hysteria*. Neural Central blatt, Nos 1 and 3. See also: **Halligan, P., Bass, C. and Marshall, J.** (eds) (2001) *Hysterical Conversion: Clinical and Theoretical Perspectives*. Oxford: Oxford University Press.

Brewer, N.T., Chapman, G.B., Brownlee, S. and Leventhal, E.A. (2002) Cholesterol control, medication adherence and illness cognition, *British Journal of Health Psychology*, **7**: 433–47.

Brickell, T.A., Chatzisarantis, N.L. and Pretty, G.M. (2006) Using past behaviour and spontaneous implementation intentions to enhance the utility of the theory of planned behaviour in predicting exercise, *British Journal of Health Psychology*, **11**(2): 249–62.

Broadbent, E., Ellis, C.J., Thomas, J. et al. (2009) Can an illness perception intervention reduce illness anxiety in spouses on myocardial infarction patients? A randomised controlled trial, *Journal of Psychosomatic Research*, **67**: 17–23.

Broadbent, E., Petrie, K.J., Ellis, C.J. et al. (2004) A picture of health–myocardial infarction patients' drawings of their hearts and subsequent disability: a longitudinal study, *Journal of Psychosomatic Research*, **57**(6): 583–7.

Broadbent, E., Petrie, K.J., Main, J. and Weinman, J. (2006) The brief illness perception questionnaire, *Journal of Psychosomatic Research*, **60**(6): 631–7.

Broadbent, E., Wilkes, C., Koschwanez, H. et al. (2015) A systematic review and meta-analysis of the Brief Illness Perception Questionnaire, *Psychology and Health*, **30**(11): 1361–85.

Broadstock, M., Michie, S. and Marteau, T.M. (2000) Psychological consequences of predictive genetic testing: a systematic review, *European Journal of Human Genetics*, **8**: 731–8.

Brodie, D.A., Slade, P.D. and Rose, H. (1989) Reliability measures in disturbing body image, *Perceptual and Motor Skills,* **69:** 723–32.

Brody, L.R. (1999) *Gender, Emotion, and the Family.* Cambridge, MA: Harvard University Press.

Broom, A. (2004) Prostate cancer and masculinity in Australian society: a case of stolen identity? *International Journal of Men's health,* **3:** 73–91.

Broom, A. (2010) Prostate cancer and masculinities in Australia, in B. Gough and S. Robertson (eds) *Men, Masculinities and Health: Critical Perspectives.* Easingstoke: Palgrave Macmillan.

Broom, A. (2010) Prostate cancer and masculinities in Australia, in B. Gough., and S. Robertson (eds) *Men, Masculinities and Health: Critical Perspectives.* Easingstoke: Palgrave Macmillan.

Broquet, K. (1999) Psychological reactions to pregnancy loss, *Primary Care Update for Obstetrics and Gynecology,* **6:** 12–16.

Brosschot, J.F. and Van der Doef, M.P. (2006) Daily worrying and somatic health complaints: testing the effectiveness of a simple worry reduction intervention, *Psychology and Health,* **21:** 19–31.

Brotherstone, E. Miles, A.K.A., Atkin, W. and Wardle, J. (2005) The impact of illustrations on public understanding of the aim of cancer screening, *Patient Education and Counseling,* **63:** 328–35.

Brown, K., Ogden, J., Gibson, L. and Vogele, C. (2008) The role of parental control practices in explaining children's diet and BMI, *Appetite,* **50:** 252–9.

Brown, K.E., Kwah, K., Alhassan, Y. and Barrett, H. (2015) REPLACE 2: an application of a community-based behaviour change intervention framework to tackle female genital mutilation (FGM) in the EU. Paper presented at BASPCAN, 12–15 April, Edinburgh.

Brown, R. and Ogden, J. (2004) Children's eating attitudes and behaviour: a study of the modelling and control theories of parental influence, *Health Education and Research,* **19**(3): 261–71.

Brown, S.L., McRae, D., Sheils, E. et al. (2021) The effect of visual interventions on illness beliefs and medication adherence for chronic conditions: a scoping review of the literature and mapping to behaviour change techniques (BCTs), *Research in Social and Administrative Pharmacy,* **18**(8): 3239–32. Doi: 10.1016/j.sapharm.2021.11.006.

Brown, T. J., Hardeman, W., Bauld, L., Holland, R., Maskrey, V., Naughton, F., Notley, C. et al. (2019) A systematic review of behaviour change techniques within interventions to prevent return to smoking postpartum. *Addictive Behaviors,* **92:** 236–43.

Brown, T.A., Cash, T.F. and Mikulka, P.J. (1990) Attitudinal body-image assessment: factor analysis of the body self relations questionnaire, *Journal of Personality Assessment,* **55:** 135–44.

Browne, J.P., McGee, H.M. and O'Boyle, C.A. (1997) Conceptual approaches to the assessment of quality of life, *Psychology and Health,* **12:** 737–51.

Brownell, K.D., Marlatt, G.A., Lichtenstein, E. and Wilson, G.T. (1986b) Understanding and preventing relapse, *American Psychologist,* **41:** 765–82.

Brownell, K.D. (1989) Weight control and your health, in *World Book Encyclopedia.* Chicago: World Book.

Bru Garcia, S., Chałupnik, M., Irving, K. and Haselgrove, M. (2022) Increasing condom use and STI testing: creating a behaviourally informed sexual healthcare campaign using the COM-B model of behaviour change, *Behavioral Sciences,* **12**(4): 108.

Bruch, H. (1974) *Eating Disorders: Obesity, Anorexia and the Person Within.* New York: Basic Books.

Brunger, H. and Ogden, J. (2013) Adjusting to persistent post concussive symptoms following mild traumatic brain injury and subsequent psycho educational intervention: a qualitative analysis in military personnel, *Brain Injury,* **28:** 71–80.

Brunger, H., Ogden, J., Malia, et al. (2014) Adjusting to persistent post-concussive symptoms following mild traumatic brain injury and subsequent psycho-educational intervention: a qualitative analysis in military personnel, *Brain injury,* **28**(1): 71–80. Doi.org/10.3109/02699052.2013.857788

Brunger, H., Ogden, J., Malia, K. et al. (2014) Adjusting to persistent post-concussive symptoms following mild traumatic brain injury and subsequent psycho-educational intervention: a qualitative analysis in military personnel, *Brain injury,* **28**(1): 71–80. Doi.org/10.3109/02699052.2013.857788.

Bryant, K.D. (2009) Contraceptive use and attitudes among female college students, *The ABNF Journal: Official Journal of the Association of Black Nursing Faculty in Higher Education Inc.,* **20**(1): 12–16.

Buchi, S.T., Villiger, B., Sensky, T. et al. (1997) Psychosocial predictors of long term success in patient pulmonary rehabilitation of patients with COPD, *European Respiratory Journal,* **10:** 1272–7.

Buchmueller, T. and Carpenter, C. S. (2010) Disparities in health insurance coverage, access, and outcomes for individuals in same-sex versus different-sex relationships, 2000–2007, *American Journal of Public Health,* **100**(3), 489–95.

Buckelew, S.P., Baumstark, K.E., Frank, R.G., et al. (1990) Adjustment following spinal cord injury, *Rehabilitation Psychology,* **35**(2): 100–109.

Buckley, J.P., Hedge, A., Yates, T. et al. (2015) The sedentary office: an expert statement on the growing case for change towards better health and productivity, *British Journal of Sports Medicine,* **49**(21): 1357–62. doi: 10.1136/bjsports-2015-094618.

Bucknall, C.A., Morris, G.K. and Mitchell, J.R.A. (1986) Physicians' attitudes to four common problems: hypertension, atrial fibrillation, transient ischaemic attacks, and angina pectoris, *British Medical Journal*, **293**: 739–42.

Bui, L., Mullan, B. and McCaffery, K. (2013) Protection motivation theory and physical activity in the general population: a systematic literature review. *Psychology, Health and Medicine*, **18**(5): 522–42.

Bullen, B.A., Reed, R.B. and Mayer, J. (1964) Physical activity of obese and non-obese adolescent girls appraised by motion picture sampling, *American Journal of Clinical Nutrition*, **4**: 211–33.

Bundy, C., Carroll, D., Wallace, L. and Nagle, R. (1998) Stress management and exercise training in chronic stable angina pectoris, *Psychology and Health*, **13**: 147–55.

Bungener, S., de Vries, A.L., Popma, A. and Steensma, T.D. (2020) Sexual experiences of young transgender persons during and after gender-affirmative treatment, *Pediatrics*, **146**(6): e20191411.

Bunten, A., Porter, L., Gold, N. and Bogle, V. (2020) A systematic review of factors influencing NHS health check uptake: invitation methods, patient characteristics, and the impact of interventions. *BMC Public Health*, **20**(1): 1–16.

Burg, M.M., Schwartz, J.E., Kronish, I.M. et al. (2017) Does stress result in you exercising less? Or does exercising result in you being less stressed? Or is it both? Testing the bi-directional stress-exercise association at the group and person (N of 1) level. *Annals of Behavioral Medicine*, **51**(6): 799–809.

Burg, M.M., Schwartz, J.E., Kronish, I.M. et al. (2017) Does stress result in you exercising less? Or does exercising result in you being less stressed? Or is it both? Testing the bi-directional stress-exercise association at the group and person (N of 1) level, *Annals of Behavioral Medicine*, **51**(6): 799–809.

Burgmer, R., Legenbauer, T., Müller, A. et al. (2014) Psychological outcome 4 years after restrictive bariatric surgery, *Obesity Surgery*, **24**(10): 1670–8.

Burish, T.G., Carey, M.P., Krozely, M.G. and Greco, F.F. (1987) Conditioned side-effects induced by cancer chemotherapy: prevention through behavioral treatment, *Journal of Consulting and Clinical Psychology*, **55**: 42–8.

Burnett, J. (1989) *Plenty and Want: A Social History of Food in England from 1815 to the Present Day*, 3rd edn. London: Routledge.

Bury, M. (1982) Chronic illness as biographical disruption, *Sociology of Health and Illness*, **4**: 167–82.

Busetto, L., Dicker, D., Azran, C. et al. (2018) Obesity Management Task Force of the European Association for the Study of Obesity Released 'Practical Recommendations for the Post-Bariatric Surgery Medical Management', *Obesity Surgery*, **28**(7): 2117–21.

Busick, D.B., Brooks, J., Pernecky, S. et al. (2008) Parent food purchases as a measure of exposure and preschool-aged children's willingness to identify and taste fruit and vegetables, *Appetite*, **51**: 468–73.

Butler, C. and Llanedeyrn, M. (1996) Late psychological sequelae of abortion: questions from a primary care perspective, *The Journal of Family Practice*, **43**: 396–401.

Buunk, B.P., Zurriaga, R. and Gonzalez P. (2006) Social comparison, coping and depression in people with spinal cord injury, *Psychology & Health*, **21**(6): 791–807.

Byrne, D., Kazwinski, C., DeNinno, J.A. and Fisher, W.A. (1977) Negative sexual attitudes and contraception, in D. Byrne and L.A. Byrne (eds) *Exploring Human Sexuality*. New York: Crowell.

Byrne, G.J.A., Raphael, B. and Arnold, E. (1999) Alcohol consumption and psychological distress in recently widowed older men, *Australian and New Zealand Journal of Psychiatry*, **33**: 740–7.

Byrne, P.S. and Long, B.E.L. (1976) *Doctor Talking to Patient*. London: HMSO.

Byrne, S., Greiner Safi, A., Kemp, D. et al. (2019) Effects of varying color, imagery, and text of cigarette package warning labels among socioeconomically disadvantaged middle school youth and adult smokers, *Health Communication*, **34**(3): 306–16.

Caceres, B.A., Streed Jr, C.G., Corliss, H.L., Lloyd-Jones, D.M., Matthews, P.A., Mukherjee, M., et al.; American Heart Association Council on Cardiovascular and Stroke Nursing; Council on Hypertension; Council on Lifestyle and Cardiometabolic Health; Council on Peripheral Vascular Disease; and Stroke Council (2020) Assessing and addressing cardiovascular health in LGBTQ adults: a scientific statement from the American Heart Association. *Circulation*, *142*(19), e321–e332.

Cadmus-Bertram, L.A., Marcus, B.H., Patterson, R.E. et al. (2015) Randomized trial of a fitbit-based physical activity intervention for women. *American Journal of Preventive Medicine*, **49**(3): 414–18.

Cagnacci, A. and Venier, M. (2019) The controversial history of hormone replacement therapy, *Medicina*, **55**(9): 602.

Calhoun, L.M., Mirzoyants, A., Thuku, S. et al. (2022) Perceptions of peer contraceptive use and its influence on contraceptive method use and choice among young women and men in Kenya: a quantitative cross-sectional study, *Reproductive Health*, **19**(1): 1–12.

Calnan, M. (1987) *Health and Illness: The Lay Perspective*. London: Tavistock.

Cameron, L.D. and Chan, C.K.Y. (2008) Designing health communications: harnessing the power of affect, imagery, and self-regulation, *Social and Personality Psychology Compass*, **2**(1): 262–82.

Cameron, L.D. (2008) Illness risk representations and motivations to engage in protective behavior: the case of skin cancer risk, *Psychology and Health*, **23**(1): 91–112.

Cameron, L.D. (2009) Can our health behaviour models handle imagery-based processes and communications? *The European Health Psychologist*, Keynote Article 1.

Campbell, C. and Murray, M. (2004) Community health psychology: promoting analysis and action for social change, *Journal of health psychology*, **9**(2): 187–195. https://doi.org/10.1177/1359105304040886

Campbell, R., Colhoun, H.M., Scottish Diabetes Research Network Epidemiology Group et al. (2020) Socio-economic status and mortality in people with type 1 diabetes in Scotland 2006–2015: a retrospective cohort study, *Diabetic medicine: a journal of the British Diabetic Association*, **37**(12): 2081–2088. Doi.org/10.1111/dme.14239.

Campbell, R., Colhoun, Scottish Diabetes Research Network Epidemiology Group et al. (2020) Socio-economic status and mortality in people with type 1 diabetes in Scotland 2006–2015: a retrospective cohort study, *Diabetic medicine: A Journal of the British Diabetic Association*, **37**(12): 2081–88. Doi.org/10.1111/dme.14239.

Cancer Research Campaign (1991) *Smoking Policy and Prevalence Among 16–19 Year Olds*. London: HMSO.

Cancer Research UK (2011) Lung cancer incidence statistics, https://www.cancerresearchuk.org/health-professional/cancer-statistics/statistics-by-cancer-type/lung-cancer/incidence

Cancer Research UK (2006) UK prostate cancer incidence statistics, info.cancerresearchuk.org.8000/cancerstats/types/prostate/incidence/.

Cancer Research UK (2015) *Cancer Incidence for Common Cancers*. https://www.cancerresearchuk.org/health-professional/cancer-statistics/incidence/common-cancers-compared#heading-Zero

Cancer Research UK (2016) Prostate cancer statistics. https://www.cancerresearchuk.org/health-professional/cancer-statistics/statistics-by-cancer-type/prostate-cancer (accessed November 2018)

Cancer Research UK (2022) https://www.cancerresearchuk.org/health-professional/cancer-statistics/statistics-by-cancer-type/lung-cancer/incidence#Leading-Five

Cane, J., O'Connor, D. and Michie, S. (2012) Validation of the theoretical domains framework for use in behaviour change and implementation research, *Implementation Science*, **7**: 37.

Canetto, S.S. (1997) Meanings of gender and suicidal behavior among adolescents, *Suicide and Life-Threatening Behavior*, **27**: 339–51.

Cannon, W.B. (1932) *The Wisdom of the Body*. New York: Norton.

Caponnetto, P., DiPiazza, J., Aiello, M.R. and Polosa, R. (2017) Training pharmacists in the stage-of-change model of smoking cessation and motivational interviewing: a randomized controlled trial. *Health Psychology Open*, **4**(2). Doi: 10.1177/2055102917736429.

Caponnetto, P., DiPiazza, J., Aiello, M.R. and Polosa, R. (2017) Training pharmacists in the stage-of-change model of smoking cessation and motivational interviewing: a randomized controlled trial. *Health Psychology Open*, **4**(2), doi: 10.1177/2055102917736429.

Cappell, H. and Greeley, J. (1987) Alcohol and tension reduction: an update on research and theory, in H.T. Blane and K.E. Leonard (eds) *Psychological Theories of Drinking and Alcoholism*. New York: Guilford Press.

Cappuccio, F.P., Cooper, D., D'Elia, L. et al. (2011) Sleep duration predicts cardiovascular outcomes: a systematic review and meta-analysis of prospective studies, *European Heart Journal*, advance online publication. 0195–668x.

Card, K.G., Lachowsky, N.J., Armstrong, H.L. et al. (2018) The additive effects of depressive symptoms and polysubstance use on HIV risk among gay, bisexual, and other men who have sex with men, *Addictive Behaviors*, **82**: 158–65.

Carey, M.P., Kalra, D.L., Carey, K.B. et al. (1993) Stress and unaided smoking cessation: a prospective investigation, *Journal of Consulting and Clinical Psychology*, **61**: 831–8.

Carlisle, A.C.S., John, A.M.H., Fife-Shaw, C. and Lloyd, M. (2005) The self-regulatory model in women with rheumatoid arthritis: relationships between illness representations, coping strategies, and illness outcome, *British Journal of Health Psychology*, **10**: 571–87.

Carmack, M. and Martens, R. (1979) Measuring commitment to running, a survey of runners' attitudes and mental states, *Journal of Sports Psychology*, **1**: 25–42.

Carolan, M. and Wright, R.J. (2017) Miscarriage at advanced maternal age and the search for meaning. *Death Studies*, **41**(3): 144–53.

Carpenter, L.L., Carvalho, J.P., Tyrka, A.R. et al. (2007) Decreased adrenocorticotropic hormone and cortisol responses to stress in healthy adults reporting significant childhood maltreatment, *Biological Psychiatry*, **62**: 1080–87.

Carpenter, L.L., Ross, N.S., Tyrka, A.R. et al. (2009) Dex/CRH test cortisol response in outpatients with major depression and matched healthy controls, *Psychoneuroendocrinology*, **34**: 1208–13.

Carpenter, L.L., Shattuck, T.T., Tyrka, A.R. et al. (2011) Effect of childhood physical abuse on cortisol stress response, *Psychopharmacology* (Berl), **214**: 367–75.

Carrigan, T., Connell., R.W. and Lee, J. (1985) Hard and heavy: toward a new sociology of masculinity, *Theory and Society*, **14**: 551–603.

Carroll, D., Lovallo, W.R. and Phillips, A.C. (2009) Are large physiological reactions to acute psychological stress always bad for health? *Social and Personality Psychology Compass,* **3:** 725–43.

Carson, J.W., Keefe, F.J., Affleck, G. et al. (2006) A comparison of conventional pain coping skills training and pain coping skills training with a maintenance training component: a daily diary analysis of short and long-term treatment effects, *The Journal of Pain,* **7**(9): 615–25.

Carter, L. and Ogden, J. (2021) Evaluating interoceptive crossover between emotional and physical symptoms, *Psychology Health and Medicine,* **26**(8):1013–22. Doi: 10.1080/13548506.2020.1778748.

Cartwright, A., Hockey, L. and Anderson, J.L. (1973) *Life Before Death.* London: Routledge.

Carver, C.S. and Scheier, M.F. (1999) Stress, coping, and self-regulatory processes, in L. A. Pervin and J.P. Oliver (eds) *Handbook of Personality Theory and Research.* New York: Guildford Press.

Casey, R. and Rozin, P. (1989) Changing children's food preferences: parents' opinions, *Appetite,* **12:** 171–82.

Caspersen, C.J., Powell, K.E. and Christenson, G.M. (1985) Physical activity, exercise, and physical fitness: definitions and distinctions for health-related research, *Public Health Reports,* **100:** 126–31.

Castelo, M., Brown, Z., D'Abbondanza, J.A. et al. (2021) Psychological consequences of MRI-based screening among women with strong family histories of breast cancer, *Breast Cancer Research and Treatment,* **189**(2): 497–508.

Catelan, R.F., Saadeh, A., Lobato, M.I.R. et al. (2021) Condom-protected sex and minority stress: Associations with condom negotiation self-efficacy, "Passing" concerns, and experiences with misgendering among transgender men and women in Brazil, *International Journal of Environmental Research and Public Health,* **18**(9): 4850.

Cazacu, I.M., Chavez, A.A.L., Saftoiu, A. and Bhutani, M.S. (2019) Psychological impact of pancreatic cancer screening by EUS or magnetic resonance imaging in high-risk individuals: a systematic review, *Endoscopic Ultrasound,* **8**(1): 17–24.

Çelik, Z. H. and Sevi, O. M. (2020) Effectiveness of cognitive behavioral therapy for smoking cessation: a systematic review, *Current Approaches in Psychiatry,* **12**(1): 54–71.

CDC (2022) https://www.cdc.gov/coronavirus/2019-ncov/science/science-briefs/underlying-evidence-table.html

Center for American Progress (2020) *The State of the LGBTQ Community in 2020: A National Public Study.* https://www.americanprogress.org/article/state-lgbtq-community-2020/#Ca=10

Center for Disease Control (2008) Smoking-attributable mortality, years of potential life lost, and productivity losses United States, 2000–2004, *Morbidity and Mortality Weekly Reports,* **57:** 1226–8.

Centers for Disease Control and Prevention (2020) *Current Contraceptive Status Among Women Aged 15–49: United States, 2017–2019.* https://www.cdc.gov/nchs/products/databriefs/db388.htm

Centers for Disease Control and Protection (2018) *Current Cigarette Smoking Among Adults—United States, 2016.* https://www.cdc.gov/mmwr/volumes/67/wr/mm6702a1.htm

Centers for Disease Control and Protection (2018) *Current Cigarette Smoking Among Adults—United States, 2016.* https://www.cdc.gov/mmwr/volumes/67/wr/mm6702a1.htm

Centers for Disease Control and Protection (2018) *Current Cigarette Smoking Among Adults—United States, 2016.* https://www.cdc.gov/mmwr/volumes/67/wr/mm6702a1.htm

Centers for Disease Control and Protection (2021) *HIV.* https://www.cdc.gov/hiv/basics/statistics.html

Centre for Reproductive Rights https://reproductiverights.org/maps/what-if-roe-fell/

Chadwick, P. and Benelam, B. (2013) Using behaviour change taxonomies to improve service delivery: a workshop with nutritionists and dietitians. *Nutrition Bulletin,* **38**(1): 108–11.

Chalmers, J., Catalan, J., Day, A. and Fairburn, C. (1985) Anorexia nervosa presenting as morbid exercising, *Lancet,* **1:** 286–7.

Champion, V.L. (1990) Breast self-examination in women 35 and older: a prospective study, *Journal of Behavioural Medicine,* **13:** 523–38.

Chan, I.W.S., Lai, J.C.L. and Wong, K.W.N. (2006) Resilience is associated with better recovery in Chinese people diagnosed with coronary heart disease, *Psychology and Health,* **21**(3): 335–49.

Chan, J.M., Rimm, E.B., Colditz, G.A. et al. (1994) Obesity, fat distribution and weight gain as risk factors for clinical diabetes in men, *Diabetes Care,* **17:** 961–9.

Chang, T.H., Chen, Y.C., Chen, W.Y. et al. (2021) Weight gain associated with COVID-19 lockdown in children and adolescents: a systematic review and meta-analysis, *Nutrients,* **13**(10): 3668.

Chang, Y., Kang, H.Y., Lim, D. et al. (2019) Long-term trends in smoking prevalence and its socioeconomic inequalities in Korea, 1992–2016, *International Journal for Equity in Health,* **18**(1): 1–10.

Chanif, C., Petpichetchian, W. and Chongchareon, W. (2013) Does foot massage relieve acute postoperative pain? A literature review, *Nurse Media Journal of Nursing,* **3**(1): 483–97.

Chapman, C.L. and de Castro, J (1990) Running addiction: measurement and associated psychological characteristics, *The Journal of Sports Medicine and Physical Fitness,* **30:** 283–90.

Charles, S.T. and Almeida, D.M. (2006) Daily reports of symptoms and negative affect: not all symptoms are the same, *Psychology and Health*, **21**: 1–17.

Charlton, A. and Blair, V. (1989) Predicting the onset of smoking in boys and girls, *Social Science and Medicine*, **29**: 813–18.

Charlton, A. (1984) Children's opinion about smoking, *Journal of the Royal College of General Practitioners*, **34**: 483–7.

Charmaz, K. (1995) Identity dilemmas of chronically ill men, in D. Sabo and D.F. Gordon (eds) *Men's Health and Illness: Gender, Power and the Body*. Thousand Oaks, CA: Sage.

Chau, J.Y., Grunseit, A.C., Chey, T. et al. (2013) Daily sitting time and all-cause mortality: a meta-analysis. *PLoS One*, **8**(11): e80000. Doi: 10.1371/journal.pone.0080000.

Chen, S.Y., Gibson, S., Katz, M.H. et al. (2002) Continuing increases in sexual risk behavior and sexually transmitted diseases among men who have sex with men: San Francisco, Calif, 1999-2001, USA, *American Journal of Public Health*, **92**(9): 1387–8.

Chepchirchir, A., Jaoko, W. and Nyagol, J. (2018) Risk indicators and effects of hypertension on HIV/AIDS disease progression among patients seen at Kenyatta hospital HIV care center, *AIDS Care*, **30**(5): 544–50.

Cheung YT, Lee AM, Ho SY, Li ET, Lam TH, Fan SY, Yip PS. (2011). Who wants a slimmer body? The relationship between body weight status, education level and body shape dissatisfaction among young adults in Hong Kong. BMC Public Health. Oct 31;11:835. doi: 10.1186/1471-2458-11-835. Adapted from: Stunkard AJ, Sorensen T, Schulsinger F (1983). Use of the Danish adoption register for the study of obesity and thinness. The genetics of neurological and psychiatric disorders. Edited by: Kety S. New York: Raven Press, 115-20.

Chevance, G., Caudroit, J., Henry, T. et al. (2018) Do implicit attitudes toward physical activity and sedentary behavior prospectively predict objective physical activity among persons with obesity? *Journal of Behavioral Medicine*, **41**(1): 31–42.

Chew, H. and Lopez, V. (2021) Global Impact of COVID-19 on weight and weight-related behaviors in the adult population: a scoping review, *International Journal of Environmental Research and Public Health*, **18**(4): 1876. Doi.org/10.3390/ijerph18041876

Childers, J. and Arnold, B. (2019) The inner lives of doctors: physician emotion in the care of the seriously Ill, *The American Journal of Bioethics*, **19**(12): 29–34.

Chow, L.S., Manoogian, E.N.C., Alvear, A. et al. (2020) Time-restricted eating effects on body composition and metabolic measures in humans who are overweight: a feasibility study, *Obesity*, **28**: 860–869. Doi.org/10.1002/oby.22756.

Chowdhuri, R.N., Pinchoff, J., Boyer, C.B. and Ngo, T.D. (2019) Exploring gender and partner communication: theory of planned behavior predictors for condom use among urban youth in Zambia, *International Journal of Gynecology & Obstetrics*, **147**(2): 258–67.

Christakis, N.A. and Fowler, J.H. (2007) The spread of obesity in a large social network over 32 years, *New England Journal of Medicine*, **357**(4): 370–9.

Christianson, H.F., Weis, J.M. and Fouad, N.A. (2013) Cognitive adaptation theory and quality of life in late-stage cancer patients. *Journal of Psychosocial Oncology*, **31**(3): 266–81.

CIA Factbook (2009) Death rates world maps. https://commons.wikimedia.org/wiki/File:Death_rate_world_map_CIA_2009.PNG

Clifton, S., Nardone, A., Field, N. et al. (2016) HIV testing, risk perception, and behaviour in the British population, *AIDS (London, England)*, **30**(6): 943–52.

Cobb, S. and Rose, R. (1973) Hypertension, peptic ulcer and diabetes in air traffic controllers, *Journal of the American Medical Association*, **224**: 489–92.

Cockburn, J., Staples, M., Hurley, S.F. and DeLuise, T. (1994) Psychological consequences of screening mammography, *Journal of Medical Screening*, **1**: 7–12.

Coen, S.P. and Ogles, B.M. (1993) Psychological characteristics of the obligatory runner: a critical examination of the anorexic analogue hypothesis, *Journal of Sport and Exercise Psychology*, **15**: 338–54.

Cohen, F. and Lazarus, R.S. (1979) Coping with the stresses of illness, in G.C. Stone, F. Cohen and N.E. Adler (eds) *Health Psychology: A Handbook*. San Francisco, CA: Jossey-Bass.

Cohen, S., Janicki-Deverts, D., Turner, R.B. and Doyle, W.J. (2015) Does hugging provide stress-buffering social support? A study of susceptibility to upper respiratory infection and illness. *Psychological Science*, **26**(2): 135–47.

Cohen, S., Kamarck, T. and Mermelstein, R. (1983) A global measure of perceived stress, *Journal of Health and Social Behaviour*, **24**: 385–96.

Cohen, S., Tyrell, A.J. and Smith, A.P. (1991) Psychological stress and susceptibility to the common cold, *New England Journal of Medicine*, **325**: 606–12.

Colagiuri, B., Schenk, L.A., Kessler, M.D. et al. (2015) The placebo effect: from concepts to genes, *Neuroscience*, **307**: 171–90.

Cole, B.S., Hopkins, C.M., Tisak, J. et al. (2008) Assessing spiritual growth and spiritual decline following a diagnosis of cancer: reliability and validity of the spiritual transformation scale, *Psycho-Oncology*, **17**: 112–21.

Colella, T.J., Gravely, S., Marzolini, S. et al. (2015) Sex bias in referral of women to outpatient cardiac rehabilitation? A meta-analysis, *European Journal of Preventive Cardiology*, **22**(4): 423–41.

Coleman, L. and Ingham, R. (1998) Attenders at young people's clinics in Southampton: variations in contraceptive use, *British Journal of Family Planning*, **24**: 101–4.

Coleman, P.K., Reardon, D.C., Strahan, T. and Cougle, J.R. (2005) The psychology of abortion: a review and suggestions for future research, *Psychology and Health*, **20**: 237–71.

Collins, D.R., Tompson, A.C., Onakpoya, I.J., Roberts, N., Ward, A.M. and Heneghan, C.J. (2017) Global cardiovascular risk assessment in the primary prevention of cardiovascular disease in adults: systematic review of systematic reviews. *BMJ open*, **7**(3): e013650.

Collins, R.E., Lopez, L.M. and Martheau, T.M. (2011a) Emotional impact of screening: a systematic review and meta-analysis, *BMC Public Health*, **11**: 603.

Collins, R.E., Wright, A.J. and Marteau, T.M. (2011b) Impact of communicating personalized genetic risk information on perceived control over the risk: a systematic review, *Genetics in Medicine*, **13**(4): 273–7.

Collins, R.L., Taylor, S.E. and Skokan, L.A. (1990) A better world or a shattered vision? Changes in life perspective following victimization, *Social Cognition*, **8**: 263–85.

Colloca, L., Klinger, R., Flor, H. and Bingel, U. (2013) Placebo analgesia: psychological and neurobiological mechanisms, *Pain*, **154**: 511–14.

Compas, B.E., Barnez, G.A., Malcarne, V. and Worshame, N. (1991) Perceived control and coping with stress: a developmental perspective, *Journal of Social Issue*, **47**: 23–34.

Conklin, M.P. and O'Connor, B.P. (1995) Beliefs about the foetus as a moderator of post-abortion psychological well-being, *Journal of Social and Clinical Psychology*, **14**: 76–95.

Conner, M. and Armitage, C.J. (1998) Extending the theory of planned behaviour: a review and avenues for further research, *Journal of Applied Social Psychology*, **28**: 1429–64.

Conner, M., Sandberg, T., McMillan, B. and Higgins, A. (2006) Role of anticipated regret, intentions and intention stability in adolescent smoking initiation, *British Journal of Health Psychology*, **11**: 85–101.

Connor, M. and Higgins, A. R. (2010) Long-term effects of implementation intentions on prevention of smoking uptake among adolescents: a cluster randomized controlled trial, *Health Psychology*, **29**(5): 529–38.

Contento, I.R., Basch, C., Shea, S. et al. (1993) Relationship of mothers' food choice criteria to food intake of pre-school children: identification of family subgroups, *Health Education Quarterly*, **20**: 243–59.

Cook, W.W. and Medley, D.M. (1954) Proposed hostility and pharasaic virtue scales for the MMPI, *Journal of Applied Psychology*, **38**: 414–18.

Cools, J., Schotte, D.E. and McNally, R.J. (1992) Emotional arousal and overeating in restrained eaters, *Journal of Abnormal Psychology*, **101**: 348–51.

Cooper, A.F., Jackson, G., Weinman, J. and Horne, R. (2002) Factors associated with cardiac rehabilitation attendance: a systematic review of the literature, *Clinical Rehabilitation*, **16**: 541–52.

Cooper, M.L. (2002) Alcohol use and risky sexual behavior among college students and youth, *Journal of Studies on Alcohol*, **14**(suppl.): 101–17.

Cooper, P.J., Taylor, M.J., Cooper, Z. and Fairburn, C.G. (1987) The development and validation of the body shape questionnaire, *International Journal of Eating Disorders*, **6**: 485–94.

Cooper, V., Buick, D., Horne, R. et al. (2002) Perceptions of HAART among gay men who declined a treatment offer: preliminary results from an interview-based study, *AIDS Care*, **14**: 319–28.

Coopersmith, S. (1967) *The Antecedents of Self-esteem.* San Francisco, CA: WH Freeman.

Corah, W.L. and Boffa, J. (1970) Perceived control, self-observation and responses to aversive stimulation, *Journal of Personality and Social Psychology*, **16**: 1–4.

Corbin, W.R. and Fromme, K. (2002) Alcohol use and serial monogamy as risks for sexually transmitted diseases in young adults, *Health Psychology*, **21**: 229–36.

Cordova, M.J., Cunningham, L.L.C, Carlson, C.R. and Andrykowski, M.A. (2001) Posttraumatic growth following breast cancer: a controlled comparison study, *Health Psychology*, **20**(3): 176–85.

Cornwell, T.B. and McAlister, A.R. (2013) Contingent choice: exploring the relationship between sweetened beverages and vegetable consumption, *Appetite*, **62**: 203–8.

Coulter, A. (1999) Paternalism or partnership? Patients have grown up and there's no going back, *British Medical Journal*, **319**: 719–20.

Courcoulas, A.P., Christian, N.J., Belle, S.H. et al. (2013) Weight change and health outcomes at 3 years after bariatric surgery among individuals with severe obesity, *JAMA*, **310**(22): 2416–25. doi: 10.1001/jama.2013.280928.

Courtenay, W.H., McCreary, D.R. and Merighi, J.R. (2002) Gender and ethnic differences in health beliefs and behaviors, *Journal of Health Psychology*, **7**(3): 219–31.

Courtenay, W.H. (2000a) Engendering health: a social constructionist examination of men's health beliefs and behaviors, *Psychology of Men and Masculinity*, **1**: 4–15.

Courtenay, W.H. (2000b) Behavioral factors associated with disease, injury, and death among men: Evidence and implications for prevention, *The Journal of Men's Studies*, **9**: 81–142.

COVID-19 Excess Mortality Collaborators (2022) Estimating excess mortality due to the COVID-19 pandemic: a systematic analysis of COVID-19-related mortality, 2020–21. *The Lancet*, **399**(10334): 1513–36. Doi.org/10.1016/S0140-6736(21)02796-3.

Cox, K.L., Gorely, T.J., Puddey, I.B. et al. (2003) Exercise behaviour change in 40 to 65-year-old women: the SWEAT study (Sedentary Women Exercise Adherence Trial), *British Journal of Health Psychology*, **8**(4): 477–95.

Crawford, A., Muere, A., Tripp, D.A. et al. (2021) The chicken or the egg: longitudinal changes in pain and catastrophizing in women with interstitial cystitis/bladder pain syndrome, *Canadian Urological Association Journal*, **15**(10): 326–31.

Crichton, E.F., Smith, D.L. and Demanuele, F. (1978) Patients' recall of medication information, *Drug Intelligence and Clinical Pharmacy*, **12**: 591–9.

Crisp, A.H., Hsu, L., Harding, B. and Hartshorn, J. (1980) Clinical features of anorexia: a study of consecutive series of 102 female patients, *Journal of Psychosomatic Research*, **24**: 179–91.

Crombez, G., Bijttebier, P., Eccleston, C. et al. (2003) The child version of the pain catastrophizing scale (PCSC): a preliminary validation, *Pain*, **104**(3): 639–46.

Crombez, G., Eccleston, C., Baeyens, F. and Eelen, F. (1998a) Attentional disruption is enhanced by threat of pain, *Behaviour Research and Therapy*, **36**: 195–204.

Crombez, G., Eccleston, C., Baeyens, F. and Eelen, F. (1998b) When somatic information threatens, catastrophic thinking enhances attentional interference, *Pain*, **75**(2–3): 187–98.

Crombez, G., Eccleston, C., Baeyens, F. et al. (1999) Attention to chronic pain is dependent upon pain-related fear, *Journal of Psychosomatic Research*, **47**(5): 403–10.

Cropley, M. and Steptoe, A. (2005) Social support, life events and physical symptoms: a prospective study of chronic and recent life stress in men and women, *Psychology, Health & Medicine*, **10**(4): 317–25.

Cropley, M., Ayers, S. and Nokes, L. (2003) People don't exercise because they can't think of reasons to exercise: an examination of causal reasoning within the transtheoretical model, *Psychology, Health & Medicine*, **8**(4): 409–14.

Crum, A.J., Corbin, W.R., Brownell, K.D. and Salovey, P. (2011) Mind over milkshakes: mindsets, not just nutrients, determine ghrelin response, *Health Psychology*, **30**: 421–30.

Crush, E.A., Frith, E. and Loprinzi, P.D. (2018) Experimental effects of acute exercise duration and exercise recovery on mood state. *Journal of Affective Disorders*, **229**: 282–7.

Cruwys, T., Bevelander, K.E. and Hermans, R.C. (2015) Social modelling of eating: a review of when and why social influence affects food intake and choice, *Appetite*, **86**: 3–18.

Cvetkovich, G. and Grote, B. (1981) Psychosocial maturity and teenage contraceptive use: an investigation of decision-making and communication skills, *Population and Environment*, **4**: 211–26.

Czajkowska, Z., Radiotis, G., Roberts, N. and Körner, A. (2013) Cognitive adaptation to nonmelanoma skin cancer, *Journal of Psychosocial Oncology*, **31**(4): 377–92.

DAFNE Study Group (2002) Training in flexible, intensive insulin management to enable dietary freedom in people with type I diabetes: dose adjustment for normal eating (DAFNE) randomised controlled trial, *British Medical Journal*, **325**: 1–6.

Dalili, Z. and Bayazi, M.H. (2019) The effectiveness of mindfulness-based cognitive therapy on the illness perception and psychological symptoms in patients with rheumatoid arthritis, *Complementary Therapies in Clinical Practice*, **34**: 139–44.

Damron, K.R. (2017) Review of the relationships among psychosocial stress, secondhand smoke, and perinatal smoking, *Journal of Obstetric, Gynecologic & Neonatal Nursing*, **46**(3): 325–33.

Daniel, J.Z., Cropley, M. and Fife-Schaw, C. (2006) The effect of exercise in reducing desire to smoke and cigarette withdrawal symptoms is not caused by distraction, *Addiction*, **101**(8): 1187–92.

Darker, C.D. and French, D.P. (2009) What sense do people make of a theory of planned behaviour questionnaire? A think-aloud study, *Journal of Health Psychology*, **14**(7): 861–71.

Darling, K.E., Fahrenkamp, A.J., Wilson, S.M. et al. (2017) Does social support buffer the association between stress eating and weight gain during the transition to college? Differences by gender, *Behavior Modification*, **41**(3): 368–81.

Dauenhauer, B., Keating, X. and Lambdin, D. (2016) Effects of a three-tiered intervention model on physical activity and fitness levels of elementary school children. *Journal of Primary Prevention*, **37**(4): 313–27.

David, L., Bolba, A.R., Chiaroni, G. et al. (2021) Coping strategies and Irritable Bowel Syndrome: a systematic review, *Journal of Gastrointestinal and Liver Diseases*, **30**(4): 485–94.

Davies, D.L. (1962) Normal drinking in recovered alcohol addicts, *Quarterly Journal of Studies on Alcohol*, **23**: 94–104.

Davies, M.J., Heller, S., Skinner, T.C. et al. (2009) Effectiveness of the diabetes education and self-management for ongoing and newly diagnosed (DESMOND) programme for people with newly diagnosed type 2 diabetes, cluster randomised controlled trial, *British Medical Journal*, **336**: 491–5.

Davis, C. (1928) Self-selection of diets by newly weaned infants, *American Journal of Disease of Children*, **36**: 651–79.

Davis, R., Campbell, R., Hildon, Z. et al. (2015) Theories of behaviour and behaviour change across the social and behavioural sciences: a scoping review. *Health Psychology Review,* **9**(3): 323–44.

Dazeley, P. and Houston-Price, C. (2015) Exposure to foods' non-taste sensory properties: a nursery intervention to increase children's willingness to try fruit and vegetables. *Appetite,* **84**: 1–6.

de Almeida-Pititto, B., Dualib, P.M., Zajdenverg, L. et al. (2020) Severity and mortality of COVID-19 in patients with diabetes, hypertension and cardiovascular disease: a meta-analysis, *Diabetology and Metabolic Syndrome,* **12**: 75. Doi.org/10.1186/s13098-020-00586-4.

de Ridder, D., Geenen, R., Kuijer, R. and van Middendorp, H. (2008) Psychological adjustment to chronic disease, *The Lancet,* **372**(9634): 246–55.

de Ridder, D.T.D. and Schreurs, K.M.G. (2001) Developing interventions for chronically ill patients: Is coping a helpful concept? *Clinical Psychology Review,* **21**: 205–40.

De Ridder, D.T.D. (1997) What is wrong with coping assessment? A review of conceptual and methodological issues, *Psychology and Health,* **12**: 417–31.

De Zwann, M., Lancaster, K.L., Mitchell, J.E. et al. (2002) Health related quality of life in morbidly obese patients: effect of gastric bypass surgery, *Obesity Surgery,* **12**: 773–80.

Dean, C., Roberts, M.M., French, K. and Robinson, S. (1984) Psychiatric morbidity after screening for breast cancer, *Journal of Epidemiology and Community Health,* **40**: 71–5.

Dean, C. (1987) Psychiatric morbidity following mastectomy: preoperative predictors and types of illness, *Journal of Psychosomatic Research,* **31**: 385–92.

Deary, V. (2008) A precarious balance: Using a self-regulation model to conceptualize and treat chronic fatigue syndrome, *British Journal of Health Psychology,* **13**(2): 231–6.

Debro, S.C., Campbell, S.M. and Peplau, L.A. (1994) Influencing a partner to use a condom: characteristics of the situation are more important than characteristics of the individual, *Psychology, Health and Medicine,* **4**: 265–79.

Deci, E.L. and Ryan, R.M. (1985) *Intrinsic Motivation and Self-determination in Human Behavior.* New York: Plenum.

Deci, E.L. and Ryan, R.M. (2000) The 'what' and 'why' of goal pursuits: human needs and the self-determination of behavior, *Psychological Inquiry: An International Journal for the Advancement of Psychological Theory,* **11**(4): 227–68.

Decker, A.M., Kapila, Y.L. and Wang, H.L. (2021) The psychobiological links between chronic stress-related diseases, periodontal/peri-implant diseases, and wound healing, *Periodontology 2000,* **87**(1), 94–106.

deHaes, J.C.J.M., van Knippenberg, F.C. and Neigt, J.P. (1990) Measuring psychological and physical distress in cancer patients: structure and application of the Rotterdam symptom checklist, *British Journal of Cancer,* **62**: 1034–8.

Dehingia, N., Barker, K.M. and Raj, A. (2022) Relationship between adolescent friendship networks and contraceptive use and unintended pregnancies in early adulthood in the United States, *Contraception,* **110**: 36–41.

Dekker, F.W., Kaptein, A.A., van der Waart, M.A.C. and Gill, K. (1992) Quality of self-care of patients with asthma, *Journal of Asthma,* **29**: 203–8.

Deliens, T., Deforche, B., De Bourdeaudhuij, I. and Clarys, P. (2015) Determinants of physical activity and sedentary behaviour in university students: a qualitative study using focus group discussions, *BMC Public Health,* **15**(1): 201.

DeMaria, A.L., Sundstrom, B., Faria, A.A. et al. (2019) Using the theory of planned behavior and self-identity to explore women's decision-making and intention to switch from combined oral contraceptive pill (COC) to long-acting reversible contraceptive (LARC), *BMC Women's Health,* **19**(1): 1–10.

Demirbas, N., Kutlu, R. and Kurnaz, A. (2021) The relationship between mindful eating and body mass index and body compositions in adults, *Annals of Nutrition and Metabolism,* **77**(5): 262–70.

Dempster, M., Carney, R. and McClements, R. (2010) Response shift in the assessment of quality of life among people attending cardiac rehabilitation, *British Journal of Health Psychology,* **15**: 307–19.

Dempster, M., Howell, D. and McCorry, N.K. (2015) Illness perceptions and coping in physical health conditions: a meta-analysis, *Journal of Psychosomatic Research,* **79**(6): 506–13.

Department for Environment, Food and Rural Affairs (2011) *National Food Survey: Household Nutrient Data from 1940–2000.* https://webarchive.nationalarchives.gov.uk/20130103024837/http://www.defra.gov.uk/statistics/foodfarm/food/familyfood/nationalfoodsurvey/

DH (Department of Health) (1995) *Obesity: Reversing the Increasing Problem of Obesity in England: A Report from the Nutrition and Physical Activity Task Forces.* London: HMSO.

DH (Department of Health) (2001) *Hospital Inpatient Statistics,* www.doh.gov.uk/HPSSS/TBL.

DH (Department of Health) (2004) *At Least Five a Week: Evidence on the Impact of Physical Activity and its Relationship to Health. A Report From the Chief Medical Officer.* London: DH.

DH (Department of Health) (2005) *Maternity Statistics 2003–2004.* London: OPCS.

DH (Department of Health) (2011) *Start Active, Stay Active: A Report on Physical Activity for Health from* the Four Home Countries' Chief Medical Officers. London: Department of Health.

Dhabhar, F.S. (2014) Effects of stress on immune function: the good, the bad, and the beautiful, *Immunologic research,* **58**(2–3): 193–210.

DHSC (Department of Health and Social Care) (2017) *Abortion statistics, England and Wales.* https://assets.publishing.service.gov.uk/government/uploads/system/uploads/attachment_data/file/714183/2017_Abortion_Statistics_Commentary.pdf

Di Carlo, C., Savoia, F., Ferrara, C. et al. (2016) 'In patient' medical abortion versus surgical abortion: patient's satisfaction, *Gynecological Endocrinology,* **32**(8): 650–4.

Diamond, E.G., Kittle, C.F. and Crockett, J.F. (1960) Comparison of internal mammary artery ligation and sham operation for angina pectoris, *American Journal of Cardiology,* **5**: 483–6.

Dias, H., Amendoeira, J., Silva, M. and Cruz, O. (2019) The influence of peers on the experience of sexuality in adolescence: a scoping review. In P. Allebeck (ed). *European Journal of Public Health.* Oxford: Oxford University Press.

Dibb, B. (2009) Positive change with Ménière's disease, *British Journal of Health Psychology,* **14**(4): 613–24.

Dibb, B., Ellis-Hill, C., Donovan-Hall, M., Burridge, J. and Rushton, D. (2014) Exploring positive adjustment in people with spinal cord injury, *Journal of Health Psychology,* **19**(8): 1043–54.

Dibb, B., Ellis-Hill, C., Donovan-Hall, M., Burridge, J. and Rushton, D. (2014) Exploring positive adjustment in people with spinal cord injury, *Journal of Health Psychology,* **19**(8): 1043–54.

DiClemente, C.C. and Hughes, S.O. (1990) Stages of change profiles in outpatient alcoholism treatment, *Journal of Substance Abuse,* **2**: 217–35.

DiClemente, C.C. and Prochaska, J.O. (1982) Self-change and therapy change of smoking behavior: a comparison of processes of change in cessation and maintenance, *Addictive Behaviours,* **7**: 133–42.

DiClemente, C.C. and Prochaska, J.O. (1985) Processes and stages of change: coping and competence in smoking behavior change, in F. Shiffman and T.A. Wills (eds) *Coping and Substance Abuse.* New York: Academic Press.

DiClemente, C.C., Prochaska, J.O., Fairhurst, S.K. et al. (1991) The process of smoking cessation: an analysis of precontemplation, contemplation, and preparation stages of change, *Journal of Consulting and Clinical Psychology,* **59**: 295–304.

Diederiks, J.P., Bar, F.W., Hopponer, P. et al. (1991) Predictors of return to former leisure and social activities in MI patients, *Journal of Psychosomatic Research,* **35**: 687–96.

Dieng, M., Butow, P.N., Costa, D.S. et al. (2016) Psychoeducational intervention to reduce fear of cancer recurrence in people at high risk of developing another primary melanoma: results of a randomized controlled trial, *Journal of Clinical Oncology,* **34**(36): 4405–14.

Dilla, D., Ian, J., Martin, J. et al. (2020) 'I don't do it for myself, I do it for them': a grounded theory study of South Asians' experiences of making lifestyle change after myocardial infarction, *Journal of Clinical Nursing,* **29**(19–20), 3687–3700.

DiMatteo, M.R., Giordani, P.J., Lepper, H.S. and Croghan, T.W. (2002) Patient adherence and medical treatment outcomes: a meta-analysis, *Medical Care,* **40**(9): 794–811.

Dinan, J.E., Hargitai, I.A., Watson, N. et al. (2021) Pain catastrophising in the oro-facial pain population, *Journal of Oral Rehabilitation,* **48**(6): 643–53.

Diner, E., Emmons, R.A., Larson, R.J. and Griffen, S. (1985) The satisfaction with life scale, *Journal of Personality Assessment,* **49**: 71–6.

DiSantis, K.I., Birch, L.L., Davey, A. et al. (2013) Plate size and children's appetite: effects of larger dishware on self-served portions and intake, *Pediatrics,* **131**(5): 1451–8.

Dishman, R.K., Oldenburg, B., O'Neal, H. and Shephard, R. J. (1998) Worksite physical activity interventions, *American Journal of Preventive Medicine,* **15**(4): 344–61.

Dishman, R.K., Sallis, J.F. and Orenstein, D.M. (1985) The determinants of physical activity and exercise, *Public Health Reports,* **100**: 158–72.

Dishman, R.K. (1982) Compliance/adherence in health-related exercise, *Health Psychology,* **1**: 237–67.

Dodds, J. and Mercey, D. (2002) London Gay Men's Survey: 2001 results. Technical report, Department of STDs, Royal Free and University College Medical School.

Doll, R. and Hill, A.B. (1954) The mortality of doctors in relation to their smoking habits: a preliminary report, *British Medical Journal,* **1**: 1451–5.

Doll, R. and Peto, R. (1981) *The Causes of Cancer.* New York: Oxford University Press.

Dombrowski, S.U., Knittle, K., Avenell, A. et al. (2014) Long term maintenance of weight loss with non-surgical interventions in obese adults: systematic review and meta-analyses of randomised controlled trials, *BMJ,* **348:** g2646.

Downing, R.W. and Rickels, K. (1983) Physician prognosis in relation to drug and placebo response in anxious and depressed psychiatric outpatients, *The Journal of Nervous and Mental Disease,* **171**: 182–5.

Doyal, L. (1994) Changing medicine? Gender and the politics of health care, in J. Gabe, D. Kelleher and G. Williams (eds) *Challenging Medicine.* London: Routledge.

Doyal, L. (2001) Sex, gender and health: the need for a new approach, *British Medical Journal,* **323**: 1061–3.

Doyle, F., Rohde, D., Rutkowska, A. et al. (2014) Systematic review and meta-analysis of the impact of depression on subsequent smoking cessation in patients with coronary heart disease: 1990 to 2013, *Psychosomatic Medicine*, **76**(1): 44–57.

Duncker, K. (1938) Experimental modification of children's food preferences through social suggestion, *Journal of Abnormal Social Psychology*, **33**: 489–507.

Dunn, A.L., Andersen, R.E. and Jakicic, J.M. (1998) Lifestyle physical activity interventions: history, short and long-term effects and recommendation, *American Journal of Preventive Medicine*, **15**: 398–412.

Dunn, C., Deroo, L. and Rivara, F.P. (2001) The use of brief interventions adapted from motivational interviewing across behavioral domains: a systematic review, *Addiction*, **96**(12): 1725–42.

Dunn, J., Occhipinti, S., Campbell, A. et al. (2011) Benefit finding after cancer: the role of optimism, intrusive thinking and social environment, *Journal of Health Psychology*, **16**(1): 169–77.

Dunton, G.F., Rebar, A.L., Gardner, B. et al. (2022/in press). Towards consensus in conceptualizing and operationalizing physical activity maintenance, *Psychology of Sport and Exercise*. Doi.org/10.1016/j.psychsport.2022.102214

Durkin, S.J., Broun, K., Spittal, M.J. and Wakefield, M.A. (2019) Impact of a mass media campaign on participation rates in a National Bowel Cancer Screening Program: a field experiment, *BMJ Open*, **9**(1): e024267.

Dusseldorp, E., van Elderen, T., Maes, S. et al. (1999) A meta-analysis of psychoeducational programmes for coronary heart disease patients, *Health Psychology*, **18**: 506–19.

d'Ettorre, G., Ceccarelli, G., Santinelli, L. et al. (2021) Post-traumatic stress symptoms in healthcare workers dealing with the COVID-19 pandemic: a systematic review, *International Journal of Environmental Research and Public Health*, **18**(2): 601.

East Ayrshire Council (2011) Pupils earn just reward for healthy eating, www.eastayrshireschoolmeals.com/p/pupils-earn-just-reward-for-healthy-eating.

Ebrecht, M., Hextall, J., Kirtley, L.G. et al. (2004) Perceived stress and cortisol levels predict speed of wound healing in healthy male adults, *Psychoneuroendocrinology*, **29**: 798–809.

Eccleston, C. and Crombez, G. (1999) Pain demands attention: a cognitive-affective model of the interruptive function of pain, *Psychological Bulletin*, **125**(3): 356–66.

Eccleston, C., Crombez, G., Aldrich, S. and Stannard, C. (2001) Worry and chronic pain patients: a description and analysis of individual differences, *European Journal of Pain*, **5**(3): 309–18.

Eccleston, C., Fisher, E., Craig, L. et al. (2014) Psychological therapies (Internet-delivered) for the management of chronic pain in adults, *Cochrane Database of Systematic Reviews*, 2.

Eccleston, C., Moore, R.A., Derry, S. et al. (2010) Improving the quality and reporting of systematic reviews, *European Journal of Pain*, **14**: 667–9.

Eccleston, C., Palermo, T.M., Williams, A.C.D.C. et al. (2009a) Psychological therapies for the management of chronic and recurrent pain in children and adolescents, *Cochrane Database of Systematic Reviews 2009*, 2, art. no. CD003968.

Eccleston, C., Williams, A.C.D.C. and Morely, S. (2009b) Psychological therapies for the management of chronic pain (excluding headache) in aults, *Cochrane Database of Systematic Reviews 2009*, 2., art. no. CD007407.

Eccleston, C. (1994) Chronic pain and attention: a cognitive approach, *British Journal of Clinical Psychology*, **33**(4): 535–47.

Eddy, P., Heckenberg, R., Wertheim, E.H. et al. (2016) A systematic review and meta-analysis of the effort-reward imbalance model of workplace stress with indicators of immune function, *Journal of Psychosomatic Research*, **91**: 1–8.

Edelman, E.J., Cheng, D.M., Krupitsky, E.M. et al. (2015) Heroin use and HIV disease progression: results from a Pilot Study of a Russian Cohort, *AIDS and Behavior*, **19**(6): 1089–97.

Edwards, N. (1954) The theory of decision making, *Psychological Bulletin*, **51**: 380–417.

Eiser, J.R. and Cole, N. (2002) Participation in cervical screening as a function of perceived risk, barriers and need for cognitive closure, *Journal of Health Psychology*, **7**(1): 99–105.

Eisler, R.M., Skidmore, J.R. and Ward, C.H. (1988) Masculine gender-role stress: predictor of anger, anxiety and health-risk behaviour, *Journal of Personality Assessment*, **5**: 133–41.

Ekelund, U., Steene-Johannessen, J., Brown, W.J. et al. (2016). Does physical activity attenuate, or even eliminate, the detrimental association of sitting time with mortality? A harmonised meta-analysis of data from more than 1 million men and women, *Lancet*, **388**(10051): 1302–10.

Elfhag, K. and Rössner, S. (2005) Who succeeds in maintaining weight loss? A conceptual review of factors associated with weight loss maintenance and weight regain, *Obesity Reviews*, **6**(1): 67–85.

Elliott, M.A., Armitage, C. J. and Baughan, C.J. (2005) Exploring the beliefs underpinning drivers' intentions to comply with speed limits, *Transportation Research Part F: Traffic Psychology and Behaviour*, **8**(6): 459–79.

Elston, D.M. (2020) Confirmation bias in medical decision-making, *Journal of the American Academy of Dermatology*, **82**(3): 572.

Elwyn, G., Edwards, A. and Kinnersley, P. (1999) Shared decision making: the neglected second half of the consultation, *British Journal of General Practice*, **49**: 477–82.

Emmson, D. M. (2007) Medically unexplained symptoms in children and adolescents, *Clinical Psychology Review*, **27**: 855–71.

Emmons, R.A. and McCullough, M.E. (2003) Counting blessings versus burdens: an experimental investigation of gratitude and subjective well-being in daily life, *Journal of Personality and Social Psychology*, **84**: 377–89.

Engbers, L.H., van Poppel, M.N.M., Chin, A. et al. (2005) Worksite health promotion programs with environmental changes: a systematic review, *American Journal of Preventative Medicine*, **29**: 61–70.

Engel, G.L. (1977) The need for a new medical model: a challenge for biomedicine, *Science*, **196**: 129–35.

Engel, G.L. (1980) The clinical application of the bio-psychosocial model, *American Journal of Psychiatry*, **137**: 535–44.

Epiphaniou, E. and Ogden, J. (2010) Successful weight loss maintenance: from a restricted to liberated self, *International Journal of Health Psychology*, **15**: 887–96.

Epton, T., Harris, P.R., Kane, R., van Koningsbruggen, G.M. and Sheeran, P. (2015) The impact of self-affirmation on health-behavior change: a meta-analysis, *Health Psychology*, **34**(3): 187–96.

Espada, J.P., Morales, A., Guillén-Riquelme, A. et al. (2015) Predicting condom use in adolescents: a test of three socio-cognitive models using a structural equation modeling approach, *BMC Public Health*, **16**(1): 35.

Espasa, R., Murta-Nascimento, C., Bayés, R. et al. (2012) The psychological impact of a false-positive screening mammogram in Barcelona, *Journal of Cancer Education*, **27**(4): 780–5.

Eurostat (2007) *GP Utilisation*, www.euphix.org.

Evans, M., Engberg, S., Faurby, M. et al. (2022) Adherence to and persistence with antidiabetic medications and associations with clinical and economic outcomes in people with type 2 diabetes mellitus: a systematic literature review, *Diabetes, Obesity and Metabolism*, **24**(3): 377–90.

Everett, B.G., Higgins, J.A., Haider, S. and Carpenter, E. (2019) Do sexual minorities receive appropriate sexual and reproductive health care and counseling? *Journal of Women's Health*, **28**(1): 53–62.

Everson, S.A., Lynch, J.W., Chesney, M.A. et al. (1997) Interaction of workplace demands and cardiovascular reactivity in progression of carotid atherosclerosis: population-based study, *British Medical Journal*, **314**: 553–8.

Eysenck, H.J. (1990) The prediction of death from cancer by means of personality/stress questionnaire: too good to be true? *Perceptual Motor Skills*, **71**: 216–18.

Eyton, A. (1982) *The F Plan Diet*. London: Bantam Press.

Ezenwankwo, E.F., Oladoyimbo, C.A., Dogo, H.M. et al. (2021) Factors influencing help-seeking behavior in men with symptoms of prostate cancer: a qualitative study using an ecological perspective, *Cancer Investigation*, **39**(6–7): 529–38.

Földi, M., Farkas, N., KETLAK Study Group et al. (2020) Obesity is a risk factor for developing critical condition in COVID-19 patients: a systematic review and meta-analysis, *Obesity reviews: an official journal of the International Association for the Study of Obesity*, **21**(10): e13095. Doi.org/10.1111/obr.13095.

Fabricatore, A.N. and Wadden, T.A. (2006) Obesity, *Annual Review of Clinical Psychology*, **2**, SSRN: http://ssrn.com/abstract=1081451.

Fagan, M.J., Glowacki, K. and Faulkner, G. (2021) 'You get that craving and you go for a half-hour run': Exploring the acceptability of exercise as an adjunct treatment for substance use disorder, *Mental Health and Physical Activity*, **21**: 100424.

Fait, T. (2019) Menopause hormone therapy: latest developments and clinical practice, *Drugs in context*, **8**: 212551.

Fallowfield, L. (1990) *The Quality of Life: The Missing Measurement in Health Care*. London: Souvenir Press.

Fallowfield, L.J., Rodway, A. and Baum, M. (1990) What are the psychological factors influencing attendance, non-attendance and re-attendance at a breast screening centre? *Journal of the Royal Society of Medicine*, **83**: 547–51.

Fang, C.Y., Daly, M.B., Miller, S.M. et al. (2006) Coping with ovarian cancer risk: the moderating effects of perceived control on coping and adjustment, *Journal of Health Psychology*, **11**: 561–80.

Fanning, J., Mullen, S.P. and McAuley, E. (2012) Increasing physical activity with mobile devices: a meta-analysis. *Journal of Medical Internet Research*, **14**(6): e161.

Farren, J., Mitchell-Jones, N., Verbakel, J.Y., Timmerman, D., Jalmbrant, M. and Bourne, T. (2018) The psychological impact of early pregnancy loss, *Human Reproduction Update*, **24**(6): 731–49.

Faubion, S.S., Kuhle, C.L., Shuster, L.T. and Rocca, W.A. (2015) Long-term health consequences of premature or early menopause and considerations for management, *Climacteric*, **18**(4): 483–91.

Fayazi, N., Naseri-Salahshour, V., Fayazi, H. and Karimy, M. (2020) An educational intervention to improve quality of life: a single-blind randomized controlled trial on the quality of life in patients with acute coronary syndrome, *Journal of Vessels and Circulation*, **2**(1): 21–26.

Fazzino, T. L., Bjorlie, K. and Lejuez, C. W. (2019) A systematic review of reinforcement-based interventions for substance use: Efficacy, mechanisms of action, and moderators of treatment effects. *Journal of Substance Abuse Treatment*, **104**: 83–96.

Featherston, R., Downie, L.E., Vogel, A.P. and Galvin, K.L. (2020) Decision making biases in the allied health professions: a systematic scoping review, *PloS One*, **15**(10): e0240716.

Feller, L., Khammissa, R.A.G., Ballyram, R. et al. (2019) Chronic psychosocial stress in relation to cancer, *Middle East Journal of Cancer*, **10**(1): 1–8.

Fernández-Basanta, S., Van, P., Coronado, C. et al. (2021) Coping after involuntary pregnancy loss: perspectives of Spanish European women, *OMEGA-Journal of Death and Dying*, **83**(2): 310–24.

Fernandes, F.R.P., Zanini, P.B., Rezende, G.R. et al. (2015) Syphilis infection, sexual practices and bisexual behaviour among men who have sex with men and transgender women: a cross-sectional study. *Sexually Transmitted Infections*, **91**(2): 142–9.

Fernbach, M. (2002) The impact of a media campaign on cervical screening knowledge and self-efficacy, *Journal of Health Psychology*, **7**(1): 85–97.

Festinger, L. (1957) *A Theory of Cognitive Dissonance.* Evanston, IL: Row, Peterson.

Feuerstein, M., Carter, R.L. and Papciak, A.S. (1987) A prospective analysis of stress and fatigue in recurrent low back pain, *Pain*, **31**: 333–44.

Field, A.E., Cheung, L., Wolf, A.M. et al. (1999) Exposure to the mass media and weight concerns among girls. *Pediatrics*, **103**(3): e36.

Figueiras, M.J. and Alves, N.C. (2007) Lay perceptions of serious illness: an adapted version of the Revised Illness Perception Questionnaire (IPQ-R) for healthly people, *Psychology and Health*, **22**(2): 143–58.

Figueiras, M.J. and Weinman, J. (2003) Do similar patient and spouse perceptions of myocardial infarction predict recovery? *Psychology and Health*, **18**(2): 201–16.

Finkelstein-Fox, L. and Park, C.L. (2019) Control-coping goodness-of-fit and chronic illness: a systematic review of the literature, *Health Psychology Review*, **13**(2): 137–62.

Finlay, S. J. and Faulkner, G. (2005) Physical activity promotion through the mass media: inception, production, transmission and consumption, *Preventive Medicine*, **40**(2): 121–30.

Fishbein, M. (ed.) (1967) *Readings in Attitude Theory and Measurement.* New York: Wiley.

Fishbein, M. and Ajzen, I. (1975) *Belief, Attitude, Intention, and Behavior: An Introduction to Theory and Research.* Reading, MA: Addison-Wesley.

Fishbein, M., Hennessy, M., Kamb, M. et al. (2001) Project Respect Study Group: using intervention theory to model factors influencing behavior change, Project RESPECT, *Evaluation and the Health Professions*, **24**(4): 363–84.

Fisher, E., Villanueva, G., Henschke, N. et al. (2022) Efficacy and safety of pharmacological, physical, and psychological interventions for the management of chronic pain in children: a WHO systematic review and meta-analysis, *Pain*, **163**(1): e1–e19.

Fisher, J.O. and Birch, L.L. (1999) Restricting access to a palatable food affects children's behavioral response, food selection and intake, *American Journal of Clinical Nutrition*, **69**: 1264–72.

Fisher, J.O., Birch, L.L., Smiciklas-Wright, H. and Piocciano, M.F. (2000) Breastfeeding through the first year predicts maternal control in feeding and subsequent toddler energy intakes, *Journal of the American Dietician Association*, **100**: 641–6.

Fisher, W.A. (1984) Predicting contraceptive behavior among university men: the role of emotions and behavioral intentions, *Journal of Applied Social Psychology*, **14**: 104–23.

Flay, B.R. (1985) Psychosocial approaches to smoking prevention: a review of findings, *Health Psychology*, **4**: 449–88.

Fleming, T.P., Watkins, A., Velazquez, M.A. et al. (2018) Origins of lifetime health around the time of conception: causes and consequences, *The Lancet*, **391**(10132): 1842–52. Doi: 10.1016/S0140-6736(18)30312-X.

Flowers, P., Smith, J. A., Sheeran, P. and Beail, N. (1998) 'Coming out' and sexual debut: understanding the social context of HIV risk-related behaviour, *Journal of Community & Applied Social Psychology*, **8**(6): 409–21.

Flowers, P., Smith, J.A., Sheeran, P. and Beail, N. (1997) Health and romance: understanding unprotected sex in relationships between gay men, *British Journal of Health Psychology*, **2**: 73–86.

Flynn, J., Slovic, P. and Mertz, C.K. (1994) Gender, race, and perception of environmental health risks, *Risk Analysis*, **14**(6): 1101–8.

Folkman, S. and Lazarus, R.S. (1988) *Manual for the Ways of Coping Questionnaire.* Palo Alto, CA: Consulting Psychologist Press.

Folkman, S. and Moskowitz, J.T. (2000) Positive affect and the other side of coping, *American Psychologist*, **55**: 647–54.

Folkman, S., Lazarus, R.S., Pimley, S. and Novacek, J. (1987) Age differences in stress and coping processes, *Psychology and Ageing*, **2**: 171–84.

Food and Drug Administration (1997) *AIDS deaths in the US 1987–1997*, available at: https://commons.wikimedia.org/w/index.php?curid=34507909

Ford, E., Williamson, D. and Liu, S. (1997) Weight change and diabetes incidence: findings from a national cohort of US adults, *American Journal of Epidemiology*, **146**: 214–22.

Fordyce, W.E. and Steger, J.C. (1979) Chronic pain, in O.F. Pomerleau and J.P. Brady (eds) *Behavioral Medicine: Theory and Practice.* Baltimore, MD: Williams & Wilkins.

Foresight (2007) *Tackling Obesities: Future Choices—Project Report.* London: The Stationery Office, http://www.foresight.gov.uk/Obesity/obesity_final/Index.html.

Formon, S.J. (1974) *Infant Nutrition,* 2nd edn. Philadelphia, PA: WB Saunders.

Freak-Poli, R.L., Cumpston, M., Albarqouni, L. et al. (2020) Workplace pedometer interventions for increasing physical activity, *Cochrane Database of Systematic Reviews,* **7**(7): CD009209.

Fredrickson, B.L., Maynard, K.E., Helms, M.J. et al. (2000) Hostility predicts magnitude and duration of blood pressure response to anger, *Journal of Behavioural Medicine,* **23**: 229–43.

Fredrickson, B.L., Robson, A. and Ljungdell, T. (1991) Ambulatory and laboratory blood pressure in individuals with negative and positive family history of hypertension, *Health Psychology,* **10**: 371–7.

Free, C. and Ogden, J. (2005) Emergency contraception use and non use in young women: the application of a contextual and dynamic model, *British Journal of Health Psychology,* **10**: 237–53.

Freeman, C. (1995) Cognitive therapy, in G. Szmukler, C. Dare and J. Treasure (eds) *Handbook of Eating Disorders: Theory, Treatment and Research.* London: Wiley.

Freeman, E.W. and Rickels, K. (1993) *Early Childbearing: Perspectives of Black Adolescents on Pregnancy, Abortion, and Contraception.* Newbury Park, CA: Sage.

Freeman, R.F., Thomas, C.D., Solyom, L. and Hunter, M.A. (1984) A modified video camera for measuring body image distortion: technical description and reliability, *Psychological Medicine,* **14**: 411–16.

Friedman, M., Thoresen, C., Gill, J. et al. (1986) Alteration of Type A behavior and its effects on cardiac recurrences in post myocardial infarction patients: summary results of the recurrent coronary prevention project, American Heart Journal, 112: 653–65.

Freidson, E. (1970) *Profession of Medicine.* New York: Dodds Mead.

French, D. and Weinman, J. (2008) Assessing illness perceptions: beyond the IPQ, *Psychology and Health,* **23**: 5–9.

French, D.P. and Sutton, S. (2010) Reactivity of measurement in health psychology: how much of a problem is it? What can be done about it? *British Journal of Health Psychology,* **15**: 453–68.

French, D.P., Cooper, A. and Weinman, J. (2006a) Illness perceptions predict attendance at cardiac rehabilitation following acute myocardial infarction: a systematic review with meta-analysis, *Journal of Psychosomatic Research,* **61**(6): 757–67.

French, D.P., Maissi, E. and Marteau, T.M. (2004) Psychological costs of inadequate cervical smear test results, *British Journal of Cancer,* **91**: 1887–92.

French, D.P., Maissi, E. and Marteau, T.M. (2005a) The purpose of attributing cause: beliefs about the causes of myocardial infarction, *Social Science & Medicine,* **60**: 1411–21.

French, D.P., Maissi, E. and Marteau, T.M. (2006b) The psychological costs of inadequate cervical smear test results: three-month follow-up, *Psycho-oncology,* **15**: 498–508.

French, D.P., Marteau, T., Senior, V. and Weinman, J. (2002a) The structure of belief about the causes of heart attacks: a network analysis, *British Journal of Health Psychology,* **7**: 463–79.

French, D.P., Marteau, T.M., Senior, V. and Weinman, J. (2005b) How valid are measures of beliefs about the causes of illness? The example of myocardial infarction, *Psychology and Health,* **20**(5): 615–35.

French, D.P., Senior, V., Weinman, J. and Marteau, T.M. (2001) Causal attributions for heart disease: a systematic review, *Psychology and Health,* **16**: 77–98.

Friedman, M. and Rosenman, R.H. (1959) Association of specific overt behavior pattern with blood and cardiovascular findings, *Journal of the American Medical Association,* **169**: 1286–97.

Friedman, M., Thoresen, C., Gill, J. et al. (1986) Alteration of Type A behavior and its effects on cardiac recurrences in post myocardial infarction patients: summary results of the recurrent coronary prevention project, *American Heart Journal,* **112**: 653–65.

Friedman, T. and Gath, D. (1989) The psychiatric consequences of spontaneous abortion, *British Journal of Psychiatry,* **155**: 810–13.

Frith, H., Harcourt, D. and Fussell, A. (2007) Anticipating an altered appearance: women undergoing chemotherapy treatment for breast cancer, *European Journal of Oncology Nursing,* **11**: 385–91.

Fritsch, C.G., Ferreira, P.H., Prior, J.L. et al. (2020) Effects of using text message interventions for the management of musculoskeletal pain: a systematic review, *Pain,* **161**(11): 2462–75.

Frost, D.M., Lehavot, K. and Meyer, I.H. (2015) Minority stress and physical health among sexual minority individuals, *Journal of Behavioral Medicine,* **38**(1): 1–8.

Fuentes Artiles, R., Staub, K., Aldakak, L. et al. (2019) Mindful eating and common diet programs lower body weight similarly: systematic review and meta-analysis, *Obesity Reviews,* **20**(11): 1619–27.

Furnham, A. and Kirkcaldy, B. (1997) Age and sex differences in health beliefs and behaviors, *Psychological Reports,* **80**(1): 63–6.

Gabhainn, S.N., Kelleher, C.C., Naughton, A.M. et al. (1999) Socio-demographic variations in perspectives on cardiovascular disease and associated risk factors, *Health Education Research,* **14**(5): 619–28.

Galeotti, M., Mitchell, G., Tomlinson, M. and Aventin, Á. (2022) Factors affecting the emotional wellbeing of women and men who experience miscarriage in hospital settings: a scoping review, *BMC Pregnancy and Childbirth*, **22**(1): 1–24.

Gallacher, J.E.J., Hopkinson, C.A., Bennett, P. et al. (1997) Effect of stress management on angina, *Psychology and Health*, **12**: 523–32.

Galvez-Sánchez, C.M., Montoro, C.I., Moreno-Padilla, M. et al. (2021) Effectiveness of acceptance and commitment therapy in central pain sensitization syndromes: a systematic review, *Journal of Clinical Medicine*, **10**(12): 2706.

Galvin, L.R. and Godfrey, H.P.D. (2001) The impact of coping on emotional adjustment to spinal cord injury (SCI): review of the literature and application of a stress appraisal and coping formulation, *Spinal Cord*, **39**: 615–27.

Garcia, J., Hankins, W.G. and Rusiniak, K. (1974) Behavioral regulation of the milieu intern in man and rat, *Science*, **185**: 824–31.

Gardner, B., Lally, P. and Rebar, A.L. (2020) Does habit weaken the relationship between intention and behaviour? Revisiting the habit-intention interaction hypothesis, *Social and Personality Psychology Compass*, **14**(8): e12553.

Gardner, B., Rebar, A.L. and Lally, P. (2019) A matter of habit: recognizing the multiple roles of habit in health behaviour, *British Journal of Health Psychology*, **24**(2): 241–49.

Garn, S.M., Bailey, S.M., Solomon, M.A. and Hopkins, P.J. (1981) Effects of remaining family members on fatness prediction, *American Journal of Clinical Nutrition*, **34**: 148–53.

Garner, D.M. (1991) *EDI-2: Professional Manual.* Odessa, FL: Psychological Assessment Resources Inc.

Garrow, J. (1997) Treatment of obesity IV: surgical treatments, in J. Garrow, *Obesity.* Blackwell: British Nutrition Foundation.

Gates, M., Hartling, L., Shulhan-Kilroy, J. et al. (2020) Digital technology distraction for acute pain in children: a meta-analysis, *Pediatrics*, **145**(2): e20191139.

Gavey, N., Schmidt, J., Braun, V. et al. (2009) Unsafe, unwanted: sexual coercion as a barrier to safer sex among men who have sex with men, *Journal of Health Psychology*, **14**(7): 1021–6.

Gellaitry, G., Cooper, V., Davis, C. et al. (2005) Patients' perception of information about HAART: impact on treatment decisions, *AIDS Care*, **7**(3): 367–76.

George, M. and Bender, B. (2019) New insights to improve treatment adherence in asthma and COPD, *Patient Preference and Adherence*, **13**: 1325–34.

George, W.H. and Marlatt, G.A. (1983) Alcoholism: the evolution of a behavioral perspective, in M. Galanter (ed.) *Recent Developments in Alcoholism*, New York: Plenum Press.

Germain, D., Wakefield, M.A. and Durkin, S.J. (2010) Adolescents' perceptions of cigarette brand image: does plain packaging make a difference? *Journal of Adolescent Health*, **46**: 385–92.

Gerrard, M., Gibbons, F.X., Benthin, A.C. and Hessling, R.M. (1996) A longitudinal study of the reciprocal nature of risk behaviors and cognitions in adolescents: what you do shapes what you think and vice versa, *Health Psychology*, **15**: 344–54.

Ghiassi, S. and Morton, J.M. (2020) Safety and efficacy of bariatric and metabolic surgery, *Current Obesity Reports*, **9**(2): 159–164.

Giannetti, V.J., Reynolds, J. and Rihen, T. (1985) Factors which differentiate smokers from ex-smokers among cardiovascular patients: a discriminant analysis, *Social Science and Medicine*, **20**: 241–5.

Gibson Miller, J., Hartman, T.K., Levita, L. et al. (2020) Capability, opportunity, and motivation to enact hygienic practices in the early stages of the COVID-19 outbreak in the United Kingdom, *British Journal of Health Psychology*, **25**(4): 856–64.

Gibson, B. (2008) Can evaluative conditioning change attitudes towards mature brands? New evidence from the implicit association test, *Journal of Consumer Research*, **35**: 178–88.

Gidlow, C.J., Ellis, N.J., Riley, V. et al. (2019) Randomised controlled trial comparing uptake of NHS Health Check in response to standard letters, risk-personalised letters and telephone invitations, *BMC Public Health*, **19**(1): 1–11.

Gijsbers van Wijk, C.M. and Kolk, A.M. (1997) Sex differences in physical symptoms: the contribution of symptom perception theory, *Social Science and Medicine*, **45**: 231–46.

Gijsbers van Wijk, C.M., Huisman, H. and Kolk, A.M. (1999) Gender differences in physical symptoms and illness behaviour: a health diary study, *Social Science and Medicine*, **49**: 1061–74.

Gil, K.M., Anthony, K.K., Carson, J.W. et al. (2001) Daily coping practice predicts treatment effects in children with sickle cell disease, *Journal of Pediatric Psychology*, **26**(3): 163–73.

Gill, J.J., Price, V.A. and Friedman, M. (1985) Reduction of type A behavior in healthy middle-aged American military officers, *American Heart Journal*, **110**: 503–14.

Gillespie, I.J., Armstrong, H.L. and Ingham, R. (2022) Exploring reflections, motivations, and experiential outcomes of first same-sex/gender sexual experiences among lesbian, gay, bisexual and other sexual minority individuals, *The Journal of Sex Research*, **59**:1, 26–38. DOI: 10.1080/00224499.2021.1960944

Gillibrand, R. and Stevenson, J. (2006) The extended health belief model applied to the experience of diabetes in young people, *British Journal of Health Psychology*, **11**: 155–69.

Gillies, P.A. and Galt, M. (1990) Teenage smoking–fun or coping? in J.A.M. Wimbust and S. Maes (eds) *Lifestyles and Health: New Developments in Health Psychology.* Leiden: DSWO/Leiden University Press.

Gillon, R. (2001) Is there a 'new ethics of abortion'? *Journal of Medical Ethics*, **27**(suppl. II): ii5–9.

Girão, W.B.A., Filizola, M.C., Brazão, G. et al. (2019) The relationship between anxiety and pain disorders: an integrative review, *International Journal of Psychological Research and Reviews*, **2**: 20. DOI: 10.28933/ijprr-2019-08-2005.

Glass, D.C. and Singer, J.E. (1972) *Urban Stress*. New York: Academic Press.

Gleghorn, A.A., Penner, L.A., Powers, P.S. and Schulman, R. (1987) The psychometric properties of several measures of body image, *Journal of Psychopathology and Behavioral Assessment*, **9**: 203–18.

Global Burden of Disease (2016) *Global Burden of Diseases, Injuries, and Risk Factors*. https://vizhub.healthdata.org/gbd-compare/#

Global Burden of Disease Project (2019) https://www.healthdata.org/gbd/2019

Gloy, V.L., Briel, M., Bhatt, D.L. et al. (2013) Bariatric surgery versus non-surgical treatment for obesity: a systematic review and meta-analysis of randomised controlled trials, *BMJ (Clinical Research ed.)*, **347**: 1–16.

Goddard, E. (1990) *Why Children Start Smoking*. London: HMSO.

Godin, G., Belanger-Gravel, A., Gagne, C. and Blondeau, D. (2008a) Factors predictive of signed consent for posthumous organ donation, *Progress in Transplantation*, **18**(2): 109–17.

Godin, G., Conner, M., Sheeran, P. et al. (2007) Determinants of repeated blood donation among new and experienced blood donors, *Transfusion*, **47**(9): 1307–15.

Godin, G., Sheeran, P., Conner, M. and Germain, M. (2008b) Asking questions changes behavior: mere measurement effects on frequency of blood donation, *Health Psychology*, **27**: 179–84.

Godin, G., Sheeran, P., Conner, M. et al. (2010) Which survey questions change behavior? Randomized controlled trial of mere measurement interventions, *Health Psychology*, **29**(6): 636–44.

Godin, G., Valois, P., Lepage, L. and Desharnais, R. (1992) Predictors of smoking behaviour: an application of Ajzen's theory of planned behaviour, *British Journal of Addiction*, **87**: 1335–43.

Goldberg, D.P. (1978) *Manual of the General Health Questionnaire*. Windsor: NFER-Nelson.

Goldberg, I.R. (1999) A broad-bandwidth, public-domain, personality inventory measuring the lower-level facets of several five-factor models, in I. Merveilde, I. Deary, F. De Fryt and F. Ostendorf (eds) *Personality Psychology in Europe: Vol. 7*. Tilburg: Tilburg University Press.

Golden, A. and Kessler, C. (2020) Obesity and genetics, *Journal of the American Association of Nurse Practitioners*, **32**(7): 493–96.

Goldschneider, A. (1920) *Das Schmerz Problem*. Berlin: Springer.

Gollwitzer, P.M. and Sheeran, P. (2006) Implementation intentions and goal achievement: a meta-analysis of effects and processes, *Advances in Experimental Social Psychology*, **38**: 69–119.

Gollwitzer, P.M. (1993) Goal achievement: the role of intentions, *European Review of Social Psychology*, **4**: 141–85.

Good, G.E., Dell, D.M., and Mintz, L.B. (1989) Male role and gender role conflict: relations to help seeking in men, *Journal of Counselling Psychology*, **36**: 295–300.

Goodwin, P. and Ogden, J. (2007) Women's reflections about their past abortions: an exploration of how emotional reactions change over time, *Psychology and Health*, **22**: 231–48.

Gordon, D.F. (1995) Testicular cancer and masculinity, in D. Sabo and D.F. Gordon (eds) *Men's Health and Illness: Gender, Power and the Body*. Thousand Oaks, CA: Sage.

Gough, B. and Robertson, S. (eds) (2010) *Men, Masculinities and Health: Critical Perspectives*. Basingstoke: Palgrave Macmillan.

Gourlan, M., Bernard, P., Bortolon, C. et al. (2016) Efficacy of theory-based interventions to promote physical activity. A meta-analysis of randomised controlled trials. *Health Psychology Review*, **10**(1): 50–66.

Gouvier, W.D., Cubic, B., Jones G. et al. (1992) Postconcussion symptoms and daily stress in normal and head-injured college populations, *Archives of Clinical Neuropsychology*, **7**: 193–211.

GOV.UK (2017) *National LGBT Survey*. https://www.gov.uk/government/consultations/national-lgbt-survey

Gracely, R.H., Dubner, R., Deeter, W.R. and Wolskee, P.J. (1985) Clinical expectations influence placebo analgesia, *Lancet*, **i**: 43.

Grant, M., Padilla, G.V., Ferrell, B.R. and Rhiner, M. (1990) Assessment of quality of life with a single instrument, *Seminars in Oncology Nursing*, **6**: 260–70.

Gratton, L., Povey, R. and Clark-Carter, D. (2007) Promoting children's fruit and vegetable consumption: interventions using the theory of planned behaviour as a framework, *British Journal of Health Psychology*, **12**: 639–50.

Graven, L.J. and Grant, J.S. (2014) Social support and self-care behaviors in individuals with heart failure: an integrative review. *International Journal of Nursing Studies*, **51**(2): 320–33.

Greaves, C., Poltawski, L., Garside, R. and Briscoe, S. (2017) Understanding the challenge of weight loss maintenance: a systematic review and synthesis of qualitative research on weight loss maintenance, *Health Psychology Review*, April 7: 1–19.

Green, E., Griffiths, F. and Thompson, D. (2006) 'Are my bones normal, doctor?' The role of technology in understanding and communicating health risks for midlife women, *Sociological Research Online*, **11**(4).

Greeno, C.G. and Wing, R.R. (1994) Stress-induced eating, *Psychological Bulletin*, **115**: 444–64.

Greenwood, J. (2001) The new ethics of abortion, *Journal of Medical Ethics*, **27**(suppl. II): ii2–4.

Greer, S., Moorey, S., Baruch, J.D.R. et al. (1992) Adjuvant psychological therapy for patients with cancer: a prospective randomised trial, *British Medical Journal*, **304**: 675–80.

Greer, S., Morris, T.E. and Pettingale, K.W. (1979) Psychological responses to breast cancer: effect on outcome, *Lancet*, **2**: 785–7.

Grey, M., Boland, E.A., Davidson, M. et al. (2000) Coping skills training for youth with diabetes mellitus has long-lasting effects on metabolic control and quality of life, *The Journal of Pediatrics*, **137**(1): 107–13.

Grimley, C.E., Kato, P.M. and Grunfeld, E.A. (2020) Health and health belief factors associated with screening and help-seeking behaviours for breast cancer: a systematic review and meta-analysis of the European evidence, *British Journal of Health Psychology*, **25**(1): 107–28.

Groesz, L.M., Levine, M.P. and Murnen, S.K. (2002) The effect of experimental presentation of thin media images on body satisfaction: a meta-analytical review, *International Journal of Eating Disorders*, **31**: 1–16.

Grogan, S., Walker, L., McChesney, G., Gee, I., Gough, B. and Cordero, M. I. (2022) How has COVID-19 lockdown impacted smoking? A thematic analysis of written accounts from UK smokers, *Psychology & Health*, **37**(1): 17–33.

Grogan, S. (2016) *Body Image: Understanding Body Dissatisfaction in Men, Women and Children*, 3rd edn. London: Routledge.

Grunfeld, E., Mant, D., Yudkin, P. et al. (1996) Routine follow up of breast cancer in primary care: randomised trial, *British Medical Journal*, **313**: 665–9.

Guadagnoli, E. and Ward, P. (1998) Patient participation on decision making, *Social Science and Medicine*, **47**: 329–39.

Gudmundsdottir, H., Johnston, M., Johnston, D. and Foulkes, J. (2001) Spontaneous, elicited and cued casual attribution in the year following a first myocardial infarction, *British Journal of Health Psychology*, **6**: 81–96.

Gum, A., Snyder, C.R. and Duncan, P.W. (2006) Hopeful thinking, participation, and depressive symptoms three months after stroke, *Psychology & Health*, **21**(3): 319–34.

Guraya, A., Rakita, U., Porter, C.L. and Feldman, S.R. (2021) A narrative review of systematic reviews on adherence to psoriasis treatments, *Dermatological Reviews*, **2**(5): 251–61.

Gureje, O., Simon, G.E., Ustun, T.B. and Goldberg, D.P. (1997) Somatisation in cross-cultural perspective: a World Health Organization study in primary care, *American Journal of Psychiatry*, **154**: 989–95.

Gustafson, P.E. (1998) Gender differences in risk perception: theoretical and methodological perspectives, *Risk Analysis*, **18**(6): 805–11.

Guthold, R., Stevens, G.A., Riley, L.M. and Bull, F.C. (2018) Worldwide trends in insufficient physical activity from 2001 to 2016: a pooled analysis of 358 population-based surveys with 1.9 million participants, *The Lancet Global Health*, **6**(10): e1077–e1086.

Guttmacher Institute (2018) www.guttmacher.org/fact-sheet/induced-abortion-worldwide

Guyll, M. and Contrada, R.J. (1998) Trait hostility and ambulatory cardiovascular activity: response to social interaction, *Health Psychology*, **17**: 30–9.

Gwozdz, W., Reisch, L., Eiben, G. et al. (2020) The effect of smileys as motivational incentives on children's fruit and vegetable choice, consumption and waste: A field experiment in schools in five European countries, *Food Policy*, **96**: 101852.

Höfer, S., Benzer, W. and Oldridge, N. (2014) Change in health-related quality of life in patients with coronary artery disease predicts 4-year mortality, *International Journal of Cardiology*, **174**(1): 7–12.

Haas, H., Fink, H. and Hartfelder, G. (1959) Das Placeboproblem, *Fortschritte der Arzneimittelforschung*, **1**: 279–354.

Haasova, M., Warren, F.C., Ussher, M. et al. (2013) The acute effects of physical activity on cigarette cravings: systematic review and meta-analysis with individual participant data, *Addiction*, **108**(1): 26–37. Doi: 10.1111/j.1360-0443.2012.04034.x

Hadjistavropoulos, H.D., Mehta, S., Wilhelms, A. et al. (2020) A systematic review of internet-delivered cognitive behavior therapy for alcohol misuse: study characteristics, program content and outcomes, *Cognitive behaviour therapy*, **49**(4): 327–46.

Hafeez, H., Zeshan, M., Tahir, M.A. et al. (2017) Health care disparities among lesbian, gay, bisexual, and transgender youth: a literature review, *Cureus*, **9**(4), e1184.

Hagger, M.S. and Chatzisarantis, N.L.D. (2009) Integrating the theory of planned behaviour and self-determination theory in health behaviour: a meta-analysis, *British Journal of Health Psychology*, **14**(2): 275–302.

Hagger, M.S. and Orbell, S. (2003) A meta-analytic review of the common-sense model of illness representations, *Psychology and Health*, **18**(2): 141–84.

Hale, S., Grogan, S. and Willot, S. (2007) Patterns of self-referral in men with symptoms of prostate disease, *British Journal of Health Psychology*, **12**: 403–19.

Hale, S., Grogan, S. and Willott, S. (2010) Male GPs' views on men seeking medical help: A qualitative study, *British Journal of Health Psychology*, **15**: 697–713.

Halford, J.C., Gillespie, J., Brown, V. et al. (2004) Effect on television advertisements for foods on food consumption in children, *Appetite*, **42**(2): 221–5.

Hall, A. and Brown, L.B. (1982) A comparison of the attitudes of young anorexia nervosa patients and non-patients with those of their mothers, *British Journal of Psychology*, **56**: 39–48.

Hall, E.E., Ekkekakis, P. and Petruzzello, S.J. (2002) The affective beneficence of vigorous exercise, *British Journal of Health Psychology*, **7**: 47–66.

Hall, J.A., Epstein, A.M. and McNeil, B.J. (1989) Multidimensionality of health status in an elderly population: construct validity of a measurement battery, *Medical Care*, **27**: 168–77.

Hall, S., Weinman, J. and Marteau, T.M. (2004) The motivating impact of informing women smokers of a link between smoking and cervical cancer: the role of coherence, *Health Psychology*, **23**(4): 419–24.

Hall, W.J., Jones, B.L., Witkemper, K.D. et al. (2019) State policy on school-based sex education: a content analysis focused on sexual behaviors, relationships, and identities, *American Journal of Health Behavior*, **43**(3): 506–19.

Hallal, P.C., Andersen, L.B., Bull, F.C. et al. (2012) Global physical activity levels: surveillance progress, pitfalls, and prospects, *Lancet*, **380**: 247–57.

Halliwell, E. and Dittmar, H. (2004) Does size matter? The impact of model's body size on women's body-focused anxiety and advertising effectiveness, *Journal of Social and Clinical Psychology*, **23**(1): 104–22.

Halm, E.A., Mora, P. and Leventhal, H. (2006) No symptoms, no asthma: the acute episodic disease belief is associated with poor self-management among inner-city adults with persistent asthma, *Chest*, **129**: 573–80.

Hamilton, K. and Waller, G. (1993) Media influences on body size estimation in anorexia and bulimia: an experimental study, *British Journal of Psychiatry*, **162**: 837–40.

Hamilton, K., Peden, A.E., Keech, J.J. and Hagger, M.S. (2018) Changing people's attitudes and beliefs toward driving through floodwaters: evaluation of a video infographic, *Transportation Research Part F: Traffic Psychology and Behaviour*, **53**: 50–60.

Hamm, P.B., Shekelle, R.B. and Stamler, J. (1989) Large fluctuations in body weight during young adulthood and twenty-five year risk of coronary death in men, *American Journal of Epidemiology*, **129**: 312–18.

Hammell, K.W. (2007) Quality of life after spinal cord injury: a meta-synthesis of qualitative findings, *Spinal Cord*, **45**: 124–39.

Hammond, D., Fong, G.T., McDonald, P.W. et al. (2003) Impact of the graphic Canadian warning labels on adult smoking behaviour, *Tobacco Control*, **12**: 391–5.

Han, T.S., Richmond, P., Avenell, A. and Lean, M.E.J. (1997) Waist circumference reduction and cardiovascular benefits during weight loss in women, *International Journal of Obesity*, **21**: 127–34.

Hanbury, A., Wallace, L. and Clark, M. (2009) Use of a time series design to test effectiveness of a theory-based intervention targeting adherence of health professionals to a clinical guideline, *British Journal of Health Psychology*, **14**(3): 505–18.

Hankins, M., French, D. and Horne, R. (2000) Statistical guidelines for studies of theory of reasoned action and the theory of planned behaviour, *Psychology and Health*, **15**: 151–61.

Harcourt, D. and Frith, H. (2008) Women's experience of an altered appearance during chemotherapy: an indication of cancer status, *Journal of Health Psychology*, **13**(5): 597–606.

Hardeman, W., Johnston, M., Johnston, D.W. et al. (2002) Application of the theory of planned behaviour in behaviour change interventions: a systematic review, *Psychology and Health*, **17**(2): 123–58.

Hardeman, W., Kinmonth, A.L., Michie, S. and Sutton, S. (2011) Theory of planned behaviour cognitions do not predict self-reported or objective physical activity levels or change in the ProActive trial, *British Journal of Health Psychology*, **16**: 135–50.

Hardeman, W., Sutton, S., Griffin, S. et al. (2005) A causal modeling approach to the development of theory-based behavior change programmes for trial evaluation, *Health Education Research Theory and Practice*, **20**(6): 676–87.

Harden, A. and Ogden, J. (1999a) Young women's experiences of arranging and having abortions, *Sociology of Health and Illness*, **21**: 426–44.

Harden, A., and Ogden, J. (1999b) 16–19 year olds' beliefs about contraceptive services and the intentions to use contraception, *British Journal of Family Planning*, **24**: 135–41.

Hardy, S. and Grogan, S. (2009) Preventing disability through exercise: investigating older adults' influences and motivations to engage in physical activity, *Journal of Health Psychology*, **14**(7): 1036–46.

Harland, J., White, M., Drinkwater, C. et al. (1999) The Newcastle exercise project: a randomised controlled trial of methods to promote physical activity in primary care, *British Medical Journal* (clinical research edn.), **319**(7213): 828–32.

Harne-Britner, S., Allen, M. and Fowler, K.A. (2011) Improving hand hygiene adherence among nursing staff, *Journal of Nursing Care Quality*, **26**(1): 39–48.

Harris, A.A. (2004) Supportive counselling before and after elective pregnancy termination, *Journal of Midwifery and Women's Health*, **49**: 105–12.

Harris, P.R. and Epton, T. (2009) The impact of self-affirmation on health cognition, health behaviour and other health-related responses: a narrative review, *Social and Personality Psychology Compass*, **3**(6): 962–78.

Harris, P.R. and Napper, L. (2005) Self-affirmation and the biased processing of threatening health risk information, *Personality and Social Psychology Bulletin*, **31**(9): 1250–63.

Harris, P.R. and Smith, V. (2005) When the risks are low: the impact of absolute and comparative information on disturbance and understanding in US and UK samples, *Psychology and Health*, **20**(3): 319–30.

Harris, P.R., Mayle, K., Mabbott, L. and Napper, L. (2007) Self-affirmation reduces smokers' defensiveness to graphic on-pack cigarette warning labels, *Health Psychology*, **26**: 434–46.

Harrison, K. and Cantor, J. (1997) The relationship between media consumption and eating disorders, *Journal of Communication*, **47**(1): 40–67.

Harrow, A., Wells, M., Humphries, G. et al. (2008) 'Seeing is believing, and believing is seeing': an exploration of the meaning and impact of women's mental images of breast cancer and their origin in health care communications, *Patient Education and Counseling*, **73**(2): 339–46.

Hartmann-Boyce, J., Johns, D.J., Jebb, S.A. and Aveyard, P. (2014a) Effect of behavioural techniques and delivery mode on effectiveness of weight management: systematic review, meta-analysis and meta-regression, *Obesity Reviews*, **15**(7): 598–609.

Hartmann-Boyce, J., Johns, D.J., Jebb, S.A. et al. (2014) Behavioural weight management programmes for adults assessed by trials conducted in everyday contexts: systematic review and meta-analysis, *Obesity Reviews*, **15**(11): 920–32.

Harvey, J.H., Barnett, K. and Overstreet, A. (2004) Trauma growth and other outcomes attendant to loss, *Psychological Inquiry*, **15**: 26–9.

Hatherall, B., Ingham, R., Stone, N. and McEachran, J. (2006) How, not just if, condoms are used: the timing of condom application and removal during vaginal sex among young people in England, *Sexually Transmitted Infections*, **83**(1): 68–70.

Hausenblas, H.A. and Downs, D.S. (2004) Prospective examination of the theory of planned behavior applied to exercise behavior during women's first trimester of pregnancy, *Journal of Reproductive and Infant Psychology*, **22**(3): 199–210.

Hausenblas, H.A. and Fallon, E.A. (2006) Exercise and body image: a meta-analysis, *Psychology & Health*, **21**(1): 33–47.

Hausenblas, H.A., Nigg, C.R., Dannecker, E.A. et al. (2001) A missing piece of transtheoretical model applied to exercise: development and validation of the temptationto not exercise scale, *Psychology and Health*, **16**: 381–90.

Havelock, C., Edwards, R., Cuzlick, J. and Chamberlain, J. (1988) The organisation of cervical screening in general practice, *Journal of the Royal College of General Practitioners*, **38**: 207–11.

Haynes, R.B., Sackett, D.L. and Taylor, D.W. (eds) (1979) *Compliance in Health Care*. Baltimore, MD: Johns Hopkins University Press.

Haynes, R.B., Yao, X., Degani, A. et al. (2002) Interventions to enhance medication adherence, *Cochrane Database Library*, CD000011.

Haynes, R.B. (1982) Improving patient compliance: an empirical review, in R.B. Stuart (ed.) *Adherence, Compliance and Generalisation in Behavioral Medicine*. New York: Brunner/Mazel.

Haynes, S.G., Feinleib, M. and Kannel, W.B. (1980) The relationship of psychosocial factors to coronary heart disease in the Framingham study. III: eight year incidence of coronary heart disease, *American Journal of Epidemiology*, **111**: 37–58.

Hayes, S.C, Luoma, J.B., Bond, F.W., Masuda, A. & Lillisa, J. (2006). Acceptance and commitment therapy: Model, processes and outcomes. Behaviour Research and Therapy, 44, 1–25.

Hays, R.D. and Stewart, A.L. (1990) The structure of self-reported health in chronic disease patients, *Psychological Assessment: A Journal of Consulting and Clinical Psychology*, **2**(1): 22–30.

Hayward, R. and Stynes, S. (2021) Self-efficacy as a prognostic factor and treatment moderator in chronic musculoskeletal pain patients attending pain management programmes: a systematic review, *Musculoskeletal Care*, **19**(3): 278–92.

Health Ireland. (2021). Health Ireland Survey 2021. https://www.gov.ie/en/publication/9ef45-the-healthy-ireland-survey-2021/

Health Survey for England (2018) https://digital.nhs.uk/data-and-information/publications/statistical/health-survey-for-england/2018/summary

Heatherton, T.F., Herman, C.P., Polivy, J.A. et al. (1988) The (mis)measurement of restraint: an analysis of conceptual and psychometric issues, *Journal of Abnormal Psychology*, **97**: 19–28.

Hefferon, K., Greay, M. and Mutrie, N. (2009) Post-traumatic growth and life threatening physical illness: a systematic review of the qualitative literature, *British Journal of Health Psychology*, **14**: 343–78.

Heider, F. (1958) *The Psychology of Interpersonal Relations*. New York: John Wiley.

Heijmans, M., Foets, M. and Rijken, M. (2001) Stress in chronic disease: do the perceptions of patients and their general practitioners match? *British Journal of Health Psychology*, **6**: 229–42.

Heim, C., Newport, D.J., Mletzko, T. et al. (2008) The link between childhood trauma and depression: insights from HPA axis studies in humans, *Psychoneuroendocrinology*, **33**(6): 693–710.

Heino, E., Fröjd, S., Marttunen, M. and Kaltiala, R. (2020) Normative and negative sexual experiences of transgender identifying adolescents in the community, *Scandinavian Journal of Child and Adolescent Psychiatry and Psychology*, **8**: 166–75.

Heinonen, I., Helajärvi, H., Pahkala, K., et al. (2013) Sedentary behaviours and obesity in adults: the cardiovascular risk in young Finns study, *BMJ Open*, **3**: e002901. Doi: 10.1136/bmjopen-2013-002901.

Heitmann, B.L. and Lissner, L. (1995) Dietary underreporting by obese individuals: is it specific or nonspecific? *British Medical Journal*, **311**: 986–9.

Helgeson, V.S. (1994) Relations of agency and communion to well-being: evidence and potential explanations, *Psychological Bulletin*, **116**: 412–28.

Helweg-Larsen, M., Tobias, M.R. and Cerban, B.M. (2010) Risk perception and moralization among smokers in the USA and Denmark: a qualitative approach, *British Journal of Health Psychology*, **15**: 871–66.

Hendy, H.M., Williams, K.E., and Camise, T.S. (2005) 'Kid's choice' school lunch program increases children's fruit and vegetable acceptance, *Appetite*, **45**(3): 250–63.

Heneghan, M.B., Hussain, T., Barrera, L. et al. (2020) Applying the COM-B model to patient-reported barriers to medication adherence in pediatric acute lymphoblastic leukemia, *Pediatric Blood & Cancer*, **67**(5): e28216.

Heneghan, M. B., Hussain, T., Barrera, L., Cai, S. W., Haugen, M., Duff, A., . . . & Badawy, S. M. (2020). Applying the COM-B model to patient-reported barriers to medication adherence in pediatric acute lymphoblastic leukemia. *Pediatric Blood & Cancer*, *67*(5), e28216.

Henningsen, P., Zimmerman, T. and Sattel, H. (2003) Medically unexplained physical symptoms, anxiety, and depression: a meta-analytic review, *Psychosomatic Medicine*, **65**: 528–33.

Henson, C., Truchot, D. and Canevello, A. (2021) What promotes post traumatic growth? A systematic review, *European Journal of Trauma & Dissociation*, **5**(4): 100195.

Herlitz, A., Nilsson, L.-G. and Backman, L. (1997) Gender differences in episodic memory, *Memory and Cognition*, **25**: 801–11.

Herman C.P. and Polivy, J.A. (1988) Restraint and excess in dieters and bulimics, in K.M. Pirke, W. Vandereycken and D. Ploog (eds) *The Psychobiology of Bulimia Nervosa*. Berlin: Springer Verlag.

Herman, C.P. and Polivy, J.A. (1984) A boundary model for the regulation of eating, in A.J. Stunkard and E.Stellar (eds) *Eating and its Disorders*. New York: Raven Press.

Herman, P. and Mack, D. (1975) Restrained and unrestrained eating, *Journal of Personality*, **43**: 646–60.

Hernandez, J.H, Babazadeh, S., Anglewicz, P.A. and Akilimali, P.Z. (2022) As long as (I think) my husband agrees. . .: role of perceived partner approval in contraceptive use among couples living in military camps in Kinshasa, DRC, *Reproductive Health*, **19**(1): 1–11.

Herold, E.S. and McNamee, J.E. (1982) An explanatory model of contraceptive use among young women, *Journal of Sex Research*, **18**: 289–304.

Herold, E.S. (1981) Contraceptive embarrassment and contraceptive behaviour among young single women, *Journal of Youth and Adolescence*, **10**: 233–42.

Heron, K.E. and Smyth, J.M. (2010) Ecological momentary interventions: incorporating mobile technology into psychosocial and health behaviour treatments, *British Journal of Health Psychology*, **15**(1): 1–39.

Herz, E. (1984) Psychological repercussions of pregnancy loss, *Psychiatric Annals*, **14**: 454–7.

Herzlich, C. (1973) *Health and Illness*. London: Academic Press.

Heslop, P., Smith, G.D., Carroll, D. et al. (2001) Perceived stress and coronary heart disease risk factors: the contribution of socio-economic position, *British Journal of Health Psychology*, **6**: 167–78.

Hetherington, M.M., Anderson, A.S., Norton, G.N.M. and Newson, L. (2006) Situational effects on meal intake: a comparison of eating alone and eating with others. *Physiology and Behavior*, **88**: 498–505.

Hewson-Bower, B. and Drummond, P.D. (2001) Psychological treatment for recurrent symptoms of colds and flu in children, *Journal of Psychosomatic Research*, **51**(1): 369–77.

Hibbert, M.P., Porcellato, L.A., Brett, C.E. and Hope, V.D. (2019) Associations with drug use and sexualised drug use among women who have sex with women (WSW) in the UK: findings from the LGBT Sex and Lifestyles Survey, *International Journal of Drug Policy*, **74**: 292–98.

Higgins, A. and Conner, M. (2003) Understanding adolescent smoking: the role of the theory of planned behaviour and implementation intentions, *Psychology, Health & Medicine*, **8**(2): 173–86.

Higgs, S. and Spetter, M.S. (2018) Cognitive control of eating: the role of memory in appetite and weight gain, *Current Obesity Reports*, **7**(1): 50–59.

Higgs, S. and Woodward, M. (2009). Television watching during lunch increases afternoon snack intake of young women. *Appetite*, **52**(1): 39–43.

Higgs, S., Williamson, A.C. and Attwood, A.S. (2008a) Recall of recent lunch and its effect on subsequent snack intake. *Physiology and Behavior*, **94**(3): 454–62.

Higgs, S., Williamson, A.C., Rotshein, P. and Humphreys, G.W. (2008b) Sensory-specific satiety is intact in amnesics who eat multiple meals, *Psychological Science*, **19**(7): 623–28.

Higgs, S. (2002) Memory for recent eating and its influence on subsequent food intake. *Appetite*, **39**(2): 159–66.

Higgs, S. (2005) Memory and its role in appetite regulation. *Appetite*, **85**(1): 67–72.

Higgs, S. (2008) Cognitive influences on food intake: the effects of manipulating memory for recent eating. *Physiology and Behavior*, **94**(5): 734–9.

Hill, E.M. and Frost, A. (2020) Illness perceptions, coping, and health-related quality of life among individuals experiencing chronic Lyme disease, *Chronic Illness*, **18**(2): 426–38. Doi: 10.1177/1742395320983875.

Hill, J.O., and Peters, J.C. (1998) Environmental contributions to the obesity epidemic, *Science*, **280**(5368): 1371–4.

Hirsch, J. (1998). Magic bullet for obesity. *British Medical Journal*, **317**: 1136–8.

Hite, S. (1976) *The Hite Report.* New York: Macmillan. **Hite, S.** (1981) *The Hite Report on Male Sexuality.* New York: A.A. Knopf. **Hite, S.** (1987) *The Hite Report on Women and Love.* London: Penguin.

Hodgkins, S. and Orbell, S. (1998) Can protection motivation theory predict behaviour? A longitudinal study exploring the role of previous behaviour, *Psychology and Health*, **13**: 237–50.

Holahan, C.J. and Moos, R.H. (1990) Life stressors, resistance factors and improved psychological functioning: an extension of the stress resistance paradigm, *Journal of Personality and Social Psychology*, **58**: 909–17.

Holahan, C.J., Moerkbak, M. and Suzuki, R. (2006) Social support, coping, and depressive symptoms in cardiac illness among Hispanic and non-Hispanic white cardiac patients, *Psychology & Health*, **21**(5): 615–31.

Holahan, C.J., Moos, R.H. and Schaefer, J.A. (1996) Coping, stress resistance and growth: conceptualising adaptive functioning, in M. Zeidner and N.S. Endler (eds) *Handbook of Coping.* New York: Wiley.

Holland, J., Ramazanoglu, C. and Scott, S. (1990a) Managing risk and experiencing danger: tensions between government AIDS health education policy and young women's sexuality, *Gender and Education*, **2**: 125–46.

Holland, J., Ramazanoglu, C. and Scott, S. (1990a) Managing risk and experiencing danger: tensions between government AIDS health education policy and young women's sexuality, *Gender and Education*, **2**: 125–46.

Holland, J., Ramazanoglu, C., Scott, S. et al. (1990b) Sex, gender and power: young women's sexuality in the shadow of AIDS, *Sociology of Health and Illness*, **12**: 336–50.

Holland, K.D. and Holahan, C.K. (2003) The relation of social support and coping to positive adaptation to breast cancer, *Psychology and Health*, **18**(1): 15–29.

Hollands, G.J., Hankins, M. and Marteau, T.M. (2010) Visual feedback of individuals' medical imaging results for changing health behaviour, *Cochrane Database of Systematic Reviews*, **1**: 1–56.

Hollands, G.J., Prestwich, A. and Marteau, T.M. (2011) Using aversive images to enhance healthy food choices, *Health Psychology*, **30**(2): 195–203.

Hollier, J.M., van Tilburg, M.A., Liu, Y. et al. (2019) Multiple psychological factors predict abdominal pain severity in children with irritable bowel syndrome, *Neurogastroenterology and Motility*, **31**(2): e13509.

Hollywood, A. and Ogden, J. (2016) Gaining weight whilst taking orlistat: a qualitative study of patients at 18 months follow up, *Journal of Health Psychology*, 21: 590–8.

Hollywood, A. and Ogden, J. (2010) Taking orlistat: predicting weight loss over 6 months, *Journal of Obesity*, 806896 Open Access.

Holmes, T.H. and Rahe, R.H. (1967) The social readjustment rating scale, *Journal of Psychosomatic Research*, **11**: 213–18.

Homel, J. and Warren, D. (2019) The relationship between parent drinking and adolescent drinking: differences for mothers and fathers and boys and girls, *Substance Use & Misuse*, **54**(4): 661–69.

Hope, S., Wager, E. and Rees, M. (1998) Survey of British women's views on the menopause and HRT, *Journal of the British Menopause Society*, **4**(1): 33–6.

Hoppe, R. and Ogden, J. (1996) The effect of selectively reviewing behavioural risk factors on HIV risk perception, *Psychology and Health*, **11**: 757–64.

Hoppe, R. and Ogden, J. (1997) Practice nurses' beliefs about obesity and weight related interventions in primary care, *International Journal of Obesity*, **21**: 141–6.

Horne, R. and Clatworthy, J. (2010) Adherence to advice and treatment, in D.P. French, K., Vedhara, A.A. Kaptein. and J. Weinman (eds) *Health Psychology*, 2nd edn. Oxford: Blackwell.

Horne, R. and Weinman, J. (1999) Patients' beliefs about prescribed medicines and their role in adherence to treatment in chronic physical illness, *Journal of Psychosomatic Research*, **47**(6): 555–67.

Horne, R. and Weinman, J. (2002) Self-regulation and self-management in asthma: exploring the role of illness perceptions and treatment beliefs in explaining non-adherence to preventer medication, *Psychology and Health*, **17**(1): 17–32.

Horne, R., Buick, D., Fisher, M. et al. (2004) Doubts about necessity and concerns about adverse effects: identifying the types of beliefs that are associated with non-adherence to HAART, *International Journal of STD & AIDS*, **15**(1): 38–44.

Horne, R., Chapman, S.C., Parham, R. et al. (2013) Understanding patients' adherence-related beliefs about medicines prescribed for long-term conditions:

a meta-analytic review of the Necessity-Concerns Framework, *PloS One*, **8**(12): e80633.

Horne, R., Cooper, V., Gellaitry, G. et al. (2007) Patients' perceptions of highly active antiretroviral therapy in relation to treatment uptake and adherence: the utility of the necessity-concerns framework, *Journal of Acquired Immune Deficiency Syndromes*, **45**(3): 334–41.

Horne, R., Weinman, J. and Hankins, M. (1999) The beliefs about medicines questionnaire: the development and evaluation of a new method for assessing the cognitive representation of medication, *Psychology and Health*, **14**: 1–24.

Horne, R. (1997) Representations of medication and treatment: advances in theory and measurement, in K.J. Petrie and J.A. Weinman (eds) *Perceptions of Health and Illness: Current Research and Applications.* London: Harwood Academic Press.

Horne, R. (2001) Compliance, adherence and concordance, in K. Taylor and G. Harding (eds) *Pharmacy Practice.* London: Taylor & Francis.

Horne, R. (2006) Compliance, adherence, and concordance: implications for asthma treatment, *Chest*, **130**(1): 65–72S.

Horwitz, R.I., Viscoli, C.M., Berkman, L. et al. (1990) Treatment adherence and risk of death after a myocardial infarction, *Lancet*, **336**(8714): 542–5.

Houston, B.H. and Vavak, C.R. (1991) Cynical hostility: developmental factors, psychosocial correlates and health behaviours, *Health Psychology*, **10**: 9–17.

Howie, F.L., Henshaw, R.C., Naji, S.A. et al. (1997) Medical abortion or vacuum aspiration? Two year follow up of a patient preference trial, *British Journal of Obstetrics and Gynaecology*, **104**(7): 829–33.

Howlett, N., Schulz, J., Trivedi, D. et al. (2019) A prospective study exploring the construct and predictive validity of the COM-B model for physical activity, *Journal of Health Psychology*, **24**(10): 1378–91.

Hubert, H.B., Feinleib, M., McNamara, P.M. and Castelli, W.P. (1983) Obesity as an independent risk factor for cardiovascular disease: a 26-year follow-up of participants in the Framingham Heart Study, *Circulation*, **67**(5): 968–77.

Hudson, B.F., Ogden, J. and Whiteley, M.S. (2015) Randomised controlled trial to compare the effect of simple distraction interventions on pain and anxiety experienced during minimally invasive varicose vein surgery, *European Journal of Pain*, **19**(10): 1447–55.

Hudson, B.F., Ogden. J. and Whiteley, M.S. (2015) A thematic analysis of varicose veins and minimally invasive surgery under local anesthetic, *Journal of Clinical Nursing*, **24**: 1502–12.

Huffman, C. S., Schwartz, T. A. and Swanson, K. M. (2015) Couples and miscarriage: the influence of gender and reproductive factors on the impact of miscarriage, *Women's Health Issues*, **25**(5): 570–78.

Hughson, A., Cooper, A., McArdle, C. and Smith, D. (1986) Psychological impact of adjuvant chemotherapy in the first two years after mastectomy, *British Medical Journal*, **293**: 1268–72.

Hughson, A., Cooper, A., McArdle, C. and Smith, D. (1987) Psychosocial effects of radiotherapy after mastectomy, *British Medical Journal*, **294**: 1515–16.

Hulse, G.K. and Tait, R.J. (2002) Six-month outcomes associated with a brief alcohol intervention for adult in-patients with psychiatric disorders, *Drug and Alcohol Review* **21**(2): 105–12.

Humphris, G. and Ozakinci, G. (2008) The AFTER intervention: a structured psychological approach to reduce fears of recurrence in patients with head and neck cancer, *British Journal of Health Psychology*, **13**: 223–30.

Hunt, S.M., McEwen, J. and McKenna, S.P. (1986) *Measuring Health Status.* Beckenham: Croom Helm.

Hunt, W. A., & Bespalec, D. A. (1974). Relapse rates after treatment for heroin addiction. Journal of Community Psychology, 2(1), 85-87.

Hursti, U.K.K. and Sjoden, P.O. (1997) Food and general neophobia and their relationship with self-reported food choice: familial resemblance in Swedish families with children of ages 7–17 years, *Appetite*, **29**: 89–103.

Hutti, M.H. (1986) An exploratory study of the miscarriage experience, *Health Care for Women International*, **7**: 371–89.

Huttunen-Lenz, M., Song, F. and Poland, F. (2010) Are psychoeducational smoking cessation interventions for coronary heart disease patients effective? Meta-analysis of interventions, *British Journal of Health Psychology*, **15**: 749–77.

Idler, E.L. and Benyamini, Y. (1997) Self-rated health and mortality: a review of twenty-seven community studies, *Journal of Health and Social Behaviour*, **38**: 21–37.

Idler, E.L. and Kasl, S.V. (1995) Self-ratings of health: do they predict change in function as ability? *Journal of Gerontology Series B–Psychological Sciences and Social Sciences*, **50B**: S344–53.

Ingham, R., Woodcock, A. and Stenner, K. (1991) Getting to know you . . . young people's knowledge of their partners at first intercourse, *Journal of Community and Applied Social Psychology*, **1**: 117–32.

Ingham, R. (2005) 'We didn't cover that at school': education *against* pleasure or education *for* pleasure? *Sex Education*, **5**(4): 375–88.

Ingledew, D.K. and Ferguson, E. (2007) Personality and riskier sexual behaviour: motivational mediators, *Psychology & Health*, **22**(3): 291–315.

Ingledew, D.K., Markland, D. and Medley, A.R. (1998) Exercise motives and stages of change, *Journal of Health Psychology*, **3**(4): 477–89.

Institute of Medicine (1995) Committee to develop criteria for evaluating the outcomes of approaches to prevent and treat obesity, in *Weighing the Options: Criteria for Evaluating Weight Management Programs*, www.iom.edu.

International Longevity Centre UK (2019) *Raising the equality flag: Health inequalities among older LGBT people in the UK.* https://ilcuk.org.uk/raising-the-equality-flag-health-inequalities-among-older-lgbt-people-in-the-uk/

Irmak, C., Vallen, B. and Robinson, S.R. (2011) The impact of product name on dieters' and non dieters' food evaluations and consumption, *Journal of Consumer Research*, **38**(2): 390–405.

Ironson, G., Bira, L. and Hylton, E. (2020) Positive and negative emotional expression measured from a single written essay about trauma predicts survival 17 years later in people living with HIV, *Journal of Psychosomatic Research*, **136**: 110166.

Isaka, Y., Inada, H., Hiranuma, Y. and Ichikawa, M. (2017) Psychological impact of positive cervical cancer screening results among Japanese women, *International Journal of Clinical Oncology*, **22**(1): 102–6.

Isbell, L.M., Tager, J., Beals, K. and Liu, G. (2020) Emotionally evocative patients in the emergency department: a mixed methods investigation of providers' reported emotions and implications for patient safety, *BMJ Quality & Safety*, **29**(10), 1–2.

Isen, A.M., Rosenzweig, A.S. and Young, M.J. (1991) The influence of positive affect on clinical problem solving, *Medical Decision Making*, **11**: 221–7.

Jacks, J.Z. and Cameron, K.A. (2003) Strategies for resisting persuasion, *Basic and Applied Social Psychology*, **25**: 145–61.

Jackson, C., Eliasson, L., Barber, N. and Weinman, J. (2014) Applying COM-B to medication adherence. *European Health Psychologist*, **16**: 7–17.

Jacobs, N., Hagger, M.S., Streukens, S. et al. (2011) Testing an integrated model of the theory of planned behaviour and self-determination theory for different energy balance-related behaviours and intervention intensities, *British Journal of Health Psychology*, 16: 113–34.

Jacobs, T.J. and Charles, E. (1980) Life events and the occurrence of cancer in children, *Psychosomatic Medicine*, **42**: 11–24.

Jaggers, J.R. and Hand, G.A. (2016) Health benefits of exercise for people living with HIV: a review of the literature. *American Journal of Lifestyle Medicine*, **10**(3): 184–92.

James, J.E. and Hardardottir, D. (2002) Influence of attention focus and trait anxiety on tolerance of acute pain, *British Journal of Health Psychology*, **7**: 149–62.

James, J.E. and Keane, M.A. (2007) Caffeine, sleep and wakefulness: implications of new understanding about withdrawal reversal, *Human Psychopharmacology*, **22**(8): 549–58.

James, J.E. and Rogers, P.J. (2005) Effects of caffeine on performance and mood: withdrawal reversal is the most plausible explanation, *Psychopharmacology*, **182**: 1–8.

James, J.E., Gregg, M.E., Kane M., Harte, F. (2005) Dietary caffeine, performance and mood: enhancing and restorative effects after controlling for withdrawal relief, *Neuropsychobiology*, **52**: 1–10.

James, J.E., Kristjánsson, Á.L. and Sigfúsdóttir, I.D. (2010) Adolescent substance use, sleep, and academic achievement: evidence of harm due to caffeine, *Journal of Adolescence*, 10.1016/j.adolescence.2010.09.006.

James, J.E. (1997) *Understanding Caffeine: A Biobehavioral Analysis.* Thousand Oaks, CA: Sage.

James, J.E. (2004) Critical review of dietary caffeine and blood pressure: a relationship that should be taken more seriously, *Psychosomatic Medicine*, **66**: 63–71.

James, J.E. (2010) Caffeine, in B.A. Johnson (ed.) *Addiction Medicine*, DOI 10.1007/978-1-4419-0338-9_26.

James, J.E. (2011) Editorial: a new journal to advance caffeine research, *Journal of Caffeine Research*, **1**: 1–3.

Jamner, L.D. and Tursky, B. (1987) Syndrome-specific descriptor profiling: a psychophysiological and psychophysical approach, *Health Psychology*, **6**: 417–30.

Janis, I.L. (1967) Effects of fear arousal on attitude change: recent developments in theory and experimental research, in L. Berkowitz (ed.) *Advances in Experimental Social Psychology*. San Diego, CA: Academic Press.

Janoff-Bulman, R. (2004) Posttraumatic growth: three explanatory models, *Psychological Inquiry*, **15**: 30–4.

Janssen, V., De Gucht, V., van Exel, H. and Maes, S. (2013) Changes in illness perceptions and quality of life during participation in cardiac rehabilitation, *International Journal of Behavioral Medicine*, **20**(4): 582–9.

Jarman, M., Ogden, J., Inskip, H. et al. (2015) How do mothers control their preschool children's eating habits and does this change as children grow older? A longitudinal analysis, *Appetite*, **95**: 466–74.

Jastreboff, A.M., Aronne, L.J., Ahmad, N.N. et al. (2022) Tirzepatide once weekly for the treatment of obesity, *The New England Journal of Medicine*, 10.1056/NEJMoa2206038.

Jebb, S.A., Prentice, A.M., Goldberg, G.R. et al. (1996) Changes in macronutrient balance during over feeding and under feeding assessed by 12 day continuous whole body calorimetry, *American Journal of Clinical Nutrition*, **64**: 259–66.

Jefferis, B.J., Parsons, T.J., Sartini, C. et al. (2018) Objectively measured physical activity, sedentary behaviour and all-cause mortality in older men: does volume of activity matter more than pattern of accumulation? *British Journal of Sports Medicine*, Epub ahead of print: doi: 10.1136/bjsports-2017-098733.

Jefferis, B.J., Sartini, C., Lee, I.M. et al. (2014) Adherence to physical activity guidelines in older adults, using objectively measured physical activity in a population-based study, *BMC Public Health*, **14**(1): 382.

Jeffery, R.W., Drewnowski, A., Epstein, L.H. et al. (2000) Long-term maintenance of weight loss: current status, *Health Psychology*, **19**: 5–16.

Jessop, D.C., Simmonds, L.V. and Sparks, P. (2009) Motivational and behavioral consequences of self-affirmation interventions: a study of sunscreen use among women, *Psychology and Health*, **24**: 529–44.

Jiang, X., Wang, J., Lu, Y. et al. (2019) Self-efficacy-focused education in persons with diabetes: a systematic review and meta-analysis, *Psychology Research and Behavior Management*, **12**: 67–79.

Jim, H.S. and Andersen, B.L. (2007) Meaning in life mediates the relationship between social and physical functioning and distress in cancer survivors, *British Journal of Health Psychology*, **12**(3): 363–81.

Jirojanakul, P. and Skevington, S. (2000) Developing a quality of life measure for children aged 5–8 years, *British Journal of Health Psychology*, **5**: 299–321.

Joekes, K., Maes, S. and Warrens, M. (2007) Predicting quality of life and self-management from dyadic support and overprotection after myocardial infarction, *British Journal of Health Psychology*, **12**(4): 473–89.

Johnston, D.W., Beedie, A. and Jones, M.C. (2006) Using computerized ambulatory diaries for the assessment of job characteristics and work-related stress in nurses, *Work & Stress*, **20**(2): 163–72.

Johnston, D.W., Cook, D.G. and Shaper, A.G. (1987) Type A behaviour and ischaemic heart disease in middle-aged British men, *British Medical Journal*, **295**: 86–9.

Johnston, D.W., Gold, A., Kentish, J. et al. (1993) Effect of stress management on blood pressure in mild primary hypertension, *British Medical Journal*, **306**: 963–6.

Johnston, D.W. (1989) Will stress management prevent coronary heart disease? *The Psychologist: Bulletin of British Psychological Society*, **7**: 275–8.

Johnston, D.W. (1992) The management of stress in the prevention of coronary heart disease, in S. Maes, H. Leventhal and M. Johnston (eds) *International Review of Health Psychology*. Chichester: Wiley.

Johnston, D.W. (2002) Acute and chronic psychological processes in cardiovascular disease, in K.W. Schaie, H. Leventhal and S.L. Willis (eds) *Effective Health Behaviour in Older Adults*. New York: Springer.

Johnston, D.W. (2002) Acute and chronic psychological processes in cardiovascular disease, in K.W. Schaie, H. Leventhal and S.L. Willis (eds), *Effective Health Behaviour in Older Adults*, pp. 55–64. New York: Springer.

Johnston, K.L. and White, K.M. (2003) Binge-drinking: a test of the role of group norms in the theory of planned behaviour, *Psychology and Health*, **18**(1): 63–77.

Johnston, M., Bonetti, D., Joice, S. et al. (2006) Recovery from disability after stroke as a target behavioural intervention: results of a randomized controlled trial, *Disability & Rehabilitation*, **29**(14): 1117–27.

Johnston, M., Foulkes, J., Johnston, D.W., et al. (1999b) Impact on patient and partners of inpatient and extended cardiac counselling and rehabilitation: a controlled trial, *Psychosomatic Medicine*, **61**: 225–33.

Johnston, M., Pollard, B., Morrison, V and Macwalter, R. (2004) Functional limitations of survival following stroke: psychological and clinical predictors of 3-year outcome, *International Journal of Behavioral Medicine*, **11**(4): 187–96.

Jokela, M., Batty, G.D., Hintsa, T. et al. (2014) Is personality associated with cancer incidence and mortality? An individual-participant meta-analysis of 2156 incident cancer cases among 42 843 men and women, *British Journal of Cancer*, **110**(7): 1820–4.

Jonas, K., Stroebe, W. and Eagly, A. (1993) Adherence to an exercise program, unpublished manuscript, University of Tübingen.

Jones, C.J., Smith, H. and Llewellyn, C. (2014) Evaluating the effectiveness of health belief model interventions in improving adherence: a systematic review. *Health Psychology Review*, **8**(3): 253–69.

Jones, C.J., Smith, H.E. and Llewellyn, C.D. (2016) A systematic review of the effectiveness of interventions using the common sense self-regulatory model to improve adherence behaviours, *Journal of Health Psychology*, **21**(11): 2709–24.

Jones, R.K., Purcell, A., Singh, S. and Finer, L.B. (2005) Adolescents' reports of parental knowledge of adolescents' use of sexual health services and their reactions tomandated parental notification for prescription contraception, *Journal of the American Medical Association*, **293**(3): 340–8.

Jones RK and Jerman J, Population Group Abortion Rates and Lifetime Incidence of Abortion: United States, 2008–2014, American Journal of Public Health, 2017.

Joo, N.-S. and Kim, B.-T. (2007) Mobile phone short message service messaging for behaviour modification in a community-based weight control programme in Korea, *Journal of Telemedicine and Telecare*, **13**(8): 416–20.

Junge, C., von Soest, T., Weidner, K. et al. (2018) Labor pain in women with and without severe fear of childbirth: a population-based, longitudinal study, *Birth: Issues in Perinatal Care*, doi: 10.1111/birt.12349

Kahn, E., Ramsey, L.T., Brownson R.C. et al. (2002) The effectiveness of interventions to increase physical activity: a systematic review. *American Journal of Preventive Medicine*, **22**(4S): 73–107.

Kalat, J.W. and Rozin, P. (1973) 'Learned safety' as a mechanism in long-delay taste-aversion learning in rats, *Journal of Comparative and Physiological Psychology*, **83**(2): 198–207.

Kaluza, G. (2000) Changing unbalanced coping profiles: a prospective controlled intervention trial in worksite health promotion, *Psychology and Health*, **15**: 423–33.

Kahneman D, Tversky A (1972). Subjective probability: A judgment of representativeness. *Cognitive Psychology*. **3** (3): 430–454. doi:10.1016/0010-0285(72)90016-3

Kahneman D, Tversky A (July 1996). On the reality of cognitive illusions. *Psychological Review*. **103**(3): 582–91, discussion 592–6.

Kang, J. and Lin, C.A. (2015) Effects of message framing and visual-fear appeals on smoker responses to antismoking ads, *Journal of Health Communication*, **20**(6): 647–55.

Kang, K., Gholizadeh, L. and Han, H.R. (2021) Health-related quality of life and its predictors in Korean patients with myocardial infarction in the acute phase, *Clinical Nursing Research*, **30**(2): 161–70.

Kannan, A., Kirkman, M., Ruseckaite, R. and Evans, S.M. (2019) Prostate care and prostate cancer from the perspectives of undiagnosed men: a systematic review of qualitative research, *BMJ open*, **9**(1): e022842.

Kanner, A.D., Coyne, J.C., Schaeffer, C. and Lazarus, R.S. (1981) Comparison of two modes of stress measurement: daily hassles and uplifts versus major life events, *Journal of Behavioural Medicine*, **4**: 1–39.

Kaplan, J.R., Manuck, S.B., Clarkson, T.B. et al. (1983) Social stress and atherosclerosis in normocholesterolemic monkeys, *Science*, **220**: 733–5.

Kara, W.S.K., Benedicto, M. and Mao, J. (2019) Knowledge, attitude, and practice of contraception methods among female undergraduates in Dodoma, Tanzania, *Cureus*, **11**(4): e4362.

Karamanidou, C., Weinman, J. and Horne, R. (2008) Improving haemodialysis patients' understanding of phosphate-binding medication: a pilot study of a psycho-educational intervention designed to change

patients' perceptions of the problem and treatment, *British Journal of Health Psychology*, **13**: 205–14.

Karasek, R. and Theorell, T. (1990) *Healthy Work: Stress, Productivity and the Reconstruction of Working Life*. New York: Basic Books.

Karasek, R.A., Theorell, T., Schwartz, J. et al. (1988) Job characteristics in relation to the prevalence of myocardial infarction in the U.S. HES and HANES, *American Journal of Public Health*, **78**: 910–18.

Karlsson, J., Sjöström, L. and Sullivan, M. (1998) Swedish obese subjects (SOS)–an intervention study of obesity: two-year follow-up of health related quality of life (HRQL) and eating behaviour after gastric surgery for severe obesity, *International Journal of Obesity*, **22**: 113–26.

Karmali, S., Brar, B., Shi, X. et al. (2013) Weight recidivism post-bariatric surgery: a systematic review, *Obesity Surgery*, **23**(11): 1922–33. doi: 10.1007/s11695-013-1070-4.

Kasl, S.V. and Cobb, S. (1966) Health behaviour, illness behaviour, and sick role behaviour: II. Sick role behaviour, *Archives of Environmental Health*, **12**: 531–41.

Katz, I.T., Ryu, A.E., Onuegbu, A.G. et al. (2013) Impact of HIV-related stigma on treatment adherence: systematic review and meta-synthesis, *Journal of the International AIDS Society*, **16**: 18640.

Katz, S., Downs, T.D., Cash, H.R. and Grotz, R.C. (1970) Progress in development of the index of ADL, *Gerontology*, **10**: 20–30.

Kauffman, S.E., Silver, P. and Poulin, J. (1997) Gender differences in attitudes toward alcohol, tobacco, and other drugs, *Social Work*, **42**(3): 231–41.

Kaushal, N., Rhodes, R.E., Meldrum, J.T. and Spence, J.C. (2017) The role of habit in different phases of exercise, *British Journal of Health Psychology*, **22**(3): 429–48.

Keefe, F.J., Lefebvre, J.C., Egert, J.R. et al. (2000) The relationship of gender to pain, pain behaviour and disability in osteoarthritis patients: the role of catastrophizing, *Pain*, **87**: 325–34.

Keller, I. and Abraham, C. (2005) Randomized controlled trial of a brief research-based intervention promoting fruit and vegetable consumption, *British Journal of Health Psychology*, **10**: 543–58.

Keller, J., Knoll, N., Gellert, P. et al. (2016). Self-efficacy and planning as predictors of physical activity in the context of workplace health promotion, *Applied Psychology: Health And Well-Being*, **8**(3): 301–21.

Keller, J., Knoll, N., Gellert, P. et al. (2016) Self-efficacy and planning as predictors of physical activity in the context of workplace health promotion. *Applied Psychology: Health and Well-Being*, **8**(3): 301–21.

Keller, J., Knoll, N., Gellert, P., Schneider, M. and Ernsting, A. (2016) Self-efficacy and planning as predictors of physical activity in the context of workplace health promotion, *Applied Psychology: Health And Well-Being,* **3**(3): 301–21.

Kelley, H.H. (1967) Attribution theory in social psychology, in D. Levine (ed.) *Nebraska Symposium on Motivation.* Lincoln, NE: University of Nebraska Press.

Kelley, H.H. (1971) *Attribution: Perceiving the Causes of Behaviour.* New York: General Learning Press.

Kemp, S., Morley, S. and Anderson, E. (1999) Coping with epilepsy: do illness representations play a role? *British Journal of Clinical Psychology,* **38**: 43–58.

Kennedy, P., Duff, J., Evans, M. and Beedie, A. (2003) Coping effectiveness training reduces depression and anxiety following traumatic spinal cord injuries, *British Journal of Clinical Psychology,* **42**(Pt 1): 41–52.

Kennedy, P., Lude, P., Elfström, M.L. and Smithson, E. (2010) Sense of coherence and psychological outcomes in people with spinal cord injury: appraisals and behavioural responses, *British Journal of Health Psychology,* **15**(3): 611–21.

Kero, A., Högberg, U. and Lalos, A. (2004) Wellbeing and mental growth: long-term effects of legal abortion, *Social Science and Medicine,* **58**: 2559–69.

Kerr, J., Eves, F.F. and Carroll, D. (2001) The influence of poster prompts on stair use: the effects of setting, poster size and content, *British Journal of Health Psychology,* **6**: 397–405.

Ketonen, M., Pajunen, P., Koukkunen, H. et al. (2008) Long-term prognosis after coronary artery bypass surgery, *International Journal of Cardiology,* **124**(1): 72–9.

Keyes, K.M., Jager, J., Mal-Sarkar, T. et al. (2019) Is there a recent epidemic of women's drinking? A critical review of national studies, *Alcoholism: Clinical and Experimental Research,* **43**(7): 1344–59.

Keys, A., Brozek, J., Henscel, A. et al. (1950) *The Biology of Human Starvation.* Minneapolis, MN: University of Minnesota Press.

Keys, A., Taylor, H.L., Blackburn, H. et al. (1971) Mortality and coronary heart disease among men studied for 23 years, *Archives of Internal Medicine,* **128**: 201–14.

Khaw, K.T., Wareham, N., Bingham, S. et al. (2008) Combined impact of health behaviours and mortality in men and women: the EPIC-Norfolk prospective population study, *PLos Medicine,* **5**(12).

Kidd, T. and Sheffield, D. (2005) Attachment style and symptom reporting: examining the mediating effects of anger and social support, *British Journal of Health Psychology,* **10**: 531–41.

Kiebert, G., de Haes, J. and van der Velde, C. (1991) The impact of breast conserving treatment and mastectomy on the quality of life of early stage breast cancer patients: a review, *Journal of Clinical Oncology,* **9**: 1059–70.

Kiecolt-Glaser, J.K. and Glaser, R. (1986) Psychological influences on immunity, *Psychosomatics,* **27**: 621–4.

Kiecolt-Glaser, J.K., Marucha, P.T., Malarkey, W.B. et al. (1995) Slowing wound healing by psychosocial stress, *Lancet,* **4**: 1194–6.

Killick, S. and Allen, C. (1997) 'Shifting the balance': motivational interviewing to help behaviour change in people with bulimia nervosa, *European Eating Disorders Review,* **5**(1): 33–41.

King N.S. and Kirwilliam, S. (2011) Permanent post-concussion symptoms after mild head injury, *Brain Injury,* **25**: 462–70.

King, A.C., Ahn, D.K. Oliveira, B.M. et al. (2008) Promoting physical activity through hand-held computer technology, *American Journal of Preventive Medicine,* **34**(2): 138–42.

King, A.C., Blair, S.N., Bild, D.E. et al. (1992) Determinants of physical activity and interventions in adults, *Medicine and Science in Sports and Exercise,* **24**: S221–37.

King, D., Hume, P.A., Hardaker, N. et al. (2019) Sports-related injuries in New Zealand: National Insurance (Accident Compensation Corporation) claims for five sporting codes from 2012 to 2016, *British Journal of Sports Medicine,* **53**(16): 1026–33.

King, L. and Hill, A.J. (2008) Magazine adverts for healthy and less healthy foods: effects on recall but not hunger or food choice by pre-adolescent children, *Appetite,* **51**(1): 194–7.

King, W.C., Chen, J.Y., Courcoulas, A.P. et al. (2017) Alcohol and other substance use after bariatric surgery: prospective evidence from a US multicenter cohort study, *Surgery for Obesity and Related Disease,* **13**(8): 1392–402.

Kinlay, S. (1988) High cholesterol levels: is screening the best option? *Medical Journal of Australia,* **148**: 635–7.

Kinsey, A., Pomeroy, W. and Martin, C. (1948) *Sexual Behaviour in the Human Male.* London: Saunders.

Kirsch, I. (2019) Placebo effect in the treatment of depression and anxiety, *Frontiers in Psychiatry,* **10**: 407.

Kissen, D.M. (1966) The significance of personality in lung cancer in men, *Annals of the New York Academy of Sciences,* **125**: 820–6.

Kivimaki, M., Leino-Arjas, P., Luukkonem, R. et al. (2002) Work stress and risk of cardiovascular mortality: prospective cohort study of industrial employees, *British Medical Journal,* **325**: 857–60.

Kjelsvik, M., Sekse, R.J.T., Moi, A.L. et al. (2018) Women's experiences when unsure about whether or not to have an abortion in the first trimester, *Health Care for Women International,* **39**(7): 784–807.

Klassen, A., Fitzpatrick, R., Jenkinson, C. and Goodacre, T. (1996) Should breast reduction surgery be rationed? A comparison of the health status of patients before and after treatment: postal question-naire survey, *British Medical Journal,* **313:** 454–7.

Klesges, R.C., Stein, R.J., Eck, L.H. et al. (1991) Parental influences on food selection in young children and its relationships to childhood obesity, *American Journal of Clinical Nutrition,* **53:** 859–64.

Klier, C.M., Geller, P.A. and Neugebauer, R. (2000) Minor depressive disorder in the context of miscarriage, *Journal of Affective Disorders,* **59:** 13–21.

Kneebone, I.I. and Martin, P.R. (2003) Coping and caregivers of people with dementia, *British Journal of Health Psychology,* **8:** 1–17.

Knight, R.E., Chabot, C., Carson, A. et al. (2019) Qualitative analysis of the experiences of gay, bisexual and other men who have sex with men who use GetCheckedOnline. com: a comprehensive internet-based diagnostic service for HIV and other STIs, *Sexually Transmitted Infections,* **95**(2): 145–50.

Knowles, S.R., Apputhurai, P., O'Brien et al. (2020) Exploring the relationships between illness perceptions, self-efficacy, coping strategies, psychological distress and quality of life in a cohort of adults with diabetes mellitus, *Psychology, Health & Medicine,* **25**(2): 214–28.

Koevska, V., Nikolikj-Dimitrova, E., Mitrevska, B. et al. (2019) Effect of exercises on quality of life in patients with postmenopausal osteoporosis–randomized trial, *Open Access Macedonian Journal of Medical Sciences,* **7**(7): 1160–65.

Kohlmann, C.W., Ring, C., Carroll, D. et al. (2001) Cardiac coping style, heartbeat detection, and the interpretation of cardiac events, *British Journal of Health Psychology,* **6:** 285–301.

Kolakowsky-Hayner, S.A., Gourley, E.V., Kreuter, J.S. et al. (1999) Pre-injury substance abuse among persons with brain injury and person with spinal cord injury, *Brain Injury,* **13:** 571–81.

Kolay, E., Bykowska-Derda, A., Abdulsamad, S. et al. (2021) Self-reported eating speed is associated with indicators of obesity in adults: a systematic review and meta-analysis, *Healthcare,* **9**(11): 1559.

Kolehmainen, N., Francis, J.J., Ramsay, C.R. et al. (2011) Participation in physical play and leisure: developing a theory- and evidence-based intervention for children with motor impairments, *BMC Pediatrics,* **11:** 100.

Kopelman, P. (1999) Treatment of obesity V: pharmacotherapy for obesity, in *Obesity: The Report of the British Nutrition Foundation Task Force.* Oxford: Blackwell Science.

Kposowa, A.J. (2000) Marital status and suicide in the National Longitudinal Mortality Study, *Journal of Epidemiology and Community Health,* **54:** 254–61.

Kral, J.G. (1995) Surgical interventions for obesity, in K.D. Brownell and C.G. Fairburn (eds) *Eating Disorders and Obesity.* New York: Guilford Press.

Krasnoryadtseva, A., Dalbeth, N. and Petrie, K. (2020) Does seeing personal medical images change beliefs about illness and treatment in people with gout? A randomised controlled trial, *Psychology & Health,* **35**(1): 107–23.

Kripalini, S., Yao, X. and Haynes, R.B. (2007) Interventions to enhance medication adherence in chronic medical consultations: a systematic review, *Archives of Internal Medicine,* **167:** 540–50.

Kruk, J., Aboul-Enein, B.H., Bernstein, J. and Gronostaj, M. (2019) Psychological stress and cellular aging in cancer: a meta-analysis, *Oxidative Medicine and Cellular Longevity,* doi: 10.1155/2019/1270397.

Kubicek, K., McNeeley, M. and Collins, S. (2015) Same-sex relationship in a straight world: individual and societal influences on power and control in young men's relationships, *Journal of Interpersonal Violence,* **30**(1): 83–109.

Kuh, D., Cooper, R., Moore, A. et al. (2018) Age at menopause and lifetime cognition: findings from a British birth cohort study, *Neurology,* **90**(19): e1673-e1681.

Kuh, D.J., Hardy, R. and Wadsworth, M.E.J. (2000) Social and behavioural influences on the uptake of hormone replacement therapy among younger women, *BJOG: An International Journal of Obstetrics and Gynaecology,* **107**(6): 731–9.

Kuijer, R.G. and DeRidder, D.T.D. (2003) Discrepancy in illness-related goals and quality of life in chronically ill patients: the role of self efficacy, *Psychology and Health,* **18**(3): 313–30.

Kumar, R. and Robson, K. (1987) Previous induced abortion and ante-natal depression in primiparae: preliminary report of a survey of mental health in pregnancy, *Psychological Medicine,* **8:** 711–15.

Kunkel, E., Bakker, J., Myers, R. et al. (2000) Biopsychosocial aspects of prostate cancer, *Psychosomatics,* **41:** 85–94.

Kwah, K.L., Fulton, E.A. and Brown, K.E. (2019) Accessing national health service stop smoking services in the UK: a COM-B analysis of barriers and facilitators perceived by smokers, ex-smokers and stop smoking advisors, *Public Health,* **171:** 123–30.

Kwasnicka, D., Dombrowski, S.U., White, M. and Sniehotta, F. (2016) Theoretical explanations for maintenance of behaviour change: a systematic review of behaviour theories. *Health Psychology Review,* **10**(3): 277–96.

Lachowsky, N.J., Brennan, D.J., Berlin, G.W. et al. (2021) A mixed method analysis of differential reasons for condom use and non-use among gay, bisexual, and other men who have sex with men, *The Canadian Journal of Human Sexuality,* **30**(1): 65–77.

Lachowsky, N.J., Tanner, Z., Cui, Z. et al. (2016) 'An event-level analysis of condom use during anal intercourse among self-reported human immunodeficiency virus-negative gay and bisexual men in a treatment as prevention environment', *Sexually Transmitted Diseases*, **43**(12): 765–70.

Lader, D. and Matheson, J. (1991) *Smoking Among Secondary School Children in England (1990): An Enquiry Carried out by the Social Survey Division of OPCS*. London: HMSO.

Laerum, E., Johnsen, N., Smith, P. and Larsen, S. (1988) Myocardial infarction can induce positive changes in lifestyle and in the quality of life, *Scandinavian Journal of Primary Health Care*, **6**: 67–71.

Laessle, R.G., Lehrke, S., and Dückers, S. (2007) Laboratory eating behavior in obesity, *Appetite*, **49**: 399–404.

Lalas, J., Garbers, S., Gold, M.A. et al. (2020) Young men's communication with partners and contraception use: a systematic review, *Journal of Adolescent Health*, **67**(3): 342–53.

Lam, L.T., Ross, F.I. and Cass, D.T. (1999) Children at play: the death and injury pattern in New South Wales, Australia, July 1990–June 1994, *Journal of Paediatrics and Child Health*, **35**: 572–7.

Lane, D., Carroll, D., Ring, C. et al. (2000) Effects of depression and anxiety on mortality and quality of life 4 months after myocardial infarction, *Journal of Psychosomatic Research*, **49**: 229–38.

Lane, D., Carroll, D., Ring, C. et al. (2002) The prevalence and persistence of depression and anxiety following myocardial infarction, *British Journal of Health Psychology*, **7**: 11–21.

Langer, R.D., Hodis, H.N., Lobo, R.A. and Allison, M.A. (2021) Hormone replacement therapy–where are we now? *Climacteric*, **24**(1): 3–10.

Laranjo, L., Ding, D., Heleno, B. et al. (2021) Do smartphone applications and activity trackers increase physical activity in adults? Systematic review, meta-analysis and metaregression, *British Journal of Sports Medicine*, **55**(8): 422–32.

Larsson, G., Spangberg, L., Lindgren, S. and Bohlin, A.B. (1990) Screening for HIV in pregnant women: a study of maternal opinion, *AIDS Care*, **2**: 223–8.

Larun, L., Nordheim, L.V., Ekeland, E. et al. (2006) Exercise in prevention and treatment of anxiety and depression among children and young people, *Cochrane Database of Systematic Reviews*, **3**, Art. No.: CD004691. Doi: 10.1002/14651858.CD004691.pub2.

Lashley, M.E. (1987) Predictors of breast self-examination practice among elderly women, *Advances in Nursing Science*, **9**: 25–34.

Lau, J., Lim, T.Z., Wong, G.J. and Tan, K.K. (2020) The health belief model and colorectal cancer screening in the general population: a systematic review, *Preventive Medicine Reports*, **20**: 101223.

Lau, J.F., Wu, X., Wu, A.S. et al. (2017) Relationships between illness perception and post-traumatic growth among newly diagnosed HIV-positive men who have sex with men in China. *AIDS and Behavior*, doi: 10.1007/s10461-017-1874-7

Lau, R., Bernard, J.M. and Hartman, K.A. (1989) Further explanations of common sense representations of common illnesses, *Health Psychology*, **8**: 195–219.

Lau, R. (1995) Cognitive representations of health and illness, in D. Gochman (ed.) *Handbook of Health Behavior Research*, vol. I. New York: Plenum.

Laudenslager, M.L., Ryan, S.M., Drugan, R.C. et al. (1983) Coping and immunosuppression: inescapable but not escapable shock suppresses lymphocyte proliferation, *Science*, **221**: 568–70.

Lawman, H.G. and Wilson, D.K. (2014) Associations of social and environmental supports with sedentary behavior, light and moderate-to-vigorous physical activity in obese underserved adolescents. *International Journal of Behavioral Nutrition and Physical Activity*, **11**(1): 92.

Lawson, V.L., Lyne, P.A., Bundy, C. and Harvey, J.N. (2007) The role of illness perceptions, coping and evaluation in care-seeking among people with type 1 diabetes, *Psychology and Health*, **22**(2): 175–91.

Lawton, M.P., Moss, M. and Glicksman, A. (1990) The quality of life in the last year of life of older persons, *The Millbank Quarterly*, **68**: 1–28.

Lawton, R., Conner, M. and McEachan, R. (2009) Desire or reason: predicting health behaviors from affective and cognitive attitudes, *Health Psychology*, **28**(1): 56–65.

Lazarus, R.S. and Cohen, F. (1973) Active coping processes, coping dispositions, and recovery from surgery, *Psychosomatic Medicine*, **35**: 375–89.

Lazarus, R.S. and Folkman, S. (1987) Transactional theory and research on emotions and coping, *European Journal of Personality*, **1**: 141–70.

Lazarus, R.S. and Launier, R. (1978) Stress-related transactions between person and environment, in L.A. Pervin and M. Lewis (eds) *Perspectives in International Psychology*. New York: Plenum.

Lazarus, R.S. (1975) A cognitively oriented psychologist looks at biofeedback, *American Psychologist*, **30**: 553–61.

Lea, T., Anning, M., Wagner, S. et al. (2019) Barriers to accessing HIV and sexual health services among gay men in Tasmania, Australia, *Journal of Gay & Lesbian Social Services*, **31**(2): 153–65.

Lean, M.E.J., Han, T.S. and Morrison, C.E. (1995) Waist circumference as a measure for indicating need for weight management, *British Medical Journal*, **311**: 158–61.

Leary, M.R., Rapp, S.R., Herbst, K.C. et al. (1998) Interpersonal concerns and psychological difficulties of psoriasis patients: effects of disease severity and fear of negative evaluation, *Health Psychology*, **17**: 530–6.

Lee, C. and Glynn Owens, R. (2002) *The Psychology of Men's Health*. Maidenhead: Open University Press.

Lee, C.J., Collins, K.A. and Burgess, S.E. (1999) Suicide under the age of eighteen: a 10-year retrospective study, *American Journal of Forensic Medicine and Pathology*, **20**: 27–30.

Lee, E. (2003) Tensions in the regulation of abortion in Britain, *Journal of Law and Society*, **30**: 532–53.

Lee, E., Clements, S., Ingham, R. and Stone, N. (2004) *A Matter of Choice? Explaining National Variations in Teenage Abortion and Motherhood*. York: Joseph Rowntree Foundation.

Lee, I.M., Shiroma, E.J., Lobelo, F. et al. (2012) Effect of physical inactivity on major non-communicable diseases worldwide: an analysis of burden of disease and life expectancy, *Lancet*, **380**(9838): 219–29. Doi: 10.1016/S0140-6736(12)61031-9.

Lee, S. and Waters, S.F. (2021) Asians and Asian Americans' experiences of racial discrimination during the COVID-19 pandemic: impacts on health outcomes and the buffering role of social support. *Stigma and Health*, **6**(1): 70–78.

Lee, T.J., Cameron, L.D., Wünsche, B. and Stevens, C. (2011) A randomized trial of computer-based communications using imagery and text information to alter representations of heart disease risk and motivate protective behaviour, *British Journal of Health Psychology*, **16**(1): 72–91.

Leforge, R.G., Velicer, W.F., Richmond, R.L. and Owen, N. (1999) Stage distributions for five health behaviours in the United States and Australia, *Preventive Medicine*, **28**: 61–74.

Leknes, S. and Bastian, B. (2014) The benefits of pain, *Review of Philosophy and Psychology*, **5**(1): 57–70.

Lepper, M., Sagotsky, G., Dafoe, J.L. and Greene, D. (1982) Consequences of superfluous social constraints: effects on young children's social inferences and subsequent intrinsic interest, *Journal of Personality and Social Psychology*, **42**: 51–65.

Lerman, C., Hughes, C., Croyle, R.T. et al. (2000) Prophylactic surgery and surveillance practices one year following BRCA1/2 genetic testing, *Preventative Medicine*, **1**: 75–80.

LeRoy, A.S., Murdock, K.W., Jaremka, L.M. et al. (2017) Loneliness predicts self-reported cold symptoms after a viral challenge, *Health Psychology*, **36**(5): 512–20.

Lett, H. S., Blumenthal, J. A., Babyak, M. A., Strauman, T. J., Robins, C., & Sherwood, A. (2005). Social support and coronary heart disease: epidemiologic evidence and implications for treatment. *Psychosomatic medicine*, *67*(6), 869–878. https://doi.org/10.1097/01.psy.0000188393.73571.0a

Leung, M.Y., Liang, Q. and Olomolaiye, P. (2015) Impact of job stressors and stress on the safety behavior and accidents of construction workers. *Journal of Management in Engineering*, **32**(1): 04015019.

Levenstein, J.H., McCracken, E.C., McWhinney, I.R. et al. (1986) The patient centred clinical method, part 1: a model for the doctor–patient interaction in family medicine, *Family Practice*, **3**: 24–30.

Leventhal, H. and Nerenz, D. (1985) The assessment of illness cognition, in P. Karoly (ed.) *Measurement Strategies in Health Psychology*. New York: Wiley.

Leventhal, H., Benyamini, Y. and Shafer, C. (2007b) Lay beliefs about health and illness, in S. Ayers (ed.) *Cambridge Handbook of Psychology, Health and Medicine*. Cambridge: Cambridge University Press.

Leventhal, H., Meyer, D. and Nerenz, D. (1980) The common sense representation of illness danger, *Medical Psychology*, **2**: 7–30.

Leventhal, H., Weinman, J., Leventhal, E.A. and Phillips, L.A. (2007a) Health psychology: the search for pathways between behaviour and health, *Annual Review of Psychology*, **59**: 8.1–29.

Lewer, D., Jayatunga, W., Aldridge, R.W. et al. (2020) Premature mortality attributable to socioeconomic inequality in England between 2003 and 2018: an observational study, *The Lancet. Public health*, **5**(1): e33–e41. Doi.org/10.1016/S2468-2667(19)30219-1

Ley, P. and Morris, L.A. (1984) Psychological aspects of written information for patients, in S. Rachman (ed.) *Contributions to Medical Psychology*. Oxford: Pergamon Press.

Ley, P. (1988) *Communicating with Patients*. London: Croom Helm.

Ley, P. (1989) Improving patients' understanding, recall, satisfaction and compliance, in A. Broome (ed.) *Health Psychology*. London: Chapman & Hall.

Lichtenstein, E., Weiss, S.M., Hitchcock, J.L. et al. (1986) Task force 3: patterns of smoking relapse, *Health Psychology*, **5**: 29–40.

Lifson, A., Hessol, N., Rutherford, G.W. et al. (1989) The natural history of HIV infection in a cohort of homosexual and bisexual men: clinical manifestations, 1978–1989. Paper presented to the 5th International Conference on AIDS, Montreal, September.

Lind, E., Ekkekakis, P. and Vazou, S. (2008) The affective impact of exercise intensity that slightly exceeds the preferred level, *Journal of Health Psychology*, **13**(4): 464–8.

Lindemann, C. (1977) Factors affecting the use of contraception in the nonmarital context, in R. Gemme and C.C. Wheeler (eds) *Progress in Sexology*. New York: Plenum.

Lindson, N., Thompson, T.P., Ferrey, A. et al. (2019) Motivational interviewing for smoking cessation, *Cochrane Database of Systematic Reviews*, (**7**), CD006936.

Linn, A.J., van Dijk, L., Smit, E.G. et al. (2013) May you never forget what is worth remembering: the relation between recall of medical information and medication adherence in patients with inflammatory bowel disease, *Journal of Crohn's and Colitis*, **7**(11): e543–e550.

Linton, S.J., Buer, N., Vlaeyen, J. and Hellising, A. (2000) Are fear-avoidance beliefs related to the inception of an episode of back pain? A prospective study, *Psychology and Health*, **14**: 1051–9.

Lipkus, I.M., Barefoot, J.C., Williams, R.B. and Siegler, I.C. (1994) Personality measures as predictors of smoking initiation and cessation in the UNC Alumni Heart study, *Health Psychology*, **13**: 149–55.

Lippke, S. and Plotnikoff, R.C. (2009) The protection motivation theory within the stages of the transtheoretical model–stage-specific interplay of variables and prediction of exercise stage transitions, *British Journal of Health Psychology*, **14**(2): 211–29.

Lissner, L., Odell, P.M., D'Agostino, R.B. et al. (1991) Variability of body weight and health outcomes in the Framingham population, *New England Journal of Medicine*, **324**: 1839–44.

Little, P., Griffin, S., Kelly, J. et al. (1998) Effect of educational leaflets and questions on knowledge of contraception in women taking the combined contraceptive pill: randomised control trial, *British Medical Journal*, **316**(7149): 1948–52.

Liu, J., Zhao, S., Chen, X. et al. (2017). The influence of peer behaviour as a function of social and cultural closeness: a meta-analysis of normative influence on adolescent smoking initiation and continuation. *Psychological Bulletin*, **143**(10): 1082.

Llewellyn, C.D. Miners, A.H., Lee, C.A. et al. (2003) The illness perceptions and treatment beliefs of individuals with severe haemophilia and their role in adherence to home treatment, *Psychology and Health*, **18**: 185–200.

Lohan, M. (2010) Developing a critical men's health debate in academic scholarship, in B. Gough and S. Robertson (eds) *Men, Masculinities and Health, Critical Perspectives*. Basingstoke: Palgrave Macmillan.

Lonergan, A. (2016) The effectiveness of cognitive behavioural therapy for pain in childhood and adolescence: a meta-analytic review. *Irish Journal of Psychological Medicine*, **33**(4): 251–64.

Long, S., Meye, C., Leung, N. and Wallis, D.J. (2011) Effects of distraction and focused attention on actual and perceived food intake in females with non-clinical eating psychopathology. *Appetite*, **56**: 350–6.

Lööw, J. and Nygren, M. (2019) Initiatives for increased safety in the Swedish mining industry: studying 30 years of improved accident rates, *Safety Science*, **117**, 437–46.

Loro, A.D. and Orleans, C.S. (1981) Binge eating in obesity: preliminary findings and guidelines for behavioural analysis and treatment, *Addictive Behaviours*, **7**: 155–66.

Louro, A.C., Fernández-Castro, J. and Blasco, T. (2016) Effects of a positive emotion-based adjuvant psychological therapy in colorectal cancer patients: a pilot study, *Psicooncología*, **13**(1): 113–25.

Lowe, C.S. and Radius, S.M. (1982) Young adults' contraceptive practices: an investigation of influences, *Adolescence*, **22**: 291–304.

Lowe, C.F., Dowey, A. and Horne, P. (1998) Changing what children eat, in A. Murcott (ed.) *The Nation's Diet: The Social Science of Food Choice*. Harlow: Addison-Wesley Longman.

Lowenstein, L., Deutsch, M., Gruberg, R. et al. (2006) Psychological distress symptoms in women undergoing medical vs. surgical termination of pregnancy, *General Hospital Psychiatry*, **28**(1): 43–7.

Lu, C.C., Hsiao, Y.C., Huang, H.W. et al. (2019) Effects of a nurse-led, stage-matched, tailored program for smoking cessation in health education centers: a prospective, randomized, controlled trial, *Clinical Nursing Research*, **28**(7), 812–29.

Lucas, R.E. and Gohm, C.L. (2000) Age and sex differences in subjective well-being across cultures, in E. Diner and E.M. Suh (eds) *Culture and Subjective Well-being*. Cambridge, MA: MIT Press.

Luise, C., Jermy, K., May, C. et al. (2002) Outcomes of expectant management of spontaneous first trimester miscarriage: observational study, *British Medical Journal*, **324**: 873–5.

Luker, K. (1975) *Taking Chances: Abortion and the Decision Not to Contracept*. Berkeley, CA: University of California Press.

Lunn, P.D., Belton, C.A., Lavin, C. et al. (2020) Using Behavioral Science to help fight the Coronavirus, *Journal of Behavioral Public Administration*, **3**(1).

Luo, T., Li, M.S., Williams, D. et al. (2021) Using social media for smoking cessation interventions: a systematic review, *Perspectives in Public Health*, **141**(1): 50–63.

Lupton, D. (1998) *The Emotional Self: A Sociocultural Exploration*. London: Sage.

Luszczynska, A. and Schwarzer, R. (2003) Planning and self-efficacy in the adoption and maintenance of breast self-examination: a longitudinal study on self-regulatory cognitions, *Psychology and Health*, **18**(1): 93–108.

Luszczynska, A., Goc, G., Scholz, U. et al. (2010) Enhancing intentions to attend cervical cancer screening with a stage-matched intervention, *British Journal of Health Psychology*, **16**: 33–46.

Lynch, J. (1977) *The Broken Heart: The Medical Consequences of Loneliness*. New York: Basic Books.

Lyndon, J., Dunkel-Schetter, C., Cohan, C.L. and Pierce, T. (1996) Pregnancy decision making as a significant life event: a commitment approach, *Journal of Personality and Social Psychology*, **71**: 141–51.

Ma, Q., Qiu, W., Fu, H. and Sun, X. (2018) Uncertain is worse: modulation of anxiety on pain anticipation by intensity uncertainty: evidence from the ERP study, *Neuroreport: For Rapid Communication of Neuroscience Research,* **29**(12): 1023–9.

Maass, S.W., Roorda, C., Berendsen, A.J. et al. (2015) The prevalence of long-term symptoms of depression and anxiety after breast cancer treatment: a systematic review, *Maturitas,* **82**(1): 100–8.

MacIntyre, S., Hunt, K. and Sweeting, H. (1996) Gender differences in health: are things really as simple as they seem?, *Social Science & Medicine,* **42**(4): 617–24.

MacNicol, S.A.M., Murray, S.M. and Austin, E.J. (2003) Relationships between personality, attitudes and dietary behaviour in a group of Scottish adolescents, *Personality and Individual Differences,* **35**: 1753–64.

MacWhinney, D.R. (1973) Problem solving and decision making in primary medical practice, *Proceeds of the Royal Society of Medicine,* **65**: 934–8.

MacWilliams, K., Hughes, J., Aston, M. et al. (2016) Understanding the experience of miscarriage in the emergency department. *Journal of Emergency Nursing,* **42**(6): 504–12.

Madden, M.E. (1988) Internal and external attributions following miscarriage, *Journal of Social and Clinical Psychology,* **7**: 113–21.

Madden, V.J., Bellan, V., Russek, L.N. et al. (2016) Pain by association? Experimental modulation of human pain thresholds using classical conditioning, *The Journal of Pain,* **17**(10): 1105–15.

Maeland, J.G. and Havik, O.E. (1987) Psychological predictors for return for work after a myocardial infarction, *Journal of Psychosomatic Research,* **31**: 471–81.

Maes, H.H., Neale, M.C. and Eaves, L.J. (1997) Genetic and environmental factors in relative body weight and human adiposity, *Behavior Genetics,* **27**(4): 325–51.

Magoc, D., Tomaka, J., Shamaley, A.G. and Bridges, A. (2016) Gender differences in physical activity and related beliefs among Hispanic college students. *Hispanic Journal of Behavioral Sciences,* **38**(2), 279–90.

Mahler, H.I.M., Kulik, J.A., Gerrard, M. and Gibbons, F.X. (2007) Long-term effects of appearance-based interventions on sun protection behaviors, *Health Psychology,* **26**: 350–60.

Mahler, H.I.M., Kulik, J.A., Gibbons, F.X. et al. (2003) Effects of appearance-based interventions on sun protection intentions and self-reported behaviors, *Health Psychology,* **22**: 199–209.

Major, B. and Gramzow, R.H. (1999) Abortion as stigma: cognitive and emotional implications of concealment, *Journal of Personality and Social Psychology,* **77**: 735–45.

Major, B., Cozzarelli, C., Cooper, M.L. et al. (2000) Psychological responses of women after first-trimester abortion, *Archives of General Psychiatry,* **57**: 777–84.

Maker, C. and Ogden, J. (2003) The miscarriage experience: more than just a trigger to psychological morbidity, *Psychology and Health,* **18**(3): 403–25.

Man, A.K.Y. and Yap, J.C.M. (2003) The effect of intraoperative video on patient anxiety, *Anaesthesia,* **58**(1): 64–8.

Mann, J.M., Chin, J., Piot, P. and Quinn, T. (1988) The international epidemiology of AIDS, in *The Science of AIDS,* readings from *Scientfic American,* pp. 51–61. New York: W.H. Freeman.

Manne, S.L. and Zautra, A.J. (1992) Coping with arthritis: current status and critique, *Arthritis & Rheumatism,* **35**: 1273–80.

Manning, M.M. and Wright, T.L. (1983) Self-efficacy expectancies, outcome expectancies and the persistence of pain control in child birth, *Journal of Personality and Social Psychology,* **45**: 421–31.

Mantzari, E., Rubin, G.J. and Marteau, T.M. (2020) Is risk compensation threatening public health in the Covid-19 pandemic? *BMJ,* **370**, m2913.

Manuck, S.B., Kaplan, J.R. and Matthews, K.A. (1986) Behavioural antecedents of coronary heart disease and atherosclerosis, *Arteriosclerosis,* **6**: 1–14.

Mapes, R. (ed.) (1980) *Prescribing Practice and Drug Usage.* London: Croom Helm.

Marcano-Olivier, M., Sallaway-Costello, J., McWilliams, L. et al. (2021) Changes in the nutritional content of children's lunches after the Food Dudes healthy eating programme, *Journal of Nutritional Science,* **10**:e40. Doi: 10.1017/jns.2021.31.

Marcus, B.H., Ciccola, J.T. and Sciamanna, C.N. (2009) Using electronic/computer interventions to promote physical activity, *British Journal of Sports Medicine,* **43**:102–5.

Marcus, B.H., Owen, N., Forsyth, L.A.H. et al. (1998) Physical activity interventions using mass media, print media, and information technology, *American Journal of Preventive Medicine,* **15**(4): 362–78.

Mardani, A., Pedram Razi, S., Mazaheri, R. et al. (2021) Effect of the exercise programme on the quality of life of prostate cancer survivors: a randomized controlled trial, *International Journal of Nursing Practice,* **27**(2): e12883.

Markfelder, T. and Pauli, P. (2020) Fear of pain and pain intensity: Meta-analysis and systematic review, *Psychological Bulletin,* **146**(5): 411–50.

Marlatt, G.A. and Gordon, J.R. (1985) *Relapse Prevention.* New York: Guilford Press.

Marmarà, D., Marmarà, V. and Hubbard, G. (2017) Health beliefs, illness perceptions and determinants of breast screening uptake in Malta: a cross-sectional survey, *BMC Public Health,* **17**(1): 416.

Marmot, M. and Wilkinson, R. (2005) *Social Determinants of Health,* 2nd edn. Oxford: Oxford University Press.

Marshall, S.J. and Biddle, S.J.H. (2001) The transtheortical model of behaviour change: a meta-analysis of applications to physical activity and exercise, *Annals of Behavioural Medicine*, **23**: 229–46.

Marteau, T.M. and Baum, J.D. (1984) Doctors' views on diabetes, *Archives of Disease in Childhood*, **56**: 566–70.

Marteau, T.M. and Riordan, D.C. (1992) Staff attitudes to patients the influence of causal attributions for illness, *British Journal of Clinical Psychology*, **31**: 107–10.

Marteau, T.M., French, D.P., Griffin, S.J. et al. (2010) Effects of communicating DNA-based disease risk estimates on risk-reducing behaviours (review), *The Cochrane Library*, 10, CD007275.

Marteau, T.M., Senior, V. and Sasieni, P. (2006) Women's understanding of a 'normal smear test result': experimental questionnaire based study, *British Medical Journal*, **322**(7285): 526–8.

Marteau, T.M., Senior, V., Humphries, S.E. et al. (2004) Psychological impact of genetic testing for familial hypercholesterolemia within a previously aware population: a randomized controlled trial, *American Journal of Medical Genetics*, **128** A: 285–93.

Marteau, T.M. (1993) Health related screening: psychological predictors of uptake and impact, in S. Marteau, and Baum, J.D. (1984) Doctors' views on diabetes, *Archives of Disease in Childhood*, **56**: 566–70.

Marteau, T.M., Ashcroft, R. and Oliver, A. (2009) Using financial incentives to achieve healthy behaviour, *British Medical Journal*, 338: 983–85.

Martikainen, P. and Valkonen, T. (1996) Mortality after death of spouse in relation to duration of bereavement in Finland, *Journal of Epidemiology Community Health*, **50**(3): 264–8.

Martin, J.I. (2006) Transcendence among gay men: implications for HIV prevention, *Sexualities*, **9**(2): 214–35.

Martin, M.C. and Kennedy, P.F. (1993) Advertising and social comparison: consequences for female preadolescents and adolescents, *Psychology & Marketing*, 10(6): 513–30.

Martinez-Calderon, J., Flores-Cortes, M., Morales-Asencio, J.M and Luque-Suarez, A. (2019) Pain-related fear, pain intensity and function in individuals with chronic musculoskeletal pain: a systematic review and meta-analysis, *The Journal of Pain*, **20**(12): 1394–1415.

Martinez-Calderon, J., Meeus, M., Struyf, F. and Luque-Suarez, A. (2020) The role of self-efficacy in pain intensity, function, psychological factors, health behaviors, and quality of life in people with rheumatoid arthritis: a systematic review, *Physiotherapy Theory and Practice*, **36**(1): 21–37.

Martinez-Calderon, J., Meeus, M., Struyf, F. and Luque-Suarez, A. (2020) The role of self-efficacy in

pain intensity, function, psychological factors, health behaviors, and quality of life in people with rheumatoid arthritis: a systematic review, *Physiotherapy Theory and Practice*, **36**(1): 21–37.

Marucha, P.T., Kiecolt-Glaser, J.K. and Favagehi, M. (1998) Mucosal wound healing is impaired by examination stress, *Psychosomatic Medicine*, **60**: 362–5.

Mason, J.W. (1975) A historical view of the stress field, *Journal of Human Stress*, **1**: 22–36.

Mason, T.E. and White, K.W. (2008) Applying an extended model in the theory of planned behaviour to breast self-examination, *Journal of Health Psychology*, **13**(7): 946–55.

Masters, W. and Johnson, V. (1966) *Human Sexual Response*. Boston, MA: Little Brown.

Matarazzo, J.D. (1980) Behavioral health and behavioral medicine: frontiers for a new health psychology, *American Psychologist*, **35**: 807–17.

Matarazzo, J.D. (1984) Behavioral health: a 1990 challenge for the health sciences professions, in J.D. Matarazzo, N.E. Miller, S.M. Weiss et al. (eds) *Behavioral Health: A Handbook of Health Enhancement and Disease Prevention*. New York: Wiley.

Matini, L. and Ogden, J. (2016) Patients' experiences of IBD and the process of adaptation: finding the new normal after diagnosis, *Journal of Health Psychology*. DOI: 10.1177/1359105315580463.

Matthews, K.A., Owens, J.F., Allen, M.T. and Stoney, C.M. (1992) Do cardiovascular responses to laboratory stress relate to ambulatory blood pressure levels? Yes in some of the people some of the time, *Psychosomatic Medicine*, **54**: 686–97.

Matthews, K.A., Woodall, K.L., Kenyon, K. and Jacob, T. (1996) Negative family environment as a predictor of boys' future status on measures of hostile attitudes, interview behaviour and anger expression, *Health Psychology*, **15**: 30–7.

Mazzi, M.A., Rimondini, M., Deveugele, M. et al. (2015) What do people appreciate in physicians' communication? An international study with focus groups using videotaped medical consultations, *Health Expectations*, **18**(5): 1215–26.

McCabe, M.P. and Ricciardelli, L.A. (2001) Parent, peer and media influences on body images and strategies to both increase and decrease body size among adolescent boys and girls, *Adolescence*, **36**(142): 225–40.

McCormick, N., Izzo, A. and Folcik, J. (1985) Adolescents' values, sexuality, and contraception in a rural New York county, *Adolescence*, **20**: 385–95.

McCracken, L.M. and Eccleston, C. (2003) Coping or acceptance: what to do about chronic pain? *Pain*, **105**(1–2): 197–204.

McCracken, L.M. & Eccleston, C. (2006). The relative Utility of coping-based vs acceptance-based approaches to chronic pain. European Journal of Pain, 10. 23-29.

McCusker, J., Stoddard, J.G., Zapka, M.Z. and Meyer, K.H. (1989) Predictors of AIDS preventive behaviour among homosexually active men: a longitudinal study, *AIDS*, **3**: 443–6.

McDermott, M.R., Ramsay, J.M. and Bray, C. (2001) Components of the anger-hostility complex as a risk factor for coronary artery disease severity: a multimeasure study, *Journal of Health Psychology*, **6**(3): 309–19.

McEwan, B.S. and Stellar, E. (1993) Stress and the individual: mechanisms leading to disease. *Archives of Internal Medicine*, **153**: 2093–101.

McGee, H.M., O'Boyle, C.A., Hickey, A. et al. (1991) Assessing the quality of life of the individual: the SEIQoL with a healthy and a gastroenterology unit population, *Psychological Medicine*, **21**: 749–59.

McGowan, L., Luker, K., Creed, F. and Chew-Graham, C.A. (2007) 'How do you explain a pain that can't be seen?': the narratives of women with chronic pelvic pain and their disengagement with the diagnostic cycle, *British Journal of Health Psychology*, **12**: 261–74.

McGowan, L.P.A., Clarke-Carter, D.D. and Pitts, M.K. (1998) Chronic pelvic pain: a meta-analytic review, *Psychology and Health*, **13**: 937–51.

McKee, K.J., Houston, D.M. and Barnes, S. (2002) Methods for assessing quality of life and wellbeing in frail older people, *Psychology and Health*, **17**(6): 737–51.

McKeown, T. (1979) *The Role of Medicine*. Oxford: Blackwell.

McKinlay, E. (2005) *Men and Health: A Literature Review*. Wellington: Wellington School of Medicine and Health Sciences, University of Otago.

McLachlan, E., Anderson, S., Hawkes, D. et al. (2018) Completing the cervical screening pathway: factors that facilitate the increase of self-collection uptake among under-screened and never-screened women, an Australian pilot study, *Current Oncology*, **25**(1): e17.

McMillen, J.C., Smith, E.M. and Fisher, R.H. (1997) Perceived benefit and mental health after three types of disaster, *Journal of Consulting and Clinical Psychology*, **65**(5): 733–9.

McMillen, J.C. (2004) Posttraumatic growth: what's it all about? *Psychological Inquiry*, **15**(1): 48–52.

McNeil, A.D., Jarvis, M.J., Stapleton, J.A. et al. (1988) Prospective study of factors predicting uptake of smoking in adolescents, *Journal of Epidemiology and Community Health*, **43**: 72–8.

McNeil, B.J., Pauker, S.G., Sox, H.C. and Tversky, A. (1982) On the elicitation of preferences for alternative therapies, *New England Journal of Medicine*, **306**: 1259–62.

McWhinney, I.R. (1995) Why we need a new clinical method, in M. Stewart, B.B. Brown, W.W. Weston et al. (eds) *Patient Centred Medicine: Transforming the Clinical Method*. London: Sage.

Mead, N. and Bower, P. (2000) Patient centredness: a conceptual framework and review of empirical literature, *Social Science and Medicine*, **51**: 1087–110.

Meadows, J., Jenkinson, S., Catalan, J. and Gazzard, B. (1990) Voluntary HIV testing in the antenatal clinic: differing uptake rates for individual counselling midwives, *AIDS Care*, **2**: 229–33.

Meads, C. and Moore, D. (2013) Breast cancer in lesbians and bisexual women: systematic review of incidence, prevalence and risk studies, *BMC Public Health*, **13**(1), 1–11.

Mechanic, D. (1962) *Students Under Stress: A Study in the Social Psychology of Adaptation*. Glencoe, IL: Free Press of Glencoe.

Meenan, R.F., Gertman, P.M. and Mason, J.H. (1980) Measuring health status in arthritis: the arthritis impact measurement scales, *Arthritis & Rheumatology*, **23**: 146–52.

Meijer, A., Conradi, H.J., Bos, E.H. et al. (2011) Prognostic association of depression following myocardial infarction with mortality and cardiovascular events: a meta-analysis of 25 years of research, *General Hospital Psychiatry*, **33**(3): 203–16.

Meints, S.M., Mawla, I., Napadow, V. et al. (2019) The relationship between catastrophizing and altered pain sensitivity in patients with chronic low back pain, *Pain*, **160**(4): 833–43.

Melzack, R. and Katz, J. (2004) The gate control theory: reaching for the brain, in T. Hadjistavropoulos and K.D. Craig (eds), *Pain: Psychological Perspectives*. Mahwah, NJ: Lawrence Erlbaum.

Melzack, R. and Wall, P.D. (1965) Pain mechanisms: a new theory, *Science*, **150**: 971–9.

Melzack, R. (1975) The McGill Pain Questionnaire: major properties and scoring methods, *Pain*, **1**: 277–99.

Mercken, L., Candel, M., van Osch, L. and de Vries, H. (2011) No smoke without fire: the impact of future friends on adolescent smoking behaviour, *British Journal of Health Psychology*, **16**: 170–88.

Metcalfe, C., Smith, G.D, Wadsworth, E. et al. (2003) A contemporary validation of the Reeder Stress Inventory, *British Journal of Health Psychology*, **8**: 83–94.

Meulders, A. (2019) From fear of movement-related pain and avoidance to chronic pain disability: a state-of-the-art review, *Current Opinion in Behavioral Sciences*, **26**:130–36.

Meyer, D., Leventhal, H. and Guttman, M. (1985) Common-sense models of illness: the example of hypertension, *Health Psychology*, **4**: 115–35.

Michalopoulou, M., Ferrey, A.E., Harmer, G. et al. (2022) Effectiveness of motivational interviewing in managing overweight and obesity: A systematic review and meta-analysis, *Annals of Internal Medicine*, **175**(6): 838–50.

Michaud, C., Kann, J.P., Musse, N. et al. (1990) Relationships between a critical life event and eating behaviour in high school students, *Stress Medicine*, **6**: 57–64.

Michel, G. (2006) A multi-level decomposition of variance in somatic symptom reporting in families with adolescent children, *British Journal of Health Psychology*, **11**(2): 345–55.

Michel, G. (2007) Daily patterns of symptom reporting in families with adolescent children, *British Journal of Health Psychology*, **12**: 245–60.

Michie, S. and Wood, C.E. (2015) Health behaviour change techniques, in M. Conner and P. Norman (eds) *Predicting and Changing Health Behaviour. Research and Practice with Social Cognition Models*, pp. 358–89. New York: McGraw Hill.

Michie, S., Atkins, L. and West, R. (2014a) *The Behaviour Change Wheel: A Guide to Designing Interventions*. London: Silverback Publishing.

Michie, S., Campbell, R., Brown, J. et al. (2014) *ABC of Theories of Behaviour Change*. London: Silverback Publishing.

Michie, S., Fixsen, D., Grimshaw, J. and Eccles, M. (2009) Specifying and reporting complex behaviour change interventions: the need for a scientific method, *Implementation Science*, **4**(1): 40.

Michie, S., Johnston, M., Abraham, C. et al. (2005) Making psychological theory useful for implementing evidence based practice: a consensus approach, *Quality and Safety in Health Care*, **14**(1): 26–33.

Michie, S., Richardson, M., Johnston, M. et al. (2013) The behavior change technique taxonomy (v1) of 93 hierarchically clustered techniques: building an international consensus for the reporting of behavior change interventions, *Annals of Behavioral Medicine*, **46**(1): 81–95.

Michie, S., Smith, J.A., Senior, V. and Marteau, T.M. (2003) Understanding why negative genetic test results sometimes fail to reassure, *American Journal of Medical Genetics*, **119**(A): 340–7.

Michie, S., van Stralen, M.M. and West, R. (2011b) The behaviour change wheel: a new method for characterising and designing behaviour change interventions, *Implementation Science*, **6**(1): 42.

Michie, S., van Stralen, M.M. and West, R. (2011) The behaviour change wheel: a new method for characterising and designing behaviour change interventions. *Implementation Science*, **6**(1): 42.

Michie, S., Weinman, J., Miller, J. et al. (2002) Predictive genetic testing: high risk expectations in the face of low risk information, *Journal of Behavioural Medicine*, **25**: 33–50.

Michie, S., West, R., Campbell, R. et al. (2014b) *ABC of Theories of Behaviour Change*. London: Silverback Publishing.

Milam, J. (2006) Posttraumatic growth and HIV disease progression, *Journal of Consulting and Clinical Psychology*, **74**(5): 817–27.

Miller, S.M., Brody, D.S. and Summerton, J. (1987) Styles of coping with threat: implications for health, *Journal of Personality and Social Psychology*, **54**: 142–8.

Miller, T.Q., Smith, T.W., Turner, C.W. et al. (1996) A meta-analytic review of research on hostility and physical health, *Psychological Bulletin*, **119**: 322–48.

Miller, W. and Rollnick, S. (2002) *Motivational Interviewing: Preparing People to Change Addictive Behaviour*. New York: Guilford Press.

Minian, N., Corrin, T., Lingam, M. et al. (2020) Identifying contexts and mechanisms in multiple behavior change interventions affecting smoking cessation success: a rapid realist review, *BMC Public Health*, **20**(1): 1–26.

Minian, N., Corrin, T., Lingam, M., deRuiter, W.K., Rodak, T., Taylor, V.H., Selby, P. et al. (2020) Identifying contexts and mechanisms in multiple behavior change interventions affecting smoking cessation success: a rapid realist review. *BMC Public Health*, **20**(1): 1–26.

Minsky, S., Vega, W., Miskimen, T. et al. (2003) Diagnostic patterns in Latino, African American and European American psychiatric patients, *Archives of General Psychiatry*, **60**: 637–44.

Mintel (1990) *Eggs. Market Intelligence*. London: Mintel.

Minuchin, S., Rosman, B.L. and Baker, L. (1978) *The Anorectic Family in Psychosomatic Families: Anorexia Nervosa in Context*. London: Harvard University Press.

Misra, A. and Ganda, O.P. (2007) Migration and its impact on adiposity and type 2 diabetes, *Nutrition*, **23**(9): 696–708.

Misselbrook, D. and Armstrong, D. (2000) How do patients respond to presentation of risk information? A survey in general practice of willingness to accept treatment for hypertension, *British Journal of General Practice*, **51**: 276–9.

Moatti, J.-P., Le Gales, C., Seror, J. et al. (1990) Social acceptability of HIV screening among pregnant women, *AIDS Care*, **2**: 213–22.

Moatti, J.P., Carrieri, M.P., Spire, B., Gastaut, J.A., Cassuto, J.P., & Moreau, J. (2000) Adherence to HAART in French HIV-infected injecting drug users: the contribution of buprenorphine drug maintenance treatment. The Manif 2000 study group. *AIDS*, **14**, 151–5.

Mocroft, A., Vella, S., Benfield, T.L. et al. (1998) Changing patterns of mortality across Europe inpatients infected with HIV-1, EuroSIDA Study Group, *Lancet*, **352**(9142): 1725–30.

Mokdad, A.H., Marks, J.S., Stroup, D.F. and Gerberding, J.L. (2004) Actual causes of death in the United States, *Journal of the American Medical Association,* **10**(29): 1238–45.

Mokdad, A.H., Marks, J.S., Stroup, D.F. and Gerberding, J.L. Actual causes of death in the United States, 2000. JAMA. 2004 Mar 10;291(10):1238–45. Review. Erratum in: JAMA. 2005 Jan 19;293(3):298. JAMA. 2005 Jan 19;293(3):293-4.

Moller, J., Hallqvist, J., Diderichensen, F. et al. (1999) Do episodes of anger trigger myocardial infarction? A case-crossover analysis in the Stockholm heart epidemiology program (SHEEP), *Psychosomatic Medicine,* **61**: 842–9.

Molloy, G.J., Dixon, D., Hamer, M. and Sniehotta, F.F. (2010) Social support and regular physical activity: does planning mediate this link? *British Journal of Health Psychology,* **15**: 859–970.

Momani, T.G. and Berry, D.L. (2017) Integrative therapeutic approaches for the management and control of nausea in children undergoing cancer treatment: a systematic review of literature, *Journal of Pediatric Oncology Nursing,* **34**(3): 173–84.

Montanaro, E.A. and Bryan, A.D. (2014) Comparing theory-based condom interventions: health belief model versus theory of planned behavior, *Health Psychology,* **33**(10), 1251–60.

Moons, L., Mariman, A., Vermeir, P. et al. (2020) Sociodemographic factors and strategies in colorectal cancer screening: a narrative review and practical recommendations, *Acta Clinica Belgica,* **75**(1): 33–41.

Moore, R.A., Eccleston, C., Derry, S. et al. (2010) 'Evidence' in chronic pain–establishing best practice in the reporting of systematic reviews, *PAIN,* **150**: 386–9.

Moore, S.C., Mayne, S.T., Graubard, B.I. et al. (2008) Past body mass index and risk of mortality among women, *International Journal of Obesity,* **32**(5): 730–9.

Moorhead, J. (1997) *New Generations: 40 Years of Birth in Britain* (National Childbirth Trust Guides). London: The Stationery Office.

Moos, R.H. and Schaefer, J.A. (1984) The crisis of physical illness: an overview and conceptual approach, in R.H. Moos (ed.) *Coping with Physical Illness: New Perspectives, 2.* New York: Plenum.

Mora, P.A., Halm, E., Leventhal, H. and Ceric, F. (2007) Elucidating the relationship between negative affectivity and symptoms: the role of illness specific affective responses, *Annals of Behavioural Medicine,* **34**(1): 77–86.

Moray, J., Fu, A., Brill, K. and Mayoral, M.S. (2007) Viewing television while eating impairs the ability to accurately estimate total amount of food consumed. *Bariatric Nursing and Surgical Patient Care,* **2**: 71–6.

Morison, L.A., Cozzolino, P.J. and Orbell, S. (2010) Temporal perspective and parental intention to accept the human papillomaviris vaccination for their daughter, *British Journal of Health Psychology,* **15**: 151–65.

Morrison, D.M. (1985) Adolescent contraceptive behaviour: a review, *Psychological Bulletin,* **98**: 538–68.

Morton, K., Beauchamp, M., Prothero, A. et al. (2015) The effectiveness of motivational interviewing for health behaviour change in primary care settings: a systematic review. *Health Psychology Review,* **9**(2): 205–23.

Mosher, W., Martinez, G., Chandra, A. et al. (2004) Use of contraception and use of family planning services in the United States, 1982–2002, *Advance Data,* **350** (December).

Moss-Morris, R., Humphrey, K., Johnson, M.H. and Petrie, K.J. (2007) Patients' perceptions of their pain condition across a multidisciplinary pain management programme: do they change and if so does it matter? *Clinical Journal of Pain,* **23**: 558–64.

Moss-Morris, R., Weinman, J., Petrie, K.J. et al. (2002) The revised illness perception questionnaire (IPQ-R), *Psychology and Health,* **17**: 1–16.

Mottram, R., Knerr, W.L., Gallacher, D. et al. (2021) Factors associated with attendance at screening for breast cancer: a systematic review and meta-analysis, *BMJ Open,* **11**(11): e046660.

Moyer, A. (1997) Psychosocial outcomes of breast conserving surgery versus mastectomy: a meta analytic review, *Health Pysychology,* **16**: 284–98.

Moynihan, J.A. and Ader, R. (1996) Psychoneuroimmunology: animal models of disease, *Psychosomatic Medicine,* **58**: 546–58.

Muñoz-Silva, A., Sanchez-Garcia, M., Nunes, C. and Martins, A. (2007) Gender differences in condom use prediction with theory of reasoned action and planned behaviour: the role of self-efficacy and control, *AIDS Care,* **19**: 1177–81.

Muellmann, S., Forberger, S., Möllers, T., Bröring, E., Zeeb, H. and Pischke, C. R. (2018) Effectiveness of eHealth interventions for the promotion of physical activity in older adults: a systematic review, *Preventive Medicine,* **108**: 93–110.

Muldoon, M.F., Barger, S.D., Flory, J.D. and Manuck, S.B. (1998) What are quality of life measurements measuring? *British Medical Journal,* **316**: 542–5.

Mullen, P.D., Green, L.W. and Persinger, G.S. (1985) Clinical trials of patient education for chronic conditions: a comparative meta-analysis of intervention types, *Preventive Medicine,* **14**: 753–81.

Muller, J.E., Abela, G.S., Nesto, R.W. and Tofler, G.H. (1994) Triggers, acute risk factors and vulnerable plaques: the lexicon of a new frontier, *Journal of American College of Cardiology,* **23**: 809–13.

Muraleetharan, V. and Brault, M.A. (2021) Friends as informal educators: The role of peer relationships in promotion of sexual health services among college students, *International Quarterly of Community Health Education*, 0272684X211034661.

Murgio, A., Fernandez Mila, J., Manolio, A. et al. (1999) Minor head injury at paediatric age in Argentina, *Journal of Neurosurgical Sciences*, **43**: 15–23.

Murray, M., Swan, A.V., Bewley, B.R. and Johnson, M.R.D. (1984) The development of smoking during adolescence: the MRC/Derbyshire smoking study, *International Journal of Epidemiology*, **12**: 185–92.

Muschetto, T. and Siegel, J.T. (2019) Attribution theory and support for individuals with depression: the impact of controllability, stability, and interpersonal relationship, *Stigma and Health*, **4** (2): 126–35.

Mwaba, S.O., Menon, A.J. and Kusanthan, T. (2020) Perceived risk of contracting HIV and AIDS among sexually active unmarried young people in Zambia, *International STD Research & Reviews*, **9**(1): 46–57.

Myers, L.B. (2000) Identifying repressors: a methodological issue for health psychology, *Psychology and Health*, **15**: 205–14.

Nanton, V., Docherty, A., Meystre, C. and Dale, J. (2009) Finding a pathway: information and uncertainty along the prostate cancer patient journey, *British Journal of Health Psychology*, 14: 437–58.

Nash, H.L. (1987) Do compulsive runners and anorectic patients share common bonds? *The Physician and Sportsmedicine*, **15**(12): 163–7.

Natarajan, M. (Ed.). (2011). Crime Opportunity Theories: Routine Activity, Rational Choice and their Variants (1st ed.). Routledge. https://doi.org/10.4324/9781315095301

National Center for Health Statistics (2009) *Health, United States, 2008*. Hyattsville, MD: National Center for Health Statistics.

National Centre for Health Outcomes Development (2011) *Compendium of Population Health Indicators*, https://digital.nhs.uk/data-and-information/publications/ci-hub/compendium-indicators

National Institute on Minority Health and Health Disparities (2016) *Director's message 10-06-16*. https://www.nimhd.nih.gov/about/directors-corner/messages/message_10-06-16.html

National Institutes of Health (1998) Clinical guidelines on the identification, evaluation, and treatment of overweight and obesity in adults: the evidence report, *Obesity Research*, **6**(suppl. 2): 51–209S.

National Statistics Online (2006) *GP Consultations*.

National Statistics (2005) www.statistics.gov.uk.

NCASA (National Center on Addiction and Substance Abuse at Columbia University) (2011) *Adolescent substance use: America's #1 public health problem*, http://www.casacolumbia.org/upload/2011/2110629adolescentsubstanceuse.pdf.

NCD Risk Factor Collaboration (NCD-RisC) (2017). Worldwide trends in body-mass index, underweight, overweight, and obesity from 1975 to 2016: a pooled analysis of 2416 population-based measurement studies in 128·9 million children, adolescents, and adults. *Lancet (London, England)*, *390*(10113), 2627–2642. https://doi.org/10.1016/S0140-6736(17)32129-3

Neame, R. and Hammond, A. (2005) Beliefs about medications: a questionnaire survey of people with rheumatoid arthritis, *Rheumatology*, **44**: 762–7.

Neel, J.V. (1999) The 'thrifty genotype' in 1998, *Nutrition Reviews, 57*(5 Pt 2): S2–9.

Neighbour, R. (1987) *The Inner Consultation*. London: Petroc Press.

Neilson, S. and Hahlin, M. (1985) Expectant management of first trimester miscarriage, *Lancet*, **345**: 84–6.

Neter, E., Glass-Marmor, L., Wolkowitz, A. et al. (2021) Beliefs about medication as predictors of medication adherence in a prospective cohort study among persons with multiple sclerosis, *BMC Neurology, 21*(1): 1–9.

Newell, A. and Simon, H.A. (1972) *Human Problem Solving*. Englewood Cliffs, NJ: Prentice Hall.

Newman, S., Fitzpatrick, R., Revenson, T.A. et al. (1996) *Understanding Rheumatoid Arthritis*. London: Routledge.

NHS (2018) https://www.nhs.uk/conditions/menopause/

NHS Centre for Reviews and Dissemination (1997) *Systematic Review of Interventions in the Treatment and Prevention of Obesity*. York: University of York.

NHS Digital (2016) *Sexual and Reproductive Health Services England, 2015–16*. https://digital.nhs.uk/data-and-information/publications/statistical/sexual-and-reproductive-health-services/sexual-and-reproductive-health-services-england-2015-16

NHS Digital (2016) https://digital.nhs.uk/data-and-information/publications/statistical/sexual-and-reproductive-health-services/sexual-and-reproductive-health-services-england-2015-16

NHS Information Centre (2009) *Health Survey for England—2008: Physical Activity and Fitness.* https://digital.nhs.uk/data-and-information/publications/statistical/health-survey-for-england/health-survey-for-england-2008-physical-activity-and-fitness

NICE (National Institute for Health and Clinical Excellence) (2009) *Costing Statement: Medicines Adherence: Involving Patients in Decisions About Prescribed Medicines and Supporting Adherence.* London: NICE.

Nie, B., Chapman, S.C., Chen, Z. et al. (2019) Utilization of the beliefs about medicine questionnaire and prediction of medication adherence in China: a systematic review and meta-analysis, *Journal of Psychosomatic Research*, **122**, 54–68.

Nipp, R.D., El-Jawahri, A., Fishbein, J.N. et al. (2016) The relationship between coping strategies, quality of life, and mood in patients with incurable cancer, *Cancer*, **122**(13): 2110–16.

Noar, S.M., Moroko., P.J. and Harlow, L.L. (2002) Condom negotiation in heterosexually active men and women: development and validation of a condom influence strategy questionnaire, *Psychology and Health*, **17**(6): 711–35.

Norman, P. and Bennett, P. (1995) Health locus of control and health behaviours, in M. Conner and P. Norman (eds) *Predicting Health Behaviour: Research and Practice with Social Cognition Models*. Buckingham: Open University Press.

Norman, P. and Conner, M. (1993) The role of social cognition models in predicting attendance at health checks, *Psychology and Health*, **8**: 447–62.

Norman, P. and Conner, M. (1996) The role of social cognition models in predicting health behaviours: future directions, in M. Conner and P. Norman (eds) *Predicting Health Behaviour: Research and Practice with Social Cognition Models*. Buckingham: Open University Press.

Norman, P. and Conner, M. (2006) The role of social cognition models in predicting health behaviours: future directions, in M. Conner and P. Norman (eds) *Predicting Health Behaviour: Research and Practice with Social Cognition Models*, 2nd edn. Maidenhead: Open University Press.

Norman, P. and Fitter, M. (1989) Intention to attend a health screening appointment: some implications for general practice, *Counselling Psychology Quarterly*, **2**: 261–72.

Norman, P. and Smith, L. (1995) The theory of planned behaviour and exercise: an investigation into the role of prior behaviour, behavioural intentions and attitude variability, *European Journal of Social Psychology*, **25**: 403–15.

Norman, P. and Wrona-Clarke, A. (2016) Combining self-affirmation and implementation intentions to reduce heavy episodic drinking in university students. *Psychology of Addictive Behaviors*, **30**(4): 434.

Norman, P., Conner, M. and Bell, R. (1999) The theory of planned behavior and smoking cessation, *Health Psychology*, **18**: 89–94.

Norman, P., Searle, A., Harrad, R. and Vedhara, K. (2003) Predicting adherence to eye patching in children with amblyopia: an application of protection motivation theory, *British Journal of Health Psychology*, **8**: 67–82.

North East Essex NHS Trust (2009) Food vouchers incentives to pregnant smokers, press release, 21 January, www.northeastessexpct.nhs.uk/news/newsitem.asp?news_?id=272.

Nourisaeed, A., Ghorban-Shiroudi, S. and Salari, A. (2021) Comparison of the effect of cognitive-behavioral therapy and dialectical behavioral therapy on perceived stress and coping skills in patients after myocardial infarction, *ARYA Atherosclerosis*, **17**: 2188.

Oakley, A. (1984) *The Captured Womb*. Oxford: Blackwell.

Oakley, A. (1992) *Social Support and Motherhood*. Oxford: Blackwell.

O'Boyle, C., McGee, H., Hickey, A. et al. (1992) Individual quality of life in patients undergoing hip replacements, *Lancet*, **339**: 1088–91.

O'Brien, P.E., McPhail, T., Chaston, T.B. and Dixon, J.B. (2006) Systematic review of medium-term weight loss after bariatric operations, *Obesity Surgery*, **16**: 1032–40.

O'Brien, S. and Lee, L. (1990) Effects of videotape intervention on pap smear knowledge, attitudes and behavior, special issue, *Behavioural Research in Cancer, Behaviour Changes*, **7**: 143–50.

O'Conner, D.B., Jones, F., Conner, M. et al. (2008) Effects of daily hassles and eating style on eating behaviour, *Health Psychology*, **27**(1): S2–31.

O'Connor, D.B., Conner, M., Jones, F. et al. (2009) Exploring the benefits of conscientiousness: an investigation of the role of daily stressors and health behaviors, *Annals of Behavioral Medicine*, **37**: 184–96.

O'Connor, R. C., Armitage, C. J. and Gray, L. (2006) The role of clinical and social cognitive variables in parasuicide, *British Journal of Clinical Psychology*, **45**(4): 465–81. (doi:10.1348/014466505X82315) (PMID:17076958)

O'Donnell, L., Stueve, A., Duran, R. et al. (2008) Parenting practices, parents' underestimation of daughters' risks, and alcohol and sexual behaviors of urban girls, *Journal of Adolescent Health*, **42**(5): 496–502.

O'Donovan, B., Mooney, T., Rimmer, B. et al. (2021) Advancing understanding of influences on cervical screening (non)-participation among younger and older women: a qualitative study using the theoretical domains framework and the COM-B model, *Health Expectations*, **24**(6): 2023–35.

Office for National Statistics (2020). Alcohol specific deaths. Statistics, https://www.ons.gov.uk/peoplepopulationandcommunity/healthandsocialcare/causesofdeath/bulletins/alcoholrelateddeathsintheunitedkingdom/registeredin2020

Office for National Statistics (2017) *Opinions and Lifestyle Survey*. https://www.ons.gov.uk

Office for National Statistics (2017c) *Statistics on Obesity, Physical Activity and Diet–England, 2017*. https://www.gov.uk/government/statistics/statistics-on-obesity-physical-activity-and-diet-england-2017

Office for National Statistics (2018) *Adult drinking habits in the UK: 2018*. https://www.ons.gov.uk

Office for National Statistics (2019) *Adult Smoking Habits in the UK: 2019*. https://www.ons.gov.uk

Office for National Statistics (2009) *Contraception and Sexual Health, 2008–9*. https://data.gov.uk/dataset/7d82e0e2-4533-4c0d-bfc1-7ecd1a3c674d/contraception-and-sexual-health

Office for National Statistics (2013) *Contraception and Sexual Health.* https://data.gov.uk/dataset/7d32e0e2-4533-4c0d-bfc1-7ecd1a3c674d/contraception-and-sexual-health

Office for National Statistics (2016) *Annual Extract of Registered Deaths.* https://www.ons.gov.uk

Office for National Statistics (2020) Life expectancy at birth for males and females, UK, between 1980 to 1982 and 2018 to 2020 https://www.ons.gov.uk/peoplepopulationandcommunity/birthsdeathsandmarriages/lifeexpectancies/bulletins/nationallifetablesunitedkingdom/2018to2020#national-life-tables-life-expectancy-in-the-uk-2018-to-2020-data

Ogden, J (2014). Attacks on the nanny state are propped up by vested interests. The Conversation. Attacks on 'nanny state' are propped up by vested interests (theconversation.com)

Ogden, J. (2016a) Celebrating variability and a call to end a systematising approach to research: the example of the Behaviour Change Taxonomy and the Behaviour Change Wheel (with 5 commentaries), *Health Psychology Review*, 10(3): 245–50.

Ogden, J. (2015) Time to retire the TPB? One of us will have to go! *Health Psychology Review*, 9(2): 165–67. Doi: 10.1080/17437199.2014.898679

Ogden, J. and Bridge, L. (2022) How a diagnosis of Polycystic Ovarian Syndrome (PCOS) is communicated impacts well-being, *BJGP Open*, 2022 Apr 29:BJGPO.2022.0014. Doi: 10.3399/BJGPO.2022.0014.

Ogden, J. and Clementi, C. (2011) The experience of being obese and the many consequences of stigma, *Journal of Obesity*, 429098, open access.

Ogden, J. and Elder, C. (1998) The role of family status and ethnic group on body image and eating behaviour, *International Journal of Eating Disorders*, 23: 309–15.

Ogden, J. and Greville, L. (1993) Cognitive changes to preloading in restrained and unrestrained eaters as measured by the Stroop task, *International Journal of Eating Disorders*, 14: 185–95.

Ogden, J. and Hills, L. (2008) Understanding sustained changes in behaviour: the role of life events and the process of reinvention, *Health: An International Journal*, 12: 419–37.

Ogden, J. and Lo, J. (2012) How meaningful are data from Likert scales?: an evaluation of how ratings are made and the role of the response shift in the socially disadvantaged *International Journal of Health Psychology*, 12: 350–61.

Ogden, J. and Maker, C. (2004) Expectant or surgical management: a qualitative study of miscarriage, *British Journal of Obstetrics and Gynaecology*, 111: 463–7.

Ogden, J. and Mundray, K. (1996) The effect of the media on body satisfaction: the role of gender and size, *European Eating Disorders Review*, 4: 171–82.

Ogden, J. and Roy Stanley, C. (2020) How do children make food choices? A think aloud methodology of the transition into agency, *Appetite, (1)* 147:104551. Doi: 10.1016/j.appet.2019.104551.

Ogden, J. and Sherwood, F. (2008) Reducing the impact of media images: an evaluation of the effectiveness of an air-brushing educational intervention on body dissatisfaction, *Health Education*, 108(6): 489–500.

Ogden, J. and Sidhu, S. (2006) Adherence, behaviour change and visualisation: a qualitative study of patients' experiences of obesity medication, *The Journal of Psychosomatic Research*, 62: 545–552.

Ogden, J. and Sidhu, S. (2006) Adherence, behaviour change and visualisation: a qualitative study of patient's experiences of obesity medication, *The Journal of Psychosomatic Research*, 61: 545–52.

Ogden, J. and Steward, J. (2000) The role of the mother–daughter relationship in explaining weight concern, *International Journal of Eating Disorders*, 28: 78–83.

Ogden, J. and Wardle, J. (1990a) Control of eating and attributional style, *British Journal of Clinical Psychology*, 29: 445–6.

Ogden, J. and Wardle, J. (1990b) Cognitive restraint and sensitivity to cues for hunger and satiety, *Physiology and Behaviour*, 47: 477–81.

Ogden, J. and Wardle, J. (1991) Cognitive and emotional responses to food, *International Journal of Eating Disorders*, 10: 297–311.

Ogden, J. and Zoukas, S. (2009) Generating physical symptoms from visual cues: an experimental study, *Psychology, Health and Medicine*, 14: 695–704.

Ogden, J. and Zoukas, S. (2009) Generating physical symptoms from visual cues: an experimental study, *Psychology, Health and Medicine*, 14: 695–704.

Ogden, J., Ambrose, L., Khadra, A. et al. (2002) A questionnaire study of GPs' and patients' belief about the different components of patient centredness, *Patient Education and Counselling*, 47: 223–7.

Ogden, J., Avenell, S. and Ellis, G. (2011) Negotiating control: patients' experiences of unsuccessful weight-loss surgery, *Psychology and Health*, 26(7): 949–64.

Ogden, J., Baig, S., Earnshaw, G. et al. (2001a) What is health? Where GPs' and patients' worlds collide, *Patient Education and Counselling*, 45: 265–9.

Ogden, J., Bandara, I., Cohen, H. et al. (2001b) GPs' and patients' models of obesity: whose problem is it anyway? *Patient Education and Counselling*, 40: 227–33.

Ogden, J., Biliraki, C., Ellis, A. et al. (2021) The impact of active or passive food preparation versus distraction on eating behaviour: an experimental study, *Appetite*, 160:105072. Doi: 10.1016/j.appet.2020.105072.

Ogden, J., Boden, J., Caird, R. et al. (1999) You're depressed; no I'm not: GPs' and patients' different models of depression, *British Journal of General Practice*, **49**: 123–4.

Ogden, J., Branson, R., Bryett, A. et al. (2003) What's in a name? An experimental study of patients' view of the impact and function of a diagnosis, *Family Practice*, **20**(3): 248–53.

Ogden, J., Clementi, C. and Aylwin, S. (2006a) The impact of obesity surgery and the paradox of control: a qualitative study, *Psychology and Health*, **21**(2): 273–93.

Ogden, J., Clementi, C., and Aylwin, S. (2006a) Having obesity surgery: a qualitative study and the paradox of control, *Psychology and Health*, **21**: 273–93.

Ogden, J., Clementi, C., Aylwin, S. and Patel, A. (2005) Exploring the impact of obesity surgery on patients' health status: a quantitative and qualitative study, *Obesity Surgery*, **15**: 266–72.

Ogden, J., Coop, N., Cousins, C. et al. (2013b) Distraction, the desire to eat and food intake: towards an expanded model of mindless eating, *Appetite*, **62**: 119–26.

Ogden, J., Cordey, P., Cutler, L. and Thomas, H. (2013a) Parental restriction and children's diets: the chocolate coin and easter egg experiments, Appetite, **61**: 36–44.

Ogden, J., Gosling, C., Hazelwood, M. and Atkins, E. (2020) Exposure to body diversity images as a buffer against the thin-ideal: an experimental study, *Psychology Health and Medicine*, **25**(10):1165–78. Doi: 10.1080/13548506.2020.1734219

Ogden, J., Heinrich, J., Potter, J. et al. (2009) The impact of viewing a hysteroscopy on a screen on the patient's experience: a randomised trial, *BJOG*, **116**: 286–92.

Ogden, J., Liakopoloulou, E., Antilliou, G. and Gough, G. (2012) The meaning of food (MOF): The development of a new measurement tool. *European Eating Disorders Review*, **20**: 423–6.

Ogden, J., Maxwell, H. and Wong, A. (2019) The development and feasibility study of a low cost evidence based app (ladle) on weight loss and behaviour change. Peer J, 7; e6907 https://doi.org/10.7717/peerj.6907

Ogden, J., Oikonomou, E. and Alemany, G. (2015) Distraction, restrained eating and disinhibition: an experimental study of food intake and the impact of 'eating on the go'. *Journal of Health Psychology*, **22**(1): 39–50.

Ogden, J., Ratcliffe, D. and Snowden-Carr, V. (2019) British Obesity Metabolic Surgery Society endorsed guidelines for the provision of psychological support pre- and post bariatric surgery, *Clinical Obesity*, **9**(6): e12339. Doi: 10.1111/cob.12339.

Ogden, J., Ratcliffe, D. and Snowdon-Carr, V. (2019) BOMSS endorsed guidelines for psychological support pre and post bariatric surgery, *Clinical Obesity*; **9**; e12339. Doi.org/10.1111/cob.12339

Ogden, J., Reynolds, R. and Smith, A. (2006b) Expanding the concept of parental control: a role for overt and covert control in children's snacking behaviour, *Appetite*, **47**: 100–6.

Ogden, J., Smith, L., Nolan, H. et al. (2011) The impact of an educational intervention to protect women against the influence of media images, *Health Education*, **111**: 412–24.

Ogden, J., Veale, D., Summers, Z. (1997) The development and validation of the Exercise Dependence Questionnaire, *Addiction Research*. **5**: 343–56.

Ogden, J., Wood, C., Payne, E. et al. (2018) 'Snack' versus 'meal': the impact of label and presentation on food intake, *Appetite*, **120**: 666–72.

Ogden, J. (1995) Cognitive and motivational consequence of dieting, *European Eating Disorders Review*, **24**: 228–41.

Ogden, J. (2000) The correlates of long-term weight loss: a group comparison study of obesity, *International Journal of Obesity*, **24**: 1018–25.

Ogden, J. (2003) Some problems with social cognition models: a pragmatic and conceptual analysis, *Health Psychology*, **22**, 424–28.

Ogden, J. (2003) Some problems with social cognition models: a pragmatic and conceptual analysis, *Health Psychology*, **22**(4): 424–8.

Ogden, J. (2010) *The Psychology of Eating: From Healthy to Disordered Behaviour*. Chichester: Wiley-Blackwell.

Ogden, J. (2016b) Theories, timing and choice of audience: some key tensions in health psychology and a response to commentaries on Ogden (2016), *Health Psychology Review*, **10**(3): 274–6.

Ogden, J. (2016c) Do no harm: balancing the costs and benefits of patient outcomes in health psychology research and practice, *Journal of Health Psychology*, doi: 10.1177/1359105316648760

Ogden, J. (2018) *The Psychology of Dieting*. London: Routledge.

Ogden, J. (2019) *Thinking Critically about Research: A Step by Step Guide*. London: Routledge.

Okie, S. (2005) Traumatic brain injury in the war zone, *New England Journal of Medicine*, **352**: 2043–47.

Oksuzyan, A., Dańko, M.J., Caputo, J. et al. (2019) Is the story about sensitive women and stoical men true? Gender differences in health after adjustment for reporting behavior, *Social Science & Medicine*, **228**: 41–50.

ölander, F., Thøgersen, J. Understanding of consumer behaviour as a prerequisite for environmental protection. *J Consum Policy* **18**, 345–385 (1995). https://doi.org/10.1007/BF01024160

Oldham-Cooper, R.E., Hardman, C.A., Nicoll, C.E. et al. (2011). Playing a computer game during lunch affects fullness, memory for lunch, and later snack intake. *American Journal of Clinical Nutrition,* **95**(2): 308–13.

Oliver, K.L. (2001) Images of the body from popular culture: engaging adolescent girls in critical inquiry, *Sport, Education and Society,* **6:** 143–64.

Olivera, S.A., Ellison, R.C., Moore, L.L. et al. (1992) Parent–child relationships in nutrient intake: the Framingham Children's Study, *American Journal of Clinical Nutrition,* **56:** 593–8.

ONS (2020) E-Cigarette use in Great Britain, https://www.ons.gov.uk/peoplepopulationandcommunity/healthandsocialcare/drugusealcoholandsmoking/datasets/ecigaretteuseingreatbritain

OPCS (Office of Population, Censuses and Surveys) (1992) *General Household Survey.* London: OPCS.

OPCS (Office of Population, Censuses and Surveys) (1994) *General Household Survey.* London: OPCS.

Orford, J. and Velleman, R. (1991) The environmental intergenerational transmission of alcohol problems: a comparison of two hypotheses, *British Journal of Medical Psychology,* **64:** 189–200.

Orford, J. (2002) *Excessive Appetites: A Psychological View of Addictions,* 2nd edn. Chichester: Wiley.

Ortega, F.B., Cadenas-Sanchez, C., Migueles, J.H. et al. (2018) Role of physical activity and fitness in the characterization and prognosis of the metabolically healthy obesity phenotype: a systematic review and meta-analysis. *Progress in Cardiovascular Diseases,* **61**(2): 190–205.

Ortega, F.B., Cadenas-Sanchez, C., Migueles, J.H. et al. (2018) Role of physical activity and fitness in the characterization and prognosis of the metabolically healthy obesity phenotype: a systematic review and meta-analysis, *Progress in Cardiovascular Diseases,* **61**(2): 190–205.

Orton, M., Fitzpatrick, R., Fuller, A. et al. (1991) Factors affecting women's responses to an invitation to attend for a second breast cancer screening examination, *British Journal of General Practice,* **41:** 320–3.

Osborn, M. and Smith, J.A. (1998) The professional experience of chronic benign lower back pain: an interpretative phenomenological analysis, *Journal of Health Psychology,* **3:** 65–83.

Osorio, C.D., Gallinaro, A.L., Lorenzi-Filho, G. and Lage, L.V. (2006) Sleep quality in patients with fibromyalgia using the Pittsburgh Sleep Quality Index, *Journal of Rheumatology,* **33:**1863–65.

Ouellette, J. and Wood, W. (1998) Habit and intention in everyday life: the multiple processes by which past behaviour predicts future behaviour, *Psychological Bulletin,* **124:** 54–74.

Our World in Data (2022) https://ourworldindata.org/covid-cases

Our World in Data (2022) https://ourworldindata.org/covid-vaccinations

Our World in Data (2022) https://ourworldindata.org/hiv-aids

O'Neil, J.M., Good, G.E. and Holmes, S. (1995) Fifteen years of theory and research on men's gender role conflict: new paradigms for empirical research, in R.F. Levant, and W.S. Pollack (eds) *A New Psychology of Men.* New York: Basic Books.

Paffenbarger, R.S. and Hale, W.E. (1975) Work activity and coronary heart mortality, *New England Journal of Medicine,* **292:** 545–50.

Paffenbarger, R.S., Hyde, R.T., Wing, A.L. and Hsieh, C.C. (1986) Physical activity, all-cause mortality, and longevity of college alumni, *New England Journal of Medicine,* **314:** 605–13.

Paixão, C., Dias, C.M., Jorge, R. et al. (2020) Successful weight loss maintenance: a systematic review of weight control registries, *Obesity Reviews,* **21**(5): e13003.

Pakenham, K., Pruss, M. and Clutton, S. (2000) The utility of socio-demographics, knowledge and health belief model variables in predicting reattendance for mammography screening: a brief report, *Psychology and Health,* **15:** 585–91.

Panagiotakos, D.B., Pitsavos, C.H., Chrysohoou, C. et al. (2003) Status and management of hypertension in Greece; role of the adoption of a Mediterranean diet: the Attica study, *Journal of Hypertension,* **21:** 1483–9.

Panhale, V.P., Walankar, P.P. and Khedekar, S.S. (2021) Chronic pain and fear-avoidance beliefs: a narrative review, *International Journal of Health Sciences and Research,* **11**(6): 219–25.

Panhale, V.P., Walankar, P.P. and Khedekar, S.S. (2021) Chronic pain and fear-avoidance beliefs: a narrative review, *International Journal of Health Sciences and Research,* **11**(6): 219–25.

Parameshwaran, V., Cockbain, B.C., Hillyard, M. and Price, J.R. (2017) Is the lack of specific lesbian, gay, bisexual, transgender and queer/questioning (LGBTQ) health care education in medical school a cause for concern? Evidence from a survey of knowledge and practice among UK medical students, *Journal of Homosexuality,* **64**(3): 367–81.

Parfitt, G., Rose, E.A. and Burgess, W.M. (2006) The psychological and physiological responses of sedentary individuals to prescribed and preferred intensity exercise, *British Journal of Health Psychology,* **11:** 39–53.

Park, C.J. (2004) The notion of growth following stressful life experiences: problems and prospects, *Psychological Inquiry,* **15**(1): 69–76.

Park, C.L. and Folkman, S. (1997) The role of meaning in the context of stress and coping, *General Review of Psychology,* **2:** 115–44.

Park, C.L., Cohen, L.H. and Murch, R.L. (1996) Assessment and prediction of stress-related growth, *Journal of Personality*, **64**: 71–105.

Park, C.L., Edmonson, D., Fenster, J.A. and Blank, T.O. (2008) Positive and negative health behavior changes in cancer survivors: a stress and coping perspective, *Journal of Health Psychology*, **13**(8): 1198–1206.

Park, L.C. and Covi, L. (1965) Non-blind placebo trial: an exploration of neurotic patients' responses to placebo when its inert content is disclosed, *Archives of General Psychiatry*, **12**: 336–45.

Parker, L. L. and Harriger, J. A. (2020) Eating disorders and disordered eating behaviors in the LGBT population: a review of the literature, *Journal of Eating Disorders*, **8**(1): 1–20.

Parkes, K.R. (2006) Physical activity and self-rated health: interactive effects of activity in work and leisure domains, *British Journal of Health Psychology*, **11**: 533–50.

Parsons, T. (1951) *The Social System*. New York: The Free Press.

Parswani, M.J., Sharma, M.P. and Iyengar, S.S. (2013) Mindfulness-based stress reduction program in coronary heart disease: a randomized control trial, *International Journal of Yoga*, **6**(2): 111.

Partridge, C.J. and Johnston, M. (1989) Perceived control and recovery from physical disability, *British Journal of Clinical Psychology*, **28**: 53–60.

Pasman, L. and Thompson, J.K. (1988) Body image and eating disturbance in obligatory runners, obligatory weightlifters and sedentary individuals, *International Journal of Eating Disorders*, **7**: 759–69.

Patel, P., Bush, T., Kojic, E.M. et al. (2018) Prevalence, incidence, and clearance of anal high-risk human papillomavirus infection among HIV-infected men in the SUN study, *The Journal of Infectious Diseases*, **217**(6): 953–63.

Patel, P., Bush, T., Kojic, E.M. et al. (2018) Prevalence, incidence, and clearance of anal high-risk human papillomavirus infection among HIV-infected men in the SUN study, *The Journal of Infectious Diseases*, **217**(6): 953–63.

Patrick, D.L. and Ericson, P.E. (1993) *Health Status and Health Policy: Allocating Resources to Health Care*. Oxford: Oxford University Press.

Pavlin, D.J., Sullivan, M.J., Freund, P.R. and Roesen, K. (2005) Catastrophising: a risk factor for post-surgical pain, *The Clinical Journal of Pain*, **21**(1): 83–90.

Paxton, S.J., Browning, C.J. and O'Connell, G. (1997) Predictors of exercise program participation in older women, *Psychology and Health*, **12**: 543–52.

Pearce, E., Jolly, K., Harris, I.M. et al. (2022) What is the effectiveness of community-based health promotion campaigns on chlamydia screening uptake in young people and what barriers and facilitators have been identified? A mixed-methods systematic review, *Sexually Transmitted Infections*, **98**(1): 62–69.

Pearl, R.L. and Puhl, R.M. (2018) Weight bias internalization and health: a systematic review, *Obesity Reviews*, **19**(8): 1141–63.

Pearson, N., Biddle, S.J., and Gorely, T. (2009) Family correlates of breakfast consumption among children and adolescents: a systematic review, *Appetite*, **52**(1): 1–7.

Pearte, C.A., Furberg, C.D., O'Meara, E. S. et al. (2006) Characteristics and baseline clinical predictors of future fatal versus nonfatal coronary heart disease events in older adults: the Cardiovascular Health Study, *Circulation*, **113**(18): 2177–35.

Pendleton, D., Schofield, T., Tate, P. and Havelock, P. (1984) *The Consultation: An Approach to Learning and Teaching*. Oxford: Oxford Medical Publications.

Pennebaker, J.W. and Smyth, J. (2016) *Opening Up by Writing it Down: The Healing Power of Expressive Writing* (3rd edn). New York: Guilford Press.

Pennebaker, J.W. (1982) *The Psychology of Physical Symptoms*. New York: Springer-Verlag.

Pennebaker, J.W. (1983) Accuracy of symptom perception, in A. Baum, S.E. Taylor and J. Singer (eds) *Handbook of Psychology and Health*, vol. 4. Hillsdale, NJ: Erlbaum.

Pennebaker, J.W. (1993) Putting stress into words: health, linguistic, and therapeutic implications, *Behaviour Research and Therapy*, **31**: 539–48.

Pennebaker, J.W. (1997) Writing about emotional experiences as a therapeutic process, *Psychological Science*, **8**(3): 162–6.

Pepper, J.K., Emery, S.L., Ribisl, K.M. et al. (2015) How risky is it to use e-cigarettes? Smokers' beliefs about their health risks from using novel and traditional tobacco products. *Journal of Behavioral Medicine*, **38**(2): 318–26.

Pereira, D.B., Antoni, M.H., Danielson, A. et al. (2003) Life stress and cervical squamous intraepithelial lesions in women with human papillomavirus and human immunodeficiency virus, *Psychosomatic Medicine*, **65**(1): 1–8.

Pereira-Miranda, E., Costa, P.R., Queiroz, V.A. et al. (2017) Overweight and obesity associated with higher depression prevalence in adults: a systematic review and meta-analysis, *Journal of American College of Nutrition*, **10**: 1–11.

Perna, F.M. and McDowell, S.L. (1995) Role of psychological stress in cortisol recovery from exhaustive exercise among elite athletes, *International Journal of Behavioural Medicine*, **2**: 13–26.

Peters, E.M., Schedlowski, M., Watzl, C. and Gimsa, U. (2021) To stress or not to stress: Brain-behavior-immune interaction may weaken or promote the immune response to SARS-CoV-2, *Neurobiology of Stress*, **14**, 100296.

Petersen, A. (1998) *Unmasking the Masculine: 'Men' and 'Identity' in a Sceptical Age.* London: Sage.

Peto, R., Lopez, A.D., Boreham, J. et al. (1994) *Mortality from Smoking in Developed Countries 1950–2000.* Oxford: Oxford University Press.

Petrie, K.J., Cameron, L.D., Ellis, C.J. et al. (2002) Changing illness perceptions after myocardial infarction: an early intervention randomized controlled trial, *Psychosomatic Medicine*, **64**: 580–6.

Petrie, K.J., Weinman, J.A., Sharpe, N. and Buckley, J. (1996) Role of patients' view of their illness in predicting return to work and functioning after myocardial infarction: longitudinal study, *British Medical Journal*, **312**: 1191–4.

Petronis, V.M., Carver, C.S., Antoni, M.H. and Weiss, S. (2003) Investment in body image and psychosocial well-being among women treated for early stage breast cancer: partial replication and extension, *Psychology and Health*, **18**(1): 1–13.

Petticrew, M., Fraser, J.M. and Regan, M. (1999) Adverse life-events and risk of breast cancer: a meta-analysis, *British Journal of Health Psychology*, **4**: 1–17.

Petty, R.E. and Cacioppo, J.T. (1986) The elaboration likelihood model of persuasion, in L. Berkowitz (ed.) *Advances in Experimental Social Psychology*, vol. 19. New York: Academic Press.

Petty, R.E. and Cacioppo, J.T. (1997) The elaboration likelihood model of persuasion, Journal of School Psychology, 35; 107-136

Phelan, S.M., Burgess, D.J., Yeazel, M.W. et al. (2015) Impact of weight bias and stigma on quality of care and outcomes for patients with obesity, *Obesity Reviews*, **16**(4): 319–26.

Phelps, J., Velez-Dalla Tor, M., Chen, C. and Shalikar, H. (2021) In patients with obesity, does treatment with weight loss medication lead to clinically significant weight loss? *Evidence-Based Practice*, **24**(5): 48–49.

Phillips, A.C., Der, G. and Carroll, D. (2008) Stressful life-events exposure is associated with 17-year mortality, but it is health-related events that prove predictive, *British Journal of Health Psychology*, **13**(4): 647–57.

Phillips, A.C., Der, G. and Carroll, D. (2010) Self-reported health, self-reported fitness and all-cause mortality: prospective cohort study, *British Journal of Health Psychology*, **15**: 337–46.

Phillips, A.L. and Mullan, B.A. (2022) Ramifications of behavioural complexity for habit conceptualization, promotion, and measurement, *Health Psychology Review*, 1–31. DOI: 10.1080/17437199.2022.2060849

Phillips, J., Ogden, J. and Copland, C. (2015) Using drawings of pain-related images to understand the experience of chronic pain: a qualitative study, *British Journal of Occupational Therapy*, **78**, 404–11.

Piccinelli, M. and Simon, G. (1997) Gender and cross-cultural differences in somatic symptoms associated withemotion distress: an international study in primary care, *Psychological Medicine*, **27**(2): 433–44.

Picot, J., Jones, J., Colquitt, J.L. et al. (2009) The clinical effectiveness and cost-effectiveness of bariatric (weight loss) surgery for obesity: a systematic review and economic evaluation, *Health Technology Assessment*, **13**: 41.

Pienaar, K., Murphy, D., Race, K. and Lea, T. (2020) Sexualities and intoxication: "To be intoxicated is to still be me, just a little blurry"—Drugs, enhancement and transformation in lesbian, gay, bisexual, transgender and queer cultures. In F. Hutton (ed), *Cultures of Intoxication* (pp. 139–63). Cham, Switzerland: Springer Nature/ Palgrave Macmillan.

Pinder, K.L., Ramierz, A.J., Black, M.E. et al. (1993) Psychiatric disorder in patients with advanced breast cancer: prevalence and associated factors, *European Journal of Cancer*, **29 A**: 524–7.

Platek, S.M., Mohamed, F.B. and Gallup Jr., G.G. (2005) Contagious yawning and the brain, *Cognitive Brain Research*, **23**: 448–52.

Pliner, P. and Loewen, E.R. (1997) Temperament and food neophobia in children and their mothers, *Appetite*, **28**: 239–54.

Plotnikoff, R.C., Lippke, S., Trinh, L. et al. (2010) Protection motivation theory and the prediction of physical activity among adults with type 1 or type 2 diabetes in a large population sample, *British Journal of Health Psychology*, **15**(3): 643–61.

Plotnikoff, R.C., Rhodes, R.E. and Trinh, L. (2009) Protection motivation theory and physical activity: a longitudinal test among a representative population sample of Canadian adults, *Journal of Health Psychology*, **14**(8): 1119–34.

Pocock, S., Brieger, D.B., Owen, R. et al. (2021) Health-related quality of life 1–3 years post-myocardial infarction: its impact on prognosis, *Open Heart*, **8**(1): e001499. Doi:10.1136/ openhrt-2020-001499.

Pocock, S., Brieger, D.B., Owen, R. et al.(2021) Health-related quality of life 1–3 years post-myocardial infarction: its impact on prognosis, *Open Heart*, **8**(1): e001499.

Polivy, J. and Herman, C.P. (1983) *Breaking the Diet Habit.* New York: Basic Books.

Polivy, J. and Herman, C.P. (1999) Distress and eating: why do dieters overeat? *International Journal of Eating Disorders*, **26**(2): 153–64.

Polivy, J., Herman, C.P., Hackett, R. and Kuleshnyk, I. (1986). The effects of self-attention and public attention on eating in restrained and unrestrained subjects. *Journal of Personality and Social Psychology*, **50**, 1253–60.

Pollard, C., and Kennedy, P. (2007) A longitudinal analysis of emotional impact, coping strategies and post-traumatic psychological growth following spinal cord injury: a 10-year review, *British Journal of Health Psychology*, **12**: 347–62.

Pomerleau, O.F. and Brady, J.P. (1979) *Behavioral Medicine: Theory and Practice.* Baltimore, MD: Williams & Wilkins.

Posavac, S.S. and Posavac, H.D. (2002) Predictors of women's concern with body weight: the roles of perceived self-media ideal discrepancies and self-esteem, *Eating Disorders*, **10**(2): 153–60.

Potthoff, S., Rasul, O., Sniehotta, F.F. et al. (2019) The relationship between habit and healthcare professional behaviour in clinical practice: a systematic review and meta-analysis, *Health Psychology Review*, **13**(1): 73–90.

Povey, R., Conner, M., Sparks, P. et al. (2000) The theory of planned behaviour and healthy eating: examining additive and moderating effects of social influence variables, *Psychology and Health*, **14**: 991–1006.

Prentice, A. (1999) Aetiology of obesity I: Introduction, in *Obesity: The Report of the British Nutrition Foundation Task Force.* Oxford: Blackwell Science.

Prentice, A.M. and Jebb, S.A. (1995) Obesity in Britain: gluttony or sloth? *British Medical Journal*, **311**: 437–9.

Prentice, A.M., Black, A.E., Goldberg, G.R. et al. (1986) High levels of energy expenditure in obese women, *British Medical Journal*, **292**: 983–7.

Prentice, A.M. (1995) Are all calories equal? in R. Cottrell (ed.) *Weight Control: The Current Perspective.* London: Chapman & Hall.

Prettyman, R.J., Cordle, C.J. and Cook, G.D. (1993) A three-month follow-up of psychological morbidity after early miscarriage, *British Journal of Medical Psychology*, **66**: 363–72.

Prinsen, S., Evers, C. and de Ridder, D.T.D. (2016) Oops I did it again: examining self-licensing effects in a subsequent self-regulation dilemma, *Applied Psychology: Health and Well-Being*, **8**(1): 104–26.

Prochaska, J.O. and DiClemente, C.C. (1982) Transtheoretical therapy: toward a more integrative model of change, *Psychotherapy: Theory Research and Practice*, **19**: 276–88.

Prochaska, J.O. and DiClemente, C.C. (1984) *The Transtheoretical Approach: Crossing Traditional Boundaries of Therapy.* Homewood, IL: Dow Jones Irwin.

Prochaska, J.O. and Velicer, W.F. (1997) The transtheoretical model of health behaviour change, *American Journal of Health Promotion*, **12**: 38–48.

Provencher, V., Polivy, J. and Herman, C.P. (2009) Perceived healthiness of food: if its healthy, you can eat more! *Appetite*, **52**(2): 340–4.

Prugger, C., Wellman, J., Heidrich, J. et al. (2008) Cardiovascular risk factors and mortality in patients with coronary heart disease, *European Journal of Epidemiology*, **23**(11): 731–7.

Public Health England (2016) *Eatwell Guide.* https://assets.publishing.service.gov.uk/government/uploads/system/uploads/attachment_data/file/528193/Eatwell_guide_colour.pdf

Public Health England (2017) Campaign to protect young people from STIs by using condoms. https://www.gov.uk/government/news/campaign-to-protect-young-people-from-stis-by-using-condoms

Public Health England (2018) *Progress towards Ending the HIV Epidemic in the United Kingdom.* https://assets.publishing.service.gov.uk/government/uploads/system/uploads/attachment_data/file/759408/HIV_annual_report_2018.pdf

Public Health England. (2021). *National Diet and Nutrition Survey.* https://www.gov.uk/government/statistics/ndns-diet-and-physical-activity-a-follow-up-study-during-covid-19

Puntillo, K. and Weiss, S.J. (1994) Pain: its mediators and associated morbidity in critically ill cardiovascular surgical patients, *Nursing Research*, **43**: 31–6.

Putnam, R.D. (1993) The prosperous community: social capital and public life, *American Prospect*, **4**: 13.

Quaife, S.L., Janes, S.M. and Brain, K.E. (2021) The person behind the nodule: a narrative review of the psychological impact of lung cancer screening, *Translational Lung Cancer Research*, **10**(5): 2427–40.

Quine, L., Rutter, D.R. and Arnold, L. (1998) Predicting safety helmet use among schoolboy cyclists: a comparison of the theory of planned behaviour and the health belief model, *Psychology and Health*, **13**: 251–69.

Rüther, T., Kiss, A., Eberhardt, K. et al. (2018) Evaluation of the cognitive behavioral smoking reduction program 'Smoke_less': a randomized controlled trial. *European Archives of Psychiatry and Clinical Neuroscience*, **268**(3): 269–77.

Raats, M.M., Shepherd, R. and Sparks, P. (1995) Including moral dimensions of choice within the structure of the theory of planned behavior, *Journal of Applied Social Psychology*, **25**: 484–94.

Rabbitte, M. and Enriquez, M. (2019) The role of policy on sexual health education in schools, *The Journal of School Nursing*, **35**(1): 27–38.

Rabiau, M., Knäuper, B. and Miquelon, P. (2006) The eternal quest for optimal balance between maximizing pleasure and minimizing harm: the compensatory health benefits model, *British Journal of Health Psychology*, **11**: 139–53.

Radley, A. (1984) The embodiment of social relation in coronary heart disease, *Social Science and Medicine*, **19**: 1227–34.

Radley, A. (1989) *Prospects of Heart Surgery: Psychological Adjustment to Coronary Bypass Grafting.* New York: Springer Verlag.

Radnitz, C., Byrne, S., Goldman, R. et al. (2009) Food cues in children's television programs, *Appetite*, 52(1): 230–3.

Radtke, T., Scholz, U., Keller, R. et al. (2011) Smoking-specific compensatory health beliefs and the readiness to stop smoking in adolescents, *British Journal of Health Psychology*, 16: 610–25.

Rafanelli, C., Gostoli, S., Tully, P.J. and Roncuzzi, R (2016) Hostility and the clinical course of outpatients with congestive heart failure, *Psychology and Health*, 31(2): 228–38.

Rains, P. (1971) *Becoming an Unwed Mother*. Chicago: Aldine.

Rajiah, K. and Venaktaraman, R. (2019) The effect of demographic and social factors on the decision-making of community pharmacists in ethical dilemmas, *Journal of Research in Pharmacy Practice*, 8(3), 174–77.

Rakowski, W. (1986) Personal health practices, health status, and expected control over future health, *Journal of Community Health*, 11(3): 189–203.

Ramirez, A.J., Craig, T.J.K., Watson, J.P. et al. (1989) Stress and relapse of breast cancer, *British Medical Journal* 298: 291–3.

Ramirez, A.J., Watson, J.P., Richards, M.A. et al. (1992) Life events and breast cancer prognosis: letter to the editor, *British Medical Journal*, 304: 1632.

Ramos-Jaraba, S.M., Berbesí-Fernández, D.Y., Bedoya-Mejía, S. et al. (2021) Factors associated with the perception of HIV vulnerability among transgender women in three Colombian cities, *Revista Peruana de Medicina Experimental y Salud Pública*, 38: 232–39.

Ramsay, J.M., McDermott, M.R. and Bray, C. (2001) Components of anger-hostility complex and symptom reporting in patient with coronary artery disease: a multi-measure study, *Journal of Health Psychology*, 6(6): 713–29.

Rankin, K., Le, D. and Sweeny, K. (2020) Preemptively finding benefit in a breast cancer diagnosis, *Psychology & Health*, 35(5): 613–28.

Rapkin, B.D. and Schwartz, C.E. (2004) Towards a theoretical model of quality of life appraisal: implications of findings from studies of response shift, *Health and Quality of Life Outcomes*, 2: 14.

Rathert, C., Wyrwich, M.D. and Boren, S.A. (2013) Patient-centered care and outcomes: a systematic review of the literature, *Medical Care Research and Review*, 70(4): 351–79.

Ratner, P.A., Johnson, J.L., Shoveller, J.A. et al. (2003) Non-consensual sex experienced by men who have sex with men: prevalence and association with mental health, *Patient Education and Counseling*, 49(1): 67–74.

Rauber, F., Steele, E.M., Louzada, M.L.D.C. et al. (2020) Ultra-processed food consumption and indicators of obesity in the United Kingdom population (2008–2016), *PLoS One*, 15(5): e0232676.

Rebar, A.L., Rhodes, R.E. and Gardner, B. (2019) How we are misinterpreting physical activity intention–behavior relations and what to do about it, *International Journal of Behavioral Nutrition and Physical Activity*, 16(1): 1–13.

Rector, T.S., Kubo, S.H. and Cohn, J.N. (1993) Validity of the Minnesota Living with Heart Failure Questionnaire as a measure of therapeutic response: effects of enalapril and placebo, *American Journal of Cardiology*, 71: 1006–7.

Redd, W.H. (1982) Behavioural analysis and control of psychosomatic symptoms in patients receiving intensive cancer treatment, *British Journal of Clinical Psychology*, 21: 351–8.

Reed, G.M., Kemeny, M.E., Taylor, S.E. and Visscher, B.R. (1999) Negative HIV-specific expectancies and AIDS-related bereavement as predictors of symptom onset in asymptomatic HIV positive gay men, *Health Psychology*, 18: 354–63.

Reed, G.M., Kemeny, M.E., Taylor, S.E. et al. (1994) Realistic acceptance as a predictor of decreased survival time in gay men with AIDS, *Health Psychology*, 13: 299–307.

Rees, K., Bennett, P., West, R. et al. (2004) Psychological interventions for coronary heary disease, *Cochrane Database of Systematic Reviews*, 2, art no. CD002902.

Reime, B., Novak, P., Born, J. et al. (2000) Eating habits, health status and concern about health: a study among 1641 employees in the German metal industry, *Preventive Medicine*, 30: 295–301.

Reisi, M., Javadzade, S.H., Shahnazi, H. et al. (2014). Factors affecting cigarette smoking based on health-belief model structures in pre-university students in Isfahan, Iran. *Journal of Education and Health Promotion*, 3: 31–5.

Remien, R.H., Stirratt, M.J., Nguyen, N. et al. (2019) Mental health and HIV/AIDS: the need for an integrated response, *AIDS (London, England)*, 33(9): 1411–20.

Repetti, R.L. (1993) Short-term effects of occupational stressors on daily mood and health complaints, *Health Psychology*, 12: 125–31.

Resnicow, K., Jackson, A., Wang, T. et al. (2001). A motivational interviewing intervention to increase fruit and vegetable intake through black churches: results of the Eat for Life trial, *American Journal of Public Health*, 91(10): 1686–93.

Reyes Fernández, B., Knoll, N., Hamilton, K., and Schwarzer, R. (2016) Social-cognitive antecedents of hand washing: action control bridges the planning–behaviour gap. *Psychology & Health*, 31(8): 993–1004.

Richard, R. and van der Pligt, J. (1991) Factors affecting condom use among adolescents, *Journal of Community and Applied Social Psychology,* **1**: 105–16.

Ridge, D. T. (2004) 'It was an incredible thrill': the social meanings and dynamics of younger gay men's experiences of barebacking in Melbourne, *Sexualities,* **7**(3): 259–79.

Riebl, S.K., Estabrooks, P. A., Dunsmore, J.C. et al. (2015) A systematic literature review and meta-analysis: The Theory of Planned Behavior's application to understand and predict nutrition-related behaviors in youth. *Eating Behaviors,* **18**: 160–78.

Riedl, D. and Schuessler, G. (2021) Prevalence of depression and cancer–a systematic review, *Zeitschrift für Psychosomatische Medizin und Psychotherapie,* **67**, OA11.

Rief, W. and Broadbent, E. (2007) Explaining medically unexplained symptoms-models and mechanisms, *Clinical Psychology Review,* **27**(7): 821–41.

Riegel, B.J. (1993) Contributions to cardiac invalidism after acute myocardial infarction, *Coronary Artery Disease,* **4**: 569–78.

Rimer, B.K., Trock, B., Lermon, C. et al. (1991) Why do some women get regular mammograms? *American Journal of Preventative Medicine,* **7**: 69–74.

Rimer, J., Dwan, K., Lawlor, D.A. et al. (2012) Exercise for depression. *Cochrane Database of Systematic Reviews,* **7**, Ar t. No.: CD004366. Doi: 10.1002/14651858.CD004366.pub5.

Riper, H., Andersson, G., Hunter, S. B., de Wit, J., Berking, M. and Cuijpers, P. (2014) Treatment of comorbid alcohol use disorders and depression with cognitive-behavioural therapy and motivational interviewing: a meta-analysis, *Addiction,* **109**(3): 394–406.

Risdon, A., Eccleston, C., Crombez, G. and McCracken, L. (2003) How can we learn to live with pain? A Q-methodological analysis of the diverse understandings of acceptance of chronic pain, *Social Science and Medicine,* **56**(2): 375–86.

Rise, J., Kovac, V., Kraft, P. and Moan, I.S. (2008) Predicting the intention to quit smoking and quitting behaviour: extending the theory of planned behaviour, *British Journal of Health Psychology,* **13**: 291–310.

Rissanen, A.M., Heliovaara, M., Knekt, P. et al. (1991) Determinants of weight gain and overweight in adult Finns, *European Journal of Clinical Nutrition,* **45**: 419–30.

Rizza, F., Gison, A., Bonassi, S. et al. (2017) 'Locus of control', health-related quality of life, emotional distress and disability in Parkinson's disease, *Journal of Health Psychology,* **22**(7): 844–52.

Robertson S. and Williamson P. (2005) Men and health promotion in the UK: ten years further on? *Health Education Journal,* **64**: 293–301.

Robertson, S. (2007) The current context of men's health and the role of masculinities, in S. Robertson, *Understanding Men and Health: Masculinities, Identity and Well-being.* Maidenhead: Open University Press.

Robinson, B.B.E., Bockting, W.O., Rosser, B.R.S. et al. (2002) The sexual health model: application of a sexological approach to HIV prevention, *Health Education Research,* **17**(1): 43–57.

Robinson, E., Aveyard, P., Daley, A. et al. (2013). Eating attentively: a systematic review and meta-analysis of the effect of food intake memory and awareness on eating. *American Journal of Clinical Nutrition,* **97**(4): 728–42.

Robinson, E., Oldham, M., Cuckson, I. et al. (2016) Visual exposure to large and small portion sizes and perceptions of portion size normality: three experimental studies, *Appetite,* **98**: 28–34. doi: 10.1016/j.appet.2015.12.010

Rocholl, M., Ludewig, M., Brakemeier, C. et al. (2021) Illness perceptions of adults with eczematous skin diseases: a systematic mixed studies review, *Systematic Reviews,* **10**(1): 1–15.

Rockliffe, L., Peters, S., Smith, D.M. et al. (2022) Investigating the utility of the COM-B and TM model to explain changes in eating behaviour during pregnancy: a longitudinal cohort study, *British Journal of Health Psychology,* **27**(3): 1077–99. Doi: 10.1111/bjhp.12590.

Rogers, R.W. (1975) A protection motivation theory of fear appeals and attitude change, *Journal of Psychology,* **91**: 93–114.

Rogers, R.W. (1985) Attitude change and information integration in fear appeals, *Psychological Reports,* **56**: 179–82.

Rohde, K., Keller, M., la Cour Poulsen, L. et al. (2019) Genetics and epigenetics in obesity, *Metabolism,* **92**: 37–50.

Romero-Corral, A.R., Montori, V.M., Somers, V.K. et al. (2006) Association of body weight with total mortality and with cardiovascular events in coronary artery disease: a systematic review of cohort studies, *Lancet,* **368**: 666–78.

Rona, R.J., Jones M., Fear, N.T. et al. (2012) Mild traumatic brain injury in UK military personnel returning from Afghanistan and Iraq: cohort and cross-sectional analyses, *The Journal of Head Trauma Rehabilitation,* **27**:33–44.

Rooney, B., Smalley, K., Larson, J. and Havens, S. (2003) Is knowing enough? Increasing physical activity by wearing a pedometer, *Wisconsin Medical Journal,* **102**(4): 31–6.

Rosário, F., Santos, M.I., Angus, K. et al. (2021) Factors influencing the implementation of screening and brief interventions for alcohol use in primary care practices: a systematic review using the COM-B system and Theoretical Domains Framework, *Implementation Science,* **16**(1): 1–25.

Rosen, C.J. and Ingelfinger, J.R. (2022) Shifting tides offer new hope for obesity, *The New England Journal of Medicine*, 10.1056/NEJMe2206939. Advance online publication.Doi.org/10.1056/NEJMe2206939.

Rosen, C.S. (2000) Is the sequencing of change processes by stage consistent across health problems? A meta-analysis, *Health Psychology*, **19**: 593–604.

Rosenberg, M. (1965) *Society and the Adolescent Self-image*. Princeton, NJ: Princeton University Press.

Rosenfeld, J.A. (1992) Emotional responses to therapeutic abortion, *American Family Physician*, **45**: 137–40.

Rosenman, R.H., Brand, R.J., Jenkins, C.D. et al. (1975) Coronary heart disease in the western collaborative heart study: final follow-up experience of 8½ years, *Journal of the American Medical Association*, **233**: 872–7.

Rosenman, R.H. (1978) Role of type A pattern in the pathogenesis of ischaemic heart disease and modification for prevention, *Advances in Cardiology*, **25**: 34–46.

Rosenstock, I.M. (1966) Why people use health services, *Millbank Memorial Fund Quarterly*, **44**: 94–124.

Roske, K., Schumann, A., Hannover, W. et al. (2008) Postpartum smoking cessation and relapse prevention intervention: a structural equation modelling application to behavioural and non-behavioural outcomes of a randomized controlled trial, *Journal of Health Psychology*, 13(4), 556–8.

Roskies, E., Seraganian, P., Oseasohn, R. et al. (1986) The Montreal type A intervention project: major findings, *Health Psychology*, **5**: 45–69.

Ross, C.E., and Bird, C.E. (1994) Sex stratification and health lifestyle: consequences of men's and women's perceived health, *Journal of Health and Social Behavior*, **35**: 161–78.

Ross, M. and Olson, J.M. (1981) An expectancy attribution model of the effects of placebos, *Psychological Review*, **88**: 408–37.

Rosser, B.A., Vowels, K.E., Keogh, E. et al. (2009) Technologically-assisted behaviour change: a systematic review of studies of novel technologies for the management of chronic illness, *Journal of Telemedicine and Telecare*, **15**: 327–38.

Rossner, S., Sjostrom, L., Noak, R. et al. (2000) Weight loss, weight maintenance and improved cardiovascular risk factors after 2 years' treatment with Orlistat for obesity, *Obesity Research*, **8**: 49–61.

Roter, D.L., Steward, M., Putnam, S.M. et al. (1997) Communication pattern of primary care physicians, *Journal of the American Medical Association*, **277**: 350–6.

Roth, G.A., Johnson, C.O., Abate, K.H., Global Burden of Cardiovascular Diseases Collaboration et al. (2018) The burden of cardiovascular diseases among US states, 1990–2016. *JAMA cardiology*, 3(5): 375–389. Doi.org/10.1001/jamacardio.2018.0385.

Roth, S. and Cohen, L.J. (1986) Approach avoidance and coping with stress, *American Psychologist*, **41**: 813–19.

Rouyard, T., Kent, S., Baskerville, R. et al. (2017) Perceptions of risks for diabetes-related complications in Type 2 diabetes populations: a systematic review. *Diabetic Medicine*, 34(4): 467–77.

Rozin, P. (1976) *The Selection of Foods by Rats, Humans, and Other Animas: Advances in the Study of Behavior*. New York: Academic Press.

Rubak, S., Sandbæk, A., Lauritzen, T. and Christensen, B. (2005) Motivational interviewing: a systematic review and meta-analysis, *The British Journal of General Practice*, **55**(513): 305–12.

Rubin, R. and Quine, L. (1995) Women's attitudes to the menopause and the use of hormone replacement therapy. Paper presented at the conference of the British Psychological Society, London.

Ruble, D.N. (1977) Premenstrual symptoms: a reinterpretation, *Science*, **197**: 291–2.

Rugg, C.D., Malzacher, T., Ausserer, J. et al. (2021) Gender differences in snowboarding accidents in Austria: a 2005–2018 registry analysis, *BMJ Open*, **11**(10): e053413.

Ruini, C. and Vescovelli, F. (2013) The role of gratitude in breast cancer: its relationships with post-traumatic growth, psychological well-being and distress, *Journal of Happiness Studies*, **14**(1): 263–74.

Ruiter, R.A.C., Abraham, C. and Kok, G. (2001) Scary warnings and rational precautions: a review of the psychology of fear appeals, *Psychology and Health*, **16**(6): 613–30.

Russo, N.F. and Zierk, K.I. (1992) Abortion, childbearing, and women's well-being, *Professional Psychology: Research and Practice*, **23**: 269–80.

Söderberg, H., Janzon, L. and Sjöberg, N.O. (1998) Emotional distress following induced abortion: a study of its incidence and determinants among abortees in Malmö, Sweden, *European Journal of Obstetrics and Gynecology, and Reproductive Biology*, **79**: 173–8.

Sable, M.R., Libbus, M.K. and Chiu, J.E. (2000) Factors affecting contraceptive use in women seeking pregnancy tests: Missouri, 1997, *Family Planning Perspectives*, **32**(3):124–31.

Sacco, P., Bucholz, K.K. and Harrington, D. (2014) Gender differences in stressful life events, social support, perceived stress, and alcohol use among older adults: results from a national survey, *Substance Use & Misuse*, **49**(4): 456–65.

Safren, S.A., O'Cleirigh, C.M., Bullis, J.R. et al. (2012) Cognitive behavioral therapy for adherence and depression (CBT-AD) in HIV-infected injection drug users: a randomized controlled trial. *Journal of Consulting and Clinical Psychology*, **80**(3): 404–15.

Sahin, C., Courtney, K. L., Naylor, P. J. and E Rhodes, R. (2019) Tailored mobile text messaging interventions targeting type 2 diabetes self-management: a systematic review and a meta-analysis, *Digital Health*, **5**, 2055207619845279.

Sairam, S., Khare, M., Michailidis, G. and Thilaganathan, B. (2001) The role of ultrasound in the expectant management of early pregnancy loss, *Ultrasound in Obstetrics and Gynecology*, **17**: 506–9.

Sait, M., Aljarbou, A., Almannie, R. and Binsaleh, S. (2021) Knowledge, attitudes, and perception patterns of contraception methods: Cross-sectional study among Saudi males, *Urology Annals*, **13**(3): 243–53.

Sajobi, T.T., Speechley, K.N., Liang, Z. et al. (2017) Response shift in parents' assessment of health-related quality of life of children with new-onset epilepsy, *Epilepsy and Behavior*, **75**: 97–101.

Sala, F., Krupat, E. and Rother, D. (2002) Satisfaction and the use of humour by physicians and patients, *Psychology and Health*, **17**: 269–80.

Sallis, J.F., Haskell, W.L., Fortmann, S.P. et al. (1986) Predictors of adoption and maintenance of physical activity in a community sample, *Preventive Medicine*, **15**: 331–41.

Salvy, S.J., Romero, N., Paluch, R., and Epstein, L.H. (2007) Peer influence on pre-adolescent girls' snack intake: effects on weight status, *Appetite*, **49**(1): 177–82.

Salvy, S.J., Vartanian, L.R., Coelho, J.S. et al. (2008) The role of familiarity on modeling of eating and food consumption in children, *Appetite*, **50**: 514–18.

Samwel, H.J.A., Kraaimaat, F.W., Crul, B.J.P. et al. (2009) Multidisciplinary allocation of chronic pain treatment: effects and cognitive-behavioural predictors of outcome, *British Journal of Health Psychology*, **14**(3): 405–21.

Sanchez, E.K., Speizer, I.S., Tolley, E. et al. (2020) Influences on seeking a contraceptive method among adolescent women in three cities in Nigeria, *Reproductive Health*, **17**(1): 1–11.

Sandberg, T. and Conner, M. (2009) A mere measurement effect for anticipated regret: impacts on cervical screening attendance, *British Journal of Social Psychology*, **48**: 221–36.

Sanders, A.E., Slade, G.D., Fillingim, R.B. et al. (2020) Effect of treatment expectation on placebo response and analgesic efficacy: a secondary aim in a randomized clinical trial, *JAMA Network Open*, **3**(4): e202907–e202907.

Sanders, C., Egger, M., Donovan, J. et al. (1998) Reporting on quality of life in randomised controlled trials: bibliographic study, *British Medical Journal*, **317**: 1191–4.

Sanderson, C.A. and Yopyk, D.J.A. (2007) Improving condom use intentions and behavior by changing perceived partner norms: an evaluation of condom promotion videos for college students, *Health Psychology*, **26**(4): 481–7.

Sanjuán, P., Molero, F., Fuster, M.J. and Nouvilas, E. (2013) Coping with HIV related stigma and well-being, *Journal of Happiness Studies*, **14**(2): 709–22.

Santi, S., Best, J.A., Brown, K.S. and Cargo, M. (1991) Social environment and smoking initiation, *International Journal of the Addictions*, **25**: 881–903.

Santos, I., Sniehotta, F.F., Marques, M.M. et al. (2017) Prevalence of personal weight control attempts in adults: a systematic review and meta-analysis, *Obesity Reviews*, **18**(1): 32–50.

Sarason, I.G., Levine, H.M., Basham, R.B. et al. (1983) Assessing social support: the social support questionnaire, *Journal of Personality and Social Psychology*, **44**: 127–39.

Sarason, I.G., Sarason, B.R., Shearin, E.N. and Pierce, G.R. (1987) A brief measure of social support: practical and theoretical implications, *Journal of Social and Personal Relationships*, **4**: 497–510.

Sarnak, D.O., Wood, S.N., Zimmerman, L.A. et al. (2021) The role of partner influence in contraceptive adoption, discontinuation, and switching in a nationally representative cohort of Ugandan women, *PLoS One*, **16**(1): e0238662.

Savage, I. (1993) Demographic influences on risk perceptions, *Risk Analysis*, **13**: 413–20.

Savage, R. and Armstrong, D. (1990) Effect of a general practitioner's consulting style on patients' satisfaction: a controlled study, *British Medical Journal*, **301**: 968–70.

Scambler, A., Scambler, G. and Craig, D. (1981) Kinship and friendship networks and women's demands for primary care, *Journal of the Royal College of General Practice*, **26**: 746–50.

Schachter, S. and Gross, L. (1968) Manipulated time and eating behaviour, *Journal of Personality and Social Psychology*, **10**: 98–106.

Schachter, S. and Rodin, J. (1974) *Obese Humans and Rats*. Potomac, MD: Erlbaum.

Schaefer, C., Quesenberry, C.P. Jr and Wi, S. (1995) Mortality following conjugal bereavement and the effects of a shared environment, *American Journal of Epidemiology*, **141**: 1142–52.

Schafer, S.M., Colloca, L. and Wager, T.D. (2015) Conditioned placebo analgesia persists when subjects know they are receiving a placebo, *The Journal of Pain*, **16**(5): 412–20.

Schappert, S.M. (1999) Ambulatory care visits to physician offices, hospital out-patient departments, and emergency departments: United States 1997, *Vital and Health Statistics–Series 13: Data from the National Health Survey*, November: 1–39.

Schmidt, L.R. and Frohling, H. (2000) Lay concepts of health and illness from a developmental perspective, *Psychology and Health*, **15**: 229–38.

Schmidt, R.A., Genois, R., Jin, J. et al. (2021) The early impact of COVID-19 on the incidence, prevalence, and severity of alcohol use and other drugs: a systematic review, *Drug and Alcohol Dependence*, **228**:109065.

Schaarrs, P.W., Jones, S.S., Parsons, J.T. et al. (2021) Sexual subcultures and HIV prevention methods: An assessment of condom use, PrEP, and TasP among gay, bisexual, and other men who have sex with men using a social and sexual networking smartphone application, *Archives of Sexual Behavior*, **50**(4): 1781–92.

Scholz, U., Schüz, B., Ziegelmann, J.P. et al. (2008) Beyond behavioural intentions: planning mediates between intentions and physical activity, *British Journal of Health Psychology*, **13**(3): 479–94.

Schurman, M., Hesse, M.D., Stephan, K.E. et al. (2005) Yearning to yawn: the neural basis of contagious yawning. *Neuro Image*, **24**: 1260–4.

Schwartz, G.E. and Weiss, S.M. (1977) *Yale Conference on Behavioral Medicine*. Washington, DC: Department of Health, Education and Welfare; National Heart, Lung, and Blood Institute.

Schwarzer, R. (ed.) (1992) *Self Efficacy: Thought Control of Action*. Washington, DC: Hemisphere.

Scott, E.J., Eves, F.F., French, D.P. and Hoppe, R. (2007) The theory of planned behaviour predicts self-reports of walking, but does not predict step count, *British Journal of Health Psychology*, **12**: 601–20.

Scott, S.E., Grunfeld, E.A., Auyeung, V. and McGurk, M. (2009) Barriers and triggers to seeking help for potentially malignant oral symptoms: implications for interventions, *Journal of Public Health Dentistry*, **69**(1) 34–40.

Scott, W., Hann, K.E. and McCracken, L.M. (2016) A comprehensive examination of changes in psychological flexibility following acceptance and commitment therapy for chronic pain, *Journal of Contemporary Psychotherapy*, **46**(3): 139–48.

Searle, A., Norman, P., Thompson, R. and Vedhara, K. (2007) A prospective examination of illness beliefs and coping in patients with type 2 diabetes, *British Journal of Health Psychology*, **12**(4): 621–38.

Seoregts, E.H.W.J., Falger, P.R.J. and Bar, F.W.H.M. (2000) Risk factor modification through nonpharmacological interventions in patients with coronary heart disease, *Journal of Psychosomatic Research*, **48**: 425–41.

Segal, L. (1994) *Straight Sex: The Politics of Pleasure*. London: Virago.

Seligman, F. and Nemeroff, C.B. (2015) The interface of depression and cardiovascular disease: therapeutic implications *Annals of the New York Academy of Sciences*, **1345**, 25–35. Doi.org/10.1111/nyas.12738

Seligman, M.E.P. and Csikszentmihalyi, M. (2000) Positive psychology: an introduction, *American Psychology*, **55**: 5–14.

Seligman, M.E.P. and Visintainer, M.A. (1985) Turnout rejection and early experience of uncontrollable shock in the rat, in F.R. Brush and J.B. Overmier (eds) *Affect Conditioning and Cognition: Essays on the Determinants of Behavior*. Hillsdale, NJ: Erlbaum.

Sell, K., Oliver, K. and Meiksin, R. (2021) Comprehensive sex education addressing gender and power: a systematic review to investigate implementation and mechanisms of impact, *Sexuality Research and Social Policy*, 1–17. DOI:10.1007/s13178-021-00674-8

Selye, H. (1956) *The Stress of Life*. New York: McGraw-Hill.

Semlyen, J., King, M., Varney, J. and Hagger-Johnson, G. (2016) Sexual orientation and symptoms of common mental disorder or low wellbeing: combined meta-analysis of 12 UK population health surveys, *BMC Psychiatry*, **16**(1), 1–9.

Senior, V., Marteau, T.M. and Weinman, J. (2000) Impact of genetic testing on causal models of heart disease and arthritis: an analogue study, *Psychology and Health*, **14**: 1077–88.

Seydel, E., Taal, E. and Wiegman, O. (1990) Risk appraisal, outcome and self efficacy expectancies: cognitive factors in preventative behaviour related to cancer, *Psychology and Health*, **4**: 99–109.

Shahab, L., Hall, S. and Marteau, T.M. (2007) Showing smokers with vascular disease images of their arteries to motivate cessation: a pilot study, *British Journal of Health Psychology*, **12**: 275–83.

Shand, L.K., Cowlishaw, S., Brooker, J.E. et al. (2015) Correlates of post-traumatic stress symptoms and growth in cancer patients: A systematic review and meta-analysis. *Psycho-Oncology*, **24**(6): 624–34.

Sheeran, P. and Orbell, S. (1998) Implementation intentions and repeated behaviour: augmenting the predictive validity of the theory of planned behaviour, *European Journal of Social Psychology*, **28**: 1–21.

Sheeran, P., White, D. and Phillips, K. (1991) Premarital contraceptive use: a review of the psychological literature, *Journal of Reproductive and Infant Psychology*, **9**: 253–69.

Sheldrick, R., Tarrier, N., Berry, E. and Kincey, J. (2006) Post-traumatic stress disorder and illness perceptions over time following myocardial infarction and subarachnoid haemorrhage, *British Journal of Health Psychology*, **11**: 387–400.

Shenassa, E.D., Frye, M., Braubach, M., and Daskalakis, C. (2008) Routine stair climbing in place of residence and body mass index: a pan-European population based study, *International Journal of Obesity*, **32**(3): 490–4.

Shenefelt, P.D. (2013) Anxiety reduction using hypnotic induction and self guided imagery for relaxation during dermatologic procedures, *International Journal of Clinical and Experimental Hypnosis*, **61**(3): 305–18.

Shepherd, J.M., Fogle, B., Garey, L. et al. (2021) Worry about COVID-19 in relation to cognitive-affective smoking processes among daily adult combustible cigarette smokers, *Cognitive Behaviour Therapy*, **50**(4): 336–50.

Shepherd, R. and Farleigh, C.A. (1986) Attitudes and personality related to salt intake, *Appetite*, **7**: 343–54.

Shepherd, R. and Stockley, L. (1985) Fat consumption and attitudes towards food with a high fat content, *Human Nutrition: Applied Nutrition*, **39A**: 431–42.

Shepherd, R. (1988) Belief structure in relation to low-fat milk consumption, *Journal of Human Nutrition and Dietetics*, **1**: 421–8.

Shepperd, S., Harwood, D., Jenkinson, C. et al. (1998) Randomised controlled trial comparing hospital at home care with inpatient hospital care. I: three-month follow-up of health outcomes, *British Medical Journal*, **316**: 1786–91.

Sherman, D.A.K., Nelson, L.D. and Steele, C.M. (2000) Do messages about health risks threaten the self? Increasing the acceptance of threatening health messages via self-affirmation, *Personality and Social Psychology Bulletin*, **26**: 1046–58.

Shinar, D., Schechtman, E. and Compton, R. (1999) Trends in safe driving behaviors and in relation to trends in health maintenance behaviors in the USA: 1985–1995, *Accident: Analysis and Prevention*, **31**(5): 497–503.

Siegel, K., Raveis, V.H., Krauss, J. et al. (1992) Factors associated with gay men's treatment initiation decisions for HIV-infection, *AIDS Education and Prevention*, **4**(2): 135–42.

Siegman, A.W. and Snow, S.C. (1997) The outward expression of anger, the inward experience of anger and CVR: the role of vocal expression, *Journal of Behavioural Medicine*, **20**: 29–46.

Siegman, A.W., Townsend, S.T., Civelek, A.C. and Blumenthal, R.S. (2000) Antagonistic behaviour, dominance, hostility and coronary heart disease, *Psychosomatic Medicine*, **62**: 248–57.

Silton, N.R., Flannelly, K.J. and Lutjen, L.J. (2013) It pays to forgive! Aging, forgiveness, hostility, and health, *Journal of Adult Development*, **20**(4): 222–31.

Silva, A. F. D. and Lopes, M. H. B. D. M. (2020) Locus of control, knowledge, attitude and practice for contraception among adolescents, *Revista Brasileira de Enfermagem*, **73**(2), e20170604.

Simpson, S.H., Eurich, D.T., Majumdar, S.R. et al. (2006) A meta-analysis of the association between adherence to drug therapy and mortality, *British Medical Journal*, **333**(7557): 15.

Simpson, W.M., Johnston, M. and McEwan, S.R. (1997) Screening for risk factors for cardiovascular disease: a psychological perspective, *Scottish Medical Journal*, **42**: 178–81.

Sirriyeh, R., Lawton, R. and Ward, J. (2010) Physical activity and adolescents: an exploratory randomized controlled trial investigating the influence of affective and instrumental text messages, *British Journal of Health Psychology*, **15**(4): 825–40.

Siu, W.H.S., Li, P.R. and See, L.C. (2021) Rate of condom use among sexually active adolescents: a nationwide cross-sectional study in Taiwan from 2012 to 2016, *BMJ Open*, **11**(8): e047727.

Sjostrom, L., Rissanen, A., Andersen, T. et al. (1998) Randomised placebo controlled trial of orlistat for weight loss and prevention of weight regain in obese patients, *Lancet*, **352**: 167–72.

Skar, S., Sniehotta, F.F., Araujo-Soares, V. and Molloy, G.J. (2008) Prediction of behaviour vs. prediction of behaviour change: the role of motivational moderators in the theory of planned behaviour, *Applied Psychology: An International Review*, **57**: 609–27.

Skelton, J.A. and Pennebaker, J.W. (1982) The psychology of physical symptoms and sensations, in G.S. Sanders and J. Suls (eds) *Social Psychology of Health and Illness*. Hillsdale, NJ: Erlbaum.

Skevington, S. and O'Connell, K. (2003) Measuring quality of life in HIV and AIDS: a review of the recent literature, *Psychology and Health*, **18**(3): 331–50.

Skevington, S., O'Connell, K.A. and the WHOQoL Group (2004a) Can we identify the poorest quality of life? Assessing the importance of quality of life using the WHOQoL-100, *Quality of Life Research*, **13**: 23–34.

Skevington, S., Sortarius, N., Amir, M. and the WHOQoL Group (2004b) Developing methods for assessing quality of life in different cultural settings, *Social Psychiatry and Psychiatric Epidemiology*, **39**: 1–8.

Skinner, T.C., Carey, M.E., Cradock, S. et al (2006) Diabetes education and self-management for ongoing and newly diagnosed (DESOND): process modelling of pilot study, *Patient Education and Counselling*, **64**: 369–77.

Slade, P. and Russell, G.F.M. (1973) Awareness of body dimensions in anorexia nervosa: cross-sectional and longitudinal studies, *Psychological Medicine*, **3**: 188–99.

Slade, P., Heke, S., Fletcher, J. and Stewart, P. (1998) A comparison of medical and surgical termination of pregnancy: choice, emotional impact and satisfaction with care, *British Journal of Obstetrics and Gynaecology*, **105**(12): 1288–95.

Smedslund, G. (2000) A pragmatic basis for judging models and theories in health psychology: the axiomatic method, *Journal of Health Psychology*, **5**: 133–49.

Smit, K., Voogt, C., Otten, R. et al. (2019) Exposure to parental alcohol use rather than parental drinking shapes offspring's alcohol expectancies, *Alcoholism: Clinical and Experimental Research*, **43**(9): 1967–77.

Smith, J.A. and Osborn, M. (2003) Interpretative phenomenological analysis, in J.A. Smith (ed.) *Qualitative Psychology*. London: Sage.

Smith, J.A., Michie, S., Stephenson, M. and Quarrell, O. (2002) Risk perception and decision-making processes in candidates for genetic testing for Huntington's disease: an interpretative phenomenological analysis, *Journal of Health Psychology*, **7**(3): 131–44.

Smith, Jonathan A. and Flowers, P. and Larkin, M. (2009) *Interpretative Phenomenological Analysis: Theory, method and research*. London: Sage.

Smith, L.M., Mullis, R.L. and Hill, W.E. (1995) Identity strivings within the mother–daughter relationship, *Psychological Reports*, **76**: 495–503.

Smith, R.A., Williams, D.K., Silbert, J.R. and Harper, P.S. (1990) Attitudes of mothers to neonatal screening for Duchenne muscular dystrophy, *British Medical Journal* **300**: 1112.

Snedecor, M.R., Boudreau, C.F., Ellis, B.E. et al. (2000) U.S. air force recruit injury and health study, *American Journal of Preventive Medicine*, **18**(3, suppl.): 129–40.

Sniehotta, F.F. (2009) Towards a theory of intentional behaviour change: plans, planning, and self-regulation, *British Journal of Health Psychology*, **14**(2): 261–73.

Sniehotta, F.F., Presseau, J. and Araújo-Soares, V. (2014) Time to retire the Theory of Planned Behaviour, *Health Psychology Review*, **8**(1): 1–7. Doi: 10.1080/17437199.2013.869710

Sniehotta, F.F., Scholz, U. and Schwarzer, R. (2005) Bridging the intention-behaviour gap: planning, self-efficacy, and action control in the adoption and maintenance of physical exercise, *Psychology and Health*, **20**(2): 143–60.

Sniehotta, F.F., Scholz, U. and Schwarzer, R. (2006) Action plans and coping plans for physical exercise: a longitudinal intervention study in cardiac rehabilitation, *British Journal of Health Psychology*, **11**: 23–37.

Snoek, H.M., Engels, R.C., Janssens, J.M., and van Strien, T. (2007) Parental behaviour and adolescents' emotional eating, *Appetite*, 49(1): 223–30.

Sobel, M.B. and Sobel, L.C. (1978) *Behavioral Treatment of Alcohol Problems*. New York: Plenum.

Sodergren, S.C., Hyland, M.E., Singh, S.J. and Sewell, L. (2002) The effect of rehabilitation on positive interpretations of illness, *Psychology and Health*, **17**(6): 753–60.

Soetens, B., Braet, C., Dejonckheere, P. and Roets, A. (2006) When suppression backfires: the ironic effects of suppressing eating-related thoughts, *Journal of Health Psychology*, **11**(5): 655–68.

Sogg, S., Lauretti, J. and West-Smith, L. (2016) Recommendations for the presurgical psychosocial evaluation of bariatric surgery patients, *Surgery for Obesity and Related Diseases*, **12**(4): 731–49.

Sohlberg, T. and Bergmark, K.H. (2020) Lifestyle and long-term smoking cessation, *Tobacco Use Insights*, 13, 1179173X20963062.

Solano, L., Costa, M., Temoshok, L. et al. (2002) An emotionally inexpressive (type C) coping style

influences HIV disease progression at six and twelve month follow-up, *Psychology and Health*, **17**(5): 641–55.

Solano, L., Montella, F., Salvati, S. et al. (2001) Expression and processing of emotions: relationship with CD4+ levels in 42 HIV-positive asymptomatic individuals, *Psychology and Health*, **16**: 689–98.

Solomon, G.F. and Temoshok, L. (1987) A psychoneuroimmunologic perspective on AIDS research: questions, preliminary findings, and suggestions, *Journal of Applied Social Psychology*, **17**: 286–308.

Solomon, G.F., Temoshok, L., O'Leary, A. and Zich, J.A. (1987) An intensive psychoimmunologic study of long-surviving persons with AIDS: pilot work background studies, hypotheses, and methods, *Annals of the New York Academy of Sciences*, **46**: 647–55.

Sommer, M., de Rijike, J.M., van Kleef, M. et al. (2010) Predictors of acute postoperative pain after elective surgery, *Clinical Journal of Pain*, **26**(2): 87–94.

Song, T., Qian, S. and Yu, P. (2019) Mobile health interventions for self-control of unhealthy alcohol use: systematic review, *JMIR mHealth and uHealth*, **7**(1): e10899.

Sparks, P., Hedderley, D. and Shepherd, R. (1992) An investigation into the relationship between perceived control, attitude variability and the consumption of two common foods, *European Journal of Social Psychology*, **22**: 55–71.

Speisman, J.C., Lazarus, R.S., Mordko, A. and Davison, L. (1964) Experimental reduction of stress based on ego defense theory, *Journal of Abnormal and Social Psychology*, **68**: 367–80.

Spitzer, L. and Rodin, J. (1981) Human eating behaviour: a critical review of studies in normal weight and overweight individuals, *Appetite*, **2**: 293–329.

Sport England (2013) *Who Plays Sport?* http://www.sportengland.org/research/who-plays-sport/

Sport Participation in England (2017) House of Commons Library, Briefing Paper CBP 8181. http://www.parliament.uk/commons-library

Stanton, R., To, Q. G., Khalesi, S., Williams, S. L., Alley, S. J., Thwaite, T. L., Vandelanotte, C. et al. (2020) Depression, anxiety and stress during COVID-19: associations with changes in physical activity, sleep, tobacco and alcohol use in Australian adults, *International Journal of Environmental Research and Public Health*, **17**(11): 4065.

Stanton, R., To, Q.G., Khalesi, S. et al. (2020) Depression, anxiety and stress during COVID-19: associations with changes in physical activity, sleep, tobacco and alcohol use in Australian adults, *International Journal of Environmental Research and Public Health*, **17**(11): 4065.

Stead, M., Hastings, G. and Eadie, D. (2002) The challenge of evaluating complex interventions: a framework for evaluating media advocacy, *Health Education Research*, **17**(3): 351–64.

Steele, C.M. (1988) The psychology of self-affirmation: sustaining the integrity of the self, in L. Berkowitz (ed.) *Advances in Experimental Social Psychology*. New York: Academic Press.

Steer, C., Campbell, S., Davies, M. et al. (1989) Spontaneous abortion rates after natural and assisted conception, *British Medical Journal*, **299**: 1317–18.

Stegen, K., Van Diest, I., Van De Woestijne, K.P. and Van Den Berch, O. (2000) Negative affectivity and bodily sensations induced by 5.5% CO2 enriched air inhalation: is there a bias to interpret bodily sensations negatively in persons with negative affect? *Psychology and Health*, **15**: 513–25.

Steiger, H., Stotland, S., Ghadirian, A.M. and Whitehead, V. (1994) Controlled study of eating concerns and psychopathological traits in relatives of eating-disordered probands: do familial traits exist? *International Journal of Eating Disorders*, **18**: 107–18.

Steinberg, J. (2001) Many undertreated HIV-infected patients decline potent antiretroviral therapy, *AIDS Patient Care*, **15**: 185–91.

Stephens, D., Kentaka, E., Varpa, K. et al. I. (2007) Positive experiences associated with Ménière's disorder, *Otology and Neurology*, 28: 982–87.

Stern, J.S. (1984) Is obesity a disease of inactivity? in A.J. Stunkard and E. Stellar (eds) *Eating and Its Disorders*. New York: Raven Press.

Stewart, A.L. and Ware, J.E. (eds) (1992) *Measuring Functioning and Well Being: The Medical Outcomes Study Approach*. Durham, NC: Duke University Press.

Stewart, S.F. and Ogden, J. (2021) The impact of body diversity vs thin-idealistic media messaging on health outcomes: an experimental study, *Psychology Health and Medicine*, **26**(5):631–43. Doi: 10.1080/13548506.2020.1859565.

Stewart, T.L., Chipperfield, J.G., Perry, R.P. and Hamm, J.M. (2016) Attributing heart attack and stroke to 'old age': implications for subsequent health outcomes among older adults, *Journal of Health Psychology*, **21**(1): 40–9.

Stewart, W.F., Lipton, R.B. and Liberman, J. (1996) Variation in migraine prevalence by race, *Neurology*, **47**: 52–9.

Stice, E., Schupak-Neuberg, E., Shaw, H.E. and Stein, R.L. (1994) Relation of media exposure to eating disorders symptomatology: an examination of mediation mechanisms, *Journal of Abnormal Psychology*, **103**: 836–40.

Stiles, W.B. (1978) Verbal response models and dimensions of interpersonal roles: a method of discourse analysis, *Journal of Personality and Social Psychology*, **36**: 693–703.

Stoate, H. (1989) Can health screening damage your health? *Journal of the Royal College of General Practitioners*, **39**: 193–5.

Stokes, J. and Rigotti, N. (1988) The health consequences of cigarette smoking and the internist's role in smoking cessation, *Annals of Internal Medicine*, **33**: 431–60.

Stone, A.A. and Brownell, K.D. (1994) The stress-eating paradox: multiple daily measurements in adult males and females, *Psychology and Health*, **9**: 425–36.

Stone, A.A. and Neale, J.M. (1984) New measure of daily coping: development and preliminary results, *Journal of Personality and Social Psychology*, **46**: 892–906.

Stone, K.E. Lamphear, B.P., Pomerantz, W.J. and Khoury, J. (2000) Childhood injuries and deaths due to falls from windows, *Journal of Urban Health*, **77**: 26–33.

Stone, N. and Ingham, R. (2000) *Young People's Sex Advice Services: Delays, Triggers and Contraceptive Use*. London: Brook Publications.

Stone, N. and Ingham, R. (2002) Factors affecting British teenagers' contraceptive use at first intercourse: the importance of partner communication, *Perspectives on Sexual and Reproductive Health*, **34**(4): 191–7.

Stone, N. and Ingham, R. (2003) When and why do young people in the United Kingdom first use sexual health services? *Perspectives on Sexual and Reproductive Health*, **35**(3): 114–20.

Stone, N., Hatherall, B., Ingham, R. and McEachran, J. (2006) Oral sex and condom use among young people in the United Kingdom, *Perspectives on Sexual and Reproductive Health*, **38**(1): 6–12.

Stonewall (2018) *LGBT in Britain*, https://www.stonewall.org.uk/lgbt-britain-health.

Stormer, S.M. and Thompson, J.K. (1996) Explanations of body-image disturbances: a test of maturational status, negative verbal commentary, social comparison, and sociocultural hypotheses, *International Journal of Eating Disorders*, **19**(2): 193–202.

Stovitz, S.D., VanWormer, J.J., Center, B.A. and Bremer, K.L. (2005) Pedometers as a means to increase ambulatory activity for patients seen at a family medicine clinic, *The Journal of the American Board of Family Medicine*, **18**(5): 335–43.

Strain, G.W., Kolotkin, R.L., Dakin, G.F. et al. (2014) The effects of weight loss after bariatric surgery on health-related quality of life and depression, *Nutrition and Diabetes*, **4**(9): e132.

Stratton, G., Fairclough, S.J. and Ridgers, N.D. (2008) Physical activity levels during the school day, in A.L. Smith and S.J.H. Biddle (eds) *Youth Physical Activity and Sedentary Behaviour: Challenges and Solutions*. Champaign, IL: Human Kinetics.

Strickhouser, J.E., Zell, E. and Krizan, Z. (2017) Does personality predict health and well-being? A metasynthesis, *Health Psychology*, **36**(8): 797–810.

Stroebele, N. and de Castro, J.M. (2004) Effect of ambience on food intake and food choice, *Nutrition*, 20(9): 821–38.

Stroebele, N. and de Castro, J.M. (2006) Listening to music while eating is related to increases in people's food intake and meal duration. *Appetite*, 47(3): 285–9.

Stronegger, W.J. Freidl, W. and Rasky, E. (1997) Health behaviour and risk behaviour: socioeconomic differences in an Austrian rural county, *Social Science and Medicine*, 44: 423–6.

Stuart, R.B. and Davis, B. (1972) *Slim Chance in a Fat World: Behavioral Control of Obesity*. Champaign, IL: Research Press.

Stubbs, J., Whybrow, S., Teixeira, P. et al. (2011) Problems in identifying predictors and correlates of weight loss and maintenance: implications for weight control therapies based on behaviour change, *Obesity Reviews*, 12(9): 688–708.

Stunkard, A.J. and Messick, S. (1985) The three factor eating questionnaire to measure dietary restraint, disinhibition and hunger, *Journal of Psychosomatic Research*, 29: 71–8.

Stunkard, A.J., Harris, J.R., Pedersen, N.L. and McClearn, G.E. (1990) A separated twin study of body mass index, *New England Journal of Medicine*, 322: 1483–7.

Stunkard, A.J., Sorenson, T.I.A., Hanis, C. et al. (1986) An adoption study of human obesity, *New England Journal of Medicine*, 314: 193–8.

Stunkard, A.J. (1958) The management of obesity, *New York State Journal of Medicine*, 58: 79–87.

Stunkard, A.J. (1984) The current status of treatment for obesity in adults, in A.J. Stunkard and E. Stellar (eds) *Eating and its Disorders*. New York: Raven Press.

Suarez, E.C, Williams, R.B., Kuhn, C.M. et al. (1991) Biobehavioural basis of coronary-prone behaviour in middle-aged men: part II, serum cholesterol, the type A behaviour pattern and hostility as interactive modulators of physiological reactivity, *Psychosomatic Medicine*, 53: 528–37.

Sim, W.H.S., Li, F.R. and See, L.C. (2021) Rate of condom use among sexually active adolescents: a nationwide cross-sectional study in Taiwan from 2012 to 2016, BMJ Open, 11(8): e047727.

Suicides in the UK: 2016 registrations. (2016) Office for National Statistics https://www.ons.gov.uk/people populationandcommunity/birthsdeathsandmarriages/deaths/bulletins/suicidesintheunitedkingdom/2016reg istrations

Sullivan, M.J.L. Thorn, B., Haythornthwaite, J.A. et al. (2001) Theoretical perspectives on the relation between catastrophising and pain, *Clinical Journal of Pain*, 17: 53–61.

Sutherland, K., Christianson, J.B. and Leatherman, S. (2008) Impact of targeted financial incentives on personal health behaviour: a review of literature, *Medical Care Research and Review*, 65: 36S–78S.

Sutton, L.S., and White, K.M. (2016) Predicting sun-protective intentions and behaviours using the theory of planned behaviour: a systematic review and meta-analysis. *Psychology and Health*, 31(11): 1272–92.

Sutton, S., Saidi, G., Bickler, G. and Hunter, J. (1995) Does routine screening for breast cancer raise anxiety? Results from a three wave prospective study in England, *Journal of Epidemiology and Community Health*, 49: 413–18.

Sutton, S., Wardle, J., Taylor, T. et al. (2000) Predictors of attendance in United Kingdom flexible sigmoidoscopy screening trial, *Journal of Medical Screening*, 7: 99–104.

Sutton, S. (1998a) Predicting and explaining intentions and behavior: how well are we doing? *Journal of Applied Social Psychology*, 28: 1317–38.

Sutton, S. (1999) The psychological costs of screening, in J.S. Tobias and I.C. Henderson (eds) *New Horizons in Breast Cancer: Current Controversies, Future Directions*. London: Chapman & Hall.

Sutton, S. (2000) Interpreting cross-sectional data on stages of change, *Psychology and Health*, 15: 163–71.

Sutton, S. (2002a) Testing attitude-behaviour theories using non-experimental data: an examination of some hidden assumptions, *European Review of Social Psychology*, 13: 293–323.

Sutton, S. (2005) Stage theories of health behaviour., in M. Conner and P. Norman (eds) *Predicting Health Behaviour*, 2nd edn. Maidenhead: Open University Press.

Sutton, S. (2010) Using social cognition models to develop health behavior interventions: the theory of planned behavior as an example, in D. French, K. Vedhara, A. Kaptein and J. Weinman (eds) *Health Psychology*, 2nd edn. Oxford: Blackwell.

Sutton, S.R. and Hallett, R. (1989) Understanding the effect of fear-arousing communications: the role of cognitive factors and amount of fear aroused, *Journal of Behavioral Medicine*, 11: 353–60.

Sutton, S. (2002b) Using social cognition models to develop health behaviour interventions: problems and assumptions, in D. Rutter and L. Quine (eds) *Changing Health Behaviour: Intervention and Research with Social Cognition Models*. Maidenhead: Open University Press.

Svensson, T., Inoue, M., Sawada, N. et al. (2016) Coping strategies and cancer incidence and mortality: the Japan Public Health Center-based prospective study, *Cancer Epidemiology*, 40: 126–33.

Swann, G., Newcomb, M.E., Crosby, S. et al. (2019) Historical and developmental changes in condom use among young men who have sex with men using a multiple-cohort, accelerated longitudinal design, *Archives of Sexual Behavior*, 48(4): 1099–1110.

Swindle, R.E. Jr and Moos, R.H. (1992) Life domains in stressors, coping and adjustment, in W.B. Walsh, R. Price and K.B. Crack (eds) *Person Environment Psychology: Models and Perspectoves*. Mahwah, NJ: Erlbaum.

Świątoniowska-Lonc, N., Tański, W., Polański, J. et al. (2021) Psychosocial determinants of treatment adherence in patients with type 2 diabetes–a review, *Diabetes, Metabolic Syndrome and Obesity: Targets and Therapy*, **14**: 2701–15.

Syrjala, K.L., Jensen, M.P., Mendoza, M.E. et al. (2014) Psychological and behavioral approaches to cancer pain management, *Journal of Clinical Oncology*, **32**(16): 1703–11.

Sysko, R., Walsh, T.B., and Wilson, G.T. (2007) Expectancies, dietary restraint, and test meal intake among undergraduate women, *Appetite*, **49**: 30–7.

Szasz, T. (1961) *The Myth of Mental Illness*. New York: Harper & Row.

Tan, R.K.J., Kaur, N., Chen, M.I.C. and Wong, C.S. (2020) Individual, interpersonal, and situational factors influencing HIV and other STI risk perception among gay, bisexual, and other men who have sex with men: a qualitative study, *AIDS Care*, **32**(12): 1538–43.

Tan, R.K.J., Kaur, N., Kumar, P.A. et al. (2020) Clinics as spaces of costly disclosure: HIV/STI testing and anticipated stigma among gay, bisexual and queer men, *Culture, Health & Sexuality*, **22**(3): 307–20.

Tanielian, T. and Jaycox, L.H. (eds) (2008) *Invisible wounds of war: psychological and cognitive injuries, their consequences, and services to assist recovery*. Santa Monica, CA: RAND Corporation.

Tannenbaum, M.B., Hepler, J., Zimmerman, R.S. et al. (2015) Appealing to fear: a meta-analysis of fear appeal effectiveness and theories, *Psychological Bulletin*, **141**(6): 1178–204.

Tardy, C.H. (1985) Social support measurement. *American Journal of Community Psychology*, **13**: 187–203.

Tayler, M. and Ogden, J. (2005) Doctors' use of euphemisms and their impact on patients' beliefs about their illness, *Patient Education and Counselling*, **57**: 321–6.

Taylor, L., Ranaldi, H., Amirova, A. et al. (2022) Using virtual representations in mHealth application interventions for health-related behaviour change: a systematic review, *Cogent Psychology*, **9**(1): 2069906.

Taylor, N., Lawton, R. and Conner, M. (2013) Development and initial validation of the determinants of physical activity questionnaire, *International Journal of Behavioral Nutrition and Physical Activity*, **10**: 74.

Taylor, R., Morrell, S., Slaytor, E. and Ford, P. (1998) Suicide in urban New South Wales, Australia 1985–1994: socio-economic and migrant interactions, *Social Science and Medicine*, **47**: 1677–86.

Taylor, R.E., Mann, A.H., White, N.J. and Goldberg, D.P. (2000) Attachment style in patients with medically unexplained physical complaints, *Psychological Medicine*, **30**: 931–41.

Taylor, S., Kemeny, M., Reed, G. and Bower, J. (1998) Psychosocial influence on course of disease: predictors of HIV progression, *Health Psychology Update*, **34**: 7–12.

Taylor, S.E., Lichtman, R.R. and Wood, J.V. (1984) Attributions, beliefs about control, and adjustment to breast cancer, *Journal of Personality and Social Psychology*, **46**: 489–502.

Taylor, S.E. (1983) Adjustment to threatening events: a theory of cognitive adaptation, *American Psychologist*, **38**: 1161–73.

Tedeschi, R.D. and Calhoun, L.G. (2004) Posttraumatic growth: conceptual foundations and empirical evidence, *Psychological Inquiry*, **15**(1): 1–18.

Tedeschi, R.D. and Calhoun, L.G. (2006) Foundations of post traumatic growth, in R.G. Tedeschi and L.G. Calhoun (eds) *Handbook of Post Traumatic Growth*. Hillsdale, NJ: Erlbaum.

Teixeira, P.J., Carraça, E.V., Marques, M.M. et al. (2015) Successful behavior change in obesity interventions in adults: a systematic review of self-regulation mediators, *BMC Medicine*, **13**: 84.

Temoshok, L. and Fox, B.H. (1984) Coping styles and other psychosocial factors related to medical status and to prognosis in patients with cutaneous malignant melanoma, in B.H. Fox and B.H. Newberry (eds) *Impact of Psychoendocrine Systems in Cancer and Immunity*. Toronto: C.J. Hogrefe.

Tennen, H. and Affleck, G. (1999) Finding benefits in adversity, in C.R. Snyder (ed.) *Coping: The Psychology of What Works*. New York: Oxford University Press.

Tennen, H., Affleck, G., Armeli, S. and Carney, M.A. (2000) A daily process approach to coping: linking theory, research and practice, *American Psychologist*, **55**: 626–36.

Teo, C.H., Ng, C.J., Booth, A. and White, A. (2016) Barriers and facilitators to health screening in men: a systematic review, *Social Science and Medicine*, **165**: 168–76.

Teo, I., Krishnan, A. and Lee, G.L. (2019) Psychosocial interventions for advanced cancer patients: a systematic review, *Psycho-oncology*, **28**(7): 1394–1407.

Teo, I., Reece, G.P., Christie, I.C. et al. (2016) Body image and quality of life of breast cancer patients: influence of timing and stage of breast reconstruction, *Psycho-Oncology*, **25**(9): 1106–12.

Terrin, N., Rodday, A.M. and Parsons, S.K. (2015) Joint models for predicting transplant-related mortality from quality of life data, *Quality of Life Research: An International Journal of Quality of Life Aspects of Treatment, Care and Rehabilitation*, **24**(1): 31–9.

Terry, D.J. (1994) Determinants of coping: The role of stable and situational factors, *Journal of Personality and Social Psychology*, **66**(5): 895–910.

Thames Valley Police (2015) Tea and consent. https://www.youtube.com/watch?v=pZwvrxVavnQ

Thames Valley Police (2015) Tea and sex. https://www.youtube.com/watch?v=pZwvrxVavnQ

Thapar, A.K. and Thapar, A. (1992) Psychological sequelae of miscarriage: a controlled study using the general health questionnaire and hospital anxiety and depression scale, *British Journal of General Practice*, 42: 94–5.

Theadom, A. and Cropley, M. (2010) 'This constant being woken up is the worst thing'–experiences of sleep in fibromyalgia syndrome, *Disability and Rehabilitation*, 32(23): 1939–47.

Theadom, A., Cropley, M. and Humphrey, K.L. (2007) Exploring the role of sleep and coping in quality of life in fibromyalgia, *Journal of Psychosomatic Research*, 62(2): 145–51.

Theadom, A., Cropley, M. and Kantermann, T. (2015a) Daytime napping associated with increased symptom severity in fibromyalgia syndrome, *BMC Musculoskeletal Disorders*, 16(1): 1–9.

Theadom, A., Cropley, M., BIONIC Research Group et al. (2015) Sleep difficulties one year following mild traumatic brain injury in a population-based study, *Sleep Medicine*, 16(8): 926–32.

Theadom, A., Cropley, M., Smith, H.E. et al. (2015b) Mind and body therapy for fibromyalgia, *Cochrane Database of Systematic Reviews*, (4). Doi: 10.1002/14651858.

Thomas, J.G., Bond, D.S., Phelan, S. et al. (2014) Weight-loss maintenance for 10 years in the National Weight Control Registry, *American Journal of Preventive Medicine*, 46(1): 17–23.

Thompson, J.K. and Heinberg, L.J. (1999) The media's influence on body image disturbance and eating disorders: we've reviled them, now we can rehabilitate them? *Journal of Social Issues*, 55(2): 339–53.

Thompson, J.P. Palmer, R.L. and Petersen, S.A. (1988) Is there a metabolic component to counterregulation? *International Journal of Eating Disorders*, 7: 307–19.

Thompson, S.C. (1986) Will it hurt less if I can control it? A complex answer to a simple question, *Psychological Bulletin*, 90: 89–101.

Thomson, P., Angus, N.J., Andreis, F. et al. (2020) Longitudinal evaluation of the effects of illness perceptions and beliefs about cardiac rehabilitation on quality of life of patients with coronary artery disease and their caregivers, *BMC Health and Quality of Life Outcomes*, 18(1): 1–14.

Tiggemann, M. and McGill, B. (2004) The role of social comparison in the effect of magazine advertisements on women's mood and body dissatisfaction, *Journal of Social and Clinical Psychology*, 23(1): 23–44.

Timio, M., Verdecchia, P., Venanzi, S. et al. (1988) Age and blood pressure changes: a 20-year follow-up study in nuns in a secluded order, *Hypertension*, 12: 457–61.

Timlin, D., McCormack, J.M. and Simpson, E.E. (2021) Using the COM-B model to identify barriers and facilitators towards adoption of a diet associated with cognitive function (MIND diet), *Public Health Nutrition*, 24(7): 1657–70.

Tollow, P. and Ogden, J. (2016) Patients' experiences of superficial venous surgery for leg ulceration: hope, investment and agency, *Journal of Health Psychology*, doi: 10.1177/1359105316643380.

Tollow, P., Ogden, J., McCabe, C. and Harcourt, D. (2020) The role and relevance of appearance in the wellbeing of adults with incurable cancer: a thematic analysis of patient's experiences, *BMJ Supportive & Palliative Care*, Nov 27:bmjspcare-2020-002632. Doi: 10.1136/bmjspcare-2020-002632.

Torgerson, J.S. and Sjostrom, L. (2001) The Swedish Obese Subjects (SOS) study: rationale and results, *International Journal of Obesity*, May 25(suppl. 1): S2–4.

Totman, R.G. (1987) *The Social Causes of Illness*. London: Souvenir Press.

Trafimow, D., Sheeran, P., Conner, M. and Finlay, K.A. (2002) Evidence that perceived behavioural control is a multidimensional construct: perceived control and perceived difficulty, *British Journal of Social Psychology*, 41: 101–21.

Trafimow, D. (2000) Habit as both a direct cause of intention to use a condom and as a moderator of the attitude-intention and subjective norm intention relations, *Psychology and Health*, 15: 383–93.

Tremblay, M.S., LeBlanc, A.G., Kho, M.E. et al. (2011) Systematic review of sedentary behaviour and health indicators in school-aged children and youth, *International Journal of Behavioral Nutrition and Physical Activity*, 8: 98. Doi: 10.1186/1479-5868-8-98.

Tremolada, M., Taverna, L., Bonichini, S., Putti, M.C., Pillon, M. and Biffi, A. (2020) Health locus of control in parents of children with leukemia and associations with their life perceptions and depression symptomatology, *Children*, 7(5): 40.

Trogen, B. and Caplan, A. (2021) Risk compensation and COVID-19 vaccines, *Annals of Internal Medicine*, 174(6): 858–59.

Troiano, R.P., Berrigan, D., Dodd, K.W. et al. (2008) Physical activity in the United States measured by accelerometer. *Medicine and Science in Sports and Exercise*, 40: 181–8.

Trostle, J.A. (1988) Medical compliance as an ideology, *Social Science and Medicine*, 27: 1299–308.

Tuckett, D., Boulton, M., Olson, C. and Williams, A. (1985) *Meetings Between Experts*. London: Tavistock.

Tudor-Locke, C., Ainsworth, B. E. and Popkin, B. M. (2001) Active commuting to school: an overlooked source of children's physical activity? *Sports Medicine*, 31(5): 309–13.

Tunaley, J.R., Slade, P. and Duncan, S. (1993) Cognitive processes in psychological adaptation to miscarriage: a preliminary report, *Psychology and Health*, **9**: 369–81.

Turk, D.C., Meichenbaum, D. and Genest, M. (1983) *Pain and Behavioral Medicine*. New York: Guilford Press.

Turk, D.C., Wack, J.T. and Kerns, R.D. (1985) An empirical examination of the 'pain-behaviour' construct, *Journal of Behavioral Medicine*, **8**: 119–30.

Turner, A.I., Smyth, N., Hall, S.J. et al. (2020) Psychological stress reactivity and future health and disease outcomes: A systematic review of prospective evidence, *Psychoneuroendocrinology*, **114**: 104599.

Tversky A, Kahneman D (1983). Extensional versus intuitive reasoning: The conjunction fallacy in probability judgement. *Psychological Review*. **90** (4): 293–315. doi:10.1037/0033-295X.90.4.293.

Uitenbroek, D.G., Kerekovska, A. and Festchieva, N. (1996) Health lifestyle behaviour and socio-demographic characteristics: a study of Varna, Glasgow and Edinburgh, *Social Science and Medicine*, **34**: 907–17.

Unicef (2020) https://data.unicef.org/resources/data_explorer

United Nations (2019) *Contraceptive Use by Method*. https://www.un.org/development/desa/pd/content/contraceptive-use-method-2019

Unruh, A.M., Ritchie, J. and Merskey, H. (1999) Does gender affect appraisal of pain and pain coping strategies? *Clinical Journal of Pain*, **15**: 31–40.

Urits, I., Hubble, A., Peterson, E. et al. (2019) An update on cognitive therapy for the management of chronic pain: a comprehensive review, *Current Pain and Headache Reports*, **23**(8): 1–7.

US Environmental Protection Agency (1992) *Respiratory Health Effects of Passive Smoking: Lung Cancer and Other Disorders*. Washington, DC: US Environmental Protection Agency.

USDA (1998/1999) *Continuing Survey of Food Intakes by Individuals (1994–6)*, www.ars.usda.gov.

Ussher, M., Nunziata, P. and Cropley, M. (2001) Effect of a short bout of exercise on tobacco withdrawal symptoms and desire to smoke, *Psychopharmacology*, **158**: 66–72.

Valanis, B.G., Bowen, D.J., Bassford, T. et al. (2000) Sexual orientation and health: comparisons in the women's health initiative sample, *Archives of Family Medicine*, **9**(9): 843–53.

Van Damme, S., Crombez, G. and Eccleston, C. (2002) Retarded disengagement from pain cues: the effect of pain catastrophizing and pain expectancy, *Pain*, **100**(1–2): 111–18.

van de Pligt, J., Zeelenberg, M., van Dijk, W.W. et al. (1998) Affect, attitudes and decisions: let's be more specific, *European Review of Social Psychology*, **8**: 33–66.

Van den Akker, K., Havermans, R.C. and Jansen, A. (2017) Appetitive conditioning to specific times of day, *Appetite*, **116**: 232–8.

Van den Berg, A.E. and Custers, M.H. (2011) Gardening promotes neuroendocrine and affective restoration from stress, *Journal of Health Psychology*, **16**(1): 3–11.

van den Berg, H., Manstead, A.S.R., van der Pligt, J. and Wigboldus, D. (2005) The role of affect in attitudes toward organ donation and donar relevant decisions, *Psychology and Health*, **20**: 789–802.

van Elderen, T. and Dusseldorp, E. (2001) Lifestyle effects of group health education for patients with coronary heart disease, *Psychology and Health*, **16**: 327–41.

van Elderen, T., Maes, S. and van den Broek, Y. (1994) Effects of a health education programme with telephone follow-up during cardiac rehabilitation, *British Journal of Clinical Psychology*, **33**: 367–78.

van Griensven, G.J.P., Teilman, R.A.P., Goudsmit, J. et al. (1986) Riskofaktoren en prevalentie van LAV/HTLV III antistoffen bij homoseksuele mannen in Nederland, *Tijdschrift voor Sociale Gezondheidszorg*, **64**: 100–7.

Van Leeuwen, C.M.C., Kraaijeveld, S., Lindeman, E. and Post, M.W. (2012) Association between psychological factors and quality of life ratings in persons with spinal cord injury: a systematic review, *Spinal Cord*, **50**(3): 174–187.

Van Loey, N., Klein-König, I., Jong, A. et al. (2018) Catastrophizing, pain and traumatic stress symptoms following burns: a prospective study, *European Journal of Pain*, doi: 10.1002/ejp.1203.

Van Mierlo, M.L., van Heugten, C.M., Post, M.W.M. et al. (2015) Life satisfaction post stroke: the role of illness cognitions, *Journal of Psychosomatic Research*, **79**(2): 137–42.

van Strien, T., Frijters, J.E., Bergers, G.P. and Defares, P.B. (1986) Dutch eating behaviour questionnaire for the assessment of restrained, emotional, and external eating behaviour, *International Journal of Eating Disorders*, **5**: 295–315.

van Strien, T., Herman, C.P. and Verheijden, M.W. (2009) Eating style, overeating, and overweight in a representative Dutch sample: does external eating play a role? *Appetite*, **52**(2): 380–7.

van Tulder, M.W., Ostelo, R., Vleeyen, J.W.S. et al. (2000) Behavioural treatment for chronic low back pain, *Spine*, **25**(20): 2688–9.

van Zuuren, F.J. (1998) The effects of information, distraction and coping style on symptom reporting during preterm labor, *Psychology and Health*, **13**: 49–54.

Van Asbeck, F.W.A., Post, M.W.M. and Pangalila, R.F. (2000) An epidemiological description of spinal cord injury in The Netherlands in 1994, *Spinal Cord*, **38**: 420–4.

Vandelanotte, C., Spathonis, K.M., Eakin, E.G. and Owen, N. (2007) Website-delivered physical activity interventions: a review of the literature, *American Journal of Preventive Medicine*, **33**(1): 54–64.

Vanderlinden, J. Adriaensen, A., Vancampfort, D., Pieters, G., Probst, M. and Vansteelandt, K. (2012) A cognitive-behavioral therapeutic program for patients with obesity and binge eating disorder: short-and long-term follow-up data of a prospective study. *Behavior Modification*, **36**(5): 670–86.

Veale, D. (1987) Exercise dependence, *British Journal of Addiction*, **82**: 735–40.

Vedhara, K. (2012) Psychoneuroimmunology: the whole and the sum of its parts, *Brain, Behavior, and Immunity*, **26**(2): 210–1.

Veenstra, G. (2000) Social capital, SES and health: an individual-level analysis, *Social Science & Medicine*, **50**(5): 619–29.

Venturini, F., Romero, M. and Tognoni, G. (1999) Patterns of practice for acute myocardial infarction in a population from ten countries, *European Journal of Clinical Pharmacology*, **54**(11): 877–86.

Verbeke, W., and Vackier, I. (2005) Individual determinants of fish consumption: application of the theory of planned behaviour, *Appetite*, **44**: 67–82.

Verplanken, B. and Aarts, H. (1999) Habit, attitude, and planned behaviour: is habit an empty construct or an interesting case of automaticity? *European Review of Social Psychology*, **10**: 101–34.

Verplanken, B., Aarts, H., van Knippenberg, A. and van Knippenberg, C. (1994) Attitude versus general habit: antecedents of travel mode choice, *Journal of Applied Social Psychology*, **24**: 285–300.

Verplanken, B., Walker, I., Davis, A. and Jurasek, M. (2008) Combining the habit discontinuity and self-activation hypotheses in explaining travel mode choices, *Journal of Environmental Psychology*, **28**: 121–27.

Villanti, A.C., West, J.C., Klemperer, E.M. et al. (2020) Smoking-cessation interventions for US young adults: updated systematic review, *American Journal of Preventive Medicine*, **59**(1): 123–36.

Vinci, C. (2020) Cognitive behavioral and mindfulness-based interventions for smoking cessation: A review of the recent literature, *Current Oncology Reports*, **22**(6): 1–8.

Violanti, J., Marshall, J. and Howe, B. (1983) Police occupational demands, psychological distress and the coping function of alcohol, *Journal of Occupational Medicine*, **25**: 455–8.

Viswanathan, S., Detels, R., Mehta, S.H. et al. (2015) Level of adherence and HIV RNA suppression in the current era of highly active antiretroviral therapy (HAART), *AIDS and Behavior*, **19**(4): 601–11.

Vitaliano, P.P., Maiuro, R.D., Russo, J. et al. (1990) Coping profiles associated with psychiatric, physical health, work and family problems, *Health Psychology*, **9**: 348–76.

Vitaliano, P.P., Russo, J., Bailey, S.L. et al. (1993) Psychosocial factors associated with cardiovascular reactivity in old adults, *Psychosomatic Medicine*, **55**(2): 164–77.

Vlaeyen, J.W.S. and Linton, S. (2000) Fear-avoidance and its consequences in chronic musculoskeletal pain: a state of the art, *Pain*, **85**: 317–32.

Volgsten, H., Jansson, C., Svanberg, A.S. et al. (2018) Longitudinal study of emotional experiences, grief and depressive symptoms in women and men after miscarriage, *Midwifery*, **64**: 23–8.

Volgsten, H., Jansson, C., Svanberg, A.S., Darj, E. and Stavreus-Evers, A. (2018) Longitudinal study of emotional experiences, grief and depressive symptoms in women and men after miscarriage. *Midwifery*, **64**: 23–28.

Von Frey, M. (1895) *Untersuchungen über die Sinnesfunctionen der menschlichen Haut erste Abhandlung: Druck-empfindung und Schmerz.* Leipzig: Hirzel.

Vos, J. (2021) Cardiovascular disease and meaning in life: a systematic literature review and conceptual model, *Palliative & Supportive Care*, **9**(3): 367–76.

Wadden, T.A., Stunkard, A.J. and Smoller, W.S. (1986) Dieting and depression: a methodological study, *Journal of Consulting and Clinical Psychology*, **64**: 869–71.

Wadsworth, M.E.J. and Kuh, D.J. (1997) Childhood influences on adult health: a review of recent work from the British 1946 National Birth Cohort Study, the MRC National Survey of Health and Development, *Paediatric and Perinatal Epidemiology*, **11**: 2–20.

Wadsworth, M.E.J. (1991) *The Imprint of Time: Childhood History and Adult Life.* Oxford: Oxford University Press.

Walburn, J., Vedhara, K., Hankins, M. et al. (2009) Psychological stress and wound healing in humans: a systematic review and meta-analysis, *Journal of Psychosomatic Research*, **67**(3): 253–71.

Walker, I., Thomas, G.O. and Verplanken, B. (2015) Old habits die hard: travel habit formation and decay in a pro-environmental organization's employees during an office relocation, *Environment & Behavior*, **47**: 1089–1106.

Waller, D., Agass, M., Mant, D. et al. (1990) Health checks in general practice: another example of inverse care? *British Medical Journal*, **300**: 1115–18.

Waller, G., Hamilton, K. and Shaw, J. (1992) Media influences on body size estimation in eating disordered and comparison subjects, *British Review of Bulimia and Anorexia Nervosa*, **6**: 81–7.

Waller, K., Kaprio, J., and Kujala, U.M. (2008) Associations between long-term physical activity, waist circumference and weight gain: a 30-year longitudinal twin study, *International Journal of Obesity*, **32**(2): 353–61.

Wallsten, T.S. (1978) Three biases in the cognitive processing of diagnostic information, unpublished paper, Psychometric Laboratory, University of North Carolina, Chapel Hill, NC.

Wallston, B.S., Alagna, S.W., Devellis, B.M. and Devellis, R.F. (1983) Social support and physical illness, *Health Psychology*, **2**: 367–91.

Wallston, K.A. and Wallston, B.S. (1982) Who is responsible for your health? The construct of health locus of control, in G.S. Sanders and J. Suls (eds) *Social Psychology of Health and Illness*. Hillsdale, NJ: Erlbaum.

Walton, A.J. and Eves, F. (2001) Exploring drug users' illness representations of HIV, hepatitis B and hepatitis C using repertory grids, *Psychology and Health*, **16**: 489–500.

Wang, H., Chang, R., Shen, Q. et al. (2020) Information-motivation-behavioral skills model of consistent condom use among transgender women in Shenyang, China, *BMC Public Health*, **20**(1): 1–9.

Wang, S.J., Liu, H.C., Fuh, J.L. et al. (1997) Prevalence of headaches in a Chinese elderly population in Kinmen: age and gender effect and cross-cultural comparisons, *Neurology*, **49**: 195–200.

Wang, Y.H., Li, J.Q., Shi, J.F. et al. (2020) Depression and anxiety in relation to cancer incidence and mortality: a systematic review and meta-analysis of cohort studies, *Molecular Psychiatry*, **25**(7): 1487–99.

Wansink, B. and Sobal, J. (2007) Mindless eating: the 200 daily food decisions we overlook, *Environment and Behavior*, **39**(1): 106–23.

Wansink, B., Painter, J. E. and Lee, Y. K. (2006a) The office candy dish: proximity's influence on estimated and actual consumption. *International Journal of Obesity*, **30**: 871–5.

Wansink, B., Van Ittersum, K. and Painter, J.E. (2006) Ice cream illusions: bowls, spoons, and self-served portion sizes. *American Journal of Preventive Medicine*, **31**(3): 240–3.

Wansink, B. (2009) *Mindless Eating: Why We Eat More Than We Think* (2nd edn). London: Hay House.

Ward, N. and Ogden, J. (2019) 'Damned if we do or don't' Bariatric surgeons' reflections on patients sub optimal outcomes post weight loss surgery, *Psychology and Health*, DOI: 10.1080/08870446.2018.1529314.

Wardle, J., Cooke, L.J., Gibson, E.L. et al. (2003) Increasing children's acceptance of vegetables: a randomized trial of parent-led exposure, *Appetite*, **40**(2): 155–62.

Wardle, J., Sanderson, S., Guthrie, C.A., Rapoport, L. and Plomin, R. (2002) Parental feeding style and the intergenerational transmission of obesity risk, *Obesity Research*, **10**: 453–62.

Wardle, J., Steptoe, A., Bellisle, F. et al. (1997) Health dietary practices among European students, *Health Psychology*, **16**: 443–50.

Wardle, J. (1995) Parental influences on children's diets, *Proceedings of the Nutrition Society*, **54**: 747–58.

Ware, J.E. and Sherbourne, C.D. (1992) The MOS 36-item short form health survey (SF-36): conceptual framework and item selection, *Medical Care*, **30**: 473–83.

Warren, C. and Cooper, P.J. (1988) Psychological effects of dieting, *British Journal of Clinical Psychology*, **27**: 269–70.

Wason, P.C. (1974) The psychology of deceptive problems, *New Scientist*, 15 August: 382–5.

Watson, J. (2000) *Male Bodies: Health, Culture and Identity*. Buckingham: Open University Press.

Watson, W.L. and Ozanne-Smith, J. (2000) Injury surveillance in Victoria, Australia: developing comprehensive injury incidence estimates, *Accident Analysis and Prevention*, **32**: 277–86.

Wearden, A. and Peters, S. (2008) Therapeutic techniques for interventions based on Leventhal's common sense model, *British Journal of Health Psychology*, **13**: 189–93.

Wearden, A., Cook, L. and Vaughan-Jones, J. (2003) Adult attachment, alexithymia, symptom reporting, and health related coping, *Journal of Psychosomatic Research*, **55**(4): 341–7.

Weatherburn, P., Hunt, A.J., Davies, P.M. et al. (1991) Condom use in a large cohort of homosexually active men in England and Wales, *AIDS Care*, **3**: 31–41.

Webb, J., Fife-Schaw, C. and Ogden, J. (2019) A randomised control trial and cost-consequence analysis to examine the effects of a print-based intervention supported by internet tools on the physical activity of UK cancer survivors, *Public health*, **171**: 106–115. Doi.org/10.1016/j.puhe.2019.04.006

Weg, R.B. (1983) Changing physiology of aging, in D.S. Woodruff and J.E. Birren (eds) *Ageing: Scientific Perspectives and Social Issues*, 2nd edn. Monterey, CA: Brooks/Cole.

Wegner, D.M., Schneider, D.J., Cater, S.R. and White, T.L. (1987) Paradoxical effects of thought suppression, *Journal of Personality and Social Psychology*, **53**: 5–13.

Wegner, D.M. (1994) Ironic processes of mental control, *Psychological Review*, **101**: 34–52.

Weidner, G., Rice, T., Knox, S.S. et al. (2000) Familiar resemblance for hostility: the National Heart, Lung, and Blood Institute Family Heart Study, *Psychosomatic Medicine*, **62**: 197–204.

Weiner, B. (1986) *An Attributional Theory of Motivation and Emotion*. New York: Springer-Verlag.

Weinman, J., Petrie, K.J., Moss-Morris, R. and Horne, R. (1996) The Illness Perception Questionnaire: a new method for assessing the cognitive representation of illness, *Psychology and Health*, **11**: 431–46.

Weinman, J., Yusuf, G., Berks, R. et al. (2009) How accurate is patients' anatomical knowledge: a cross-sectional, questionnaire study of six patient groups and a general public sample, *BMC Family Practice*, **10**: 43.

Weinstein, N., Rothman, A.J. and Sutton, S.R. (1998) Stage theories of health behavior: conceptual and methodological issues, *Health Psychology*, **17**: 290–9.

Weinstein, N. (1983) Reducing unrealistic optimism about illness susceptibility, *Health Psychology*, **2**: 11–20.

Weinstock, M.A. Rossi, J.S., Redding, C.A. et al. (2000) Sun protection behaviors and stages of change for the primary prevention of skin cancers among beachgoers in southeastern New England, *Annals of Behavioral Medicine*, **22**(4): 286–93.

Weisman, C.S., Plichta, S., Nathanson, C.A. et al. (1991) Consistency of condom use for disease prevention among adolescent users of oral contraceptives, *Family Planning Perspective*, **23**: 71–4.

Weiss, G.L. and Larson, D.L. (1990) Health value, health locus of control and the prediction of health protective behaviours, *Social Behaviour and Personality*, **18**: 121–36.

Weisse, C.S., Turbiasz, A.A. and Whitney, D.J. (1995) Behavioral training and AIDS risk reduction: overcoming barriers to condom use, *AIDS Education and Prevention*, **7**(1): 50–9.

Weller, S.S. (1984) Cross-cultural concepts of illness: variables and validation, *American Anthropologist*, **86**: 341–51.

Wellings, K., Field, J., Johnson, A.M. and Wadsworth, J (1994) *Sexual Behaviour in Britain: The National Survey of Sexual Attitudes and Lifestyles*. Harmondsworth: Penguin.

Wen, C.P., Wai, J.P., Tsai, M.K. et al. (2011). Minimum amount of physical activity for reduced mortality and extended life expectancy: a prospective cohort study, *Lancet*, **378**: 1244–53.

Wen, Y., Yang, Y., Shen, J. et al. (2021) Anxiety and prognosis of patients with myocardial infarction: a meta-analysis, *Clinical Cardiology*, **44**(6): 761–70.

Wenzlaff, R.M. and Wegner, D.M. (2000) Thought suppression, *Annual Review of Psychology*, **51**: 59–91.

West, R. (2006) *Theory of Addiction*. Oxford: Blackwell.

West, R. and Michie, S. (2015) Applying the Behaviour Change Wheel: a very brief guide, https://www.ucl.ac.uk/behaviour-change/files/bcw-summary.pdf

West, R. and Shiffman, S. (2004) *Smoking Cessation*. Oxford: Health Press.

West, R. and Sohal, T. (2006) 'Catastrophic' pathways to smoking cessation: findings from a national survey, *British Medical Journal*, **332**(7539): 458–60.

West, R., Michie, S., Rubin, G.J. and Amlôt, R. (2020) Applying principles of behaviour change to reduce SARS-CoV-2 transmission, *Nature Human Behaviour*, **4**(5): 451–59.

West, R., Walia, A., Hyder, N. et al. (2010) Behavior change techniques used by the English Stop Smoking Services and their associations with short-term quit outcomes, *Nicotine & Tobacco Research*, **12**(7): 742–7.

Westhaver, R. (2005) 'Coming out of your skin': circuit parties, pleasure and the subject, *Sexualities*, **8**(3): 347–74.

Weston, S.J., Hill, P.L. and Jackson, J.J. (2015) Personality traits predict the onset of disease, *Social Psychological and Personality Science*, **6**(3): 309–17.

White, A. M., Slater, M. E., Ng, G., Hingson, R. and Breslow, R. (2018) Trends in alcohol-related emergency department visits in the United States: results from the Nationwide Emergency Department Sample, 2006 to 2014, *Alcoholism: Clinical and Experimental Research*, **42**(2): 352–59.

White, A.M. (2020) Gender differences in the epidemiology of alcohol use and related harms in the United States, *Alcohol Research: Current Reviews*, **40**(2): 01.

White, I.R., Altmann, D.R. and Nanchahal, K. (2002) Alcohol consumption and mortality: modelling risks for men and women at different ages, *British Medical Journal*, **27**(325): 191.

White, K.M., Robinson, N.G., Young, R.M. et al. (2008) Testing an extended theory of planned behaviour to predict young people's sun safety in a high risk area, *British Journal of Health Psychology*, **13**(3): 435–48.

White, P.D., Goldsmith, K.A., Johnson, A.L. et al. (2011) Comparison of adaptive pacing therapy, cognitive behaviour therapy, graded exercise therapy, and specialist medical care for chronic fatigue syndrome (PACE): a randomised trial, *Lancet*, **377**(9768): 823–36.

Whitley, B.E. and Schofield, J.W. (1986) A meta-analysis of research on adolescent contraceptive use, *Population and Environment*, **8**: 173–203.

Whittaker, R., McRobbie, H., Bullen, C., Rodgers, A., Gu, Y. and Dobson, R. (2019) Mobile phone text messaging and app-based interventions for smoking cessation, *Cochrane Database of Systematic Reviews*, 10(10):CD006611.

WHO cardiovascular disease fact sheet (2015) https://www.who.int/health-topics/cardiovascular-diseases/#tab=tab_1 / https://publichealth.wustl.edu/global-cardiovascular-disease/

WHO (2016). Key abortion facts. https://www.who.int/reproductivehealth/news/440KeyAbortionFactsFinal.pdf

WHO (2018) www.who.int/news-room/detail/28-09-2017-worldwide-an-estimated-25-million-unsafe-abortions-occur-each-year

WHO (2008). Unsafe abortions. http://apps.who.int/iris/bitstream/handle/10665/44529/9789241501118_eng.pdf;jsessionid=0B650EBD879FDDBEDF27AD52639D2780?sequence=1

WHO (World Health Organization) (1996) *Research on the Menopause in the 1990s.* Geneva: WHO.

WHO (World Health Organization) (1947) *Constitution of the World Health Organization.* Geneva: WHO.

WHO (World Health Organization) (2003) *Adherence to Long-term Therapies: Evidence for Action.* Geneva: WHO.

WHO (World Health Organization) (2006) *Sexual and Reproductive Health: Defining Sexual Health,* http://www.who.int/reproductivehealth/topics/sexual_health/sh_definitions/en/index.html

WHO (World Health Organization) (2016) *Obesity and Overweight,* https://www.who.int/news-room/fact-sheets/detail/obesity-and-overweight

WHO (2018) *Life Expectancy.* http://www.who.int/gho/mortality_burden_disease/life_tables/situation_trends/en/

WHO (2020) https://www.who.int/en/news-room/fact-sheets/detail/noncommunicable-diseases

WHO Global InfoBase (online tool) https://www.who.int/ncd_surveillance/infobase/en/

WHO (2017) *Prevalence of Tobacco Use.* http://www.who.int/gho/tobacco/use/en/

WHO (2017) https://www.who.int/images/default-source/maps/hiv_deaths_2016.png?sfvrsn=f6e230db_0 or https://www.who.int/images/default-source/maps/hiv_deaths_2016.png?sfvrsn=f6e230db_0

WHO (2020) https://covid19.who.int/

WHO (2020) https://www.who.int/en/news-room/fact-sheets/detail/noncommunicable-diseases

WHOQoL Group (1993) *Measuring Quality of Life: The Development of a World Health Organization Quality of Life Instrument (WHOQoL).* Geneva: WHO.

Wickramasekera, I. (1980) A conditioned response model of the placebo effect: predictions from the model, *Biofeedback and Self Regulation,* **5:** 5–18.

Wiczinski, E., Döring, A., John, J. and von Lengerke, T. (2009) Obesity and health-related quality of life: does social support moderate existing associations? *British Journal of Health Psychology,* **14:** 717–34.

Widman, L., Choukas-Bradley, S., Noar, S.M. et al. (2016) Parent-adolescent sexual communication and adolescent safer sex behavior: a meta-analysis. *JAMA Pediatrics,* **170**(1): 52–61.

Wiebe, D.J. and McCallum, D.M. (1986) Health practices and hardiness as mediators in the stress–illness relationship, *Health Psychology,* **5:** 425–38.

Wild, B., Erb, M. and Batels, M. (2001) Are emotions contagious? Evoked emotions while viewing emotionally expressive faces: quality, quantity, time course and gender differences, *Psychiatry Research,* **102:** 109–24.

Wilding, J.P., Batterham, R.L., Calanna, S., et al. (2021) Once-weekly semaglutide in adults with overweight or obesity, *New England Journal of Medicine,* **384:** 989–1002.

Wilkinson, A.V., Holahan, C.J. and Drane-Edmundson, E.W. (2002) Predicting safer sex practices: the interactive role of partner cooperation and cognitive factors, *Psychology and Health,* **17**(6): 697–709.

Wilkinson, C., Jones, J.M. and McBride, J. (1990) Anxiety caused by abnormal result of cervical smear test: a controlled trial, *British Medical Journal,* **300:** 440.

Wilkinson, D. and Abraham, C. (2004) Constructing an integrated model of the antecedents of adolescent smoking, *British Journal of Health Psychology,* **9:** 315–33.

Willems, R.A., Bolman, C.A., Lechner, L. et al. (2020) Online interventions aimed at reducing psychological distress in cancer patients: evidence update and suggestions for future directions, *Current Opinion in Supportive and Palliative Care,* **14**(1): 27–39.

Willer, C.J., Speliotes, E.K., Loos, R.J. et al. (2009) Six new loci associated with body mass index highlight a neuronal influence on body weight regulation, *Nature Genetics,* **41**(1): 25–34. Doi: 10.1038/ng.287.

Willett, W.C., Manson, J.E., Stampfer, M.J. et al. (1995) Weight, weight change and coronary heart disease in women: risk within the 'normal' weight range, *Journal of the American Medical Association,* **273:** 461–5.

Williams, A.C. (2002) Facial expression of pain: an evolutionary account, *Behaviour and Brain Sciences,* **25**(4): 439–55.

Williams, K.E., Paul, C., Pizzo, B. and Riegel, K (2008) Practice does make perfect: a longitudinal look at repeated taste exposure, *Appetite,* **51**(3): 739–42.

Williams, S., Weinman, J.A., Dale, J. and Newman, S. (1995) Patient expectations: what do primary care patients want from their GP and how far does meeting expectations affect patient satisfaction? *Journal of Family Practice,* **12:** 193–201.

Willmott, T. J., Pang, B. and Rundle-Thiele, S. (2021) Capability, opportunity, and motivation: an across contexts empirical examination of the COM-B model, *BMC Public Health*, **21**(1): 1–17.

Wills, T.A. (1985) Supportive functions of interpersonal relationships, in S. Cohen and S.L. Syme (eds) *Social Support and Health*. Orlando, FL: Academic Press.

Wilson, J.M.G. (1965) Screening criteria, in G. Teeling-Smith (ed.) *Surveillance and Early Diagnosis in General Practice*. London: Office of Health Economics.

Wimmelmann, C.L., Dela, F. and Mortensen, E.L. (2014a) Psychological predictors of weight loss after bariatric surgery: a review of the recent research, *Obesity Research and Clinical Practice*, **8**(4): 299–313.

Wimmelmann, C.L., Dela, F. and Mortensen, E.L. (2014b) Psychological predictors of mental health and health-related quality of life after bariatric surgery: a review of the recent research, *Obesity Research and Clinical Practice*, **8**(4): 314–24.

Winefield, H., Murrell, T., Clifford, J. and Farmer, E. (1996) The search for reliable and valid measures of patient centredness, *Psychology and Health*, **11**: 811–24.

Winfield, E.B. and Whaley, A.L. (2002) A comprehensive test of the health belief model in the prediction of condom use among African American college students, *Journal of Black Psychology*, **28**: 330–46.

Wing, R.R. and Phelan, S. (2005) Long-term weight loss maintenance. *American Journal of Clinical Nutrition*, **82**(Supplement 1): 222S–225S.

Wing, R.R., Koeske, R., Epstein, L.H. et al. (1987) Long term effects of modest weight loss in type II diabetic patients, *Archives of Internal Medicine*, **147**: 1749–53.

Wing, R.R., Papandonatos, G., Fava, J.L. et al. (2008) Maintaining large weight losses: the role of behavioral and psychological factors, *Journal of Consulting and Clinical Psychology*, **76**(6): 1015–21.

Winger, J.G., Adams, R.N. and Mosher, C.E. (2016) Relations of meaning in life and sense of coherence to distress in cancer patients: a meta-analysis, *Psycho-Oncology*, **25**(1): 2–10.

Wong, C.L. and Mullan, B.A. (2009) Predicting breakfast consumption: an application of the theory of planned behaviour and the investigation of past behaviour and executive function, *British Journal of Health Psychology*, **14**: 489–504.

Wong, M. and Kaloupek, D.G. (1986) Coping with dental treatment: the potential impact of situational demands, *Journal of Behavioural Medicine*, **9**: 579–98.

Woodcock, A., Stenner, K. and Ingham, R. (1992) Young people talking about HIV and AIDS: interpretations of personal risk of infection, *Health Education Research: Theory and Practice*, **7**: 229–47.

Woods, E.R., Lin, Y.G. and Middleman, A. (1997) The associations of suicide attempts in adolescents, *Pediatrics*, **99**: 791–6.

Wooley, S.C. and Wooley, O.W. (1984) Should obesity be treated at all? in A.J. Stunkard and E. Stellar (eds) *Eating and Its Disorders*. New York: Raven Press.

World Bank (2008) World Bank backs anti-AIDS experiment, press reviews 28 April, http://web.worldbank.org/WBSITE/EXTERNAL/NEWS/0,date:2008-04-28~menuPK:34461~pagePK:34392~piPK:64256810~theSitePK:4607,00.html.

World Health Organization (2020) WHO Director-General's opening remarks at the media briefing on COVID-19, 5 June 2020. https://www.who.int/director-general/speeches/detail/who-director-general-s-opening-remarks-at-the-media-briefing-on-covid-19---5-june-2020

Wright, C.E., Ebrecht, M., Mitchell, R. et al. (2005) The effect of psychological stress on symptom severity and perception in patients with gastro-oesophageal reflux, *Journal of Psychosomatic Research*, **59**: 415–24.

Wright, J.A., Weinman, J. and Marteau, T.M. (2003) The impact of learning of a genetic predisposition to nicotine dependence: an analogue study, *Tobacco Control*, **12**: 227–30.

Writing Group for the Women's Health Initiative Investigators (2002) Risks and benefits of oestrogen plus progesterone in healthy post-menopausal women, *Journal of the American Medical Association*, **288**(3): 321–33.

Wu, T., Wong, S.K.H., Law, B.T.T. et al. (2020) Five-year effectiveness of bariatric surgery on disease remission, weight loss, and changes of metabolic parameters in obese patients with type 2 diabetes: a population-based propensity score-matched cohort study. *Diabetes/Metabolism Research and Reviews*, **36**(3): e3236.

Wyper, M.A. (1990) Breast self-examination and health belief model, *Research in Nursing and Health*, **13**: 421–8.

Yan, Y., Bayham, J., Richter, A. and Fenichel, E.P. (2021) Risk compensation and face mask mandates during the COVID-19 pandemic, *Scientific Reports*, **11**(1): 1–11.

Yan, Z.H., Lin, J., Xiao, W.J. et al. (2019) Identity, stigma, and HIV risk among transgender women: a qualitative study in Jiangsu Province, China, *Infectious Diseases of Poverty*, **8**: 94.

Yang, J., Hanna-Pladdy, B., Gruber-Baldini, A.L. et al. (2017) Response shift: the experience of disease progression in Parkinson disease, *Parkinsonism and Related Disorders*, **36**: 52–6.

Yang, Y., Shields, G.S., Wu, Q. et al. (2019) Cognitive training on eating behaviour and weight loss: a meta-analysis and systematic review, *Obesity Reviews,* **20**(11): 1628–41.

Yao, E. and Siegel, J.T. (2021) The influence of perceptions of intentionality and controllability on perceived responsibility: applying attribution theory to people's responses to social transgression in the COVID-19 pandemic, *Motivation Science,* 7(2): 199–206.

Yardley, L. (1994) *Vertigo and dizziness.* London: Routledge.

Yardley, L., Dibb, B. and Osborne, G. (2003) Factors associated with quality of life in Meniere's disease, *Clinical Otolaryngology,* 28: 436–41.

Yardley, L., Masson, E., Verschuur, C., et al. (1992) Symptoms, anxiety and handicap in dizzy patients: development of the vertigo symptom scale, *Journal of Psychosomatic Research,* **36:** 731–41.

Yi, S., Plant, A., Tuot, S. et al. (2019) Factors associated with condom use with non-commercial partners among sexually-active transgender women in Cambodia: findings from a national survey using respondent-driven sampling, *BMC Public Health,* **19**(1): 1–11.

Yi-Frazier, J.P., Yaptangco, M., Semana, S. et al. (2015) The association of personal resilience with stress, coping, and diabetes outcomes in adolescents with type 1 diabetes: variable-and person-focused approaches, *Journal of Health Psychology,* **20**(9): 1196–206.

Yip, P.S., Callanan, C. and Yuen, H.P. (2000) Urban/rural and gender differentials in suicide rates: east and west, *Journal of Affective Disorders,* **57:** 99–106.

Young B. and Robb K.A. (2021) Understanding patient factors to increase uptake of cancer screening: a review, *Future Oncology,* **17**(28):3757–75. Doi: 10.2217/fon-2020-1078.

Yousaf, O., Grunfeld, E.A. and Hunter, M.S. (2015) A systematic review of the factors associated with delays in medical and psychological help-seeking among men, *Health Psychology Review,* 9(2): 264–76.

Yousaf, O., Grunfeld, E. A., & Hunter, M. S. (2015). A systematic review of the factors associated with delays in medical and psychological help-seeking among men. *Health psychology review,* 9(2), 264-276.

Yousuf, A., Arifin, S.R.M. and Ramli Musa, M.L.M. (2019) Depression and HIV disease progression: a mini-review, *Clinical Practice and Epidemiology in Mental Health,* **15:**153–59.

Yzer, M.C., Siero, F.W. and Buunk, B. (2001) Bringing up condom use and using condoms with new sexual partners: intentional or habitual? *Psychology and Health,* **16:** 409–21.

Zaman, A., Ellingson, L., Sunken, A. et al. (2021) Determinants of exercise behaviour in persons with Parkinson's disease, *Disability and Rehabilitation,* **43**(5): 696–702.

Zeiser, K., Hammel, G., Kirchberger, I. and Traidl-Hoffmann, C. (2021) Social and psychosocial effects on atopic eczema symptom severity–a scoping review of observational studies published from 1989 to 2019, *Journal of the European Academy of Dermatology and Venereology,* **35**(4): 835–43.

Zhai, L., Zhang, Y. and Zhang, D. (2015) Sedentary behaviour and the risk of depression: a meta-analysis. *British Journal of Sports Medicine,* **49**(11): 705–9.

Zhang, L., Lu, X., Bi, Y. and Hu, L. (2019) Pavlov's pain: the effect of classical conditioning on pain perception and its clinical implications, *Current Pain and Headache Reports,* **23**(3): 1–12.

Zhang, M., Liu, S., Yang, L. et al.(2019) Prevalence of smoking and knowledge about the hazards of smoking among 170 000 Chinese adults, 2013–2014, *Nicotine and Tobacco Research,* **21**(12): 1644–51.

Zhou, S., Shapiro, M.A. and Wansink, B. (2017) The audience eats more if a movie character keeps eating: an unconscious mechanism for media influence on eating behaviors, *Appetite,* **108***:* 407–15.

Zhu, L., Shi, Q., Zeng, Y. et al.(2022) Use of health locus of control on self-management and HbA1c in patients with type 2 diabetes, *Nursing Open,* **9**(2): 1028–39.

Ziegler, D.K. (1990) Headache: public health problem, *Neurologic Clinics,* **8:** 781–91.

Zigmond, A.S. and Snaith, R.P. (1983) The Hospital Anxiety and Depression Scale, *Acta Psychiatrica Scandinavica,* **67:** 361–70.

Zola, I.K. (1973). Pathways to the doctor: from person to patient, *Social Science and Medicine,* **7:** 677–89.

Zolese, G. and Blacker, C.V.R. (1992) The psychological complications of therapeutic abortion, *British Journal of Psychiatry,* **160:** 742–9.

Zsigmond, O., Vargay, A., Józsa, E. and Bányai, É. (2019) Factors contributing to post-traumatic growth following breast cancer: results from a randomized longitudinal clinical trial containing psychological interventions, *Developments in Health Sciences,* **2**(2): 29–35.

Index for health psychology

Page numbers in italics are figures; with 't' are tables.

Cruwys, T. 98–9
cue exposure 176
Curry, Edwina 195
Cvetkovich, G. 149
Czajkowska, Z. 227

D

DAFNE study group 435
Dalli, Z. 234
Daniel, J.Z. 130
Darker, C.D. 52
Darling, K.E. 295
Dannenhuer, B. 135
David, L. 224–5
Davis, B. 389
Davis, C. 95
Dazeley, P. 96
de Almeida-Pititto B. 428–9
Dean, C. 260
Deoro, S.C. 159
Deci, E.L. 36–7
decision-making
   shared 270
   theory 11, *12*
decisional control 309
decisions, doctors making 263–7, *264–6*
Decker, A.M. 294
delay in help-seeking *243*, 249–54, *250*
delete, ABCDE system 177
Deliens, T. 174
DeMaria, A.L. 150
demographics
   and CHD 405
   and exercise 130–1, *130*
   and illness cognitions 217
   and screening uptake *256*, 257
Dempster, M. 231, 438
depression
   and cancer 363
   and CHD 401–2, 406, 407
   and exercise 128
   and LGBTQ+ 473
   and miscarriage 449
DESMOND (diabetes education and self-management
      for ongoing and newly-diagnosed) 234
d'Ettorre, G. 307
developmental model, eating behaviour 95–101, 111
Dhabhar, F.S. 294, 299
Di Carlo, C. 458
Dialectical Behavioural Therapy (DBT) 405
Diamond, E.G. 356
diaries 176
Dias, H. 165
Dibb, B. 359, 397
DiClemente, C.C. 77–8
Dieng, M. 366
dieting 106–9, *107–8*, 389–91
differences in theories 14
DiMatteo, M.R. 273
direct/indirect pathways between psychology and
      health 10, *11*
disease model of addiction 66, 68, 69–73
Dishman, R.K. 130, 136
disinhibition, and dieting 107

dissonance 179
distorted body size estimation 101
distraction techniques 176
'doing as you're told' 340
Doll, R. 62
Dormandy, E. 257
Downing, R.W. 340
drinking 60–4, *61–2, 64*
   and gender 464–5
   stages of substance use 73–80, *74, 79*
   and stress 295, 296
drinking water 247, *247*
Dunn, J. 229
Dunton, G.F. 136
Durkin, S.J. 259
Dusseldorp, E. 404

E

eating behaviour 88
   cognitive models *92*, 93–5
   critical approaches 109
   critical thinking about 110–11
   developmental model 95–101
   and health 90
   healthy diets 88–9, *89*, 90–2, *91–2*
   and obesity 384–7, *385–6*
   and stress 295, 297
   weight concern model 101–9, *102, 104–5, 107–8*
Eccleston, C. 329, 333, 334
ecological momentary interventions (EMIs) 194–5
Eddy, P. 294
Edelman, E.J. 354
education, sex 162–5
Eiser, J.R. 258
Ekelund, U. 125
elaboration likelihood model (ELM) 197–8, *198*
Elder, C. 105
elderly
   and diet 91, *91*
   and exercise 120, *120–1, 123–4*, 136
Elliott, M.A. 181, 182
Elston, D.M. 267
emotion
   and adherence 278–9
   and eating 387, 395
   and exercise 133
   and screening uptake 258
   see also affect
emotion-focused coping 304–5
emotional expression
   and HIV/AIDS 356–8
   and men 464, *464*, 469, 472
Engel, G.L. 9
Enhancing Positive Emotions Procedure
      (EPEP) 367
Enrique, M. 188
environmental factors, and health 246–7, *246–7*
Epton, T. 189
Espada, J.P. 150
evaluate, ABCDE system 177
evaluative conditioning 174
Evans, M. 274
events, stress 292–3
Everson, S.A. 301